FIELD GUIDE TO LARGE ANIMAL INTERNAL MEDICINE

FIELD GUIDE TO LARGE ANIMAL INTERNAL MEDICINE

BRADFORD P. SMITH, DVM, Dipl ACVIM
Professor, Department of Medicine and Epidemiology
Director, Veterinary Medical Teaching Hospital
Associate Dean for Clinical Programs
School of Veterinary Medicine
University of California, Davis, California

Prepared by
Christine King, BVSc, MACVSc, MVetClinStud

Mosby
A Harcourt Health Sciences Company
St. Louis London Philadelphia Sydney Toronto

Mosby

A Harcourt Health Sciences Company

Editor-in-Chief: John A. Schrefer
Editorial Manager: Linda L. Duncan
Senior Developmental Editor: Teri Merchant
Project Manager: John Rogers
Project Specialist: Beth Hayes
Designer: Teresa Breckwoldt

FIRST EDITION

NOTICE
Pharmacology is an ever-changing field. Standard safety precautions must be followed, but as new research and clinical experience broaden our knowledge, changes in treatment and drug therapy may become necessary or appropriate. Readers are advised to check the most current product information provided by the manufacturer of each drug to be administered to verify the recommended dose, the method and duration of administration, and contraindications. It is the responsibility of the treating veterinarian, relying on experience and knowledge of the patient, to determine dosages and the best treatment for each individual patient. Neither the Publisher nor the editor assumes any liability for any injury and/or damage to persons or property arising from this publication.

Mosby, Inc.
A Harcourt Health Sciences Company
11830 Westline Industrial Drive
St. Louis, Missouri 63146

Printed in the United States of America

Library of Congress Cataloging in Publication Data

Smith, Bradford P.
Field guide to large animal internal medicine / Bradford P. Smith ; prepared by Christine King.–1st ed.
p. ; cm.
Handbook to accompany: Large animal internal medicine / [edited by] Bradford P. Smith. 3rd ed. 2001.
ISBN 0-323-00978-6
1. Veterinary internal medicine. I. King, Christine, II. Large animal internal medicine. III. Title.
[DNLM: 1. Veterinary Medicine–methods–Handbooks. 2. Animal Diseases–Handbooks. 3. Horses–Handbooks. 4. Ruminants–Handbooks.
SF 745 S643f2002]
SF745 .S57 2002
636.089′6–dc21 2001030759

01 02 03 04 05 GW/RRD-W 9 8 7 6 5 4 3 2 1

Contributors

MONICA R. ALEMAN, MVZ, Dipl ACVIM

TREVOR R. AMES, DVM, MS, Dipl ACVIM

JOHN ANGELOS, DVM, MS

JANE E. AXON, BVSc, MACVSc

JOHN C. BAKER, DVM, PhD, Dipl ACVIM

GEORGE M. BARRINGTON, DVM, PhD, Dipl ACVIM

JILL BEECH, VMD, Dipl ACVIM

STEVEN L. BERRY, DVM, MPVM

CHRISTINE F. BERTHELIN-BAKER, DVM, Dip ACVIM (Neurology)

JILL McCLURE BLACKMER, DVM, MS, Dipl ACVIM, ABVP

J. TRAVIS BLACKWELDER, MS, DVM

TERRY L. BLANCHARD, DVM, MS, Dipl ACT

ANTHONY T. BLIKSLAGER, DVM, PhD, Dipl ACVS

RICHARD BOWEN, DVM, PhD

JAMES P. BRENDEMUEHL, DVM, PhD, Dipl ACT

GORDON W. BRUMBAUGH, DVM, PhD, Dipl ACVIM

T. DOUGLAS BYARS, DVM, Dipl ACVIM, ACVECC

GARY P. CARLSON, DVM, PhD, Dipl ACVIM, ACVP

ELIZABETH A. CARR, DVM, PhD, Dipl ACVIM

STAN W. CASTEEL, DVM, PhD, Dipl ABVT

H. MICHAEL CHADDOCK, DVM

ERIN CHAMPAGNE, DVM, Dipl ACVO

NOAH D. COHEN, VMD, MPH, PhD, Dipl ACVIM

ANTHONY W. CONFER, DVM, MS, PhD, Dipl ACVP

VANESSA L. COOK, MA, VetMB, MS, MRCVS, Dipl ACVS

RICK CORBETT, BSc, MSc, PAg

KEVIN CORLEY, BSc, BVM&S, PhD, MRCVS

VICTOR S. CORTESE, DVM, PhD, Dipl ABVP (Dairy)

JAMES S. CULLOR, DVM, PhD

ROBIN M. DABAREINER, DVM, PhD, Dipl ACVS

ANDREW DART, BVSc, DVCS, MACVSc, Dipl ACVS, ECVS

ERIC W. DAVIS, DVM, MS, Dipl ACVIM, ACVS

FABIO DEL PIERO, DVM, Dipl ACVP

JOSEPH DiPIETRO, DVM, MS

THOMAS J. DIVERS, DVM, Dipl ACVIM, ACVECC

LORRAINE DOEPEL, BSc

BRETT DOLENTE, VMD

MAARTEN DROST, DVM, Dipl ACT

GERALD E. DUHAMEL, DMV, PhD, Dipl ACVP

NOËL O. DYBDAL, DVM, PhD, Dipl ACVIM

JOAN DZIEZYC, DVM, Dipl ACVO

JACK EASLEY, DVM, MS, Dipl ABVP (Equine)

NANCY E. EAST, DVM, MPVM

ANITA J. EDMONDSON, BVM&S, MPVM, MRCVS

JOHN A. ELLIS, DVM, PhD, Dipl ACVP, ACVM

ROBERT V. ENGLISH, DVM, PhD

ANNE G. EVANS, DVM, MBA, Dipl ACVD

JAMES F. EVERMANN, MS, PhD

SUSAN L. EWART, DVM, PhD, Dipl ACVIM

GILLES FECTEAU, DMV, Dipl ACVIM

ANDREW T. FISCHER, Jr., DVM, Dipl ACVS

SHERRILL A. FLEMING, DVM, Dipl ABVP (Food Animal), ACVIM

ROBERT W. FULTON, DVM, PhD, Dipl ACVM

FRANCIS D. GALEY, DVM, PhD, Dipl ABVT

FRANKLYN GARRY, DVM, MS, Dipl ACVIM

LISLE W. GEORGE, DVM, PhD, Dipl ACVIM

TERRY C. GERROS, DVM, Dipl ACVIM

CAROL L. GILLIS, DVM, PhD

MARY BELLE GLAZE, DVM, MS, Dipl ACVO

DAVID P. GNAD, DVM

DANIEL GOULD, DVM, PhD, Dipl ACVP

DAN GROOMS, DVM, PhD, Dipl ACVIM

CHARLES GUARD, DVM, PhD

SPRING K. HALLAND, DVM

KEVIN HAUSSLER, DVM, DC, PhD

A. JUDSON HEINRICHS, MS, PhD

NANCY L. HESTERS, DVM, MBA

MELISSA T. HINES, DVM, PhD, Dipl ACVIM

HAROLD F. HINTZ, PhD

DWIGHT C. HIRSH, DVM, PhD

CHARLES A. HJERPE, DVM

DAVID R. HODGSON, DVM, PhD, Dipl ACVIM, FACSM

PATRICIA A. HOGAN, VMD

CLIFFORD M. HONNAS, DVM, Dipl ACVS

R. NEIL HOOPER, DVM, MS, Dipl ACVS

JOHN K. HOUSE, BVMS, PhD, Dipl ACVIM

ELAINE HUNT, DVM, Dipl ACVIM

JANET K. JOHNSTON, DVM, Dipl ACVIM

ROBERT L. JONES, DVM, PhD, Dipl ACVM

SAMUEL L. JONES, DVM, PhD, Dipl ACVIM

CARTER E. JUDY, DVM

STEVEN G. KAMERLING, RPh, PhD

ANDRIS J. KANEPS, DVM, PhD, Dipl ACVS

VERNON C. LANGSTON, DVM, PhD, Dipl ACVCP

RICHARD A. LeCOUTEUR, BVSc, PhD, Dipl ACVIM (Neurology)

GUY D. LESTER, BVMS, Dipl ACVIM

STUART LINCOLN, DVM, PhD, Dipl ACVP

ROBERT L. LINFORD, DVM, PhD, Dipl ACVS

MICHAEL A. LIVESAY, BVMS, Dipl ACVS

K.C. KENT LLOYD, DVM, PhD

JEANNE LOFSTEDT, BVSc, MS, Dipl ACVIM

GUY LONERAGAN, BVSc (Hons), MS

JOHN MAAS, DVM, MS, Dipl ACVN, ACVIM

MELINDA H. MacDONALD, DVM, PhD, Dipl ACVS

ROBERT J. MacKAY, BVSc, PhD, Dipl ACVIM

JOHN E. MADIGAN, DVM, MS, Dipl ACVIM

K. GARY MAGDESIAN, DVM, Dipl ACVECC

DAVID J. MAGGS, BVSc (Hons), Dipl ACVO

JOHN B. MALONE, DVM, PhD

PEGGY MARSH, DVM

PATRICK M. McCUE, DVM, PhD, Dipl ACT

LAURIE A. McDUFFEE, DVM, PhD, Dipl ACVS

SHEILA M. McGUIRK, DVM, PhD, Dipl ACVIM

DENNIS M. MEAGHER, DVM, PhD, Dipl ACVS

NAT T. MESSER IV, DVM, Dipl ABVP

PAUL G.E. MICHELSEN, MS, DVM

NICHOLAS J. MILLICHAMP, BVetMed, PhD, MRCVS, Dipl ACVO

CECIL P. MOORE, DVM, MS, Dipl ACVO

JAMES N. MOORE, DVM, PhD, Dipl ACVS

DEBRA DEEM MORRIS, DVM, MS, Dipl ACVIM

DEREK MOSIER, DVM, PhD, Dipl ACVP

MICHAEL MURPHY, DVM, PhD, Dipl ABVT

MICHAEL J. MURRAY, DVM, MS, Dipl ACVIM

MARK P. NASISSE, DVM, Dipl ACVO

JONATHAN M. NAYLOR, BSC, BVSc, PhD, Dipl ACVIM, ACVN

JAMES A. ORSINI, DVM, Dipl ACVS

GUY H. PALMER, DVM, PhD, Dipl ACVP

MARY ROSE PARADIS, DVM, MS, Dipl ACVIM

STEVEN M. PARISH, DVM, Dipl ACVIM

JOHN R. PASCOE, BVSc, PhD, Dipl ACVS

ERWIN G. PEARSON, DVM, MS, Dipl ACVIM

ARLENA B. PIPKIN, DMV

KONNIE H. PLUMLEE, DVM, MS, Dipl ABVT, ACVIM

KIMBERLY D. RAGER, DVM

VIRGINIA B. REEF, DVM, Dipl ACVIM

CRAIG R. REINEMEYER, DVM, PhD

DAVID G. RENTER, DVM

JAMES P. REYNOLDS, DVM, MPVM

STEVEN M. ROBERTS, DVM, MS, Dipl ACVO

JOAN DEAN ROWE, DVM, MPVM, PhD

BONNIE R. RUSH, DVM, MS, Dipl ACVIM

GUY ST. JEAN, DMV, MS, Dipl ACVS

GEORGE SAPERSTEIN, DVM

WILLIAM J.A. SAVILLE, DVM, PhD, Dipl ACVIM

JOHN SCHLIPF, DVM, MS, Dipl ACVIM

HAROLD C. SCHOTT II, DVM, PhD, Dipl ACVIM

LOREN G. SCHULTZ, DVM

BRAD SEGUIN, DVM, MS, PhD, Dipl ACT

DEBRA C. SELLON, DVM, PhD, Dipl ACVIM

NATHAN M. SLOVIS, DVM, Dipl ACVIM

BRADFORD P. SMITH, DVM, Dipl ACVIM

JOHN A. SMITH, DVM, MS, MAM, Dipl ACVIM (Large Animal), ACPV

MARY O. SMITH, BVM&S, PhD, Dipl ACVIM (Neurology)

JOSEPH HOYT (JOE) SNYDER, DVM

STANLEY P. SNYDER, DVM, PhD, Dipl ACVP

J. GLENN SONGER, PhD

SHARON J. SPIER, DVM, PhD, Dipl ACVIM

†ANTHONY A. STANNARD, DVM, PhD, Dipl ACVD

SUSAN M. STOVER, DVM, PhD, Dipl ACVS

GEORGE M. STRAIN, PhD

CORINNE R. SWEENEY, DVM, Dipl ACVIM

RAYMOND W. SWEENEY, VMD, Dipl ACVIM

RONALD L. TERRA, DVM, MS, Dipl ABVP

PHILIP G.A. THOMAS, PhD, Dipl ACT

MARK C. THURMOND, DVM, PhD

MATS H.T. TROEDSSON, DVM, PhD, Dipl ACT

---

†Deceased.

JAMES R. TURK, DVM, PhD, Dipl ACVP

JEFF W. TYLER, DVM, MPVM, PhD, Dipl ACVIM

CHRISTINE A. UHLINGER, VMD, MPH, Dipl ABVP

WENDY E. VAALA, VMD, Dipl ACVIM

STEPHANIE J. VALBERG, DVM, PhD, Dipl ACVIM

STEVEN D. VAN CAMP, DVM, Dipl ACT

DAVID C. VAN METRE, DVM, Dipl ACVIM

DICKSON D. VARNER, DVM, Dipl ACT

PAMELA WAGNER VON MATTHIESSEN, DVM, MD, Dipl ACVS

KRISTINA R. VYGANTAS, DVM

ANGELINE E. WARNER, DVM, DSc, Dipl ACVIM

JEFFREY P. WATKINS, DVM, MS, Dipl ACVS

JOHANNA L. WATSON, DVM, PhD, Dipl ACVIM

EUGENE C. WHITE, DVM

NATHANIEL A. WHITE II, DVM, MS, Dipl ACVD

STEPHEN D. WHITE, DVM, Dipl ACVD

SUSAN L. WHITE, DVM, MS, Dipl ACVIM

JAMI L. WHITING, DVM

R. DAVID WHITLEY, DVM, MS, Dipl ACVO

ROBERT H. WHITLOCK, DVM, PhD, Dipl ACVIM

STEVEN E. WIKSE, DVM, Dipl ACVP

PAMELA A. WILKINS, DVM, PhD, Dipl ACVIM

W. DAVID WILSON, BVMS, MS, MRCVS

ANNE M. ZAJAC, DVM, PhD

JERRY L. ZAUGG, DVM, PhD

STEVEN C. ZICKER, DVM, PhD, Dipl ACVIM, ACVN

Preface

Field Guide to Large Animal Internal Medicine is designed as a handy, current reference for use by veterinarians, veterinary students, veterinary technicians, and other clinic staff. The goal of this field guide is to provide readers with fast, helpful information on assessment, diagnosis, and treatment of the most common problems encountered in large animals. In no way is it an exhaustive work; it is best used in conjunction with the third edition of *Large Animal Internal Medicine,* in which the reader will find more detailed discussions of relevant physiology, pathophysiology, diagnostic testing, procedures, and underlying rationales for treatment options, as well as hundreds of supporting illustrations and extensive reference lists.

This book emphasizes two major sections of the parent text. First, because of the extensive amount of reduction that has been done, we have focused foremost on what has come to be known as a hallmark of the Smith text: discussion of clinical signs. This section helps guide the reader toward diagnosis and treatment based on presenting manifestations. The second major section features brief monograph-like discussions on an array of common problems, organized by organ system. Specific disorders include discussions of assessment, diagnosis, and medical management. This book also includes several helpful summary tables and an indispensable section on poisoning, including monographs of toxic plants, animals, metals, and pesticides; industrial toxicants; drug overdose; and feed additives. Helpful page cross-references to the parent text have been provided throughout the field guide to direct readers to more detailed information.

Field Guide to Large Animal Internal Medicine is your indispensable clinical quick reference!

BRADFORD P. SMITH

Contents

PART I

History, Physical Examination, and Medical Records

1

Ruminant History, Physical Examination, and Records

Consulting Editor RONALD L. TERRA

PHYSICAL EXAMINATION *(Text pp. 3-13)*

The first step in the diagnostic approach to a sick ruminant is collection of a thorough history. A systematic and complete examination should then be performed, beginning with visual assessment of the patient and its herdmates from a distance. Physical examination is discussed in Chapter 1 of *Large Animal Internal Medicine,* third edition. Following are some examination techniques and findings specific to ruminant species.

Urine Collection

Obtaining a sample for urinalysis is most productive when performed while the animal is relaxed, that is, before the physical examination begins. Specific methods vary with species and gender. Stroking the perineum often elicits urination in cows but is only occasionally effective in ewes and does. In male cattle, massaging the prepucial orifice often stimulates urination, but in male sheep and goats it is often unrewarding. In sheep and goats of either gender, urination can usually be stimulated at the end of the physical examination by preventing the animal from breathing until it urinates. (NOTE: This technique should not be used on severely compromised patients.)

Rectal Temperature

Normal temperature ranges for each species are as follows:

- Cattle–adults 38°-39° C (100.5°-102.5° F); calves 39°-40.5° C (101.5°-103° F)
- Sheep–adults 39°-40° C (102°-103.5° F); lambs 39.5°-40.5° C (102.5°-104° F)
- Goats–adults 38.5°-39.5° C (101.5°-103.5° F); kids 39°-40.5° C (102°-104° F)

These are not absolute values; the upper limits should be adjusted to account for ambient temperature and housing.

Abdominal Ballottement and Palpation

The abdomen should be ballotted, checking for an increase in fluid (e.g., ruminal or intestinal stasis, peritonitis, ruptured bladder) and for masses (e.g., fetus, impacted abomasum, abscess, tumor). Deep palpation of the paralumbar fossa also may reveal masses. In goats the abdominal fat pad is prominent and tends to obscure any significant findings on ballottement. In goats, lambs, and calves, two hands can be used to palpate the abdomen; the normal, freely movable left kidney usually is readily palpable.

Rumen palpation and auscultation

Normally the rumen has a doughy texture with a small gas cap dorsally; it usually is not distended above a plane level with the most lateral aspect of the last rib. Rumen contractions should be observed, ausculted, and counted. Normally, primary rumen contractions occur 1.5 to 3 times per minute. Hypocalcemia and peritonitis can result in weak or absent contractions. Hypermotility is rare but may be seen with vagal indigestion.

Abdominal "Pings"

Gas-distended abdominal viscera are identified by a pinging sound, heard while simultaneously auscultating and flicking the finger against the thoracic and abdominal walls. Localizing the pings to certain areas helps in identifying the structure involved.

Right side

Pings on the right side involve one of the following structures:

- *Cecum*–The ping is located dorsally in the paralumbar fossa and can extend caudally to the tuber coxae and cranially under the ribcage.
  - The size of the area can vary from 6 inches (15 cm) with cecal displacement to 3 feet (1 m) in length with cecal torsion.
- *Spiral colon*–Typically the ping is localized to the dorsocranial paralumbar fossa.
  - The area is round, 10 inches or less (25 cm) in diameter, and centered high under the last rib; rarely does it extend further forward than the tenth intercostal space.
  - This ping is common in anorectic cattle and has no specific diagnostic significance.
- *Right-sided abomasal displacement (RDA) or torsion*–The ping can extend as far cranially as the ninth intercostal space and caudally into the paralumbar fossa.
  - The size of the area ranges from 18 inches (45 cm) with abomasal displacement, up to 3 feet (1 m) with torsion.
  - In simple RDA or dilation, the only finding may be a small gas ping in a cow with a depressed appetite and decreased milk production.
  - Abomasal torsion or volvulus also causes depression, dehydration, scleral injection, and colic.

Left side

Pings on the left side involve one of the following structures:

- *Rumen*–Ruminal tympany can cause pings that occupy the whole of the left paralumbar fossa.
  - These pings generally do not extend to the right side and rarely extend as far cranial as the eleventh rib. They tend to be monotone.
- *Left-sided abomasal displacement (LDA)*–There is a ping over the eleventh rib, on a line from the hip to the elbow; it is 12 to 18 inches (30 to 45 cm) wide and easily outlined. They tend to be variable in pitch and intensity.
  - Generally the caudal extent is the thirteenth rib, although the ping can extend into the paralumbar fossa, in which case the outline of the abomasum is palpable.
  - Intermittent gas bubbling or "toilet flushing" sounds are often heard over the abomasum; identification of a fluid line within the displacement aids diagnosis.

Both sides

Pings that are found dorsally on both sides of the abdomen most likely indicate free gas within the peritoneal cavity (pneumoperitoneum). These pings can extend from the thoracolumbar junction caudally to the retroperitoneal space.

Cardiac Auscultation

Heart rate and rhythm should be determined during thoracic auscultation. Normal resting heart rates vary with species and age:

- Cattle–adults 40-80 (average 60) beats/min; calves 100-140 (average 120) beats/min
- Sheep–adults 60-120 (average 75) beats/min; lambs 120-160 (average 140) beats/min
- Goats–adults 70-110 (average 85) beats/min; kids 120-160 (average 140) beats/min

Abnormalities of rate and rhythm

Tachycardia can be seen with stress or excitement (e.g., restraint), fever, inflammation, pain, hypocalcemia, or hypovolemia. Bradycardia is seen with conduction disorders and with some metabolic diseases (e.g., uremia, hypokalemia). The most common causes of arrhythmias are atrial fibrillation in adult cattle and hyperkalemia in diarrheic neonates. While the heart is being auscultated, the peripheral pulse should be evaluated. The most convenient artery for palpation usually is the external maxillary artery.

Abnormal heart sounds

Muffling or displacement of the heart sounds can indicate space-occupying lesions within the thorax or pericardial disease. Cranial displacement of the heart sounds is also found with distention of the ruminoreticulum.

Thoracic Auscultation

Respiratory rate and pattern should be noted during thoracic auscultation. Normal resting respiratory rates vary with ambient temperature, species, and age:

- Cattle–adults 12-36 (average 24) breaths/min; calves 30-60 (average 48) breaths/min
- Sheep–adults 12-72 (average 36) breaths/min; lambs 30-70 (average 50) breaths/min
- Goats–adults 15-40 (average 28) breaths/min; kids 40-65 (average 50) breaths/min

Breath sounds

In sheep, goats, and calves, inspiratory sounds can be heard ventrally and over the large airways, but expiratory sounds are minimal (except in sheep, in which they are often audible). In larger cattle, only very faint inspiratory sounds are normally heard. Thus significant pulmonary disease may be present in ruminants without any auscultable abnormalities. Percussion of the chest wall to determine the ventral lung border is most useful in goats and calves.

Testing for Ventral Thoracic or Abdominal Pain

There are two methods for detecting ventral thoracic/abdominal pain:

- Withers pinch test–The trachea is auscultated while the examiner squeezes and presses over the patient's withers.
  - Painful lesions cause the animal to resist normal ventroflexion of the spine or to emit a grunt or hold its breath.
- Ballottement of the xiphoid–The trachea is auscultated while the examiner applies pressure to the patient's xiphoid region with the knee or fist.
  - A grunt indicates that the maneuver caused the animal pain.
  - NOTE: Some animals kick when this procedure is performed.

Rectal Palpation

Rectal palpation generally is not possible in small ruminants, so the following pertains to cattle. The pelvic wall is palpated for retroperitoneal abscesses and pelvic fractures. The left kidney and rumen normally are readily palpable, as are the preiliac (internal iliac) lymph nodes along the craniodorsal surface of the ilium, and the reproductive organs.

DIAGNOSTIC TESTS IN THE FIELD

Laboratory procedures that can be performed in the field include the following:

- California mastitis test (CMT) for detection of subclinical mastitis (see Chapter 34)
- Dipstick urinalysis (see Chapter 10)
- Measurement of rumen pH for diagnosis of lactic acidosis
  - Rumen fluid is collected via stomach tube and tested with standard pH paper.
  - A rumen pH less than 5.5 is indicative of lactic acidosis.

- Liptac test (percutaneous centesis over a left-sided "ping"), used to differentiate between ruminal distention and LDA
  - Fluid from an LDA has a pH less than 4; ruminal fluid has a pH of 6 or greater.
- Serum chemistries (using portable analyzers)

INSURANCE, PREPURCHASE, AND INTERSTATE HEALTH EXAMINATIONS *(Text pp. 13-14)*

A complete physical examination is necessary for insurance and prepurchase examinations. For prepurchase examinations, a complete blood count and serum chemistry panel should also be performed and appropriate samples tested for brucellosis and bovine leukosis. TB test should be performed. Additional laboratory tests for anaplasmosis and bluetongue may also be indicated.

Interstate Health Certificates

When the number of animals presented for interstate health examinations is large, visual inspection of all animals in the group is performed and those showing abnormalities of behavior, physical condition, gait, or posture are examined more thoroughly. *It is essential that the veterinarian signing the health certificate has examined the livestock sufficiently to be confident that no infectious diseases are present in the consigned group.*

2

Equine History, Physical Examination, and Records

Consulting Editors T. DOUGLAS BYARS • JAMI L. WHITING

Physical examination begins with a detailed medical history, which should be directed toward the clinical problem. An overall assessment of the patient should then be made at a distance. Basic information obtained during the physical examination should include rectal temperature, pulse rate, and respiratory rate, which are best determined while the patient is relaxed.

EVALUATION OF BODY SYSTEMS *(Text pp. 15-23)*

Evaluation of specific body systems is outlined in the following sections. All pertinent findings should be noted in the patient's medical record.

Circulatory System

Evaluation of the circulatory system involves assessment of the following:

- Heart rate, rhythm, and heart sounds
  - The heart should be auscultated bilaterally and any murmurs graded (I-V or I-VI) and the valvular site and phase of the cardiac cycle described.
  - Arrhythmias should be evaluated with electrocardiogram, except for common findings such as second-degree atrioventricular block in calm, asymptomatic horses.
- Mucous membrane color, capillary refill time, and presence of scleral injection
- Temperature of the extremities (ears and distal limbs)
- Any abnormalities found, such as jugular pulsation, subcutaneous edema, and lymphadenopathy/lymphangitis

Alterations in the cardiovascular system are discussed in Chapter 6.

Respiratory System

The respiratory system is evaluated by the following methods:

- Measuring the respiratory rate and assessing mucous membrane color
- Auscultating both the upper (larynx and trachea) and lower airways
  - Both sides of the thorax should be ausculted and abnormalities characterized regarding the location or absence of sounds and the phase of respiration involved.
- Assessing nasal airflow
  - Wet the hands and gently hold them over the nostrils to evaluate both intensity and equality of air movement.
- Smelling the breath for fetid odors
- Inspecting the internal nares (septal mucosa) using a penlight
- Percussing the paranasal sinuses, listening for dullness

- Percussing the thorax in suspected cases of abscessation, tumor, or pleural effusion
  - A pleximeter and tablespoon or direct finger percussion can be used.

Evaluation of patients with respiratory disease is discussed in Chapter 29.

Gastrointestinal System

The gastrointestinal system is examined by bilateral auscultation of the abdomen for intestinal sounds. If the clinical complaint involves the abdomen, checking for gastric reflux and performing a rectal examination may also be indicated. Evaluation of the alimentary tract is discussed in Chapter 30.

Integument

The type, distribution, number, and site layer of involvement of skin lesions are readily evaluated (see Chapter 11). The mucous membranes should be evaluated as an extension of the integumentary system.

Musculoskeletal System

For most medical cases a cursory evaluation of the musculoskeletal system is sufficient. The approach to diagnosis of lameness or stiffness in horses is discussed in Chapter 13 of *Large Animal Internal Medicine,* third edition.

Urogenital System

The urogenital system is examined by manual palpation, rectal palpation, vaginoscopy (speculum examination), endoscopy, and ultrasonography. Samples for culture or urinalysis should be obtained before any contaminating procedures are performed.

Eyes

Use of a penlight allows examination of the anterior segment of the eye, as well as the pupillary light response (direct and consensual). The menace response should also be evaluated. The posterior segment of the eye should be examined with an ophthalmoscope whenever vision deficits are part of the primary complaint. This and other diagnostic procedures, including fluorescein staining, are discussed in Chapter 37.

Nervous System

The patient's attitude, posture, and head carriage should be assessed at a distance. Further examination of the neurologic system involves evaluation of the cranial nerves, spinal reflexes, tail tone, postural responses, and gait (see Chapter 8).

PART II

Manifestations of Disease

3

Pain

Consulting Editor JAMES N. MOORE

Contributor STEVEN G. KAMERLING

The anatomic and physiologic basis of pain and the pathophysiologic effects of pain are discussed in Chapter 3 of *Large Animal Internal Medicine,* third edition. General diagnostic approaches to localized or regional pain are also discussed in that chapter. Specific tests and procedures for diagnosis of the diseases listed in the following sections are discussed in the relevant chapters.

ABDOMINAL PAIN *(Text pp. 31-32)*

Manifestations of abdominal pain include tail swishing, bruxism, pawing, stamping of the feet, stretching, looking or kicking at the abdomen, lying down, treading of the hind feet, splinting, tachycardia, tachypnea, sweating, rolling, grunting, decreased milk production, ketosis, anorexia, and depression.

Causes of Abdominal Pain

Horses

Common causes of abdominal pain in horses include the following:

- Tympany (accumulation of gas)
- Intestinal obstruction
- Intestinal muscle spasm ("cramps")
- Gastric ulcers (foals)
- Meconium impaction (neonates)
- Parturition

Ruminants

Common causes of abdominal pain in ruminants include the following:

- Abomasal gas (calves)
- Abomasal volvulus
- Abomasal ulcer
- Accumulation of gas ("bloat")
- Cecal displacement/torsion
- Intestinal torsion/volvulus
- Intussusception
- Peritonitis
- Traumatic reticuloperitonitis
- Urolithiasis
- Uterine tear with peritonitis/adhesions
- Vaginal indigestion

Less common and uncommon causes of abdominal pain in horses and ruminants are listed on p. 32 of *Large Animal Internal Medicine,* third edition.

CHEST PAIN *(Text pp. 32-33)*

Manifestations of chest pain include reluctance to move; rapid, shallow respiration; splinting of the thorax; grunting; abduction of the elbows; weight loss; and hemoptysis.

Causes of Chest Pain

Horses

Common causes of chest pain in horses include the following:

- Lung abscess
- Pleuritis
- Pleuropneumonia
- Pneumonia

Ruminants

Common causes of chest pain in ruminants include the following:

- Pleuropneumonia or pneumonia
- "Shipping fever" complex
- Thrombosis of the caudal vena cava
- Traumatic reticuloperitonitis-pericarditis

Less common causes of chest pain in horses and ruminants are listed on p. 33 of *Large Animal Internal Medicine,* third edition.

PAIN IN THE EXTREMITIES *(Text pp. 33-34)*

Manifestations of extremity pain include reluctance to move, abnormal gait, swelling, skin abrasions/lacerations, weight loss, decubital sores, and exudation.

Causes of Extremity Pain

Horses

Common causes of pain in the extremities in horses include the following:

- Degenerative joint disease
- Hoof wall defects
- Improper trimming/shoeing
- Lacerations
- Ligamentous strain ("sprain")
- Navicular disease
- Sole bruise or abscess
- Synovitis

Ruminants

Common causes of pain in the extremities in ruminants include the following:

- Degenerative arthritis
- Foot rot
- Interdigital fibroma
- Lacerations and foreign bodies
- Laminitis (horizontal fissures of the hoof wall)
- Sole abscess, bruise, ulceration, or puncture wounds
- Traumatic gonitis
- Vertical fissure of hoof wall (sand crack)

Less common and uncommon causes of extremity pain in horses and ruminants are listed on pp. 33-34 of *Large Animal Internal Medicine,* third edition.

BACK AND NECK PAIN *(Text p. 34)*

Manifestations of back and neck pain include reluctance to move, reluctance to bend the neck, pain on palpation, reduced performance, recumbency, and straining.

Causes of Back and Neck Pain

Horses

Common causes of back and neck pain in horses include the following:

- Exertional rhabdomyolysis
- Fractures of the dorsal spinous processes
- Ligamentous strain
- Muscular damage
- Overriding dorsal spinous processes
- Thrombophlebitis

Ruminants

Common causes of back and neck pain in ruminants include the following:

- Meningitis
- Muscle injury
- Tuber coxae fractures
- Urolithiasis
- Vertebral/sacral fractures
- White muscle disease
- Vertebral/spinal abscess

Less common and uncommon causes of back and neck pain in horses and ruminants are listed on p. 34 of *Large Animal Internal Medicine,* third edition.

PAIN ON URINATION *(Text pp. 34-35)*

Manifestations of painful urination (dysuria) include straining, prolonged urination, dripping urine, grunting, restlessness, estrus behavior, arching of the back, kicking at the abdomen, tail swishing, treading, recumbency, and abnormal discharges.

Causes of Pain on Urination

In horses the most common cause of pain on urination is bladder calculi. In foals, it is ruptured bladder. Less common causes include cystitis, neoplasia, urethritis, urethral calculi, and vaginitis. In ruminants the most common cause is urolithiasis. Less common causes include cystitis, prepucial prolapse, pyelonephritis, prepucial injury or infection, and vaginitis.

4

Alterations in Body Temperature

Consulting Editor SUSAN L. WHITE

The general diagnostic approach to hyperthermia and fever are discussed in Chapter 4 of *Large Animal Internal Medicine,* third edition. Specific tests and procedures for diagnosis of the diseases listed in the following sections are discussed in the relevant chapters.

HYPERTHERMIA *(Text p. 37)*

Causes of increased body temperature, other than fever, include the following:

- Sustained exercise
- Tonic-clonic seizure activity
- Malignant hyperthermia (see Chapter 40)
- Ergopeptine alkaloids (found in endophyte-infected fescue or ryegrass)
- Heat stroke (more common in ruminants than in horses)
- Anhidrosis (inability to sweat in horses; see Chapter 39)
- Central nervous system (CNS) disease that damages the hypothalamus
  - CNS disease may result in hyperthermia (most common) or hypothermia.
  - Central hyperthermia is characterized by lack of diurnal variation, anhidrosis, resistance to antipyretic drugs, and excessive response to external cooling.
- Certain drugs and toxins

Drugs Associated With Hyperthermia/Fever

Drugs that most commonly cause hyperthermia include the following:

- Antimicrobials–amphotericin B, erythromycin, penicillins, sulfonamides
- Antiarrhythmics–procainamide, quinidine
- Other drugs–antihistamines, phenothiazines

Drugs that occasionally cause hyperthermia include cephalosporins, cimetidine, furazolidone, iodides, levamisole, and rifampin.

Toxic Causes of Hyperthermia/Fever

Toxic causes of hyperthermia include the following:

- All species–selenium, arsenic, mercury, chlorinated hydrocarbons, dinitrophenol, propylene glycol, trichloroethylene-extracted feed, pyrrolizidine alkaloids, algae, castor bean (*Ricinus* spp.), water hemlock (*Cicuta* spp.), Jimson weed *(Datura stramonium)*
- Horses–blister beetle (cantharidin), mycotoxins
- Ruminants–zinc, iodine, paraquat, crude oil, kerosene, coal oil, ergot, bracken fern, milkweed (*Asclepias* spp.; cattle, sheep), *Brassica* spp. (mustards, crucifers, cress)

- Cattle–fescue toxicosis, gossypol toxicity (cottonseed)
- Sheep and goats–rhododendron, buttercup (*Calthapalustris* and *Ranunculus* spp.; sheep), halothane (goats)

FEVER *(Text pp. 38-43)*

Infectious Causes of Fever

Horses

Common infectious causes of fever in horses include the following:

- Respiratory–viral upper respiratory tract infection, strangles (*Streptococcus equi* infection), pneumonia (bacterial or viral), pleuropneumonia
- Gastrointestinal (GI)–enteritis, salmonellosis, proximal duodenitis-jejunitis, rotavirus diarrhea (foals), endotoxemia from GI disorders, internal parasites
- Urogenital–urachal abscess (foals), metritis (mares)
- Musculoskeletal–septic arthritis, osteomyelitis (foals), traumatic tenosynovitis, cellulitis
- Systemic–septicemia (foals), equine monocytic ehrlichiosis (Potomac horse fever)
- Other–peritonitis, tetanus, localized occult abscesses (thorax, abdomen, upper respiratory tract)

Less common and uncommon infectious causes of fever in horses are listed on p. 40 of *Large Animal Internal Medicine,* third edition.

Ruminants

Common infectious causes of fever in ruminants include the following:

- Respiratory–pneumonia (viral, mycoplasma, bacterial), verminous pneumonia (cattle)
- GI–enteritis, traumatic reticuloperitonitis (cattle), toxemia from GI disorders, bovine viral diarrhea/mucosal disease (cattle)
- Musculoskeletal–osteomyelitis, septic arthritis, *Mycoplasma* spp. arthritis (goats)
- Urogenital–metritis, balanoposthitis (sheep), leptospirosis
- CNS–*Haemophilus somnus* infection (thromboembolic meningoencephalomyelitis), listeriosis
- Systemic–clostridial infections (blackleg *[C. chauvoei], C. perfringens* types A or D [sheep, goats]), anaplasmosis, septicemia, *Mycoplasma* spp. septicemia (goats)
- Other–mastitis, otitis media/interna, contagious ecthyma (sheep, goats), abscesses (pharyngeal, internal lymph nodes, feet), omphalophlebitis (neonates)

Less common and uncommon infectious causes of fever in ruminants are listed on p. 40 of *Large Animal Internal Medicine,* third edition.

Neoplastic and Immunologic Causes of Fever

Common neoplastic causes of fever include the following:

- Horses–metastatic melanoma, lymphosarcoma, squamous cell carcinoma, fibrosarcoma
- Ruminants–bovine leukosis (cattle), lymphosarcoma

Common immunologic causes of fever include the following:

- Horses–purpura hemorrhagica, urticaria, certain drugs
- Ruminants–drug allergies, urticaria ("milk allergy" in cattle)

Less common and uncommon neoplastic and immunologic causes of fever are listed on p. 41 of *Large Animal Internal Medicine,* third edition.

Miscellaneous Causes of Fever

Miscellaneous causes of fever include the following:

- All species–phlebitis/thrombophlebitis, ocular trauma, burns, smoke inhalation, snake bite, acute renal failure
- Horses–hyperlipidemia/hepatic lipidosis, acute hepatic necrosis (Theiler's

disease), chronic active hepatitis, cholelithiasis, recurrent uveitis, foreign body (oral or upper airway), hyperkalemic periodic paralysis (HYPP)
- Ruminants–salt toxicity/water deprivation, primary photosensitization
- Cattle–fat necrosis, cholelithiasis, acute bovine pulmonary emphysema, postparturient hemoglobinuria

Fever of Unknown Origin

Patients with febrile episodes of more than 3 weeks' duration, in which a diagnosis has not been made after routine diagnostic efforts, are considered to have fever of unknown origin (FUO). Most cases of FUO are caused by common diseases with unusual presentations. The following steps are suggested:

1. Document the fever–record the patient's rectal temperature at least twice daily.
  - *Intermittent fever* (diurnal variation >0.75° C [>1.5° F]) is most commonly caused by infection, although it can also occur with neoplasia.
  - *Remittent fever* (febrile cycles of days rather than hours) is characteristic of brucellosis, equine infectious anemia (EIA), and blood-borne protozoal diseases such as babesiosis.
  - *Sustained fever* is most often caused by drugs or toxins.
2. Review the history, especially for environmental causes such as poor ventilation and high humidity, toxic plants, pesticides/herbicides, and drug administration.
3. Perform or repeat a thorough physical examination, evaluating all body systems.
4. Obtain a minimum database consisting of a complete blood count (including fibrinogen), serum biochemistry panel, and urinalysis.
  - In horses, add an EIA titer.
  - In neonates, add blood culture and measurement of serum immunoglobulin G (IgG).

If the fever persists for more than 48 hours after appropriate environmental changes have been made and drug therapy is discontinued, repeat the physical examination and database. If no abnormalities are found on physical or laboratory evaluations, consider additional tests (e.g., abdominocentesis, blood culture, serology, ultrasonography, radiography) and treat symptomatically. However, therapeutic trials of antimicrobials should be restricted to cases in which strong evidence of bacterial infection exists.

HYPOTHERMIA *(Text pp. 44-45)*

Severely hypothermic animals (core temperature <30° C [<86° F]) are profoundly depressed and have marked hypoventilation, absence of muscle activity, and poor reflexes. Decreased blood volume and depressed cardiac function lead to hypoxia, acidosis, and cardiac arrhythmias; hypothermic neonates are often hypoglycemic and have potassium imbalances.

Management of Hypothermia

Hypothermic animals should be warmed by protecting them from wind and drafts, drying them, and providing a microenvironment of high ambient temperature. Other recommendations include the following:

- Gradually warm severely hypothermic animals over 24 hours while monitoring body temperature and cardiovascular status.
  - Rapid rewarming may result in life-threatening cardiac arrhythmias and worsening of metabolic acidosis and hypoxia.
- Maintain adequate perfusion with warmed intravenous crystalloid fluids; add dextrose and monitor blood glucose in neonates.
- Consider providing warmed, humidified oxygen and performing gastric (rumen) or rectal lavage with warm fluids.

Concurrent signs of septic disease in hypothermic animals signal a guarded prognosis.

5

Alterations in Respiratory Function

Consulting Editors W. DAVID WILSON • JEANNE LOFSTEDT

Contributor STEPHANIE J. VALBERG

The diagnostic approaches to respiratory dysfunction are discussed in Chapter 5 of *Large Animal Internal Medicine,* third edition. Specific tests and procedures for diagnosis of the diseases listed in the following sections are discussed in Chapters 20 (neonates) and 29.

COUGH *(Text pp. 46-54)*

Cough is a common presenting complaint. Cough with fever usually indicates a primary infectious cause or a secondary infection superimposed on a noninfectious cause. Cough without fever is typically found in chronic obstructive pulmonary disease (COPD), abnormalities of the larynx or pharynx, parasitic pneumonia, exercise-induced pulmonary hemorrhage (EIPH), tracheobronchial foreign body, tracheal collapse, and neoplasia involving the airway.

Horses

Common causes of cough in horses include the following:

- Viral infection–equine influenza (types A1 and A2), equine herpesvirus (EHV-1 and EHV-4), rhinovirus (1, 2, and 3), reovirus
- Bacterial pneumonia, pleuritis, or pleuropneumonia
- COPD
- Mechanical irritation (e.g., dust)
- Pharyngitis, pharyngeal lymphoid hyperplasia
- Postviral hyperreactive airways

Less common, uncommon, and toxic causes of coughing in horses are listed on p. 47 of *Large Animal Internal Medicine,* third edition.

Ruminants

Common causes of cough in ruminants include the following:

- Any ruminant–*Pasteurella multocida* and *Mannheimia hemolytica* pneumonia (shipping fever, enzootic calf pneumonia), lungworm infection, chronic bacterial pneumonia with abscessation or consolidation (*Arcanobacterium pyogenes* [formerly *Actinomyces pyogenes*] and others), parainfluenza virus type 3, *Mycoplasma* spp. pneumonia, abscess (oral, lingual, retropharyngeal, pharyngeal, laryngeal), trauma (pharyngeal, laryngeal, tracheal, bronchial, chest wall), esophageal obstruction, septicemia (neonates)
- Cattle–*Haemophilus somnus* pneumonia, atypical interstitial pneumonia, infectious bovine rhinotracheitis (bovine herpesvirus type 1 [BHV-1]), bovine respiratory syncytial virus, necrotic laryngitis (calf diphtheria; also affects sheep)
- Goats–*Mycoplasma mycoides* subspecies *mycoides* infection, caprine arthritis-encephalomyelitis (CAE) pneumonia, BHV-1 infection

Less common, uncommon, and toxic causes of coughing in ruminants are listed on p. 48 of *Large Animal Internal Medicine,* third edition.

NASAL DISCHARGE *(Text pp. 54-60)*

Causes of Serous/Mucoid Nasal Discharge

Serous nasal discharge generally indicates disease affecting the nasal passages or upper respiratory tract. Unilateral nasal discharges generally originate from structures rostral to the caudal end of the nasal septum. Bilateral nasal discharges result from diseases affecting structures caudal to the nasal septum or from bilateral conditions involving the nasal passages or paranasal sinuses.

Horses

Common causes of serous or mucoid nasal discharge in horses include the following:

- Viral infection–influenza, equine herpesvirus (EHV-1, EHV-2, or EHV-4), rhinovirus, adenovirus, reovirus
- Pharyngitis, chronic pharyngeal lymphoid hyperplasia
- Nasal/paranasal sinus infection, cysts, polyps, or tumors
- Early bacterial pneumonia/pleuritis
- Early strangles *(Streptococcus equi* infection)
- Guttural pouch infection/mycosis
- Overflow of nasolacrimal ducts
- COPD

Less common and uncommon causes of serous or mucoid nasal discharge in horses are listed on p. 55 of *Large Animal Internal Medicine,* third edition.

Ruminants

Many of the common causes of serous or mucoid nasal discharge in ruminants are the same as those listed previously as common causes of coughing. In cattle, any debilitating illness that reduces lingual nose cleaning can also result in serous/mucoid nasal discharge. Infestation with nasal botflys *(Oestrus ovis)* is another cause of nasal discharge in sheep and goats. Less common, uncommon, and toxic causes of serous or mucoid nasal discharge in ruminants are listed on p.56 of *Large Animal Internal Medicine,* third edition.

Causes of Purulent Nasal Discharge

Horses

Common causes of purulent nasal discharge in horses include the following:

- Postviral bacterial respiratory tract infection
- Nasal passages (U)*–bacterial rhinitis; fungal rhinitis, nasal granuloma, nasal aspergillosis; nasal foreign body; nasal tumor, polyp, or cyst; conchal necrosis
- Paranasal sinuses (U)–infection, cyst, or tumor
- Progressive ethmoid hematoma (U)
- Pharyngeal/retropharyngeal area–pharyngitis, abscessation (e.g., *S. equi* infection [strangles]), guttural pouch empyema/chondroids or mycosis
- Lower respiratory tract–bacterial pneumonia, pleuritis, or pleuropneumonia; lung abscess
- Nasal, skull, or upper airway trauma (unilateral or bilateral discharge)

Less common and uncommon causes of purulent nasal discharge in horses are listed on p. 57 of *Large Animal Internal Medicine,* third edition.

Ruminants

Common causes of purulent nasal discharge in ruminants are similar to those described as common causes of serous/mucoid nasal discharge or coughing. Less common, exotic, and toxic causes of purulent nasal discharge in ruminants are listed on p. 57 of *Large Animal Internal Medicine,* third edition.

**U,* Unilateral discharge.

Causes of Ingesta in Nasal Discharge

Horses

Common causes of ingesta in nasal discharge in horses include the following:

- Esophageal obstruction (choke)
- Cleft palate, palatal hypoplasia (neonates)
- Pharyngitis
- Strangles (*S. equi* infection)
- Dorsal displacement of the soft palate
- Guttural pouch infection, mycosis, or neoplasia involving nerves
- Glossopharyngeal nerve damage
- Botulism ("shaker foal" syndrome)
- Retropharyngeal abscess

Less common and uncommon causes of ingesta in nasal discharge in horses are listed on p. 59 of *Large Animal Internal Medicine,* third edition.

Ruminants

Common causes of ingesta in nasal discharge in ruminants include the following:

- Esophageal obstruction, foreign body choke
- Pharyngeal or retropharyngeal abscess
- Pharyngeal trauma or foreign body
- Megaesophagus (cattle, goats)

Less common and uncommon causes of ingesta in nasal discharge in ruminants are listed on p. 59 of *Large Animal Internal Medicine,* third edition.

EPISTAXIS AND HEMOPTYSIS *(Text pp. 60-64)*

Epistaxis is blood at the external nares. *Hemoptysis* is the coughing up of blood. Although hemoptysis is the hallmark of pulmonary hemorrhage in cattle, it is rarely seen in horses.

Horses

Common causes of epistaxis in horses include the following:

- Upper airway and head–guttural pouch mycosis, progressive ethmoid hematoma, nasal trauma, pharyngeal/retropharyngeal trauma or abscess, nasal polyps, tumors (nasal, paranasal sinuses), foreign body (nasal, pharyngeal, laryngeal, tracheal)
- Lower airway–EIPH, bronchial foreign body
- Other–idiopathic thrombocytopenic purpura, immune-mediated thrombocytopenia, purpura hemorrhagica

Less common, uncommon, and toxic causes of epistaxis in horses are listed on p. 61 of *Large Animal Internal Medicine,* third edition.

Ruminants

Common causes of epistaxis in ruminants include the following:

- Any ruminant–pharyngeal/retropharyngeal trauma or abscess, paranasal sinus infection, nasal trauma, foreign body (nasal, pharyngeal, laryngeal, tracheal, bronchial)
- Cattle–lung embolus from vena cava thrombosis, dehorning (adults)
- Sheep, goats–nasal botflys *(O. ovis);* nasal adenoma, adenopapilloma, adenocarcinoma

Less common, uncommon, and toxic causes of epistaxis in ruminants are listed on p. 61 of *Large Animal Internal Medicine,* third edition.

Hemoptysis

The following conditions can cause hemoptysis in ruminants:

- Caudal vena cava thrombosis
- Aspiration pneumonia
- Pharyngeal/retropharyngeal abscess or trauma
- Thoracic trauma (fractured ribs or sternum)

- Foreign body (nasal, oropharyngeal, tracheal, bronchial)
- Pulmonary aspergillosis

RESPIRATORY DISTRESS (DYSPNEA) *(Text pp. 64-69)*

Horses

Respiratory causes

Common respiratory causes of dyspnea in horses include the following:

- Bacterial pneumonia, pleuritis, or pleuropneumonia
- Pulmonary abscessation
- COPD (housing associated or pasture associated)
- Strangles (*S. equi* infection)
- Viral pneumonia (influenza, EHV-1 or EHV-4, adenovirus, equine viral arteritis)
- Aspiration pneumonia
- Prematurity, dysmaturity, immaturity (foals)
- Neonatal septicemia (foals)
- Pharyngeal/retropharyngeal abscess or trauma

Nonrespiratory causes

Common nonrespiratory causes of dyspnea in horses include the following:

- Cardiac disease (e.g., congestive heart failure, mitral insufficiency)
- Shock (septic, cardiogenic, hypovolemic, acute blood loss)
- Endotoxemia
- Anemia (e.g., neonatal isoerythrolysis, autoimmune hemolytic anemia, blood loss)
- Pain (e.g., abdominal crisis, laminitis, myopathy, fracture)
- Hyperthermia (e.g., fever, postexhaustion syndrome, anhidrosis, heat stroke)

Less common, uncommon, and toxic causes of respiratory distress in horses are listed on pp. 65-66 of *Large Animal Internal Medicine,* third edition.

Ruminants

Respiratory causes

Common respiratory causes of dyspnea in ruminants include the following:

- Any ruminant–*Mannheimia hemolytica* (formerly *Pasteurella hemolytica*) and *Pasteurella multocida* pneumonia (shipping fever, enzootic calf pneumonia), bacterial pneumonia with consolidation/abscessation (*A. pyogenes* and others), aspiration/foreign body pneumonia (especially after hypocalcemia), respiratory syncytial virus, lungworm infection
- Cattle–*H. somnus* pneumonia, necrotic laryngitis *(Fusobacterium necrophorum),* infectious bovine rhinotracheitis (BHV-1), atypical interstitial pneumonia, acute bovine pulmonary edema and emphysema, *Micropolyspora faeni* hypersensitivity pneumonitis ("farmer's lung")
- Sheep, goats–visceral caseous lymphadenitis *(Corynebacterium pseudotuberculosis);* necrotic laryngitis (sheep); ovine progressive pneumonia virus (sheep); *Mycoplasma ovipneumoniae* (sheep); *M. mycoides* subspecies *mycoides, M. agalactiae,* and other *Mycoplasma* spp. (goats)

Nonrespiratory causes

Common nonrespiratory causes of dyspnea in ruminants include the following:

- Hyperthermia (e.g., fever, rapid rise in ambient temperature, heat stroke)
- Pain (e.g., abdominal crisis, urethral calculi, traumatic reticuloperitonitis)
- Distended abdominal viscus
- Acidosis (e.g., rumenal lactic acidosis, pregnancy toxemia)
- Electrolyte aberrations (e.g., hypocalcemia, hypomagnesemia)
- Hypovolemic, cardiac, or septic shock
- Fluid/electrolyte loss (e.g., acute diarrhea, GI obstruction)
- Endotoxemia (e.g., coliform mastitis, metritis, enteritis, salmonellosis, septicemia)
- Neonatal septicemia

- Anemia (e.g., iron deficiency, postparturient hemoglobinuria, hemolysis, anaplasmosis, eperythrozoonosis)
- White muscle disease (nutritional myodegeneration)
- Anaphylaxis/allergy

Less common, uncommon, and toxic causes of respiratory distress in ruminants are listed on pp. 66-67 of *Large Animal Internal Medicine,* third edition.

TACHYPNEA *(Text pp. 69-70)*

Tachypnea (increased respiratory rate) can be either physiologic or pathologic (in which case it is a manifestation of respiratory distress). Physiologic causes of tachypnea include pain, exertion, heat, fever, and anxiety or other stress. The following lists detail the more likely pathologic causes of tachypnea.

Horses

Respiratory causes

Common respiratory causes of tachypnea in horses are similar to those listed for dyspnea, except that patients with strangles, neonatal septicemia, or pharyngeal/retropharyngeal abscess/trauma tend to present with dyspnea rather than with tachypnea.

Nonrespiratory causes

Common nonrespiratory causes of tachypnea are similar to those listed for dyspnea; other common causes of tachypnea in horses include the following:

- Acidosis (e.g., acute enterocolitis, urinary bladder rupture, renal tubular acidosis)
- Anaphylaxis
- Blood transfusion reaction
- Gastric dilation

Less common, uncommon, and toxic causes of tachypnea in horses are listed on pp. 70-71 of *Large Animal Internal Medicine,* third edition.

Ruminants

The common respiratory and nonrespiratory causes of tachypnea in ruminants are similar to those listed for dyspnea. Less common, uncommon, and toxic causes are listed on pp. 71-72 of *Large Animal Internal Medicine,* third edition.

CYANOSIS *(Text pp. 70-76)*

Cyanosis can be classified as peripheral or central. Peripheral cyanosis occurs when blood flow through a tissue is slowed. Central cyanosis results either from inadequate oxygenation of arterial blood or from the presence of an abnormal hemoglobin derivative (e.g., methemoglobinemia).

Horses

Common causes of central cyanosis in horses include the following:

- Respiratory–bacterial pneumonia, pleuritis, or pulmonary abscessation (e.g., *Rhodococcus equi, Streptococcus* spp.); COPD; aspiration pneumonia; viral pneumonia (e.g., influenza, EHV-1 or EHV-4, adenovirus)
- Cardiac–ventricular septal defect with pulmonary hypertension; tetralogy of Fallot
- Other–prematurity, dysmaturity, or immaturity (neonates); toxic methemoglobinemia (e.g., red maple poisoning); anaphylaxis; hypovolemic, cardiac, or septic shock

Less common, uncommon, and toxic causes of central cyanosis in horses are listed on p. 73 of *Large Animal Internal Medicine,* third edition.

Ruminants

Common causes of central cyanosis in ruminants include the following:

- Bacterial pneumonia or pulmonary abscessation–*Mannheimia hemolytica, A. pyogenes, P. multocida, Corynebacterium pseudotuberculosis* (sheep, goats)
- Viral pneumonia–respiratory syncytial virus (cattle), ovine progressive pneumonia (sheep), CAE virus (goats)
- Other respiratory disorders–parasitic pneumonia (lungworm), aspiration pneumonia, pulmonary edema, acute bovine pulmonary edema and emphysema (cattle)
- Cardiac defects–tetralogy of Fallot, ventricular septal defect with pulmonary hypertension
- Other–toxic methemoglobinemia, anaphylaxis, rumenal bloat, shock (hypovolemic, cardiac, or septic)

Less common, uncommon, and toxic causes of central cyanosis in ruminants are listed on p. 74 of *Large Animal Internal Medicine,* third edition.

ABNORMAL RESPIRATORY NOISE (STRIDOR) *(Text pp. 76-80)*

Stridor is an abnormal, intense respiratory sound that is usually generated in the upper airway, most often during inspiration.

Horses

Common causes of stridor in horses include the following:

- Laryngeal–idiopathic laryngeal hemiplegia (ILH; roaring), arytenoid chondritis, epiglottic entrapment
- Pharyngeal/retropharyngeal–dorsal displacement of the soft palate, retropharyngeal abscess, chronic pharyngeal lymphoid hyperplasia
- Other–strangles (*S. equi* infection), guttural pouch empyema or mycosis, laxity of the alar cartilage

Less common, uncommon, and toxic causes of stridor in horses are listed on p. 77 of *Large Animal Internal Medicine,* third edition.

Ruminants

Common causes of stridor in ruminants include the following:

- Any ruminant–abscess (pharyngeal, laryngeal, retropharyngeal, oral), actinobacillosis (wooden tongue, nasal actinobacillosis), trauma (oral, nasal, pharyngeal, laryngeal, tracheal), anaphylaxis or drug reaction, sinusitis, foreign body (nasal, oral, pharyngeal, laryngeal, tracheal, bronchial)
- Cattle–necrotic laryngitis (calf diphtheria)
- Sheep, goats–nasal botflys *(O. ovis),* caseous lymphadenitis *(C. pseudotuberculosis);* nasal adenocarcinoma, adenopapilloma, or polyp; necrotic laryngitis (sheep)

Less common and uncommon causes of stridor in ruminants are listed on pp. 77-78 of *Large Animal Internal Medicine,* third edition.

EXERCISE INTOLERANCE AND POOR PERFORMANCE IN HORSES *(Text pp. 81-86)*

Investigation of exercise intolerance or poor athletic performance is discussed in *Large Animal Internal Medicine,* third edition. The more common causes of exercise intolerance that may be inapparent at rest include the following:

- Obstructive upper airway disease–dorsal displacement of the soft palate, dynamic pharyngeal collapse, idiopathic laryngeal hemiplegia, chronic pharyngeal lymphoid hyperplasia, epiglottic entrapment, axial deviation of the aryepiglottic folds, arytenoid chondritis, paranasal sinus empyema or cysts, guttural pouch infections

- Lower airway disease–EIPH; recurrent airway obstruction (COPD); viral infections (EHV-1 or EHV-4, influenza, adenovirus, reovirus); inflammatory lower airway disease; bacterial pneumonia, pleuritis, or pleuropneumonia
- Cardiovascular disease–atrial fibrillation, ventricular premature contractions, ventricular tachycardia, mitral or aortic insufficiency, myocardial dysfunction, pericarditis, aortoiliofemoral arteriosclerosis or thrombosis
- Musculoskeletal disease–exertional rhabdomyolysis, lameness (limbs, back, neurologic conditions), focal muscle strain
- Metabolic/systemic disease–anemia, fluid and electrolyte imbalances, anhidrosis, heat exhaustion, neoplasia, liver disease
- Other–obesity, poorly trained horse, poor genetic potential, administration of illicit medications

6

Alterations in Cardiovascular and Hemolymphatic Systems

Consulting Editors SHEILA M. McGUIRK • VIRGINIA B. REEF

The general diagnostic approaches to cardiovascular and hemolymphatic dysfunction are discussed in Chapter 6 of *Large Animal Internal Medicine,* third edition. Specific tests and procedures for diagnosis of the diseases listed below are discussed in Chapters 20 (neonates), 28 (cardiovascular system), and 35 (hemolymphatic system).

PERIPHERAL EDEMA/PLEURAL EFFUSION/ASCITES *(Text pp. 88-90)*

Edema is an abnormal accumulation of extracellular fluid in the interstitial spaces of the tissues or in body cavities (e.g., pleural effusion, ascites). It can be localized or generalized. Peripheral edema typically is cool, painless, and pitting.

Causes of Peripheral Edema/Pleural Effusion/Ascites

Horses

The more common causes of peripheral edema, pleural effusion, and ascites in horses include the following:

- Cardiac disease–chronic heart failure, valvular insufficiency (mitral, tricuspid, or aortic), vegetative endocarditis, congenital heart defects, cardiomyopathy, pericarditis
- Vascular or lymphatic disease–vasculitis, thrombophlebitis, lymphatic obstruction, ulcerative lymphangitis, lymphadenitis (e.g., *Corynebacterium pseudotuberculosis* abscesses)
- Gastrointestinal (GI) malabsorption–inflammatory bowel disease, neoplasia, parasitism
- Infectious conditions–equine infectious anemia, equine ehrlichiosis, equine viral arteritis
- Other–pleuritis, liver disease, vitamin E/selenium deficiency, hypoproteinemia, purpura hemorrhagica, trauma, lymphosarcoma

Uncommon causes of peripheral edema, pleural effusion, and ascites in horses are listed on p. 89 of *Large Animal Internal Medicine,* third edition.

Ruminants

The more common causes of peripheral edema, pleural effusion, and ascites in ruminants include the following:

- Cardiac disease–chronic heart failure, valvular insufficiency (mitral or tricuspid), vegetative endocarditis, high altitude disease ("brisket disease"), congenital heart defects, cor pulmonale, pericarditis (traumatic reticulopericarditis)

- Vascular or lymphatic disease–thrombophlebitis, lymphatic obstruction (*C. pseudotuberculosis,* lymphosarcoma)
- Renal disease–amyloidosis, glomerulonephritis, urolithiasis (ruptured urethra or bladder)
- GI malabsorption–lymphosarcoma, Johne's disease, parasitism
- Neoplasia–heart base tumors, lymphosarcoma
- Other–pleuritis, liver disease, vitamin E/selenium deficiency, hypoproteinemia

Uncommon causes of peripheral edema, pleural effusion or ascites in ruminants are listed on p. 89 of *Large Animal Internal Medicine,* third edition.

CARDIAC ARRHYTHMIAS *(Text pp. 90-92)*

Cardiac arrhythmias are abnormalities in the normal heart rate, rhythm, or conduction pattern. They are more common in horses than in other domestic animals.

Benign or Functional Arrhythmias

Horses

Horses may have arrhythmias at rest that are considered benign ("innocent," physiologic, or functional). They include second-degree atrioventricular (AV) block, sinus arrhythmia, sinus bradycardia, and sinoatrial block or arrest. Benign arrhythmias should disappear at high heart rates (e.g., during exercise, excitement, or administration of atropine or glycopyrrolate).

Ruminants

In general, cattle do not have benign arrhythmias, although sinus bradycardia or sinus arrhythmia often occurs in cattle that are held off feed for 12 to 48 hours. Sinus arrhythmia in goats is found in many normal animals and is considered benign.

Causes of Arrhythmia

It is important to determine whether an abnormal arrhythmia is primary or secondary:

- *Primary* arrhythmias are caused by pathologic heart conditions such as myocarditis, valvular disease, conduction system abnormalities, and pericarditis.
- *Secondary* arrhythmias are caused by such conditions as excitement, fever, electrolyte imbalances (especially potassium, calcium), acid-base disturbances, GI diseases, and toxemia.
    - Cattle with GI disease are more susceptible to arrhythmias, especially atrial fibrillation.
    - Lymphosarcoma, high altitude disease, foot rot, and cor pulmonale (secondary to pulmonary hypertension) are other causes of arrhythmias in cattle.

CARDIAC MURMURS *(Text pp. 92-94)*

Common Causes of Cardiac Murmurs

The more common causes of murmurs include the following:

- Physiologic–anemia, excitement, fever, youth, exercise (horses)
- Valvular disease–degenerative, vegetative, or dilatory
- Bacterial endocarditis
- Congenital heart defects
- Myocarditis
- Pericarditis (in cattle, traumatic reticulopericarditis)

Lymphosarcoma is another common cause of murmurs in cattle. Less common causes of cardiac murmurs in horses and ruminants are listed on p. 93 of *Large Animal Internal Medicine,* third edition.

Systolic Murmurs

Ejection murmurs

Ejection murmurs are caused by obstructed, increased, or turbulent flow during ventricular contraction. The point of maximum intensity is typically over the pulmonic or aortic valve. Causes include the following:

- "Innocent" murmurs (common in young animals and in horses)
- Anemia or fever
- Aortic or pulmonary stenosis
- Atrial or ventricular septal defect
- Tetralogy of Fallot

Regurgitant murmurs

Regurgitant murmurs typically begin with AV valve closure and end after pulmonic and aortic valve closure, making the second heart sound inaudible. Diagnostic considerations include mitral or tricuspid valve regurgitation, ventricular septal defect, and tetralogy of Fallot.

Diastolic Murmurs

Diastolic murmurs can occur between heart sounds S_4 and S_1 (atrial systolic murmur), between S_2 and S_3 (ventricular filling), or from S_2 to S_1 (aortic insufficiency). Atrial systolic and ventricular filling murmurs are usually functional.

Continuous Murmurs

Continuous murmurs are heard throughout the cardiac cycle. They are uncommon in large animals. The murmur associated with patent ductus arteriosus, a normal finding in foals for a short time after delivery, can be continuous but is more often systolic. Traumatic pericarditis in cattle causes a continuous "washing machine" murmur, heard most easily on the left.

MUFFLED HEART SOUNDS *(Text pp. 94-95)*

Physical factors in normal animals, such as obesity, large size, and thick chest wall, can muffle the heart sounds on auscultation. In other instances, heart sounds are muffled because of displacement of the heart from the thoracic wall by one of the following:

- Fluid–pericardial effusion
  - *Pleural* effusion in the absence of pericardial effusion causes radiating heart sounds but absence of airway sounds.
- Soft tissue mass–abscess or tumor
- Air–pneumothorax, pneumomediastinum, emphysema

Rarely is muffling of heart sounds attributed to weak cardiac contractions alone, although this can be a finding in recumbent cows with marked hypocalcemia.

EXERCISE INTOLERANCE/WEAKNESS/SYNCOPE *(Text pp. 95-96)*

Exercise intolerance, weakness, or syncope (sudden collapse with loss of consciousness; fainting) can be caused by disease in one of several body systems.

Causes of Cardiovascular Exercise Intolerance, Weakness, and Syncope

Common causes of exercise intolerance, weakness, and syncope in horses include the following:

- Cardiovascular–myocardial disease, arrhythmias, aortic or pulmonary artery rupture, aortic-iliac-femoral arteriosclerosis or thrombosis, congenital heart defects, chronic heart failure, pericardial disease
- Hyperkalemic periodic paralysis (HYPP)
- Central nervous system disturbances resulting in loss of consciousness

Common causes in ruminants include myocardial disease, cardiac arrhythmias, congenital heart defects, and chronic heart failure.

JUGULAR VENOUS DISTENTION/PULSATION *(Text pp. 96-98)*

Jugular vein pulsations are primarily a reflection of right-sided heart activity. They are observed in normal animals, but the pulse seldom radiates more than one third the way up the neck when the head is held in a normal, upright position. Abnormal jugular pulsations occur with increased resistance to right ventricular filling.

- Prominent pulsations are seen with tricuspid valve regurgitation and with atrial arrhythmias.
  - If the jugular vein is compressed near the ramus of the mandible and massaged toward the heart, refilling is indicative of tricuspid valve regurgitation.
- Distention with pulsations is seen with right-sided heart failure, constrictive pericarditis, and cardiomyopathy (rare).
- Distention without pulsations can occur with compression of the cranial vena cava by a cranial thoracic or mediastinal mass, or with jugular thrombosis.

Causes of Jugular Venous Distention/Pulsation

The more common causes of jugular venous distention and pulsations include the following:

- Cardiac–right-sided heart failure, chronic heart failure, cardiomyopathy, tricuspid insufficiency, atrial fibrillation (horses), pericarditis (cattle)
- Cranial mediastinal mass–lymphosarcoma, abscess
- Jugular phlebitis/thrombosis

In ruminants, other causes include vitamin E/selenium deficiency (white muscle disease), monensin toxicity, cor pulmonale caused by chronic pneumonia, and high altitude disease. Uncommon causes are listed on p. 97 of *Large Animal Internal Medicine,* third edition.

PAINFUL PERIPHERAL SWELLINGS *(Text p. 98)*

Peripheral vascular and lymphatic diseases can be manifested by diffuse swelling, localized swellings (papules, nodules, macules, wheals), or subcutaneous edema of the extremities. As the disease progresses, necrosis, ulceration of the skin, exudation, and lameness or a painful response to palpation are often noted.

Causes of Painful Peripheral Swellings

Horses

The more common causes of painful peripheral swelling in horses include the following:

- Vascular disease–thrombophlebitis, hypersensitivity vasculitis (complicated by skin necrosis and secondary infection), purpura hemorrhagica
- Infection–abscess (e.g., *C. pseudotuberculosis* in the western United States), cellulitis, equine viral arteritis, *E. equi* infection, equine infectious anemia, clostridial myositis
- Insect or snake bite
- Topical counterirritants, firing, or soring

Less common causes are listed on p. 98 of *Large Animal Internal Medicine,* third edition.

Ruminants

The more common causes of painful peripheral swelling in ruminants include the following:

- Thrombophlebitis

- Abscess
- Clostridial myositis (malignant edema, blackleg)
- Fescue foot, ergotism
- Cellulitis (injection site or wound)
- Insect or snake bite
- Frostbite

Less common causes are listed on p. 98 of *Large Animal Internal Medicine,* third edition.

ENLARGED LYMPH NODES *(Text pp. 97-99)*

Single or multiple lymph node enlargement (lymphadenopathy) occurs with infectious (i.e., bacterial, viral, fungal), neoplastic, and, rarely, immune-mediated diseases. Lymphadenopathy may cause obstruction to lymphatic drainage, leading to peripheral edema, pleural effusion, or ascites.

Causes of Lymphadenopathy

Common causes in horses include strangles (*Streptococcus equi* infection), lymphosarcoma, upper respiratory tract infection, and *C. pseudotuberculosis* lymphadenitis. Common causes in ruminants include caseous lymphadenitis *(C. pseudotuberculosis),* lymphosarcoma (including bovine leukosis virus), and abscess or cellulitis in the area drained by that node.

ABNORMAL PERIPHERAL PULSE *(Text pp. 99-101)*

Hyperkinetic Arterial Pulse

Hyperkinetic pulses occur in patients with one of the following:

- Increased cardiac output (e.g., during fever, exercise, excitement, pain)
- Increased stroke volume
- Bradycardia
- Conditions in which there is a rapid run-off of blood in the arterial system (e.g., aortic valve regurgitation, patent ductus arteriosus, aortic-cardiac fistulas)

Hypokinetic Arterial Pulse

Hypokinetic pulses are present in patients with diminished stroke volume caused by the following:

- Hypovolemia (e.g., dehydration, shock, toxemia)
- Left ventricular failure
- Mitral or aortic valve stenosis (rare in large animals)

Pulse Deficits

Abnormal peripheral pulses may be detected in patients with cardiac arrhythmias. With premature ventricular contractions (PVCs), there is a compensatory pause and thus a stronger pulse in the beat after the PVC. With atrial fibrillation, the strength of the peripheral pulse is variable; with this and other tachyarrhythmias, there is a palpable pulse deficit.

7

Alterations in Alimentary and Hepatic Function

Consulting Editors BRADFORD P. SMITH • K. GARY MAGDESIAN

The general diagnostic approaches to alterations in alimentary and hepatic function are discussed in Chapter 7 of *Large Animal Internal Medicine,* third edition. Specific tests and procedures for diagnosis of the diseases listed below are discussed in Chapters 20 (neonates) and 30.

DIARRHEA *(Text pp. 102-108)*

Diarrhea may be a sign of a primary bowel disease or a nonspecific response to sepsis, toxemia, or disease of another organ system. Five major mechanisms may be involved:

1. *Malabsorption* (villus atrophy or damage), such as from rotavirus or coronavirus infection, cryptosporidiosis, salmonellosis, Johne's disease, or granulomatous bowel disease.
2. *Osmotic overload* from any disease causing maldigestion and/or malabsorption, or from cathartics such as dioctyl sodium sulfosuccinate (DSS) and magnesium phosphate or sulfate.
    - In ruminants, grain overload resulting in ruminal osmotic changes can cause diarrhea, as can changes in abomasal pH with type II ostertagiasis.
3. *Hypersecretion,* such as with enterotoxigenic *Escherichia coli, Salmonella* spp., and *Clostridium perfringens.*
4. *Hypermotility* (decreased transit time), which can occur with many bowel diseases because of bowel irritation; it may also accompany peritonitis.
5. *Increased blood-to-lumen hydraulic pressure,* such as with hypoalbuminemia, heart failure, portal hypertension associated with liver disease, and lymphosarcoma.

Causes of Diarrhea

Horses

Common causes of diarrhea in adult horses include the following:

- Colitis/typhlitis
- Salmonellosis
- Enteritis
- Potomac horse fever (equine monocytic ehrlichiosis)
- Endotoxemia/gram-negative sepsis
- Overfeeding, sudden change in diet
- *Clostridium difficile* infection

Less common causes of diarrhea in horses are listed on p. 103 of *Large Animal Internal Medicine,* third edition. Diarrhea in neonatal foals is discussed in Chapter 20.

Ruminants

Common causes of diarrhea in adult ruminants include the following:

- Internal parasites–nematodes, coccidiosis
- Enteritis or colitis/typhlitis–salmonellosis, Johne's disease, bovine viral diarrhea (BVD; cattle), winter dysentery (cattle), malignant catarrhal fever (cattle)
- Other gastrointestinal (GI) disturbances–abomasal displacement or torsion (cattle), intussusception
- Feed-related causes–indigestion (spoiled feed, overfeeding, or sudden change), grain overload (rumen acidosis), molybdenosis/copper deficiency
- Peritonitis
- Sepsis/toxemia
- Enterotoxemia
- Organ failure–heart, liver, kidney
- Drugs–xylazine (large doses), cathartics/laxatives, parasympathomimetics

Less common causes of diarrhea in ruminants are listed on p. 105 of *Large Animal Internal Medicine,* third edition. With chronic diarrhea, parasitism, Johne's disease, copper deficiency (molybdenosis), selenium deficiency, liver failure, and other diseases of individual animals (e.g., bovine leukosis virus [BLV], amyloidosis, heart failure, uremia) should be considered.

Toxic Causes of Diarrhea

The list of drugs, chemicals, and plant toxins that can cause diarrhea includes the following:

- All species–salt, propylene glycol, sulfur, phosphorus, arsenic, monensin, lasalocid, salinomycin, oak (acorn poisoning), slaframine ("slobber factor"), mycotoxins
- Horses–phenylbutazone, blister beetles (cantharidin), selenium, amitraz, DSS, reserpine, mercury, organophosphates, oleander, Japanese yew (*Taxus* sp.), castor bean, avocado, thorn apple (*Datura* sp.), algae
- Ruminants–levamisole, polybrominated biphenyl, sodium bicarbonate, aflatoxin, herbicides, zinc, copper, chlorpyrofos, lincomycin, trichothecene (T2 toxin), selenium-accumulating plants

A more complete list is found on p. 105 of *Large Animal Internal Medicine,* third edition.

COLIC *(Text pp. 108-111)*

Colic is a manifestation of visceral abdominal pain. It may be acute, chronic, or recurrent. The five basic causes of colic pain in large animals are as follows:

1. Distention of the gut with fluid, gas, or ingesta
2. Pulling on the root of the mesentery
3. Ischemia or infarction
4. Deep ulcers in the stomach or bowel
5. Peritonitis

Causes of Colic

Horses

The more common causes of colic in horses include the following:

- GI–accumulation of intestinal gas, hypermotility/intestinal spasm, feed impaction, meconium impaction (neonates), gastric ulcers, mesenteric abscess
- Urogenital–ovarian tumor, abscess, or hematoma; parturition; uterine torsion; ruptured bladder (foals)
- Other–diaphragmatic hernia, acute hepatitis, hepatic lipidosis

Less common, uncommon, and toxic causes of colic in horses are listed on p. 108 of *Large Animal Internal Medicine,* third edition.

Ruminants

The more common causes of colic in ruminants include the following:

- GI–increased intestinal gas, intussusception, torsion/volvulus of the mesenteric root, intestinal foreign body/obstruction, abomasal torsion, abomasal ulcer, cecal dilation/volvulus, severe bloat
- Urogenital–urolithiasis, ruptured bladder, acute pyelonephritis
- Peritonitis

Less common, uncommon, and toxic causes of colic in ruminants are listed on p. 109 of *Large Animal Internal Medicine,* third edition.

MELENA *(Text pp. 111-112)*

Melena (dark, tarry feces) is caused by blood in the lumen of the stomach or proximal intestinal tract. Usually, melena results from ulceration in the stomach or abomasum, but it may also result from ingestion of blood, oral or pharyngeal bleeding, or coughing up of blood that is then swallowed. Fairly large amounts of blood (1 to 2 L) are required to produce a positive fecal occult blood test in horses.

Causes of Melena

Common causes of melena in horses include gastric or duodenal ulcers, gastric squamous cell carcinoma (especially in old horses), and swallowing of coughed-up blood. In ruminants, abomasal ulcers and intussusception are the main differentials to be considered. Intussusception should be suspected if the animal is passing dark red feces and showing signs of colic. Consideration should also be given to clotting abnormalities (e.g., disseminated intravascular coagulation, warfarin poisoning). Less common and uncommon causes of melena in horses and ruminants are listed on p. 112 of *Large Animal Internal Medicine,* third edition.

BLOOD, FIBRIN, OR MUCUS IN FECES *(Text pp. 112-113)*

Blood (Dysentery)

Dysentery refers to bloody diarrhea. Fresh blood or clots in the feces (hematochezia) is the result of bleeding into the distal intestinal tract. Occasionally, blood from the female reproductive tract appears in or on the feces. Frank blood in feces without diarrhea or other evidence of GI dysfunction or systemic illness may be a result of a bleeding disorder, a traumatic foreign body, rectal examination or other iatrogenic trauma, or rectal trauma in a mare from a stallion penetrating the rectum.

Fibrin or Mucus

Fibrin in or on the feces appears as casts, chunks of yellow-gray material, or mucosa-like sheets. It indicates severe inflammatory bowel disease. Mucus in or on the feces increases with inflammatory bowel disease, although it is common when fecal volume is small, such as in anorectic animals.

Causes of Blood, Fibrin, or Mucus in the Feces

Common causes of blood, fibrin, or mucus feces in horses include the following:

- Foreign body
- Rectal tear/trauma
- Intussusception
- Blister beetle (cantharidin) toxicity
- Colitis (fibrin)
- Salmonellosis (fibrin)

Common causes in ruminants include foreign body, intussusception, coccidiosis, and salmonellosis. Less common and uncommon causes of blood or fibrin/mucus in the feces are listed on p. 113 of *Large Animal Internal Medicine,* third edition.

ABDOMINAL DISTENTION/CONSTIPATION *(Text pp. 113-114)*

Abdominal distention may be caused by feed, fluid, gas, feces, or neoplasm. Pregnancy or extreme obesity also result in abdominal enlargement. Constipation is usually a secondary problem.

Causes of Abdominal Distention

Horses

Common causes of abdominal distention in horses include the following:

- GI–ileus, intestinal foreign body (e.g., enterolith), intestinal impaction or tympany, necrotizing enterocolitis (foals), torsion or volvulus of the bowel
- Peritonitis
- Sudden decrease in exercise

Less common and uncommon causes are listed on p. 113 of *Large Animal Internal Medicine,* third edition.

Ruminants

Common causes of abdominal distention in ruminants include the following:

- Physiologic–pregnancy, obesity
- GI–vagal indigestion, grain overload, bloat, ileus, cecal volvulus or dilation, fat necrosis involving the colon or rectum, intestinal obstruction, reticulo-omasal orifice obstruction/foreign body
- Other–hypocalcemia, peritonitis, ruptured bladder (uroperitoneum), pelvic mass (abscess, tumor)

Less common and uncommon causes are listed on p. 114 of *Large Animal Internal Medicine,* third edition.

REGURGITATION/VOMITING *(Text pp. 114-116)*

Regurgitation is the reflux of esophageal, gastric, or ruminal contents into the mouth or nose. Vomiting is a coordinated, centrally mediated event, usually preceded by nausea (inappetence), hypersalivation, or retching. Vomiting is unusual in both ruminants and horses. Horses have such marked tone at the cardiac sphincter that vomiting occurs only when intragastric pressure is extreme. Thus vomiting in horses is often associated with gastric rupture.

Causes of Regurgitation/Vomiting

Horses

Common causes of regurgitation in horses include the following:

- Choke (esophageal obstruction)
- Esophageal trauma, foreign body, or diverticulum
- Foreign body in the pharynx or trachea
- Guttural pouch infection with pharyngeal paresis
- Gastric dilation/rupture (vomiting)

Less common, uncommon, and toxic causes of regurgitation/vomiting in horses are listed on p. 115 of *Large Animal Internal Medicine,* third edition.

Ruminants

Common causes of regurgitation in ruminants include the following:

- Esophageal trauma or foreign body
- Oral/pharyngeal foreign body, abscess, or trauma
- Salt toxicity (water deprivation followed by unrestricted access) (vomiting)
- Tumor, papilloma, or other mass in the rumen or esophagus
- Toxins and poisonous plants (vomiting)

Less common, uncommon, and toxic causes of regurgitation/vomiting in ruminants are listed on p. 115 of *Large Animal Internal Medicine,* third edition.

DYSPHAGIA *(Text pp. 116-118)*

Dysphagia describes abnormalities of prehension, mastication, and swallowing. It is associated with diseases of the mouth, pharynx, esophagus, mandible, and masseter muscles. Dysphagia may also be associated with central or peripheral neurologic lesions resulting in malfunction in these areas.

When dysphagia causes loss of large amounts of saliva, acid-base and electrolyte disorders may develop. Cattle and sheep may experience hypovolemia and severe metabolic acidosis, whereas horses may have a transient metabolic alkalosis following massive saliva loss.

Causes of Dysphagia

Causes of dysphagia can be divided into three categories:

1. Pain (probably the most common cause of dysphagia in large animals)
   - Pain can be caused by oral lesions or foreign bodies, dental problems (especially in horses, sheep, and goats), mandibular fractures, pharyngeal injuries from balling guns.
2. Neurologic or neuromuscular
   - In horses, guttural pouch disease resulting in pharyngeal paresis is a common cause of dysphagia; botulism can also cause pharyngeal paresis.
   - In ruminants, listeriosis often causes facial paralysis and dysphagia.
   - Rabies is an important differential in any species.
3. Obstructive
   - Common obstructive causes include choking (esophageal obstruction) in horses, pharyngeal lesions, and retropharyngeal lesions (e.g., strangles abscess in horses).

Mechanical interference with prehension, chewing, or swallowing can also cause dysphagia. Comprehensive lists of possible causes of dysphagia in horses and ruminants are found on p. 117 of *Large Animal Internal Medicine,* third edition.

ORAL VESICLES, EROSIONS, ULCERS, AND GROWTHS *(Text pp. 118-119)*

Most of the infectious diseases causing oral lesions also cause other lesions or symptoms; they are often divided into those also causing diarrhea and those not causing diarrhea. Of those in North America not associated with diarrhea, vesicular stomatitis is most common in cattle and horses, bluetongue in sheep, and contagious ecthyma in sheep and goats. The two most common diseases that cause oral lesions and diarrhea in cattle are bovine viral diarrhea/mucosal disease (BVD/MD) and malignant catarrhal fever.

Table 7-1 in *Large Animal Internal Medicine,* third edition, lists the infectious diseases associated with oral lesions in large animals and describes the typical oral lesions and other types of lesions found.

Causes of Oral Lesions

Horses

Common causes of oral vesicles, erosions, ulcers, or growths in horses include the following:

- Vesicular stomatitis
- Phenylbutazone toxicity
- Yellow bristle grass (*Setaria* spp.) or other plant awn stomatitis
- Oral foreign bodies

Less common causes include irritant or caustic chemicals, periodontal gingivitis, blister beetle (cantharidin) toxicity, and uremia.

Ruminants

Common causes of oral vesicles, erosions, ulcers, or growths in ruminants include the following:

- Any ruminant–vesicular stomatitis, traumatic or irritant stomatitis, bristle

grass ulcers or other plant awn stomatitis, oral foreign body, actinobacillosis ("woody tongue")
- Cattle–BVD/MD, bovine papular stomatitis
- Sheep and goats–bluetongue (sheep), contagious ecthyma (orf virus)

Less common and uncommon causes are listed on p. 118 of *Large Animal Internal Medicine,* third edition.

ICTERUS (JAUNDICE) *(Text pp. 120-121)*

Icterus and *jaundice* are synonymous and refer to yellow discoloration in the sclera and mucous membranes. Icterus results from increased amounts of bilirubin in tissues and increased serum bilirubin levels. It usually indicates decreased excretion of bilirubin with liver or biliary tract disease or increased production of bilirubin with hemolytic anemia. The most pronounced jaundice is usually seen with hepatic or obstructive biliary disease because conjugated bilirubin stains connective tissue most avidly. However, it is possible to have liver disease without icterus.

Causes of Icterus

Horses

The more common causes of icterus in horses include the following:
- Hepatic–pyrrolizidine alkaloid toxicity, serum-associated hepatitis, hepatitis (acute or chronic active), cholangitis or cholangiohepatitis, bile stones or other biliary obstruction, anorexia (fasting hyperbilirubinemia)
- Hemolytic–immune-mediated hemolytic anemia, *Ehrlichia equi* infection, neonatal isoerythrolysis

Less common and uncommon causes of icterus in horses are listed on p. 120 of *Large Animal Internal Medicine,* third edition.

Ruminants

Common hepatic causes icterus in ruminants include pyrrolizidine alkaloid toxicity, aflatoxicosis, and fat cow syndrome (fatty liver). Common hemolytic causes include leptospirosis, anaplasmosis, and bacillary hemoglobinuria *(Clostridium haemolyticum).* Less common and uncommon causes of icterus in ruminants are listed on p. 121 of *Large Animal Internal Medicine,* third edition.

8

Localization and Differentiation of Neurologic Diseases

Consulting Editor MARY O. SMITH

Contributor LISLE W. GEORGE

Diagnosis of neurologic disease must begin with careful evaluation of the patient's signalment, history, diet, environment, vaccination and infectious disease history, and reproductive status (specifically, stage of pregnancy or lactation). A thorough physical examination should be performed before or with the neurologic examination to identify systemic or regional disease that may underlie the neurologic problem.

NEUROLOGIC EXAMINATION *(Text pp. 128-139)*

The objectives of the neurologic examination are to determine whether the animal has a neurologic disease and, if so, where the lesion is located. The diagnostic plan is then made on the basis of lesion location and most likely differential diagnoses. A recommended approach to the neurologic examination is to begin with procedures that require minimal handling of the animal; then proceed to those that require manipulation:

- Mentation and behavior
- Gait–observe the animal walking in a straight line, on a circle, over an obstacle (e.g., a curb or ground pole), on a slope; back up the animal; perform the tail pull test
- Conscious proprioception and postural reactions–response to placement of the limbs in an abnormal position (e.g., abduction, crossing of the limbs)
    - Additional postural reactions, such as hopping and hemiwalking, can be tested in small ruminants, calves, and some foals.
- Abnormalities of posture and righting response (most easily tested in small ruminants and recumbent animals)
- Spinal reflexes
    - Myotactic or tendon reflexes (recumbent animals only) involve the triceps tendon, biceps muscle, middle patellar ligament, and cranial tibial muscle.
    - Flexor reflexes produce a withdrawal response to painful stimulus applied to the distal limb. Perform this test only in recumbent animals.
    - Perineal reflex is demonstrated by anal sphincter constriction and tail clamping in response to pinching of the anus.
    - Panniculus or cutaneous reflex is a wrinkling or flinching of the skin over the trunk in response to light touch or pinching.

Cervical reflex in horses is demonstrated by local skin twitch in response to tapping or pinching of the skin in the caudal half of the neck.
Cervicoauricular reflex in horses is an ear twitch in response to lightly tapping the skin over C1 to C3 vertebrae.
"Slap" test or laryngeal adductor reflex is a contraction of the dorsal cricoarytenoid muscle in response to a sharp slap applied to the saddle region on the opposite side of the horse.

- Muscle mass and tone
- Cranial nerves (CNs) (see following discussion)

Neurologic examination is described in detail in *Large Animal Internal Medicine,* third edition.

Cranial Nerves

Following is a brief review of CN function:

- CN I (olfactory nerve)–sense of smell; difficult to objectively assess
- CN II (optic nerve)–vision; assessed by response to visual cues, menace response, pupillary light reflex, and negotiating an obstacle course
- CN III, IV, and VI (oculomotor, trochlear, and abducens nerves)–eye position in the orbit
  - CN III dysfunction results in ventrolateral strabismus; ptosis; and a dilated, unresponsive pupil.
  - CN IV dysfunction results in dorsomedial strabismus.
  - CN VI dysfunction results in medial strabismus and inability to retract the globe.
- CN V (trigeminal nerve)–facial sensation and motor function to the masticatory muscles
  - Sensory function is tested by lightly stimulating the face with the tip of a closed hemostat.
  - The palpebral reflex (brisk closure of the eyelids in response to light touch in the periorbital area) tests both sensory function of CN V and motor function of CN VII.
  - Opening the jaw assesses the strength of the masticatory muscles and thus the motor component of CN V; bilateral motor paralysis results in a dropped jaw.
  - Note: Rabies is an important differential in animals with a dropped jaw.
- CN VII (facial nerve)–innervates the muscles of facial expression; assessed by evaluating muscle tone in the ears, lips, eyelids, and muzzle
  - Facial nerve dysfunction results in facial paresis or paralysis, loss of sensation on medial aspect of the pinna, decreased tear production, and decreased salivation.
- CN VIII (acoustic nerve)–contributes to the vestibular system and to hearing; assessed by evaluating gait, extensor tone, head posture, and eye position and movement
  - CN VIII can also be evaluated using brainstem auditory evoked potentials (see text).
- CN IX, X, and XI (glossopharyngeal, vagus, and accessory nerves)–motor function to the muscles of the neck, pharynx, and palate
  - The vagus nerve also stimulates secretion from glands of the visceral and respiratory mucosae and controls forestomach motility in ruminants.
  - Dysfunction causes dysphagia (IX and X), laryngeal paresis or paralysis (X), and atrophy of the sternocephalicus, brachiocephalicus, and trapezius muscles (XI).
- CN XII (hypoglossal nerve)–motor function to the tongue and geniohyoideus muscle; tested by pulling the patient's tongue out and assessing tone and retractability

Examination of Neonates

Following are some differences between neonatal foals and adult horses that may affect interpretation of the neurologic examination:

- Muscle tone and spinal reflexes–in foals less than 3 weeks of age limbs are hypertonic and hyperreflexic (more pronounced in the rear limbs)
  - Some foals demonstrate myoclonus after percussion of the patellar or triceps tendons.
  - When restrained, newborn foals relax into a trancelike state, periodically awakening and struggling violently before becoming passive again.
- Menace response–absent in foals for up to 2 weeks after birth

LOCALIZATION OF CENTRAL NERVOUS SYSTEM LESIONS *(Text p. 139)*

Localization of lesions within the nervous system is the first and the key step in developing a differential diagnosis list for any animal presenting with signs of neurologic disease. Neurologic lesions can be localized to one of seven regions: (1) cerebral cortex and thalamus, (2) midbrain, (3) cerebellum, (4) medulla oblongata, (5) spinal cord, (6) peripheral nerve (cranial nerves or spinal nerves), or (7) muscle. Once the anatomic site of the lesion has been determined, diagnostic tests such as cerebrospinal fluid analysis, radiography, myelography, and serology can be performed to further characterize the disease.

Following is a summary of central nervous system (CNS) signs and the likely locations of the lesion:

Symptom	Usual lesion location
Changes in gait and locomotion	
Ataxia	Nonspecific; any area of CNS
Conscious proprioceptive deficit	Nonspecific; any area of CNS except cerebellum
Hypermetria	Cerebellum or peduncles, spinocerebellar tracts
Circling or falling to one side	Basal ganglia, cortex, vestibular nuclei, cerebellum
Paraplegia/hemiplegia	Nonspecific
Changes in sensorium and behavior	
Coma or semicoma	Brainstem, thalamus, cortex
Depression	Brainstem, thalamus, cortex
Convulsions	Brainstem, thalamus, cortex
Head pressing, propulsive walking	Cortex (frontal lobe), limbic system
Aggression/rage	Limbic system, frontal lobe, amygdala
Inappropriate sexuality	Limbic system
Hyperphagia or hypophagia	Hypothalamus
Diabetes insipidus	Hypothalamus
Head shaking	Unknown, probably peripheral neuropathy
Changes in head posture	
Stiff neck	Meninges, cervical spine
Head tilt	Thalamus, cerebral cortex, medulla, cerebellum
Head tremor	Cerebellum, basal ganglia
Opisthotonus	Cerebellum, rostral brainstem, cerebrum, acoustic nerve (CN VIII)
Cranial nerve dysfunction	
Amaurosis (central blindness)	Cortex, internal capsule, optic chiasm, optic nerve (CN II), eye
Anisocoria	Cervical spine, vagosympathetic trunk, brainstem (oculomotor nerve nucleus), cranial cervical ganglion, ciliary ganglion, oculomotor nerve (CN III)
Mydriasis	Oculomotor nerve (CN III), brain stem, eye
Miosis	Vagosympathetic trunk, ciliary ganglia, tectum, brain stem, cervical spinal cord
Ptosis	Facial nerve (CN VII), vagosympathetic trunk, ciliary ganglion, brainstem, cervical spinal cord

Symptom	Usual lesion location
Strabismus:	
Ventrolateral	Cerebellum, vestibular nucleus, oculomotor nerve (CN III)
Dorsomedial	Trochlear nerve (CN IV)
Medial	Abducens nerve (CN VI)
Nystagmus:	
Horizontal	Facial nerve (CN VII; peripheral)
Vertical/rotary	Vestibular nuclei, peripheral vestibular receptor, cerebellum, auditory nerve (CN VIII)
Jaw drop	Metencephalon, trigeminal motor nucleus, trigeminal nerve (CN V)
Flaccid tongue	Medulla, hypoglossal nerve (CN XII), hypoglossal nucleus, tongue muscle
Facial paralysis	Medulla, facial nerve (CN VII), facial muscles
Facial analgesia	Trigeminal nerve (CN V; sensory component)
Dry eye	Facial nerve (CN VII), before entering the petrous temporal bone
Abnormal spinal reflexes	
Patellar reflex	Spinal cord segments L4 to L6, femoral nerve, quadriceps femoris muscles
Forelimb flexors	Spinal cord segments C5 to T2; radial, ulnar, musculocutaneous, and median nerves; innervated muscles
Hindlimb flexors	Spinal cord segments L6 to S2; femoral, ischiatic, peroneal, and tibial nerves; flexor and extensor muscles
Triceps reflex	Spinal cord segments C6 to T1, radial nerve, triceps muscle
Panniculus reflex	Spinal cord segment C8, thoracodorsal nerve, dorsal column of thoracic spinal cord
Anal reflex	Spinal cord segments S1 to S5, pudendal nerve
Ear twitch	Dorsal columns of spinal cord segments C1 to C3, facial nerve, facial nucleus, ear muscles
Urine dribbling	Spinal cord, pons, pelvic nerves, bladder wall

LESIONS OF THE CEREBRUM, BASAL GANGLIA, AND THALAMUS *(Text pp. 139-144)*

Clinical Manifestations

Signs of disease involving the telencephalon (cerebrum, basal ganglia) and diencephalon (thalamus) include the following:

- Changes in behavior and level of consciousness–dullness/depression, stupor, narcolepsy, coma, excitement/mania, seizures
- Vision disturbance–bilateral blindness (amaurosis), contralateral blindness (hemianopsia), menace reflex deficit, change in pupil size (small to pinpoint)
- Circling and/or head turn (toward the lesion side)
- Abnormal postural reactions (contralateral)–decreased or absent conscious proprioception
- Abnormal spinal reflexes (hyperreflexia), altered muscle tone (spasticity), tremors
- Urinary incontinence (upper motor neuron)

The gait usually is normal; obvious ataxia or paresis/paralysis is rare.

Diseases Producing Cortical/Thalamic Signs

Horses

The following diseases can produce cortical signs in horses:

- Bacterial, fungal, or protozoal infection–brain abscess/meningitis, leukoencephalomalacia, equine protozoal myeloencephalitis
- Viral infection–rabies; Eastern, Western, or Venezuelan equine encephalomyelitis; Near Eastern encephalitis; equine herpesvirus type 1; West Nile virus; borna
- Other–hepatic or renal encephalopathy, parasitic migration, hydrocephalus, idiopathic epilepsy, narcolepsy, brain tumor, trauma/hematoma

Predominant clinical signs associated with each of these diseases are listed in Table 8-8 of *Large Animal Internal Medicine,* third edition.

Ruminants

The following diseases can cause cortical or thalamic signs in ruminants:

- Infection–rabies, pseudorabies, bovine spongiform encephalopathy (cattle), malignant catarrhal fever (cattle), sporadic bovine encephalomyelitis (cattle), *Sarcocystis* spp. (cattle), scrapie (sheep, goats), border disease (sheep, goats), caprine arthritis-encephalitis (goats), maedi-visna (sheep)
- Nutritional or toxic–polioencephalomalacia, sulfur poisoning, lead poisoning, salt poisoning, vitamin A deficiency, nitrofurazone toxicosis (cattle), grass staggers, plant poisonings (see text)
- Other–trauma/hematoma/brain edema, brain abscess/meningitis, brain tumor

Predominant clinical signs associated with each of these diseases are listed in Table 8-7 of *Large Animal Internal Medicine,* third edition.

LESIONS OF THE BRAINSTEM AND CRANIAL NERVES *(Text pp. 144-147)*

Clinical Manifestations

Midbrain

Signs of disease involving the mesencephalon (midbrain) include the following:

- Changes in level of consciousness–dullness/depression, stupor, narcolepsy, coma
- Abnormal posture–opisthotonus, decerebrate posture
- Abnormal visual or ocular function–bilateral or contralateral blindness, change in pupil size (small pupils with early/mild lesions; dilated, nonresponsive pupils with severe lesions), menace reflex deficit (contralateral), anisocoria (asymmetric lesions)
- Circling, head turn (toward lesion side)
- Gait abnormalities (contralateral)–decreased or absent conscious proprioception, ataxia, paresis, paralysis
- Abnormal spinal reflexes (hyperreflexia), altered muscle tone (spasticity)
- Urinary incontinence (upper motor neuron)

Pons and cerebellum

Signs of disease involving the metencephalon (pons, cerebellum) include the following:

- Abnormal posture–head tilt, decerebellate posture
- Circling, head turn (usually away from lesion side)
- Nystagmus (variable)
- Gait abnormalities–ataxia, hypermetria or dysmetria
- Abnormal spinal reflexes (occasional hyperreflexia), altered muscle tone (ipsilateral hypotonus, contralateral spasticity)
- Urinary incontinence (rare)

Medulla oblongata

Signs of disease involving the medulla oblongata include the following:

- Change in level of consciousness–dullness/depression

- Abnormal posture–head tilt, circling, head turn toward lesion side
- Strabismus, nystagmus (spontaneous, abnormal), menace reflex deficit
- Dysphagia; jaw weakness; tongue weakness, deviation, or paralysis
- Facial anesthesia/analgesia, facial paresis/paralysis
- Roaring, snoring, dysphonia
- Gait abnormalities (ipsilateral)–decreased or absent conscious proprioception, ataxia, paresis, paralysis
- Abnormal spinal reflexes (hyperreflexia), altered muscle tone (normal or increased tone)
- Urinary incontinence

Diseases Causing Spasticity or Tremors

The following diseases cause spasticity or tremors:

- Hereditary and congenital conditions–cerebellar hypoplasia (ruminants), cerebellar abiotrophy (horses, cattle), daft lambs (sheep), lysosomal storage disease (cattle, goats), hereditary neuraxial edema (cattle), bovine familial convulsions and ataxia (cattle), maple syrup urine disease (cattle)
    - Specific causes of cerebellar hypoplasia include bovine viral diarrhea, bluetongue, Akabane virus, border disease, Wesselbron disease, and hereditary factors.
- Nutritional or toxic conditions–grass staggers (ruminants), hypomagnesemia (horses, cattle), locoism and *Swainsonia* poisoning, *Solanum dimidiatum* poisoning (cattle)
    - Specific causes of grass staggers include Bermuda, Kikuyu, rye, canary, and Dallis grasses and mycotic tremorgens.

Predominant clinical signs associated with each of these diseases are listed in Table 8-9 of *Large Animal Internal Medicine,* third edition.

Diseases Involving the Brainstem and Cranial Nerves

Following is a list of diseases that affect the brainstem and cranial nerves and the primary area(s) involved:

- Viral encephalomyelitis (rabies, malignant catarrhal fever in cattle)–multifocal brainstem, particularly the medulla oblongata
- Listeriosis (cattle)–multifocal brainstem, particularly the basal ganglia, metencephalon, and medulla oblongata
- Thromboembolic meningoencephalomyelitis (cattle)–multifocal brainstem and cortex
- Peripheral vestibular disease–auditory nerve (CN VIII); can also involve the facial nerve (CN VII)
- Verminous migration–multifocal brainstem, most commonly the thalamus and diencephalon
- Space-occupying mass (tumor, abscess)–cerebellopontine angle; CN V, VII, and VIII
- Horner's syndrome (see below)–C8 to T1 motor neurons (gray matter), spinal roots, vagosympathetic trunk, sympathetic spinal cord tracts, periorbita
- Guttural pouch mycosis (horses)–guttural pouch

Predominant clinical signs associated with each of these diseases are listed in Table 8-11 of *Large Animal Internal Medicine,* third edition.

Horner's Syndrome

Horner's syndrome is caused by a lesion somewhere along the course of the preganglionic or postganglionic sympathetic nerves that innervate the head, in spinal cord segments T1 to T3, or (rarely) in the cervical spinal cord or brainstem. Specific causes include compressive lesions of the gray matter in spinal segments T1 to T3, neoplasia, abscessation (mediastinal, thoracic, retrobulbar, or involving the cervical sympathetic trunk), esophageal perforation, guttural pouch mycosis (horses), and otitis media/interna. Transient Horner's syndrome may occur after intravenous injection of xylazine.

Clinical signs

Signs include miosis, enophthalmia, ptosis, and increased warmth on the ipsilateral side of the face. In cattle there is loss of sweating on the ipsilateral side of the *planum nasale;* in horses there is excessive sweating on the affected side. Preganglionic and postganglionic denervation may be differentiated by instilling 1:1000 epinephrine (0.1 ml) into the eye with the miotic pupil. Pupillary dilation occurs within 20 minutes in patients with postganglionic lesions and within 40 minutes in those with preganglionic lesions.

LESIONS OF THE SPINAL CORD AND PERIPHERAL NERVES *(Text pp. 147-150)*

Clinical Manifestations

Spinal cord, C1 to C5

Signs of disease involving the cervical spinal cord segments C1 to C5 include the following:

- Gait abnormalities (ipsilateral, thoracic and pelvic limbs)–decreased or absent conscious proprioception, ataxia, paresis, paralysis
- Abnormal spinal reflexes (ipsilateral)–hyperreflexia (thoracic and pelvic limbs), decreased or absent caudal cervical and auricular reflexes, decreased or absent "slap test" (horses)
- Altered muscle tone–normal or increased tone
- Urinary incontinence

Spinal cord, C6 to T2

Signs of disease involving cervicothoracic spinal cord segments C6 to T2 include the following:

- Gait abnormalities (ipsilateral, thoracic and pelvic limbs)–decreased or absent conscious proprioception, ataxia, paresis, paralysis
- Abnormal spinal reflexes (ipsilateral)–hyporeflexia in thoracic limbs, hyperreflexia in pelvic limbs, decreased or absent caudal cervical and auricular reflexes, decreased or absent "slap test" (horses), absent panniculus reflex
- Horner's syndrome (ipsilateral)
- Altered muscle tone–decreased tone in thoracic limbs, normal or increased tone in pelvic limbs
- Urinary incontinence

Spinal cord, T3 to L2

Signs of disease involving thoracolumbar spinal cord segments T3 to L2 include the following:

- Gait abnormalities (ipsilateral, pelvic limbs only)–decreased or absent conscious proprioception, ataxia, paresis, paralysis
- Abnormal spinal reflexes (ipsilateral)–hyperreflexia in pelvic limbs, decreased panniculus reflex caudal to lesion
- Altered muscle tone (ipsilateral)–normal or increased tone in pelvic limbs
- Urinary incontinence

Spinal cord, L3 to S3

Signs of disease involving lumbosacral spinal cord segments L3 to S3 include the following:

- Gait abnormalities (ipsilateral, pelvic limbs only)–decreased or absent conscious proprioception, ataxia, paresis, paralysis
- Abnormal spinal reflexes (ipsilateral)–hyporeflexia in pelvic limbs
- Altered muscle tone–decreased tone in pelvic limbs, flaccid tail
- Urinary and fecal incontinence (lower motor neuron)

Peripheral nerve and muscle

Signs of disease involving the peripheral nerves, neuromuscular junction, or muscle include the following:

- Gait abnormalities–paresis or paralysis in affected limbs, decreased or absent conscious proprioception, ataxia, paresis, paralysis
- Abnormal spinal reflexes (ipsilateral)–hyporeflexia in affected limbs

- Altered muscle tone–decreased tone and muscle atrophy in affected limbs, flaccid tail
- Urinary and fecal incontinence (lower motor neuron)

Causes of Spinal Cord, Peripheral Nerve, or Neuromuscular Signs

Diseases involving the spinal cord, peripheral nerves, or motor end plate in large animals include the following:

- All species–vertebral fractures or dislocation, cervical spinal abscess, spinal tumor (lymphosarcoma, neurofibroma), developmental defects, verminous migration, tetanus, botulism, locoism, dying-back axonopathies, peripheral nerve injuries, ionophore toxicosis (monensin, lasalocid, salinomycin), myotonia congenita, acquired torticollis, tick paralysis
- Horses–occipitoatlantoaxial malformation, degenerative myelopathy, cervical stenotic myelopathy, cervical vertebral instability, equine herpesvirus type 1, cauda equina neuritis, ischemic myelopathy (fibrocartilaginous embolism), segmental myelitis, periodic hyperkalemia, bromide intoxication, sorghum poisoning, stringhalt
- Cattle–occipitoatlantoaxial malformation, progressive ataxia (Charolais), spastic paresis ("Elso heel"), spastic syndrome ("crampy"), periodic hyperkalemia, neosporosis (calves), cycad palm poisoning, sorghum poisoning
- Sheep–copper deficiency, ischemic myelopathy (fibrocartilaginous embolism), humpy back/Coonabarabran disease
- Goats–copper deficiency, caprine arthritis-encephalitis virus, coyotillo poisoning

Predominant clinical signs associated with each of these diseases are listed in Table 8-12 of *Large Animal Internal Medicine,* third edition.

9

Alterations in Body Weight or Size

Consulting Editor JOHN MAAS

The general diagnostic approaches to decreased growth or weight gain and to weight loss are discussed in Chapter 9 of *Large Animal Internal Medicine,* third edition. Specific tests and procedures for diagnosis of the diseases listed in the following sections are discussed in the relevant chapters.

DECREASED GROWTH/DECREASED WEIGHT GAIN *(Text pp. 152-160)*

Major pathogenic mechanisms that result in decreased growth/weight gain include (1) inadequate dietary intake, (2) toxicosis, (3) genetic or congenital abnormalities, (4) parasitism, (5) infections or inflammatory processes, and (6) environmental factors. Nutritional requirements and growth charts for horses and ruminants are found in Chapter 9 of *Large Animal Internal Medicine,* third edition.

Causes of Decreased Growth or Weight Gain

Horses

Common causes of decreased growth/decreased weight gain in horses include the following:

- Nutritional–protein-calorie malnutrition
- Parasitism
- Respiratory–bacterial pneumonia, lung abscess, pleuropneumonia, pleuritis
- Gastrointestinal (GI)–gastric ulcers, salmonellosis, diarrhea
- Prematurity, dysmaturity
- Musculoskeletal–osteomyelitis, arthritis
- Combined immunodeficiency in foals

Less common and uncommon causes are listed on p. 153 in *Large Animal Internal Medicine,* third edition.

Ruminants

Common causes of decreased growth/decreased weight gain in ruminants include the following:

- Nutritional–protein-calorie malnutrition, selenium or copper deficiency
- Parasitic–ostertagiasis I and II, coccidiosis, other GI parasites, liver flukes, lungworms, sarcoptic mange
- Respiratory–pneumonia *(Mannheimia, Pasteurella, Haemophilus)*
- GI–salmonellosis, bovine virus diarrhea (cattle), rotavirus or coronavirus diarrhea, cryptosporidiosis, enterotoxigenic *Escherichia coli,* diarrhea
- Liver disease, hepatic abscessation
- Lameness–foot rot, laminitis, foot warts (papillomatous digital dermatitis), osteomyelitis

Less common, uncommon, and toxic causes are listed on p. 153 in *Large Animal Internal Medicine,* third edition.

WEIGHT LOSS *(Text pp. 160-168)*

Weight loss is generally associated with one or more of the following circumstances:

- Anorexia (usually secondary to primary disease)
- Increased nutrient demands
  - Physiologic causes include cold weather, pregnancy, lactation, and intense exercise.
  - Pathologic causes include infection/sepsis, trauma, parasitism, and burns.
- Protein-calorie malnutrition or deficiency of essential micronutrients such as copper, cobalt (vitamin B_{12}), and vitamin A

Causes of Weight Loss

Horses

Common causes of weight loss in horses include the following:

- Nutritional–protein-calorie malnutrition
- Parasitic–internal parasites, *Strongylus vulgaris* thromboembolism, wound myiasis
- Respiratory–pneumonia/lung abscess, pleuritis, *Streptococcus equi* infection (strangles), chronic obstructive pulmonary disease, *Rhodococcus equi* infection
- GI–sand colic/impaction, gastric/duodenal ulcers, gastric squamous cell carcinoma
- Other–cribbing/wind sucking, dental or jaw abnormalities, peritonitis, abdominal abscess, septic arthritis, pituitary adenoma, neoplasia, renal failure (acute or chronic), pyrrolizidine alkaloid hepatotoxicity

Less common, uncommon, and other toxic causes are listed on pp. 160-161 in *Large Animal Internal Medicine,* third edition.

Ruminants

Common causes of weight loss in ruminants include the following:

- Nutritional–protein-calorie malnutrition, selenium or copper deficiency
- Parasitic–liver flukes, lungworms, GI parasites, sarcoptic mange, lice/ked infestation, wound myiasis
- Respiratory–bacterial pneumonia, pulmonary abscess, infectious bovine rhinotracheitis (cattle)
- GI–Johne's disease, ruminal acidosis, displaced abomasum, abomasal ulcer, diarrhea (rotavirus, coronavirus, unknown cause), vagal indigestion, traumatic reticuloperitonitis/pericarditis, winter dysentery (cattle), salmonellosis, bovine viral diarrhea (cattle), coccidiosis, enterotoxigenic colibacillosis, intussusception, cryptosporidiosis
- Musculoskeletal–foot rot, pedal osteomyelitis, sole abscess, septic arthritis, other lameness
- Systemic–bovine leukosis, actinobacillosis, actinomycosis, anaplasmosis (cattle), leptospirosis, pasteurellosis (septicemic), bluetongue
- Urinary–urolithiasis, pyelonephritis, cystitis
- Metabolic–ketosis, fat necrosis (cattle), pregnancy toxemia
- Toxic–pyrrolizidine alkaloid toxicosis, fescue toxicity (cattle)
- Other–peritonitis, hepatic abscess, pharyngeal or retropharyngeal abscess, dental abnormalities, agammaglobulinemia (neonates), mastitis (coliform or staphylococcal), mammary abscess

Less common, uncommon, and other toxic causes are listed on pp. 162-163 in *Large Animal Internal Medicine,* third edition.

OBESITY *(Text pp. 168-170)*

Obesity is a common problem in domestic species. Obese patients (especially ruminants) are at particular risk for reproductive failure or metabolic disease late in pregnancy or during lactation.

Dry cows with access to high-energy diets are predisposed to fat cow syndrome. Obese horses and ponies that rapidly lose weight or are anorectic are susceptible to hyperlipidemia and hyperlipemia. Fat cow syndrome and hyperlipidemia/hyperlipemia are discussed in Chapter 31.

PICA *(Text p. 170)*

Pica is defined as a depraved or abnormal appetite, such as chewing or eating wood (fences, trees, buildings), dirt, bones, or other nonfeedstuffs. Pica has been associated with protein-calorie malnutrition, parasitism, obesity, and deficiencies of phosphorus, salt, protein, or micronutrients. Horses may chew wood fences from boredom alone.

10

Alterations in Urinary Function

Consulting Editors THOMAS J. DIVERS • DAVID C. VAN METRE

The general diagnostic approaches to urinary dysfunction are discussed in Chapter 10 of *Large Animal Internal Medicine,* third edition. Specific tests and procedures for diagnosis of the diseases listed in the following sections are discussed in the relevant chapters.

DYSURIA/STRANGURIA *(Text pp. 171-173)*

Dysuria is difficult or painful urination; *stranguria* is slow and painful urination. Dysuria or stranguria is usually caused by urethral obstruction, inflammation of the urethra or bladder, or neurologic conditions that prevent normal bladder emptying. In foal, calves, lambs, and kids, it may also result from a urachal abscess. There are few disorders in large animals that cause urinary incontinence without stranguria or dysuria. Ectopic ureter should be considered in young animals with persistent urinary incontinence.

Causes of Dysuria or Urinary Incontinence

Horses

Causes of dysuria/stranguria or urinary incontinence in horses include the following:

- Urinary–urethral or cystic calculi, urethral injury, hemorrhage into the urinary tract (causing obstruction), cantharidin toxicosis, bladder neoplasia, urethritis, cystitis, ruptured bladder or ureter, ectopic ureter, bladder prolapse after foaling
- Genital–penile or prepucial trauma/swelling, vaginal trauma/swelling (especially after foaling), habronemiasis, smegma accumulation
- Neurologic–herpes myelitis, rabies, severe spinal cord disease, vertebral body infection or fracture, sorghum poisoning, neonatal maladjustment (foals)
- Other–prolonged recumbency, myositis,* laminitis,* colic,* peritonitis,* estrogen-responsive dysuria (rare in horses)

Ruminants

Causes of dysuria/stranguria or urinary incontinence in ruminants include the following:

- Urogenital–urethral calculi, hemorrhage into the urinary tract, urethral injury secondary to calving or breeding, penile or preputial injury, cystitis, pelvic entrapment of the bladder, urachal abscess, prolapsed bladder (accompanying vaginal prolapse), bladder neoplasia, congenital urethral disorders
- Neurologic–rabies, sacral fracture, extradural lymphosarcoma, spinal cord trauma/compression

---

*These conditions can mimic dysuria/stranguria.

Causes in sheep and goats include urethral calculi, cystitis, injury to (or swelling around) the urethra, spinal cord trauma or compression, and ulcerative posthitis. Urethral calculi should be suspected in a dysuric sheep or goat that was castrated at an early age and in castrated sheep and cattle receiving high-grain diets in feedlots, as well as in intact males.

HEMATURIA *(Text pp. 173-174)*

Hematuria is blood in the urine. It may appear as gross blood clots passed at the beginning, during, or at the end of urination or as a more uniform red discoloration throughout urination without clots. In the latter situation, it is necessary to determine that the discoloration is hematuria and not hemoglobinuria, bilirubinuria, or myoglobinuria. This is accomplished by dipstick evaluation of the urine, examination of the urine sediment for cell types and crystals, and assessment of the patient's packed cell volume and plasma protein and the color of the plasma and mucous membranes.

Causes of Hematuria

Horses

Causes of hematuria in horses include the following:

- Urethra–habronemiasis, calculi, idiopathic proximal dorsal urethral hemorrhage (males), urethritis, neoplasia (especially squamous cell carcinoma), trauma
- Bladder–calculi, cystitis, neoplasia, amorphous debris, bleeding diathesis (e.g., warfarin), blister beetle (cantharidin) toxicosis
- Kidney–calculi, trauma, nephritis, leptospirosis, vascular anomaly, parasite migration, neoplasia, vasculitis, glomerulopathy, papillary necrosis, blister beetle toxicosis, idiopathic kidney disease

Ruminants

Causes of hematuria in ruminants include the following:

- Urethra–calculi, trauma, urethritis, papilloma
- Bladder–bracken fern or other bleeding diathesis, papilloma/neoplasia, calculi, cystitis, polyps
- Kidney–pyelonephritis, trauma, infarction, malignant catarrhal fever, endotoxic shock, leptospirosis

PYURIA *(Text pp. 174-175)*

Pyuria is purulent debris in the urine. It may be a gross or microscopic observation. To be termed *pyuria* a midstream-voided or catheterized sample should have 8 white blood cells (WBCs) or more per high-power field; in septic cystitis there are 10,000 or more organisms per milliliter of urine. Pyuria may be a result of a septic disease or nonseptic inflammation. Pathogenic organisms are most often gram-negative bacteria. Gram-positive bacteria, such as *Staphylococcus, Corynebacterium,* and *Streptococcus* spp., may also cause urinary tract infections. Fever may or may not be present, but pyuria originating from the upper urinary tract often is accompanied by systemic illness. In females it is important to examine the reproductive tract to confirm that it is not the source of pyuria.

UREMIA *(Text pp. 175-179)*

Uremia refers to the presence of excessive urinary constituents in the blood and the resulting systemic effects. The predominant clinical signs in large animals are depression and anorexia. Weight loss, oral erosions, gastrointestinal ulcers, polyuria, polydipsia, melena, diarrhea, and excessive dental tartar are other signs. Coagulopathy and/or platelet dysfunction might also be seen. Uremia may be the result of either acute or chronic renal failure.

Causes of Acute Renal Failure

In animals with acute renal failure, azotemia (elevated serum creatinine and urea nitrogen) is present concurrently with a urine specific gravity less than 1.021. The predominant mechanisms causing renal failure in large animals are injury to renal tubular epithelium (e.g., inflammation, obstruction, toxic tubular nephrosis, immunologic disorders) and alterations in renal hemodynamics.

Horses

Causes of acute renal failure in horses include the following:

- Hemodynamic causes–severe hypovolemia (e.g., colitis), septic or hemorrhagic shock, heart failure, coagulopathies, adverse drug reaction
- Toxic nephrosis–aminoglycosides, tetracyclines, vitamin D, mercury, nonsteroidal antiinflammatory drugs (NSAIDs), amphotericin, pigment (hemoglobin, myoglobin) nephropathy
- Immunologic causes–drug-induced interstitial nephritis, glomerulopathy
- Sepsis–*Actinobacillus* spp., *Leptospira* spp., pyelonephritis, septic infarcts

Ruminants

Causes of acute renal failure in ruminants include the following:

- Hemodynamic causes–renal vein thrombosis, severe bloat, shock (hypovolemic or septic), heart failure
- Toxic plants–oak or acorn (*Quercus* spp.), *Halogeton glomerulatus*, greasewood *(Sarcobatus vermiculatus)*, soursob (*Oxalis* spp.), pigweed (*Amaranthus* spp.), *Kochia* spp., sorrel or dock (*Rumex* spp.), lamb's-quarter *(Chenopodium album)*, rhubarb *(Rheum rhaponticum)*, Russian thistle *(Salsola pestifer)*, *Lantana camara*, *Isotropis* spp.
- Drugs–aminoglycosides, sulfonamides, oxytetracycline, monensin
- Chemicals–arsenic, mercury, ethylene glycol, gasohol by-products, paraquat, chlorinated hydrocarbons, sodium fluoride, copper
- Endogenous substances–hemoglobin, myoglobin
- Mycotoxins–ochratoxin, citrinin
- Septic causes–pyelonephritis, septic mastitis or metritis (can cause infarction and renal necrosis)

Causes of Chronic Renal Failure

Chronic renal failure is the result of a slow and progressive loss of nephron function and/or numbers. Azotemia with isosthenuria (urine specific gravity 1.008 to 1.014) is typical, although serum creatinine may be only in the high-normal range. Chronic renal failure in large animals is usually the result of progressive glomerular disease or persistent/progressive tubulointerstitial disease.

Horses

Causes of chronic renal failure (CRF) in horses include the following:

- Tubulointerstitial–any of the causes of acute renal failure, chronic or intermittent obstruction (especially of the ureters), chronic pyelonephritis, granulomatous infiltration, neoplasia, NSAID-induced papillary necrosis (rare cause of CRF), renal dysplasia, polycystic kidney
- Glomerular–renal hypoplasia, amyloidosis, immune-mediated glomerulonephritis, glomerulosclerosis (unknown cause)

Ruminants

Causes of chronic renal failure in ruminants include the following:

- Tubulointerstitial–any of the causes of acute renal failure, chronic obstruction (urolithiasis), chronic pyelonephritis
- Glomerular–amyloidosis, glomerulonephritis (rare)

POLYURIA *(Text pp. 179-180)*

Polyuria is the passage of abnormally large volumes of urine. Causes of polyuria in large animals include the following:

- Urinary–acute or chronic renal failure, pyelitis

- Metabolic–hyperglycemia, diabetes mellitus, Cushing's syndrome (horses)
- Idiopathic–psychogenic water drinking (horses)
- Iatrogenic–steroids, fluids, diuretics
- Other–diabetes insipidus; salt deficiency or toxicity; urea toxicity; severe deficiencies of chloride, potassium

Investigating Polyuria

If urine osmolality is close to the isosthenuric range and remains similar to plasma regardless of the patient's fluid status (urine specific gravity 1.008 to 1.014), primary renal disease should be considered. If serum creatinine or other assessment of glomerular filtration is normal, a water deprivation test may be needed to determine the ability of the tubules to concentrate urine. Alternatively, fractional excretion of sodium can be determined on simultaneously collected urine and serum samples:

$$FE_{Na} = (\text{urine [Na]}/\text{serum [Na]}) \div (\text{urine [Cr]}/\text{serum [Cr]}) \times 100$$

where *[Na]* is the sodium concentration and *[Cr]* is the creatinine concentration. An FE_{Na} greater than 1% in an adult animal is highly suggestive of primary tubular disease or sodium toxicity. If the urine specific gravity or osmolality is less than 1.007, diabetes insipidus, polydipsia, and renal medullary washout should be considered.

URACHAL LEAKAGE OF URINE *(Text p. 180)*

The clinical signs of incomplete urachal closure in newborn animals are visible dripping of urine from the ventral abdomen or a wet umbilical stump and swelling of the umbilical area. It is important to determine whether improper closure is the result of a septic inflammatory disease or a less serious problem. If urachal leakage first develops when the animal is several days old, urachal infection should be strongly considered.

CRYSTALLURIA *(Text p. 180)*

Crystalluria is the presence of crystals in the urine. It may be microscopic, in which case no clinical signs may be observed, or it may be seen as crystals on the prepucial hairs. In the latter case the likelihood of urinary tract infection and the potential for obstruction should be considered. Crystalluria and pyuria may be found in the same patient.

URINE DIPSTICK ANALYSIS *(Text pp. 180-181)*

Following is a summary of significant findings on urine dipstick analysis in large animals:

- *pH*–Urine pH should be alkaline (greater than 7.4) in herbivores.
  - Acidic pH is suggestive of systemic acidosis (e.g., ruminal acidosis).
  - Acidic urine is not uncommon in cattle with systemic alkalosis (paradoxic aciduria).
  - Strongly alkaline urine in a depressed, anorexic horse is suggestive of renal tubular acidosis.
- *Protein*–Trace to 1+ protein is common in herbivores with alkaline urine (test not specific in alkaline urine).
  - Strong positive indicates severe glomerular protein leakage or, more commonly, hemorrhage, hemolysis, or myoglobinuria.
- *Blood*–A positive reaction can occur from hemoglobinuria, myoglobinuria, hematuria, and reproductive or fecal blood contamination of urine.
  - Patients with acute renal failure are often positive for blood.

- *Ketones*–In dairy cattle a strong reaction is suggestive of primary ketosis, whereas a weaker reaction may be suggestive of secondary ketosis (e.g., abomasal displacement).
  - A positive ketone reaction is rare in horses but may occur with hyperlipidemia.
- *Bilirubin*–A positive reaction is rare in cattle; in horses it usually indicates liver disease.
- *Glucose*–Glycosuria can occur with stress (especially in horses), glucose therapy, Cushing's syndrome (horses), rabies, enterotoxemia, renal disease, various metabolic disturbances (e.g., diabetes mellitus, hyperammonemia), and xylazine administration (in cattle).

11

Alterations in the Skin

Consulting Editors STEPHEN D. WHITE • ANNE G. EVANS

The diagnostic approaches to skin conditions are discussed in Chapter 11 of *Large Animal Internal Medicine,* third edition. The specific diseases listed below are discussed in Chapter 38 (skin) and other relevant chapters.

DIAGNOSTIC PROCEDURES *(Text pp. 182-197)*

In addition to a detailed history and thorough physical examination, the following diagnostic procedures may be useful:

- Skin scrapings (for mites)
- Acetate tape preparations (for *Oxyuris equi* or *Chorioptes* spp.)
- Dermatophyte culture and KOH preparation (for fungi and others)
- *Dermatophilus* preparation
  - Crusts are minced, mixed with several drops of saline on a glass slide, air dried, heat fixed, then stained with Gram, Giemsa, or Wright stain.
  - *Dermatophilus congolensis* are gram-positive, filamentous cocci that branch horizontally and longitudinally, forming parallel rows like railroad tracks.
- Microfilarial preparation (for cutaneous onchocerciasis in horses, stephanofilariasis in cattle, and elaephorosis and parelaphostrongylosis in sheep and goats)
  - Punch biopsy specimens are halved, with one half preserved in 10% buffered formalin for histopathologic examination and the other examined fresh.
  - Fresh tissue is minced on a glass slide, and a few drops of nonbacteriostatic saline are added; after 15 minutes the slide is examined at ×4 objective for signs of movement.
- Cytologic examination (on specimens collected by fine-needle aspiration or puncture of a pustule with a sterile scalpel blade)
- Biopsy for routine histopathologic study or direct immunofluorescence testing
  - Samples for histopathologic study are preserved in 10% buffered formalin.
  - Samples for immunofluorescence testing are preserved in Michel's fixative.
- Bacterial culture and sensitivity
- Superficial and deep fungal culture
- Hypoallergenic test diet
- Intradermal skin testing

These procedures are discussed in Chapter 11 of *Large Animal Internal Medicine,* third edition.

PRURITUS *(Text pp. 197-198)*

Pruritus is the most common symptom of cutaneous disease. It may represent a manifestation of a systemic disease, a hypersensitivity reaction, or a primary skin disease. Common causes include the following:

- Flying insects–*Culicoides* hypersensitivity, stable fly, tabanids (horse fly, deer

fly), simulids (black fly, buffalo gnat), horn flies *(Lyperosia* or *Haematobia irritans),* sheep ked (*Malophagus ovinus;* sheep, goats)
- Ectoparasites–pediculosis (lice), trombiculiasis, chorioptic mange, psoroptic mange (ruminants)
- Other–pinworms (*O. equi,* horses), scrapie (sheep, goats)

Less common causes are listed in Tables 11-1 and 11-2 in *Large Animal Internal Medicine,* third edition.

NODULES, TUMORS, AND SWELLINGS *(Text pp. 198-199)*

Nodules, tumors, and swellings may arise from a variety of cutaneous disorders and, rarely, as symptoms of systemic disease (e.g., lymphosarcoma, amyloidosis, anaphylaxis). The major diagnostic considerations are hypersensitivity reactions, infectious diseases, sterile inflammatory diseases, and neoplasia.

Causes of Skin Nodules and Swellings

Common causes of skin nodules, tumors, and swellings include the following:
- Parasites–cutaneous habronemiasis (horses), warbles (*Hypoderma;* ruminants)
- Hypersensitivity–urticaria (hives), milk allergy (cattle)
- Bacteria–strangles (*Streptococcus equi;* horses), ulcerative or caseous lymphangitis *(Corynebacterium pseudotuberculosis),* folliculitis/furunculosis (*Pseudomonas* spp., *Staphylococcus* spp., *Corynebacterium* spp., *Arcanobacterium* spp.) in ruminants
- Neoplasia–papilloma, squamous cell carcinoma, sarcoidosis (horses), melanoma (horses), cutaneous lymphosarcoma (horses), mastocytoma (horses), fibroma/fibrosarcoma (ruminants)
- Other–hematoma/seroma, subcutaneous foreign body, fibropapillomatosis/papillomatosis, sporotrichosis, nodular necrobiosis (horses), aural plaques (horses), exuberant granulation tissue (proud flesh; horses)

Less common causes are listed in Tables 11-1 and 11-2 in *Large Animal Internal Medicine,* third edition.

ULCERATIONS AND EROSIONS *(Text p. 199)*

An *ulcer* is a cutaneous defect involving complete loss of epidermis and usually part of the underlying dermis. An *erosion* involves only partial loss of the epidermis. Ulcers and erosions are usually secondary skin lesions. The most common cause is pruritus. Other causes include rupture of fluid-filled lesions (e.g., pustules, vesicles), erosion of enlarging nodules or tumors, and external trauma (mechanical, heat, or chemical induced).

Causes of Ulcerations and Erosions

Common causes of cutaneous ulcerations and erosions include the following:
- Parasites–stable fly, tabanids (horse fly, deer fly), simulids (black fly, buffalo gnat), *L. irritans* (horn fly), myiasis (ruminants), cutaneous habronemiasis (horses)
- Bacteria (ruminants)–foot rot, ulcerative posthitis/vulvitis, impetigo, mammary pustular dermatitis (staphylococcal [cattle], actinobacillosis [sheep]), *C. pseudotuberculosis* abscess
- Viruses (ruminants)–pseudocowpox (cattle), ulcerative dermatosis (sheep), infectious bovine rhinotracheitis (cattle), bovine herpes mammillitis (BHV-2; cattle), mammary pustular dermatitis (BHV-3), caprine herpesvirus (goats), bovine viral diarrhea (cattle), bluetongue (sheep)
- Other–trauma (excoriations, lacerations, abrasions), pressure necrosis, squamous cell carcinoma, irritants, vasculitis, burns (thermal, chemical, frictional)

Less common causes are listed in Tables 11-1 and 11-2 in *Large Animal Internal Medicine,* third edition.

PAPULES, PUSTULES, AND VESICLES *(Text pp. 199-201)*

Papules, pustules, and vesicles are circumscribed, elevated lesions less than 1 cm in diameter. A *papule* is a solid lesion (i.e., a small nodule). A *pustule* is a fluctuant accumulation of pus (i.e., a small abscess). A *vesicle* is a small accumulation of acellular fluid. Vesicles are rarely seen clinically because of their fragility and susceptibility to rupture.

Papular lesions have the most extensive differential diagnoses, including hypersensitivity reactions (most often parasitic), irritation by ectoparasites, infectious diseases (bacterial, fungal, and viral), and neoplasia (e.g., papilloma, sarcoid). Pustules are most commonly associated with bacterial infections, although fungi and, rarely, parasites (e.g., *Demodex*) can cause pustule formation. Sterile pustular diseases are less frequently recognized (e.g., drug eruptions, sterile eosinophilic folliculitis [cattle]). Vesicles form as a result of certain viral diseases, during severe inflammatory reactions (e.g., allergic contact dermatitis), with autoimmune diseases, and with physical damage (mechanical, thermal, or chemical).

Causes of Papules, Pustules, and Vesicles

Common causes of cutaneous papules, pustules, and vesicles include the following:

- Flying insects–*Culicoides* hypersensitivity, stable fly, tabanids (horse fly, deer fly), simulids (black fly, buffalo gnat), *L. irritans* (horn fly), *Musca* spp. (ruminants), sheep ked (*M. ovinus;* sheep, goats)
- Ectoparasites–trombiculiasis, chorioptic mange, psoroptic mange (ruminants)
- Bacteria–folliculitis/furunculosis (*Staphylococcus* spp., *Pseudomonas* spp., *C. pseudotuberculosis*), impetigo
- Viruses (ruminants)–contagious ecthyma (orf; sheep, goats), bovine papular stomatitis (cattle), fibropapillomatosis/papillomatosis, pseudocowpox (cattle), BHV-2 (cattle), BHV-3, infectious bovine rhinotracheitis (cattle), caprine herpesvirus (goats)
- Neoplasia–papilloma, sarcoidosis (horses), papillomatous digital dermatitis (cattle)
- Other–dermatophytosis, irritants, papillomatosis (warts; horses), *Pemphigus foliaceus* (horses)

Less common causes are listed in Tables 11-1 and 11-2 in *Large Animal Internal Medicine,* third edition.

SCALING AND CRUSTING *(Text p. 201)*

Scale is a visible accumulation of fragments of the horny layer of the skin. *Crusts* are dried exudate that adheres to the skin surface and hair. Crusts often cover excoriations, erosions, or ulcers. All pruritic diseases can result in scale and crust formation. Viral diseases are important nonpruritic causes of scaling and crusting in ruminants; ulceration and erosion with involvement of the oral cavity and mucocutaneous junctions are common.

Causes of Scaling and Crusting

The following are causes of scaling and crusting:

- Flying insects–*Culicoides* hypersensitivity, stable fly, tabanids (horse fly, deer fly), simulids (black fly, buffalo gnat), *L. irritans* (horn fly), *Musca* spp. (ruminants), sheep ked (*M. ovinus;* sheep, goats)
- Ectoparasites–pediculosis (lice), chorioptic mange, psoroptic mange (ruminants)
- Other parasitic conditions–cutaneous onchocerciasis (horses), stephanofilariasis (cattle)
- Bacteria–dermatophilosis (rain scald), folliculitis/furunculosis (*Staphylococcus* spp., *C. pseudotuberculosis*), impetigo, mammary pustular dermatitis (staphylococcal [cattle], actinobacillosis [sheep])
- Nutritional conditions–protein-calorie starvation, zinc deficiency (ruminants)

- Other (horses)–dermatophytosis, photosensitization, pemphigus foliaceus aural plaques, anhidrosis, generalized granulomatous disease, seborrhea (mane and tail, cannon keratosis, linear keratosis, generalized), iodine, irritants, vasculitis
- Other (ruminants)–photosensitization, irritants, dermatophytosis, contagious ecthyma (orf; sheep, goats), bovine inherited parakeratosis (cattle)

Less common causes are listed in Tables 11-1 and 11-2 in *Large Animal Internal Medicine,* third edition.

ABNORMAL COAT LENGTH AND DENSITY *(Text pp. 202-204)*

Decreased coat length and density is termed *alopecia* or *hypotrichosis.* Increased coat length and density is termed *hirsutism* or *hypertrichosis.* Both alopecia and hirsutism may be complete or partial, diffuse or focal, and congenital or acquired. With alopecia, the initial step is to determine if the alopecia is congenital or acquired. If acquired, it must be determined whether it is primary or secondary to another skin condition such as pruritus or ulceration.

Causes of Abnormal Coat Length and Density

Horses

The following conditions can result in *alopecia* in horses:

- Common–self-trauma induced by pruritus, dermatophilosis (rain scald), dermatophytosis, cutaneous onchocerciasis, protein-calorie starvation, scarring after inflammation, drug eruption, telogen effluvium (high fever, severe illness, parturition)
- Less common–piedra, pemphigus foliaceus demodectic mange, photosensitization, iodine toxicity, selenosis (alkali disease), thallium toxicity, keratosis (cannon, linear, or generalized), reticulated leukotrichia, alopecia areata

The primary cause of *hirsutism* in horses is hyperadrenocorticism.

Ruminants

The more common causes of *alopecia* in ruminants include the following:

- Nutritional–protein-calorie starvation, zinc deficiency
- Infectious–dermatophilosis (rain scald), dermatophytosis
- Parasitic–stephanofilariasis (cattle)
- Other–scarring after inflammation, telogen effluvium

Hirsutism in ruminants is caused by in utero infection (border disease of lambs) or a breed-specific hereditary defect (hypertrichosis in European Friesian cattle).

ABNORMAL PIGMENTATION *(Text pp. 204-206)*

Causes of Abnormal Pigmentation in Horses

The following conditions can result in leukoderma and leukotrichia:

- Common–scarring after inflammation, cutaneous onchocerciasis, sarcoidosis
- Less common–demodectic mange, anhidrosis, hairy vetch poisoning, generalized granulomatous disease, albinism, black hair follicle dystrophy (Appaloosas), juvenile Arabian leukoderma, spotted leukotrichia (Arabians), reticulated leukotrichia (Quarter Horses), hyperesthetic leukotrichia (possibly viral)

Hyperpigmentation can result from inflammation, such as persistent cutaneous trauma caused by friction.

Causes of Abnormal Pigmentation in Ruminants

The following conditions can result in hypopigmentation in ruminants:

- Common–copper deficiency, molybdenum toxicity
- Less common–scarring after inflammation, albinism (cattle), oculocutaneous hypopigmentation (Angus cattle), Chediak-Higashi syndrome (cattle)

Hyperpigmentation can be caused by melanoma (cattle) or scarring after inflammation.

12

Alterations in Sexual Function

Consulting Editor MATS H.T. TROEDSSON

Contributors PATRICK M. McCUE • STEVEN D. VAN CAMP
JAMES P. BRENDEMUEHL

The general diagnostic approaches to alterations in sexual function are discussed in Chapter 12 of *Large Animal Internal Medicine,* third edition. The specific diseases listed in the following sections are discussed in Chapter 41 and other relevant chapters.

MALE SEXUAL DYSFUNCTION *(Text pp. 207-211)*

Sexual dysfunction in males is usually recognized by changes in sexual behavior, abnormalities or diseases of the genital organs, or decreased pregnancy rates in females bred. Sexual function may be altered by any of four major mechanisms:

- Physical abnormalities that limit reproductive ability or desire
  - Common causes include rear limb conformational defects, back problems, or foot diseases in bulls and rams and degenerative joint disease of the hocks in stallions.
- Congenital or acquired abnormalities of the genital organs (penis, prepuce, scrotum, testicles, spermatic cords, or accessory sex glands)
- Decreased libido
- Poor semen quality (volume, spermatozoa concentration, percentage of progressive motility, and percentage of morphologic abnormalities)

Specific causes of altered sexual function in stallions and male ruminants are listed on pp. 208-209 of *Large Animal Internal Medicine,* third edition.

Microbiologic Samples

Microbiologic samples should be collected when evaluating infertility in stallions and when evaluating high-risk bulls. In stallions, swabs from the urethra and fossa glandis should be cultured before and after ejaculation for potentially pathogenic organisms, especially *Taylorella equigenitalis, Pseudomonas aeruginosa,* and *Klebsiella pneumoniae.* In bulls, smegma samples should be collected from the prepuce and cultured for *Trichomonas fetus* and *Campylobacter fetus.* In rams, semen should be cultured for *Brucella ovis, Actinobacillus seminis,* and *Histophilus ovis.*

CYCLIC IRREGULARITY *(Text pp. 211-213)*

Cyclic irregularity refers to an abnormal interval from the first day of estrus until the first day of the subsequent estrus.

Causes of Cyclic Irregularity

Mares

Common causes of cyclic irregularity in mares include the following:

- Ovarian function–transitional season, diestrous ovulation, pubertal cycles, persistent corpus luteum
- Other mare factors–pneumovagina, endometritis, early embryonic death
- Human factors–erroneous heat detection, intrauterine therapy, diestrual endometrial biopsy, cervical dilation
- Endophyte-infected fescue

Less common and uncommon causes of cyclic irregularity in mares are listed on p. 212 of *Large Animal Internal Medicine,* third edition.

Cows, ewes, and does

Common causes of cyclic irregularity in cows, ewes, and does include the following:

- Human factors–erroneous heat detection, intrauterine therapy
- Systemic infection–leptospirosis, infectious bovine rhinotracheitis, bovine viral diarrhea
- Genital tract infection–campylobacteriosis, trichomoniasis
- Other dam/fetal factors–endometritis, cystic ovaries, embryonic death after maternal recognition of pregnancy
- Environmental heat stress

Uncommon causes of cyclic irregularity in ruminants are listed on p. 212 of *Large Animal Internal Medicine,* third edition.

ANESTRUS *(Text pp. 213-215)*

Anestrus (lack of estrus) may be a normal physiologic phenomenon, a sign of disease, or an indication of inefficient heat detection. Pregnancy is the most common cause of anestrus and should be ruled out before proceeding with diagnostic tests.

Causes of Anestrus

Mares

Common causes of anestrus in mares include the following:

- Ovarian factors–seasonal anestrus (fall, winter), persistent corpus luteum, diestrous ovulation
- Other maternal/fetal factors–pregnancy, early embryonic death after maternal recognition of pregnancy, fetal death after endometrial cup formation (days 35 to 40), psychologic factors, maternal behavior
- Poor heat detection

Less common and uncommon causes of anestrus in mares are listed on p. 213 of *Large Animal Internal Medicine,* third edition.

Cows, ewes, and does

Common causes of anestrus in cows, ewes, and does include the following:

- Environmental and management factors–season (spring/early summer in sheep and goats), poor heat detection, poor nutrition (especially energy intake), heat stress, poor footing (cattle)
- Maternal/fetal factors–pregnancy, luteal cysts (cattle, goats), pyometra, lactation (beef cattle and sheep, heavy lactation in any species), postpartum period, primiparity
- Other–foot and leg problems, freemartinism (cattle, goats), intersex conditions (goats), periparturient disease

The two most important causes of anestrus in a herd are poor estrus detection and inadequate nutrition. Concurrent nonreproductive disease must be considered in individual anestric animals. Less common and uncommon causes of anestrus in ruminants are listed on p. 213-214 of *Large Animal Internal Medicine,* third edition.

REPEAT BREEDER *(Text pp. 215-217)*

Repeat breeders are females that have been bred during three or more successive heat periods without becoming pregnant. The causes are numerous and include male, female, and management factors. The pathogenesis involves either fertilization failure (FF) or early embryonic death (EED). The interval between heats may help differentiate between FF and EED. Fertilization failure usually does not affect the interestrous interval, whereas the interval may be prolonged if fetal death occurs after maternal recognition of pregnancy (postestrus days 15 to 17 in cows, days 11 to 14 in mares, and days 12 to 13 in ewes and does).

When investigating a herd problem, begin by evaluating the males used or assessing the semen quality and techniques used for artificial insemination. When dealing with an individual repeat breeder, begin by evaluating the female.

Causes of Repeat Breeding

Mares

Common causes of repeat breeding in mares include the following:

- Environmental and management factors–transitional season, poor heat detection, poor artificial insemination timing, early foal heat breeding, endophyte-infested fescue
- Uterine/vaginal problems–endometritis, pneumovagina, metritis, endometrial fibrosis, uterine lymphatic lacunae, endometrial cysts, poor uterine clearance, ventral uterine sacculation
- Ovulation failure
- Twins

Less common and uncommon causes of repeat breeding in mares are listed on p. 215 of *Large Animal Internal Medicine,* third edition.

Cows, ewes, and does

Common causes of repeat breeding in cows, ewes, and does include the following:

- Environmental and management factors–poor heat detection, poor artificial insemination timing or technique, malnutrition, environmental heat stress
- Maternal factors–follicular cysts, endometritis, inadequate uterine involution after parturition
- Infection–trichomoniasis, campylobacteriosis, leptospirosis

Less common and uncommon causes of repeat breeding in ruminants are listed on p. 216 of *Large Animal Internal Medicine,* third edition.

PREGNANCY LOSS *(Text pp. 217-221)*

Pregnancy loss refers to failure of a conceptus to be maintained successfully to term. It may be classified as early embryonic death, abortion, or stillbirth.

Early Embryonic Death

Early embryonic death refers to death of a conceptus before organogenesis is complete (55 days in horses, 45 days in cattle, and 34 days in sheep). Embryo loss before maternal recognition of pregnancy results in return to estrus at the normal time (see Repeat Breeder). Embryonic loss after this period may result in persistent corpora lutea in mares, pseudopregnancy in does, and irregular return to estrus in cows.

Causes of EED in mares

Common causes of early embryonic death in mares include impaired oviductal or uterine environment (e.g., chronic endometritis, endometrial fibrosis) and embryonic defects. Less common and uncommon causes are listed on p. 219 of *Large Animal Internal Medicine,* third edition.

Causes of EED in ruminants

Common causes of EED in ruminants include the following:

- Any ruminant–embryonic defects

- Cows–campylobacteriosis, infectious bovine rhinotracheitis/pustular vulvovaginitis, trichomoniasis, bovine viral diarrhea
- Ewes and does–toxoplasmosis, border disease

Less common and uncommon causes of pregnancy loss resulting from early embryonic death in ruminants are listed on p. 219 of *Large Animal Internal Medicine,* third edition.

Abortion

Causes of abortion in mares

Common causes of abortion in mares include the following:

- Equine herpesvirus (EHV-1) infection
- Twinning
- Chronic endometritis, endometrial fibrosis
- Bacterial placentitis (*Streptococcus* spp., *Escherichia coli, Pseudomonas* spp., *Klebsiella* spp., *Staphylococcus* spp.)
- Fungal placentitis (*Aspergillus* spp.)

Less common and uncommon causes of abortion in mares are listed on p. 219 of *Large Animal Internal Medicine,* third edition.

Causes of abortion in ruminants

Common causes of abortion in ruminants include the following:

- Any ruminant–leptospirosis, brucellosis, protozoal abortion (*Neospora* spp.; cattle, goats), bacterial abortion
- Cattle–epizootic bovine abortion (western United States), *Arcanobacterium (Actinomyces) pyogenes, Bacillus* spp., infectious bovine rhinotracheitis/pustular vulvovaginitis, trichomoniasis, bovine viral diarrhea
- Sheep and goats–campylobacteriosis, toxoplasmosis, border disease, chlamydiosis

Less common and uncommon causes of abortion in ruminants are listed on p. 219 of *Large Animal Internal Medicine,* third edition.

Diagnostic approach to abortion

To maximize diagnostic success, information and samples must be collected from the fetus, placenta, dam, and herd. Ideally the entire aborted fetus and placenta should be submitted to a diagnostic laboratory for examination. If this cannot be done, a prompt necropsy should be performed and the following samples submitted:

- Fetus–chilled/frozen and fixed samples of lung, liver, kidney, spleen, thymus, skeletal muscle, and heart
  - Chilled/frozen samples of heart blood and abomasal or stomach contents
  - Fixed samples of adrenal gland, lymph node, and brain
- Placenta–chilled/frozen and fixed samples of allantochorion (cotyledons and intercotyledonary area in ruminants) and allantoamnion
  - Chilled/frozen samples of amniotic fluid and umbilical cord blood
- Dam/herd–paired serum samples, vaginal or uterine swabs

Chilled/frozen samples should be submitted for culture, virus isolation, and fluorescent antibody tests. Samples for histopathologic examination should be fixed in 10% buffered formalin or Bouin fixative. Dams that have aborted should be isolated from the remainder of the herd.

FESCUE TOXICOSIS *(Text pp. 221-223)*

Tall fescue *(Festuca arundinacea)* is a common pasture grass in the southeastern and northwestern United States. Infestation of the grass with an endophytic fungus *(Neotyphodium coenophialum)* is common. Ingestion of endophyte-infected fescue causes a variety of adverse effects in horses and ruminants.

Clinical Manifestations of Fescue Toxicity

Horses

Manifestations of fescue toxicity in horses include the following:

- Reduced fertility–decreased pregnancy rates (early embryonic death), cyclic irregularity, persistent corpora lutea
- Prolonged gestation
- Placental edema, increased placental weight
- Periparturient problems–premature placental separation, fetal oversize, dystocia, retained placenta, agalactia or hypogalactia
- Poor neonatal viability–dysmaturity despite long gestational period, reduced colostral IgG absorption, and neonatal hypoadrenalism, hypopituitarism, and hypothyroidism
- Other–hirsutism, hyperhidrosis

Ruminants

Manifestations of fescue toxicity in ruminants include the following:

- Reduced conception and calving rates (cyclic irregularity, early pregnancy loss), delayed return to cyclicity postpartum
- Dystocia
- Reduced calf birth weight
- Agalactia or hypogalactia
- Other–hyperthermia, hyperpnea, hirsutism, reduced weight gain, photosensitization, necrosis of the digits ("fescue foot") and tips of the ears and tail, fat necrosis

Management of Fescue Toxicosis in Mares

Pregnant mares with suspected endophyte exposure should be removed from the suspect pasture or hay source by day 300 of gestation and fed a high-quality hay (preferably a legume). Where removal from infected fescue is not feasible, administration of domperidone is effective in preventing and treating clinical fescue toxicosis.

PROLONGED GESTATION *(Text pp. 223-224)*

Prolonged gestation periods are those that exceed the normal gestational variation attributable to genetic, nutritional, and environmental factors. Normal gestational lengths are as follows:

- Mares–310 to 374 days (thoroughbreds)
- Cows–275 to 292 days (dairy); 271 to 310 days (beef)
- Ewes–143 to 155 days
- Does–146 to 155 days

Pathologically prolonged gestation may be attributed to genetic, infectious, or toxic factors.

Causes of Prolonged Gestation

Horses

Causes of prolonged gestation in mares include fescue toxicity, fetal mummification, and delayed embryonic development. Prolonged gestation generally is not associated with excessively large foals or dystocia, so in the absence of clinical signs that indicate a high-risk pregnancy, there is no reason to perform elective induction.

Ruminants

Causes of prolonged gestation in cows, ewes, and does include the following:

- Any ruminant–fetal mummification, fetal hypothalamic-hypophyseal-adrenal axis disorder, fescue toxicity, hydrops amnii (cattle, sheep), bluetongue virus (cattle, sheep)
- Cattle–vitamin A deficiency, *Veratrum album* toxicity (causes adrenal hypoplasia), high environmental temperature, bovine viral diarrhea, genetic disorder of Holstein and Guernsey cattle

- Sheep–*Veratrum californicum* toxicity (causes adrenal hypoplasia), border disease

DYSTOCIA *(Text pp. 224-227)*

Dystocia (difficult parturition) results from either maternal or fetal conditions that impede fetal passage through the birth canal. Fetal causes are more common than maternal causes.

Causes of Dystocia

Common causes of dystocia include the following:

- Any species–fetal malpresentation, malposition, or malposture
- Horses–abortion, arthrogryposis, twinning
- Ruminants–fetopelvic disproportion (especially in cattle), uterine torsion, lymphedema, failure of cervical dilation (cattle, sheep)
- Cattle–twins or triplets, preparturient hypocalcemia

Less common and uncommon causes of dystocia in horses and ruminants are listed on pp. 224-225 of *Large Animal Internal Medicine,* third edition.

Epidural Anesthesia

Caudal epidural anesthesia with 4 to 8 ml of 2% lidocaine can facilitate examination and resolution of dystocia, although it may cause hindlimb weakness and ataxia. Safe and effective analgesia can also be induced by epidural administration of xylazine (0.17 mg/kg, diluted in 10 ml saline) or a combination of lidocaine (0.22 mg/kg) and xylazine (0.17 mg/kg).

Sequelae of Dystocia

The most common reproductive injuries incurred by the dam during parturition are cervical, vaginal, and vulvar lacerations or hematomas, postparturient vaginal necrosis, and uterine hemorrhage. Gastrointestinal complications, such as constipation from perineal inflammation and bruising or rupture of entrapped or compressed segments of bowel, can occur in mares. Musculoskeletal and neurologic complications have been reported after parturition in cows and mares. Retained placenta, delayed uterine involution, metritis, and laminitis may result from normal parturition but are more often sequelae of dystocia.

RETAINED FETAL MEMBRANES *(Text pp. 227-228)*

Mares

This condition is present when the fetal membranes have not been expelled by 3 hours after delivery. Metritis and systemic signs of toxemia/septicemia (fever, depression, dehydration, and laminitis) may occur when fetal membranes are retained for more than 24 hours. Occasionally mares with retained fetal membranes show signs of colic.

Causes of retained fetal membranes

Common causes of retained fetal membranes in mares include the following:

- Dystocia
- Preterm or induced parturition
- Abortion, stillbirth
- Endometritis/metritis
- Twinning

Less common causes of retained fetal membranes in mares are listed on p. 227 of *Large Animal Internal Medicine,* third edition.

Ruminants

Fetal membranes are considered to be pathologically retained if they are not expelled by 8 to 12 hours after calving in cows and 24 hours after delivery in ewes and does. In cows that have calved spontaneously and without problem after a normal gestation period, little illness is associated with retained fetal membranes. However, the incidence of postpartum complications, such as metritis, pyometra, ketosis, mastitis, delayed conception, and abortion, is increased. Metritis and toxemia/septicemia occur more often when retention of fetal membranes is associated with gestation of abnormal length, dystocia, nutritional deficiencies, or certain infectious diseases.

Causes of retained fetal membranes

Common causes of retained fetal membranes in cows, ewes, and does include the following:

- Multiple births
- Induced parturition
- Placentitis (bacterial or fungal)
- Hypocalcemia
- Abortion or stillbirth
- Dystocia
- Abnormal gestational length

Less common causes of retained fetal membranes in ruminants are listed on p. 228 of *Large Animal Internal Medicine,* third edition.

ALTERATIONS IN LACTATION *(Text pp. 228-232)*

Mammary Enlargement

When examining an animal with an enlarged mammary gland, it is important to determine whether the enlargement is attributable to an infectious or noninfectious cause. Mastitis is the most common infectious cause of mammary gland inflammation (see Chapter 34). Trauma is the most common noninfectious cause.

Causes of mammary enlargement

Common causes of mammary enlargement include the following:

- Any species–mastitis, periparturient udder edema (see the following), mammary abscessation
- Mares–gland distention associated with weaning
- Ruminants–trauma (contusion, hematoma, seroma, laceration), pendulous udder (cattle, goats), blind quarters (aplastic duct; cattle)

Less common causes of mammary enlargement in horses and ruminants are listed on p. 229 of *Large Animal Internal Medicine,* third edition.

Udder Edema

Mares

Udder edema is most common in brood mares during the last 1 to 2 weeks of gestation and persists for as long as 3 days after foaling. It is accompanied by ventral edema that ranges from local swelling of the udder and adjacent subcutaneous tissues to extensive swelling from caudal to the udder forward to the axilla. Affected mares are uncomfortable and reluctant to move; some refuse to allow their foals to nurse.

Ruminants

Two forms of udder edema are seen in cattle. In the physiologic or acute form, edema of the mammary gland and adjacent abdominal and perineal areas develops during late gestation and persists into the early postpartum period. In the chronic form, affected cows develop udder edema within 6 weeks after calving, and the edema may persist for several months. The swelling may be localized in the form of plaques on the caudoventral aspect of the udder or it may involve the ventral abdominal wall. Udder edema is relatively common in dairy goats, particularly 2-year-old does kidding for the first time. Affected does usually have colostrum at parturition, but within a few hours the udder is warm, hard, and agalactic.

Causes of udder edema in ruminants include the following:

- Physiologic periparturient udder edema
- Hereditary predisposition

- Nutritional–overfeeding grain prepartum, excess dietary protein, obesity, excess dietary sodium or potassium, hypomagnesemia (chronic udder edema)
- Disturbances in udder blood and lymphatic circulation
- Excessively long dry period
- Anemia

Agalactia

Agalactia (failure of lactation after parturition) may be attributable to a primary endocrinologic or mammary gland problem, or it may be secondary to any of the multitude of systemic diseases. Agalactia should not be confused with failure of milk ejection (milk letdown). Administration of oxytocin can enhance milk letdown but has no effect on milk production.

Causes of agalactia

Common causes of agalactia or hypogalactia include the following:

- All species–mammary aplasia or hypoplasia, mastitis, mammary abscessation
- Mares–abortion, premature birth, postpartum complications, fescue toxicosis
- Sheep and goats–caseous lymphadenitis with udder involvement, ovine progressive pneumonia virus contagious arthritis-encephalitis (hard udder)

Less common causes of agalactia in horses and ruminants are listed on p. 230 of *Large Animal Internal Medicine,* third edition.

Galactorrhea

Galactorrhea is the abnormal manifestation of lactation. It occasionally occurs in young animals, both males and females, possibly as a result of transplacental transmission of maternal steroids. Precocious mammary development and galactorrhea occur in pregnant and nonpregnant mares and in nonpregnant doelings and heifers being suckled by other young animals. Gynecomastia (mammary development in a male) can occur in bucks.

Causes of galactorrhea

The most common cause of galactorrhea is abortion. Lactation may commence before or even without expulsion of the dead fetus. Lactation during pregnancy has also been observed in association with multiple fetuses, in utero death of one twin fetus, placentitis, placental separation, pseudopregnancy in goats, ovarian tumors, and zearalenone toxicity.

13

Musculoskeletal Abnormalities

Consulting Editor JOHN MASS

Contributors CARTER E. JUDY • RICHARD A. LeCOUTEUR

The general diagnostic approaches to musculoskeletal abnormalities are discussed in Chapter 13 of *Large Animal Internal Medicine,* third edition. The specific diseases listed in the following sections are discussed in Chapters 36 (bones, joints, and connective tissues) and 40 (muscles).

LAMENESS AND STIFFNESS *(Text pp. 233-237)*

Generally lameness is characterized by an inability to maintain a normal gait, manifested by asymmetry in movement, apparent incoordination or weakness, and inefficient or ineffective motion of the limbs. *Stiffness* refers to a generalized restriction in freedom of movement in a limb, the neck, or the back. Most causes of lameness are associated with conditions of the musculoskeletal or nervous system; in both horses and ruminants, the forefeet are the most common site of lameness.

Causes of Lameness or Stiffness

Horses

Common causes of lameness or stiffness in horses include the following:

- Foot–infection, bruised or punctured sole, hoof wall defect, laminitis, navicular disease
- Bone–bucked shins, physitis, sesamoiditis, angular limb deformity, fracture, osteomyelitis, bone cyst
- Joint–degenerative joint disease, osteochondrosis, upward fixation of the patella (locking patella), septic arthritis, luxation/subluxation, cruciate/meniscal rupture, ankylosis
- Tendon or ligament–sprain/strain, tenosynovitis, tendonitis (bowed tendon), flexural deformity (contracted tendons), disruption of the suspensory apparatus (breakdown), tendon rupture, arthrogryposis
- Muscle–muscle injury (soreness, bruise, trauma, compartmental syndrome), rhabdomyopathy (tying up), fibrotic/ossifying myopathy, postanesthetic myasthenia
- Other–subcutaneous abscess, cellulitis, purpura hemorrhagica

Less common, uncommon, toxic, and nutritional causes of lameness or stiffness in horses are listed on p. 234 of *Large Animal Internal Medicine,* third edition.

Ruminants

Common causes of lameness or stiffness in ruminants include the following:

- Foot–infection, hoof defect, interdigital dermatitis (infectious foot rot) or fibroma, underrun heel, granuloma of the sole (Rusterholtz ulcer), laminitis,

corkscrew claw and other growth abnormalities, overgrown feet, bruised or overworn sole, foot warts
- Bone–fractures, osteomyelitis
- Joint–septic arthritis, chlamydial arthritis (sheep), caprine arthritis-encephalitis (goats), *Mycoplasma* spp., polyarthritis (sheep, goats), ligament rupture (e.g., cranial cruciate or collateral ligament in the stifle)
- Tendon or ligament–contracted tendons, arthrogryposis
- Muscle–blackleg, abscess
- Other–puncture wound

Less common, uncommon, toxic, and nutritional causes of lameness or stiffness in ruminants are listed on p. 237 of *Large Animal Internal Medicine,* third edition.

POSTURAL DEFORMITIES *(Text pp. 237-239)*

A *postural deformity* is an abnormal stance caused by a neurologic deficit, pain, or a musculoskeletal problem. Postural deformities can be congenital or acquired. Congenital deformities may be caused by tendon contracture or laxity, osseous malformation, or hypoplasia/aplasia of osseous structures or soft tissues. Acquired deformities are most often caused by trauma or disease.

Causes of Postural Deformities

Most of the listed causes of lameness or stiffness can cause postural deformities in horses and ruminants. Flexor laxity and cuboidal bone hypoplasia are other causes in foals. In ruminants the following conditions can also cause postural deformities:
- Bone–rickets, physitis/epiphysitis, osteomalacia, hypertrophic osteopathy, hyperparathyroidism
- Joint–luxation, degenerative joint disease, upward fixation of the patella
- Tendon or ligament–severed or ruptured tendon, septic tenosynovitis, ruptured peroneus tertius
- Muscle–denervation atrophy, ruptured gastrocnemius (goats)
- Congenital conditions–lupinosis (crooked calf syndrome), syndactyly, hemimelia (radial, tibial, ulnar hypoplasia), osteogenesis imperfecta, dactylomegaly (shorthorn cattle), contracted tendons, angular limb deformities, shortened longbones (acorn calves)

More complete lists of the causes of postural deformities in horses and ruminants are found on pp. 238-239 of *Large Animal Internal Medicine,* third edition.

SWELLINGS AND ENLARGEMENTS *(Text pp. 239-241)*

Soft tissue swellings and bony enlargements are most often produced by trauma, inflammation, infection, or neoplasia. Bony enlargements associated with the metaphysis and physis in young, growing animals are usually secondary to nutritional and traumatic factors. The cause of the swelling or enlargement often depends on the structures involved:
- Bone–osteophyte (degenerative joint disease), fracture, osteomyelitis, physitis/epiphysitis, osteochondroma, periosteal reaction (e.g., bucked shins), hypertrophic osteopathy
- Joint–synovial effusion, synovial herniation, hygroma, periarthritis, luxation/subluxation
- Tendon or ligament–tendonitis, desmitis, tenosynovitis, tendon or ligament rupture
- Muscle–abscess, fascial tears (herniation)
- Subcutaneous tissue or skin–hematoma, edema (inflammatory or noninflammatory), abscess, cellulitis, fibrous scar tissue, neoplasia, granuloma, granulation tissue, insect or snake bite, parasitic nodules (e.g., habronemiasis, phycomycosis), calcinosis

More comprehensive lists of the causes of swellings and enlargements in horses and ruminants are found on pp. 240-241 of *Large Animal Internal Medicine,* third edition.

PARESIS AND WEAKNESS *(Text pp. 241-244)*

Paresis is a deficit of voluntary movement. It results from disruption of voluntary motor pathways between cerebral cortex and motor unit. *Weakness* refers to a lack of physical strength and power. Weakness may occur in the absence of paresis in some neurologic disorders; it also may result from many disease processes that do not primarily involve the nervous system (e.g., heart failure, respiratory insufficiency).

Causes of Paresis and Weakness

Horses

Causes of paresis and weakness in horses include the following:

- Degenerative–equine degenerative myeloencephalopathy (EDM)
- Anomalous/congenital–hydrocephalus, vertebral and spinal cord malformations
- Metabolic–exertional rhabdomyolysis, hyperkalemic periodic paralysis (HYPP), hypothyroidism, hyperthermia, hypocalcemia, hypokalemia, hepatic lipidosis, hepatoencephalopathy
- Nutritional–malnutrition, vitamin E/selenium deficiency, vitamin A deficiency
- Neoplastic–brain or spinal cord tumor, lymphosarcoma, melanoma, leukemia
- Infectious/inflammatory–encephalitis/myelitis, equine protozoal myeloencephalitis (EPM), diskospondylitis, botulism, rabies, ehrlichiosis, tuberculosis, equine herpesvirus myeloencephalitis, cerebrospinal nematodiasis
- Toxic–snake bite, plant poisons (star thistle, oleander, moldy corn, white snake root, locoweed, larkspur, delphinium, onion, moldy sweet clover), vitamin D, phosphorus, heavy metals (lead, arsenic), tick paralysis
- Traumatic–vertebral fracture or luxation
- Vascular–postanesthetic hemorrhagic myelopathy

Ruminants

Causes of paresis and weakness in ruminants include the following:

- Anomalous/congenital–progressive degenerative myeloencephalopathy (Brown Swiss cattle), progressive ataxia (Charolais cattle), inherited progressive spinal myelinopathy (Murray Grey cattle), inherited myophosphorylase deficiency (Charolais cattle)
- Metabolic–acidosis, ketosis, vagal indigestion, urolithiasis, hypocalcemia, hypomagnesemia, anemia, hypothermia
- Nutritional–vitamin E/selenium deficiency, polioencephalomalacia (thiamine deficiency), malnutrition, water intoxication/salt poisoning
- Neoplastic–spinal vertebral neoplasia (usually lymphoma)
- Infectious/inflammatory–salmonellosis, parasitism, cryptosporidiosis, coccidiosis, colibacillosis, anaplasmosis, pneumonia, peritonitis, encephalomyelitis, mastitis, botulism, rabies, sepsis, gastrointestinal ulceration, bovine spongiform encephalopathy, viral diarrhea
- Toxic–lead poisoning, snake bite, tick paralysis
- Traumatic–lightning strike, gunshot wound, vertebral fracture or luxation

MUSCLE SPASMS AND MYOCLONUS *(Text pp. 244-245)*

Muscle spasms are sudden, transient, involuntary contractions of a muscle or group of muscles attended by pain and loss of function. *Myoclonus* is characterized by abrupt, brief, rapid, arrhythmic, asynergic, involuntary contractions involving portions of muscles, entire muscles, or groups of muscles. The movements may be single or repetitive (10 to 50/min) and either localized or generalized. Muscle spasms and myoclonus can result from dysfunction of the brain, spinal cord, peripheral nerve, neuromuscular junction, or the muscle itself.

Causes of Muscle Spasms and Myoclonus

Horses

Causes of muscle spasms and myoclonus in horses include the following:

- Anomalous/congenital–myotonia congenita
- Metabolic–hyperkalemic periodic paralysis (HYPP), hypocalcemia, hypoglycemia, hypothermia, exhaustion, shivering
- Neoplastic–insulinoma
- Infectious/inflammatory–tetanus, rabies, influenza, tick-borne encephalitis, meningitis
- Idiopathic–neonatal maladjustment syndrome
- Toxic–strychnine, organochlorines, chlorinated hydrocarbons

Ruminants

Causes of muscle spasms and myoclonus in ruminants include the following:

- Anomalous/congenital–congenital posterior paralysis (Danish red calves), inherited congenital myoclonus (formerly neuraxial edema, Polled Hereford cattle), maple syrup urine disease (Polled Herefords), lethal spasms (Jersey and Hereford calves), congenital brain edema (Hereford calves)
- Metabolic–hypomagnesemia, hypocalcemia, hypoglycemia
- Infectious/inflammatory–tetanus, rabies, pseudorabies, meningitis, coccidiosis
- Toxic–chlorinated hydrocarbons, strychnine, cocklebur, buckeye

14

Collapse/Sudden Death

Consulting Editors STAN W. CASTEEL • JAMES R. TURK

APPROACH TO DIAGNOSIS *(Text pp. 246-247)*

Collapse is a state of extreme prostration and depression. *Sudden death* is clinically unexplained, rapid death (in 12 to 24 hours) occurring in apparently healthy animals during normal activity. Generally, sudden death is associated with fatal dysfunction of the cardiovascular, nervous, respiratory, or gastrointestinal system.

Specimen Collection

Unless the cause of death is apparent, the following considerations are important for effective use of a diagnostic laboratory:

- Collect a detailed history.
- Collect the appropriate specimens.
  - Many cases of sudden death are attributed to central nervous system (CNS) dysfunction, so the brain should be removed.
  - For toxicologic examination, submit sections of gastrointestinal (GI) tract and contents, liver, and kidney.
  - 100 to 200 g of tissue or ingesta, 50 ml of urine, all fluid from both eyes, and 5 to 10 ml of blood or serum suffice for most analytic procedures.
  - When poisoning is suspected, submit samples of feed, water, baits, poisonous plants, and suspect materials; 1 kg of each usually is adequate
- Preserve all specimens correctly.
  - Samples submitted for chemical analysis should be frozen in individual containers.
  - Specimens for bacteriologic or virologic examination should be packaged separately and chilled; dry ice should not be used.
  - Tissues for histopathologic examination should be sliced 4 to 5 mm thick and fixed in 10% buffered formalin.
  - The brain should be sectioned midsagittally, with one half frozen and the other placed in 10% buffered formalin.
  - Suspected poisonous plants should be placed in a plastic bag with wet paper towels or dried between two sheets of paper.

INFECTIOUS CAUSES *(Text pp. 247-248)*

Horses

Infectious causes of collapse and sudden death in horses include the following:

- Acute colitis
- Anthrax
- Babesiosis
- Clostridial diseases–botulism,* clostridial myopathy, *Clostridium difficile* diar-

*Likely to involve several animals.

rhea, hemorrhagic enterotoxemia (*Clostridium perfringens;* foals), *Clostridium sordellii* dysentery (foals)

- Equine monocytic ehrlichiosis (Potomac fever)
- Guttural pouch mycosis (severe hemorrhage)
- Neonatal septicemia (especially *Actinobacillus equuli*) or diarrhea
- Salmonellosis*
- Tyzzer's disease (acute/peracute hepatitis in foals)

Ruminants

Infectious and parasitic causes of collapse and sudden death in ruminants include the following:

- Any ruminant–abscess rupture (liver hilus, pituitary), anthrax,* black disease (infectious necrotic hepatitis), blackleg, botulism,* *Clostridium haemolyticum* (bacillary hemoglobinuria, redwater),* *C. perfringens* enterotoxemia, coliform mastitis, endocarditis, leptospirosis, neonatal septicemia, neonatal diarrhea, pseudorabies, salmonellosis,* septic metritis
- Cattle–anaplasmosis,* lymphosarcoma (cardiac), peracute malignant catarrhal fever, thromboembolic meningoencephalomyelitis *(Haemophilus somnus)**
- Sheep and goats–listeriosis, liver fluke (sheep), *Pasteurella* septicemia* (lambs), mycoplasmosis (kids)

METABOLIC AND NUTRITIONAL CAUSES *(Text pp. 248-249)*

Horses

The two most likely metabolic and nutritional causes of collapse and sudden death in horses are hypocalcemia and vitamin E/selenium deficiency (white muscle disease).

Ruminants

Metabolic/nutritional causes of collapse or sudden death in ruminants include the following:

- Hypocalcemia–associated with onset of lactation in cattle, stress in older lactating ewes, and transport combined with fasting and weather stress
- Hypomagnesemia–develops under similar conditions as hypocalcemia, especially in cows and ewes in heavy lactation and on lush grass pastures
- Polioencephalomalacia
- Ruminal lactic acidosis in animals unaccustomed to high-carbohydrate diets
- Selenium deficiency (nutritional myodegeneration involving the heart)
- Progressive myocardial fibrosis ("falling disease" in cattle)

CARDIOVASCULAR CAUSES IN HORSES *(Text p. 249)*

Cardiovascular causes of collapse and sudden death in horses include the following:

- Heart–aortic ring/root rupture (especially stallions), endocarditis, myocarditis, traumatic pericardial rupture, coronary occlusion (from endocarditis or *Strongylus vulgaris* larvae)
- Hemorrhage–splenic rupture, uterine artery rupture, exercise-induced pulmonary hemorrhage, other causes of massive abdominal or thoracic hemorrhage
- Thromboembolism–CNS embolism (from endocarditis or intracarotid injection), thrombi of verminous origin

*Likely to involve several animals.

PHYSICAL CAUSES *(Text p. 249)*

Horses

Physical causes of collapse and sudden death in horses include the following:

- Air embolism from an open vein above the heart (e.g., open catheters, severe head wounds involving teeth and sinuses)
- Diaphragmatic rupture associated with trauma or violent exercise
- Birth trauma (neonates)
- Lightning strike, electrocution
- Gunshot wound
- Heat stroke or work stress
- Fracture of the basisphenoid or basioccipital bone after flipover injury

Ruminants

Physical causes of collapse and sudden death in ruminants include the following:

- Abomasal bloat in calves and lambs allowed to drink large quantities of warm milk replacer at infrequent intervals
- Ruminal bloat in intensively raised ruminants or after complete esophageal obstruction
- Lightning strike, electrocution
- Gunshot wound
- Heat stroke–grazing endophyte-infected fescue potentiates heat intolerance
- Traumatic reticulopericarditis (acute hemorrhage or arrhythmia after cardiac puncture)

TOXIC CAUSES *(Text pp. 249-253)*

Horses

Toxic causes of collapse and sudden death in horses include the following:

- Chemicals–4-aminopyridine (an avicide), arsenic-containing pesticides, organophosphate and carbamate insecticides
- Feed-associated toxins–cantharidin (blister beetle),* *Fusarium moniliforme*-contaminated corn (leukoencephalomalacia, moldy corn poisoning), monensin*
- Medications–intravenous overdose of insulin or potassium, ferrous fumarate (foals)
- Plants–castor bean, cyanogenic plants, Japanese yew, oleander, poison hemlock, red maple, sweet clover, tobacco, water hemlock
- Other–black flies, blue-green algae,* toxic gases (nitrogen dioxide, hydrogen sulfide, carbon monoxide)

Botanical names of toxic plants are listed with the common names on p. 250 of *Large Animal Internal Medicine,* third edition.

Ruminants

Toxic causes of collapse and sudden death in ruminants include the following:

- Chemicals–4-aminopyridine (Avitrol), anticoagulants, arsenic, chlorinated hydrocarbon pesticides, petroleum products, metaldehyde, nicotine sulfate, organophosphate and carbamate pesticides, strychnine
- Feed-associated toxins–botulism,* copper toxicity (cattle, sheep), gossypol (cotton seed),* ionophores (monensin, lasalocid),* 4-methyl-imidazole (bovine bonkers syndrome; cattle, sheep), urea*
- Other–selenium (parenteral overdose), toxic gases (carbon monoxide, hydrogen sulfide,* nitrogen dioxide*), water deprivation (salt toxicity), lead*

---

*Likely to involve several animals.

Poisonous Plants

The following plants can cause collapse or sudden death in ruminants:

- Any ruminant–blue-green algae,* cyanogenic plants, death camas, golden chain tree, inkweed, laurels, milkweed, monkshood, nightshades, nitrate-accumulating plants, oleander, perilla mint, poison hemlock, summer cypress, sweet clover, tobacco, water hemlock, yew
- Cattle–bubby bush, cocklebur, greasewood, halogeton, larkspur
- Sheep–canary grass, cocklebur, death camas, greasewood, halogeton, lupines

Botanical names of toxic plants are listed with the common names on p. 251 of *Large Animal Internal Medicine,* third edition.

MISCELLANEOUS CAUSES *(Text p. 253)*

Miscellaneous causes of collapse and sudden death include the following:

- Any large animal–allergic reactions, anaphylactic shock (penicillin, other antibiotics, drugs, vaccines, blood transfusion)
- Horses–colitis X (necrotizing typhlocolitis), GI accidents (volvulus, torsion, intussusception, incarceration, tympany, rupture), untreated uterine torsion in pregnant mares, serum sickness (acute hepatitis 50 to 90 days after administration of equine biologics)
- Cattle–perforated abomasal ulcers, tracheal edema ("honker syndrome" in feedlot cattle), sudden death syndrome in feeder cattle on high-carbohydrate diets
- Any ruminant–internal hemorrhage (e.g., uterine artery rupture during parturition), immune-mediated hemolytic anemia (neonatal isoerythrolysis), thymoma or thymic lymphosarcoma (most common in old goats)

---

*Likely to involve several animals.

PART III

Disorders and Management of the Neonate

15

The Peripartum Period

Consulting Editors WENDY E. VAALA • JOHN K. HOUSE

ASSESSMENT OF THE MARE DURING LATE GESTATION *(Text pp. 257-259)*

Mares with high-risk pregnancies should be identified early, treated appropriately, and monitored carefully through the birth process. Mares experiencing problem pregnancies may be assigned to one of three categories: (1) history of abnormal pregnancy, delivery, or newborn foal; (2) problem with the current pregnancy as a result of systemic illness or reproductive abnormality; and (3) an abnormal periparturient event.

Conditions Associated With High-Risk Foals

Maternal conditions

Maternal problems that may result in a high-risk foal include the following:

- History–foal with neonatal isoerythrolysis, neonatal maladjustment syndrome, or congenital malformation; premature foal or postterm foal that appears premature; asphyxiated foal; dystocia; premature placental separation; foal rejection; recent exposure to equine herpesvirus, equine arteritis virus, or *Leptospira* spp.
- Systemic problems–fever, anemia or hypoproteinemia, endotoxemia, intestinal crisis, malnutrition, severe systemic infection, laminitis, prolonged recumbency from neurologic or musculoskeletal problem, excessive medications, prolonged transport before parturition
- Reproductive, mammary gland, or localized problems–severe endometrial fibrosis, hydrops allantois or amnii, purulent vaginal discharge, prepubic tendon rupture, pelvic injuries, agalactia (e.g., fescue toxicity), failure to produce good quality colostrum, premature lactation

Abnormality of labor or delivery

Abnormalities of parturition in the current pregnancy that may result in a high-risk foal include the following:

- Premature parturition or abnormally long gestation
- Prolonged labor or dystocia
- Induction of labor or cesarean section
- Premature placental separation
- Umbilical cord abnormality or early cord rupture

Neonatal abnormalities

Any of the following factors can result in a high-risk foal:

- Gestational problems–placental disease (e.g., placentitis, villous atrophy, edema), twins, prematurity or dysmaturity, exposure to infectious diseases (e.g., influenza)
- Parturient problems–meconium-stained fluid or neonate
- Problems in the neonatal period–orphan; delayed or insufficient colostral intake; trauma (birth, predators, dam); adverse environmental conditions; failure to be up and nursing by 2 to 3 hours of age; weakness, poor appetite; congenital abnormalities

Monitoring Techniques

Following are some methods of evaluation during late gestation in mares:

- Serum progestogen concentration
  - Concentrations may be increased in mares with placental disease.
  - Progestogen may be very low (less than 2 ng/ml) in pregnant mares subjected to stressful conditions (e.g., colic, uterine torsion) that subsequently abort.
- Serum relaxin concentration
  - Normal levels peak at 80 to 100 ng/ml by day 175 and remain elevated until birth.
  - Low relaxin levels in late pregnancy may indicate placental insufficiency (e.g., fescue toxicosis, placentitis).
- Electrolyte concentrations in mammary secretions to predict impending parturition
  - As parturition nears, calcium and sodium increase and potassium decreases.
  - An increase in calcium to more than 40 mg/dl is the most reliable indicator of readiness for birth.
- Fetal heart rate (FHR) monitoring using Doppler ultrasonography
  - The FHR normally decreases from higher than 120 bpm before day 160 to between 60 and 90 bpm in late gestation.
  - Heart rate accelerations associated with fetal movement are normal, but persistent fetal tachycardia or bradycardia suggest fetal compromise.
- FHR and rhythm using electrocardiography (after day 150)
  - The left arm electrode is placed on the mare's dorsal midline in the lumbar region, and the left leg electrode is placed 15 to 20 cm cranial to the udder on the ventral midline.

Biophysical profile

Transabdominal ultrasonography with a 2- to 4-MHz transducer can be used to detect twins, document fetal position, and develop a biophysical profile to assess fetal well-being. The biophysical profile includes the following:

- FHR reactivity–FHR averages 60 to 90 bpm in last month of gestation
  - Transient bouts of tachycardia (+25 to +40 bpm) can occur during or after fetal activity.
- Fetal activity–increases with gestational age
  - In late gestation the fetus should demonstrate good tone and moderate activity, with only brief episodes (less than 20 minutes) of inactivity
- Fetal breathing movements
  - Regular breathing movements may be observed in late-term fetuses.
- Assessment of fetal fluid
  - Maximum ventral fluid depth averages 8 cm for amniotic fluid and 13 cm for allantoic fluid.
  - Excessive fetal fluid is observed with hydrops; markedly decreased amounts may be seen with placental dysfunction.
  - Fetal fluids increase in turbidity as gestation advances.
- Evaluation of placental integrity
  - Average uteroplacental thickness is 8 to 15 mm (mean 1.26 ± 0.33 cm).
  - Thickening may indicate placental edema, separation, or placentitis.
- Fetal size as indicated by fetal aortic diameter
  - Mean thoracic aortic diameter is 2.1 cm at 300 days and 2.7 cm at term.

PLACENTAL INSUFFICIENCY *(Text pp. 259-260)*

Uteroplacental vascular insufficiency can result in fetal asphyxia. Conditions associated with chronic asphyxia in large-animal fetuses include chronic placentitis, villous atrophy, twin or postterm pregnancies, and ingestion of endophyte-infected fescue (mares) or ponderosa pine (cows). Effects of chronic fetal hypoxia include growth retardation and an increased risk of meconium aspiration and persistent arterial hypertension, hypoglycemia, and hypothermia after birth. Immature skeletal ossification, particularly of the carpal and tarsal bones, has been associated with growth retardation in foals.

Management

Problems that should raise suspicion of chronic uteroplacental insufficiency include the following:

- Premature lactation
- Purulent vaginal discharge
- Previous history of growth-retarded foal
- Advanced maternal age
- Prolonged gestation

In these situations, labor and delivery should be attended and the neonate should be examined for evidence of growth retardation, infection (particularly in utero-acquired pneumonia secondary to placentitis), and metabolic and acid-base derangements. Ample colostrum should be administered, and body temperature and blood glucose should be monitored closely.

MANAGEMENT OF HIGH-RISK PREGNANCY IN MARES
(Text pp. 260-261)

Spontaneous vaginal delivery is generally preferred in high-risk mares because of the problems associated with the untimely delivery of a premature foal and the complications sometimes associated with induced labor or cesarean section (see Chapter 20).

Indications for Induction or Cesarean Section

Induction of parturition should be considered if there is evidence of (1) severe fetal distress; (2) premature placental separation or a history of such, associated with a dead or asphyxiated foal; (3) hydrops allantois/amnii; (4) unproductive stage I labor; (5) uterine inertia; (6) impending prepubic tendon rupture; or (7) life-threatening maternal illness.

Indications for cesarean section include (1) pelvic injury or abnormality resulting in obstruction of the birth canal, (2) gastrointestinal crisis requiring surgery, (3) severe dystocia, (4) placental thickening and insufficiency associated with fescue toxicity, and (5) catastrophic and terminal illness or injury in the mare (e.g., gut rupture or fractured limb).

Induction of Parturition

If induction of parturition or cesarean section is elected, every effort should be made to ensure that the fetus is mature. Three essential criteria are (1) gestation of longer than 330 days, (2) good-quality colostrum in the udder, and (3) softening of the cervix. If premature delivery appears unavoidable, one or two doses of corticosteroid can be administered to the mare in the hope of accelerating fetal lung maturation.

Induction protocols

Various protocols using intravenous (IV) oxytocin have been recommended to induce parturition:

- Slow, continuous infusion at a rate of 1 unit/min (usually results in delivery in 20 to 40 minutes)
- Multiple injections of 10 to 20 units (IV or intramuscularly [IM]) every 10 minutes
- 2.5 units every 15 to 20 minutes until rupture of the chorioallantois or a total dose of 20 units has been administered (may be the more physiologic method)

NOTE: Induction of parturition in mares has a higher incidence of premature placental separation and neonatal asphyxia than spontaneous delivery. Cesarean section also predisposes to neonatal asphyxia.

EVALUATION OF PERIPARTUM RUMINANTS *(Text pp. 261-264)*

Reduced fetal viability in ruminants often reflects mismanagement of maternal nutrition or the maternal environment during the last trimester of pregnancy. Common causes of perinatal death in ruminants include the following:

- Dystocia–fetopelvic incompatibility (heifers), weak labor secondary to hypocalcemia, uterine torsion, incomplete cervical dilation
- Cold stress
- Pneumonia (lambs)
- Nutritional imbalance–protein-energy deficiencies, pregnancy toxemia, copper excess/deficiency, iron excess, iodine excess/deficiency, selenium deficiency, vitamin A deficiency
- Infection–viral, bacterial, protozoal, fungal, or rickettsial (see main text)
- Other–trauma (obstetric, castration/tail docking), toxins (plants, nitrates), or genetic disorder (see main text)

Assessment of Fetal Viability

Assessment of fetal viability in ruminants includes the following procedures:

- Rectal palpation (cows)–evaluation of fetal movement, uterine blood flow, and uterine tone
  - Reduced fremitus in the uterine arteries and increased uterine tone may be palpated after fetal death.
- Visual or vaginal speculum examination for presence of vaginal discharge
- Ultrasonography (transabdominal in small ruminants, transrectal in cattle)
  - Normal FHR for full-term calves is 90 to 125 bpm and for lambs is 108 to 126 bpm.
  - FHR accelerations associated with fetal movement are a sign of fetal well-being; persistent bradycardia or tachycardia indicate fetal stress.
  - Thickening of the uterine wall, increased echogenicity of fetal fluids, altered fetal posture, altered contour of the amnion, and reduced definition and size of the caruncles may be seen after fetal death.
- Measurement of estrone sulfate in plasma or milk (see main text)

Induction of Parturition

Manipulation of parturition may be considered for maternal, fetal, or management reasons. Induction of parturition or cesarean section is often necessary to prevent mortality in small ruminants with pregnancy toxemia. Fetal viability is often improved by induction with dexamethasone; however, delivery of the fetuses via cesarean section is often necessary because of the debilitated state of the dam. Administration of flumethasone (10 mg) or dinoprost (25 mg) to pregnant cows 30 hours before elective cesarean section can improve neonatal lung function.

Induction techniques

Exogenous glucocorticoids, prostaglandin ($PGF_{2\alpha}$), or a combination of both may be used to induce parturition:

- Cattle–20 to 30 mg of dexamethasone, alone or in combination with 25 mg of $PGF_{2\alpha}$
  - Cows treated with dexamethasone prostaglandin within 14 days of the anticipated calving date usually calve within 72 hours; using the combination decreases the interval to 36 hours.
  - A lower incidence of dystocia and greater calf viability are reported in cows induced with glucocorticoids.

- Sheep and goats–10 to 20 mg of dexamethasone and/or 15 mg of $PGF_{2\alpha}$
  - Glucocorticoids are more effective than prostaglandin for inducing parturition in sheep.

Retention of fetal membranes is a common complication of induced parturition in cattle. Administration of 25 mg of triamcinolone (Opticortinol) at day 270 followed by induction with dexamethasone and $PGF_{2\alpha}$ 6 days later reduces the incidence of retained fetal membranes associated with induction in cattle.

16

Perinatal Adaptation, Asphyxia, and Resuscitation

(Text pp. 266-276)

Consulting Editors WENDY E. VAALA • JOHN K. HOUSE

ACUTE PERINATAL ASPHYXIA *(Text pp. 267-272)*

Peripartum asphyxia can occur with rapid, seemingly uncomplicated deliveries, but it is more likely with dystocia, induced delivery, cesarean section, premature placental separation and other placental abnormalities, umbilical cord abnormalities, twinning, postdated pregnancy, and severe maternal illness. Asphyxia may also occur in the neonatal period; causes include severe hemorrhage (hypovolemic shock) and severe cardiorespiratory dysfunction (e.g., pneumonia, cardiac malformations, pulmonary hypertension, airway obstruction).

Clinical signs related to asphyxial injury may not appear for hours or days after the insult. Following are some specific clinical consequences and their management.

Hypoxic Ischemic Encephalopathy

Perinatal asphyxia can result in hypoxic ischemic encephalopathy (HIE) associated with hemorrhage, edema, and necrosis of brain tissue. Mild asphyxia produces transient tissue ischemia with potentially reversible damage.

Clinical findings

Neonatal foals suffering from HIE display a wide spectrum of neurologic signs that include the following:

- Jitteriness, hyperalertness
- Stupor, somnolence, difficult to arouse
- Lethargy, hypotonia
- Clonic seizures, extensor rigidity, hypertonia, tonic posturing
- Aimless wandering, head pressing, loss of affinity for the dam, inability to find the udder
- Abnormal vocalization (barking, high-pitched cry)
- Loss of suckle, dysphagia, decreased tongue tone, odontoprisis
- Central blindness, anisocoria, mydriasis, nystagmus, eye deviation
- Head tilt, head and neck turn
- Irregular respiration, apnea, abnormally slow respiratory rate
- Proprioceptive deficits, spastic dysmetric gait
- Seizures (varying from subtle to severe)
- Coma, death

Diagnosis

Diagnosis is based on the history and exclusion of other causes of neurologic dysfunction, including the following: (1) metabolic disorders (hypocalcemia, hypomagnesemia, hyponatremia/hypernatremia, hyperlipemia, hyperglycemia, severe azotemia, hepatoencephalopathy), (2) infectious conditions (septic meningitis, septicemia/endotoxemia, EHV-1 infection), (3) malformations involving the central nervous system (CNS) or vertebral column, (4) cranial or vertebral trauma, and (5) toxins. Leukogram, serum chemistry, and cerebrospinal fluid analysis are useful in ruling out many of these conditions.

Treatment

Currently, suggested treatment includes the following:

- Anticonvulsant therapy to control seizures
  - Diazepam (0.11 to 0.44 mg/kg intravenously [IV]) is used initially.
  - Phenobarbital (2 to 10 mg/kg slowly IV every 12 hours) is used to control severe or repeated seizures; pentobarbital at the same dosage can also be used.
  - Neonates receiving high doses of anticonvulsants should be monitored closely for respiratory depression, loss of thermoregulatory control, and hypotension.
- Nursing care to prevent self-trauma
- Careful fluid therapy to prevent overhydration and either hypoglycemia or hyperglycemia
- DMSO or mannitol to control CNS edema
  - DMSO is administered at 0.5 to 1 g/kg IV as a 10% to 20% solution given slowly over 1 to 2 hours; it can be repeated every 12 hours.
  - Mannitol is given 0.25 to 1 g/kg IV as a 20% solution over 15 to 20 minutes, repeated every 12 to 24 hours.

Cardiopulmonary Effects

Hypoxia may have the following effects on the cardiopulmonary system:

- Reestablishment of fetal circulation–right-to-left flow through the ductus arteriosus and foramen ovale
- Decreased surfactant production–predisposes to atelectasis
- Central hypoventilation–causes periods of apnea or abnormal breathing patterns
- In utero passage of meconium and meconium aspiration–variably causes suffocation, regional atelectasis, interstitial emphysema and pneumothorax, and chemical pneumonitis with alveolar collapse and edema
  - Thoracic radiographs may reveal perihilar infiltrates and focal atelectasis.
- Reduced myocardial contractility, tricuspid valve insufficiency, systemic hypotension, and possibly cardiac failure

Treatment

Treatment is directed at the following:

- Correcting hypoxemia, acidosis, and hypoglycemia
  - For mild to moderate hypoxemia, increase the amount of time the foal spends in sternal recumbency or standing and administer humidified intranasal oxygen at 2 to 8 L/min.
  - Foals suffering severe hypoxemia and hypercapnea ($Pa{O_2}$ less than 40 mm Hg and $Pa{CO_2}$ greater than 65 mm Hg) require positive-pressure ventilation.
  - Caffeine (10 mg/kg orally [PO] initially, then 2.5 to 3 mg/kg PO every 24 hours) can be used to treat periodic apnea and abnormally slow breathing patterns.
- Maintaining cardiac output and blood pressure
  - Hypotension is treated with dopamine (2 to 10 μg/kg/min) or dobutamine (2 to 15 μg/kg/min) as an IV infusion.
  - Digoxin (0.02 to 0.035 mg/kg PO every 24 hours) may be indicated for cardiac failure.

Renal Effects

During asphyxia, redistribution of blood flow away from the kidneys often results in decreased renal perfusion and acute tubular necrosis. Oliguria is a common sign of acute renal failure in asphyxiated foals. Other signs include peripheral edema, elevated serum creatinine and urine γ-glutamyltransferase (GGT), and electrolyte disturbances (hyponatremia and hypochloremia).

Treatment

Fluid intake and output should be monitored carefully in oliguric neonates to prevent fluid overload. Renal blood flow and urine output may be increased with the following measures:

- Low to moderate doses of dopamine or dobutamine (2 to 10 μg/kg/min IV infusion)
  - Blood pressure and urine output should be monitored carefully during infusion.
- Diuretics
  - Furosemide can be given as a continuous IV infusion (0.25 to 2 μg/kg/hr), as a periodic IV infusion (0.25 to 0.5 mg/kg every 1 to 6 hours), or intramuscularly (IM) (1 mg/kg every 12 hours).
  - Serum electrolytes and hydration status should be monitored during frusemide therapy.
  - Mannitol (0.5 to 1 g/kg IV as a 20% solution, given slowly over 15 to 20 minutes) is an alternative.

Gastrointestinal Effects

Many asphyxiated foals demonstrate mild signs of gastrointestinal (GI) malfunction, including meconium impaction and intolerance to enteral feeding (delayed gastric emptying, abdominal distention, diarrhea, and colic). Colic, bloody diarrhea, and sudden death have been observed secondary to extensive intestinal mucosal sloughing (necrotizing enterocolitis).

Treatment

Treatment depends on the presenting complaint:

- Nasogastric decompression relieves proximal gut distention.
- Enema administration stimulates distal colonic function and encourages passage of gas.
- Prokinetics may improve gastric emptying and intestinal motility.*
  - Metoclopramide (0.25 to 0.5 mg/kg IV infusion every 6 to 8 hours)
  - Erythromycin (1 to 2 mg/kg PO or IV infusion every 6 hours)
  - Cisapride (10 mg PO every 6 to 8 hours)
- Severe large bowel distention may require percutaneous trocarization.

Exploratory celiotomy may be performed; however, multisystemic derangements often make these foals poor surgical candidates.

Feeding recommendations

After administration of colostrum, enteral feeding should be performed very cautiously, if at all, in asphyxiated foals. Foals with severe GI dysfunction should have enteral feeds withheld and should be started on parenteral nutrition until intestinal motility has returned. Reassuring signs include manure passage, normal borborygmi, and stable vital signs. Enteral feeding should be started cautiously with fresh mare's milk or colostrum.

Antiulcer medications

Because intestinal ischemia predisposes to ulceration, antiulcer medications are recommended. Options include the following:

- Sucralfate, 20 to 40 mg/kg PO every 6 hours
- Ranitidine, 5 to 10 mg/kg PO every 6 to 8 hours or 1 to 2 mg/kg IV every 8 hours
- Cimetidine, 15 mg/kg PO every 6 hours or 6.6 mg/kg IV every 6 hours
- Omeprazole, 2 mg/kg PO every 24 hours

Failure of Passive Transfer

Maladjusted foals are at increased risk for failure of passive transfer (FPT) as a result of their abnormal nursing behavior. Serum IgG levels should be evaluated and colostrum or plasma administered to treat FPT.

*It is important to rule out obstructive lesions (e.g., intussusceptions) and allow time for the damaged bowel to heal before using prokinetics in a compromised foal.

RESUSCITATION OF NEONATES *(Text pp. 272-275)*

Resuscitation of large-animal neonates should proceed as follows:

1. Clear the airway using postural drainage (suspend the patient upside down for 30 seconds) and careful nasopharyngeal suction.
2. Stimulate respiration by rubbing the patient's thorax and limbs.
3. Provide an external heat source (infrared lamps, blankets) and avoid drafts.
4. (a) If there is a heartbeat and the patient is breathing, provide supportive care.
   - Nasal insufflation of oxygen
   - Colostrum, warmth, IV fluids, and dextrose
   - Dopamine (2 to 10 μg/kg/min IV) as needed to maintain good perfusion
4. (b) If there is no heartbeat, begin external cardiac massage (60 to 80/min) and intubate.
   - Give epinephrine (0.02 mg/kg) via the endotracheal tube.
   - Insert an IV catheter and begin rapid IV infusion of warm lactated Ringer's (20 to 40 ml/kg).
   - If there is no palpable pulse and poor membrane perfusion but a spontaneous heartbeat, repeat epinephrine (0.02 mg/kg IV) and give dopamine IV as needed (see step 4a).
   - If there is no palpable pulse and no spontaneous heartbeat, change the cardiac compression technique (patient position, operator) and give epinephrine at 0.2 mg/kg IV.
   - When a pulse is palpable and capillary refill time is adequate, return to step 4a.
5. If the patient is not breathing, intubate and begin positive-pressure ventilation.
   - Preferably, use an endotracheal tube and Ambu bag at 20 breaths/min (pressure relief valve set at 42 cm H_2O).
   - Alternatively, insert an esophageal feeding tube into the proximal esophagus, occlude the muzzle and esophagus distal to tube end, and blow into tube.
   - Check electrolytes and blood gases.
   - If the patient is hypocalcemic and hyperkalemic, give calcium chloride (20 mg/kg slowly IV).
   - If the patient is acidotic despite ventilation for more than 5 minutes and acceptable perfusion, give sodium bicarbonate (1 to 2 mEq/kg slowly IV).

Postresuscitation Care

After resuscitation it is important to closely monitor cardiopulmonary function and treat accordingly:

- Give dopamine by slow IV infusion (2 to 10 μg/kg/min) if peripheral perfusion is poor (e.g., decreased capillary refill, poor pulses, cool extremities, tachycardia, oliguria).
  - NOTE: Dopamine should not be mixed with sodium bicarbonate.
- Periodically monitor serum electrolytes, blood gases, and blood glucose, and administer appropriate fluid therapy to correct any deficits.
- Position the patient in sternal recumbency and provide oxygen via nasal insufflation.
- Monitor body temperature closely, and provide heating lights and pads as necessary.
- Ensure adequate colostral intake.
  - Feed 15% of the neonate's body weight in colostrum during the first 24 hours of life; if necessary, tube feed the colostrum to avoid aspiration.
  - Passive transfer should be evaluated at 18 hours of age and plasma administered if plasma IgG is less than 400 mg/dl.

17

Initial Management and Physical Examination of the Neonate

(Text pp. 277-293)

Consulting Editors WENDY E. VAALA • JOHN K. HOUSE • JOHN E. MADIGAN

ROUTINE CARE OF NEWBORN FOALS *(Text pp. 278-279)*

The following procedures should be carried out on or considered in all newborn foals:

- Closely observe the foal's behavior and the behavior of the mare toward the foal.
- If the umbilical cord did not rupture, break it manually.
  - Place one hand on the foal's abdomen and the other on the cord distal to where it would naturally break and give a sharp pull.
- Apply disinfectant to the umbilical stump–0.5% chlorhexidine solution is preferred.
  - Disinfect the umbilicus several times during the first 48 hours or until the stump is dry.
- If the foal has not nursed effectively by 2 to 3 hours of age, give at least 20 ml/kg of good-quality colostrum by bottle or gavage feeding, ideally within the first 6 hours of life.
- Administer tetanus antitoxin (1500 U) to the foal if the foal did not receive timely immunoglobulin supplementation (colostrum or intravenous [IV] plasma).
- Administer selenium supplementation to foals born in selenium-deficient areas and whose dams did not receive selenium supplementation during pregnancy.
- Consider giving an enema to prevent discomfort and straining from meconium passage.
  - A phosphate-based enema (e.g., Fleet) or warm, diluted soapy water is acceptable.
- Perform hematologic evaluation on all high-risk foals (see Chapter 15).

Modified Apgar Score

The modified Apgar score can be used to detect early signs of peripartum asphyxia in neonatal foals. The test is best performed within 15 minutes of delivery. Five assessments are made, and the findings for each are assigned a value from 0 to 2 (Table 17-1).

TABLE 17-1
Apgar Score: Assessment of Neonatal Asphyxia

Parameter	0 Points	1 Point	2 Points
APPEARANCE	Gray/blue mucous membranes	Pale pink mucous membranes	Pink mucous membranes
PULSE (bpm)	Absent	<60, irregular	>60, regular
GRIMACE			
Nasal stimulation	No response	Grimace	Strong grimace, sneeze
Ear tickle	No response	Head/neck motion	Ear tickle, head shake
Thoracolumbar stimulus	No response	Head/neck motion	Attempt to stand with head, neck, limb motion
ATTITUDE (MUSCLE TONE)	Limp, lateral recumbency	Semisternal, some limb flexion	Sternal
RESPIRATION (breaths/min)	Absent	<30, irregular	>30, regular, can whinny

ROUTINE CARE OF RUMINANT NEONATES *(Text pp. 279-280)*

Newborn ruminants may need the following care:

- Observe the interaction between newborn and dam; intervene promptly if maternal conformation or behavior impedes the neonate's efforts to nurse.
- Collect serum before colostral intake in suspected cases of in utero infection.
  - Serum IgM and IgG may be elevated in such cases (normal values are less than 0.2 mg/ml).
- Tube feed colostrum (3 L for dairy calves) during the first 12 hours of life if free-choice consumption is questionable.
- Apply chlorhexidine solution to the umbilicus after assisted deliveries.
- Supplement neonates with vitamin E and selenium in areas where nutritional myodegeneration is common and the dam has not been supplemented during pregnancy:
  - Selenium 2.5 to 3 mg/45 kg
  - α-Tocopherol 500 IU orally (lambs and kids)

PHYSICAL EXAMINATION OF LARGE ANIMAL NEONATES *(Text pp. 280-290)*

Many high-risk neonates look relatively healthy in the first hours after birth but can rapidly deteriorate in 12 to 24 hours. The presence of one localizing sign (e.g., diarrhea) may obscure the fact that other organ systems are involved. Multiple problems in the same individual are the rule rather than the exception. Thus prompt collection of a complete database (i.e., history, physical examination, complete blood count, serum chemistries, immunoglobulin status, radiographs, and ultrasonography) is often necessary to form a realistic idea of the neonate's problems and prognosis.

Normal Parameters

An initial assessment of sick neonates should be made to determine whether there is a need for immediate intervention. Attention should also be paid to identification of congenital malformations. Normal parameters for foals and calves are as follows:

- Gestational age–327 to 365 days (average 341) in foals; 271 to 310 days in calves (average for Holsteins and Shorthorns, 278 to 282 days)
- Time to suckling reflex–2 to 20 minutes (stimulated by placing a finger in the neonate's mouth)
- Time to stand–15 to 120 minutes (average, 57) in foals; 60 to 158 minutes (up to 228 minutes without dam) in calves
- Time to nurse from dam–35 to 240 minutes (average, 111) in foals; 1 to 4 hours in calves
  - A newborn foal should be considered potentially abnormal if it takes more than 2 hours to stand or more than 3 hours to nurse from the mare.
- Body temperature–37° to 38° C (98.6° to 100.4° F)
- Heart rate–80 to 130 bpm in foals; 90 to 110 bpm in calves
- Respiratory rate (foals)–60 to 80 breaths/min within 30 minutes of foaling; 30 to 40 breaths/min by 1 hour after foaling

Normal hematologic and serum biochemical values for neonatal foals and calves are given in Tables 17-2 to 17-4.

Cardiovascular System

Peripheral pulses should be strong and regular, and the limbs should be warm. Mucous membranes should be moist and pink, and the capillary refill time should be less than 2 seconds. A loud, holosystolic or continuous murmur associated with the ductus arteriosus is normal in foals and usually disappears by 4 days of age. Pathologic causes of a persistent murmur include patent ductus arteriosus, ventricular septal defect, and valvular defects. Bacterial endocarditis should be considered if a cardiac murmur is associated with recurrent fever. Cardiac arrhythmias may

TABLE 17-2
Normal Hematology Reference Values (for Neonatal Foals)

Parameter	Gestational age (premature foals)			Postnatal age (term foals)	
	300-309 Days mean	310-319 Days mean	320-334 Days mean	1 Day mean ± SD	2-7 Days mean ± SD
RBC (× 10^6/μl)	9.6	10.1	11.3	10.5 ± 1	9.26 ± 0.8
Hb (g/dl)	13.1	14.1	13.2	14.4 ± 1.1	13.2 ± 1.2
PCV (%)	41	42	43	420 ± 3.6	36.5 ± 3.1
MCV (fl)	42.7	42.2	38.6	40.2 ± 3.6	39.4 ± 2.3
MCH (pg)	14	14.4	11.8	13.6 ± 1.1	14.5 ± 1.1
MCHC (%)	32.4	33.8	30.5	33.8 ± 2	36.2 ± 1.1
Icterus index (u)				40.0 ± 15	30.0 ± 15
Total plasma protein (g/dl)				6.1 ± 0.8	6.4 ± 0.6
Fibrinogen (mg/dl)				243 ± 74	310 ± 90
Total WBC/μl	5000	6800	4900	8632 ± 2570	9075 ± 2200
Neutrophils/μl	1230	1540	1940	6381 ± 2225	6528 ± 2000
Bands/μl				<50	>50
Lymphocytes/μl	3720	5090	2960	2021 ± 2225	2203 ± 575
Monocytes/μl				222 ± 160	305 ± 145
Eosinophils/μl				0	22
Basophils/μl				8	17
Neutrophil/lymph ratio	0.33	0.3	0.66	3.16	2.96

Hb, Hemoglobin; *MCH,* mean corpuscular hemoglobin; *MCHC,* mean corpuscular hemoglobin concentration; *MCV,* mean corpuscular volume; *PCV,* packed cell volume; *RBC,* red blood cell; *WBC,* white blood cell.

TABLE 17-3
Normal Serum Biochemical Reference Values for Normal-Term Postnursing Foals

Parameter	Age: 1 Day mean ± SD	Age: 4-7 Days mean ± SD	Parameter	Age: 1 Day mean ± SD	Age: 4-7 Days mean ± SD
Sodium (mEq/L)	139.7 ± 6	139.5 ± 4.2	Total bilirubin (mg/dl)	4.3 ± 2.2	4.4 ± 1.1
Potassium (mEq/L)	4.4 ± 0.9	4.5 ± 0.4	Direct bilirubin (mg/dl)	0.5 ± 0.2	0.8 ± 0.4
Chloride (mEq/L)	103.5 ± 3	101.3 ± 4	Indirect bilirubin (mg/dl)	3.8 ± 1.5	3.5 ± 1.1
Bicarbonate (mEq/L)	22.9 ± 3.4	24.3 ± 2.1	Alkaline phosphatase (IU/L)	2282 ± 1100	1949 ± 1100
Calcium (mg/dl)	11.7 ± 1.1	11.4 ± 0.8	GGT (IU/L)	29.6 ± 15	18.3 ± 7.3
Inorganic phosphorus (mg/dl)	5 ± 0.85	6.4 ± 0.8	SDH (IU/L)	2 ± 0.9	2 ± 0.9
Magnesium (mg/dl)	2.2 ± 0.35	2.7 ± 0.15	AST (SGOT) (IU/L)	154 ± 55	225 ± 60
Glucose (mg/dl)	136 ± 40	150 ± 30	LDH (IU/L)	487 ± 100	490 ± 100
BUN (mg/dl)	18.9 ± 4.3	13.6 ± 5.6			
Creatinine (mg/dl)	2.3 ± 0.6	1.3 ± 0.3			

AST, Aspartate transaminase (SGOT); *BUN,* blood urea nitrogen; *GGT,* γ-glutamyltransferase; *LDH,* lactate dehydrogenase; *SDH,* sorbitol dehydratase.

TABLE 17-4
Normal Hematology Reference Values (for Neonatal Calves)

Parameter	Age			
	Birth	24 hrs	48 hrs	3 weeks
Red blood cells (×10^6/µl)	9.35 ± 1.02	8.17 ± 1.34	7.72 ± 1.09	8.86 ± 0.68
Hemoglobin (g/dl)	12.86 ± 1.85	10.93 ± 2.05	10.49 ± 1.8	11.32 ± 1.02
Packed cell volume (%)	41 ± 6	34 ± 6	32 ± 6	35 ± 3
Mean corpuscular volume (fl)	43.2 ± 2.4	41 ± 2.8	41.1 ± 2.3	39.1 ± 1.9
Mean corpuscular hemoglobin concentration (g/dl)	31.3 ± 1.1	32.1 ± 0.8	32.6 ± 1.0	32.8 ± 1.6
Total WBC/µl	13.99 ± 5.73	9.81 ± 2.8	7.76 ± 1.95	8.65 ± 1.69
Neutrophils/µl	10,940 ± 5,700	6,480 ± 2,660	4,110 ± 2,040	2,920 ± 1,140
Bands/µl	100 ± 150	310 ± 460	210 ± 450	10 ± 30
Lymphocytes/µl	2,980 ± 2,730	2,730 ± 820	2,850 ± 880	5,050 ± 800
Monocytes/µl	590 ± 660	230 ± 210	350 ± 280	620 ± 330
Eosinophils/µl	0	20 ± 40	20 ± 30	20 ± 40
Basophils/µl	0	0.02 ± 0.05	0.02 ± 0.05	0.02 ± 0.04
Total protein (g/dl)	4.8 ± 0.3	6.4 ± 0.7	6.4 ± 0.7	6.4 ± 0.3
Fibrinogen (mg/dl)	258 ± 138	288 ± 105	335 ± 116	283 ± 147
Urea nitrogen (mg/dl)	6.36 ± 2.36	7.52 ± 2.13	6.93 ± 3.13	
Creatinine (mg/dl)	4.14 ± 1.27	1.69 ± 0.35	1.27 ± 0.24	
Total bilirubin	0.34 ± 0.66	1.28 ± 0.5	0.89 ± 0.41	
Sodium (mEq/L)	141 ± 3.77	135 ± 2.86	135 ± 3.68	
Potassium (mEq/L)	6.1 ± 1.86	5.46 ± 0.56	5.63 ± 0.96	
Chloride (mEq/L)	97.39	95.76	95.28	
Calcium (mg/dl)	12.24 ± 1.64	10.22 ± 1.2	10.65 ± 0.56	
Phosphorus (mg/dl)	8.16 ± 1.39	7.22 ± 0.87	7.46 ± 0.87	
Creatinine phosphokinase (U/L)	83 ± 42	531 ± 532	256 ± 364	
Aspartate aminotransferase (U/L)	18 ± 19	99 ± 18	72 ± 25	
γ-Glutamyltransferase (U/L)	8 ± 3	1761 ± 1058	846 ± 517	

From Adams R et al: *Am J Vet Res* 53:944-950, 1992; and Adams R et al: *Cornell Vet* 83:13-29, 1993.

be observed in neonates with electrolyte disturbances secondary to diarrhea or uroperitoneum.

Respiratory System

Breathing pattern and rate

The breathing pattern in standing foals should be regular, but during sleep the breathing pattern may become markedly irregular, with alternating periods of apnea and tachypnea. In conscious foals, periodic apnea and abnormally slow respiration are often the result of metabolic disturbances (e.g., hypoglycemia, hypocalcemia), hypothermia, advanced prematurity, or hypoxia-induced central respiratory suppression. Tachypnea often is a response to pain or stress.

Effort of breathing

The visible effort of breathing should be minimal, with no excessive rib retraction or grunting. A prominent sign of lung disease is increased work of breathing, characterized by nostril flare, rib retractions, and increased abdominal effort. Foals on the brink of respiratory failure may grunt at the end of expiration or develop paradoxic respiration (chest wall collapse during inspiration).

Lung sounds

Lung sounds in neonates typically are much easier to hear than in adults, but the loudness of the large airway sounds may obscure subtle abnormalities in the smaller airways. Lung sounds in neonates often do not correlate well with the severity of pulmonary disease (although increasingly obvious adventitial sounds may indicate resolution of the disease process).

Ancillary diagnostic tools

Lung disease in neonates is usually diffuse and the result of infection (acquired in utero or postpartum) or lung atelectasis associated with immaturity, recumbency, or surfactant deficiency. Because of the difficulty of accurately assessing the respiratory system with physical examination alone, thoracic radiography, ultrasonography, and arterial blood gas analysis are important diagnostic tools.

Gastrointestinal Tract and Abdomen

Borborygmi should be evident bilaterally on auscultation of the abdomen. If the neonate is relaxed, it is sometimes possible to detect impaction of the large or small colon and other masses (e.g., hairballs in the rumen in calves) by abdominal palpation. The urinary bladder may also be palpated and expressed. The inguinal rings and umbilical area should be palpated for hernias.

Meconium passage

Most newborn animals display some degree of straining associated with passage of meconium (most of which should be passed within the first 48 hours). Meconium impaction is the most common cause of colic in otherwise healthy neonatal foals; in most cases it resolves uneventfully with medical therapy. Neonates that fail to pass any meconium within the first 12 to 24 hours and on digital examination have only mucus in the rectum should be considered at high risk of having an incomplete gastrointestinal tract (e.g., atresia coli or recti).

Abdominal distention

Abdominal distention in neonates may be the result of either small or large bowel distention. Causes of abdominal distention and colic include ileus, peritonitis, enteritis, hypoxic gut damage, meconium impaction, and other intestinal obstructions (e.g., intussusception, volvulus). Abdominal radiography and ultrasonography can be very helpful in diagnosing abdominal problems in neonates. Abdominocentesis can also be useful. Normal values are as follows:

- Nucleated cell count–less than 1500 cells/μl in foals; mean of 3350 cells/μl in calves
- Total protein–2 g/dl or less in foals; mean of 2.5 g/dl in calves

Fecal consistency and pH

Passage of melena may be associated with infectious enteritis (e.g., clostridiosis, salmonellosis) and necrotizing enterocolitis as result of hypoxic ischemic bowel injury. Infectious diarrhea is a leading cause of mortality in calves 3 to 21 days of age. Fecal pH may be used to distinguish secretory diarrhea (e.g., enterotoxigenic *Escherichia coli*) from diarrhea associated with maldigestion/malabsorption. Secretory diarrhea produces an alkaline pH, whereas maldigestion/malabsorption is associated with an acidic fecal pH.

Forestomach dysfunction

Abnormal forestomach function in neonatal ruminants is often reflected by altered abdominal contour. Passage of a stomach tube helps distinguish rumenal and abomasal distention and facilitates collection of a rumen fluid sample. A putrid odor to the rumen fluid is common with putrefactive indigestion, when milk is delivered to the rumen in greater than normal quantities (escape from the esophageal groove) or via backflow from the abomasum (abomasal inflammation or obstruction). Evaluation of rumen fluid pH and chymosin (renin) activity are useful for distinguishing abomasal reflux from esophageal groove overflow:

- Rumen fluid pH is usually greater than 7 with rumen putrefaction and low with abomasal reflux.
- Renin activity in rumen fluid suggests abomasal reflux.
  - Renin activity is assessed by adding 2 ml of rumen fluid to 2 ml of whole milk on a California Mastitis Test plate; the presence of renin coagulates the milk casein.

Urogenital System

The external genitalia of both sexes should be examined for congenital malformations. A persistent frenulum prevents some colts from extending their penis to urinate during the first week of life. Rupture of the urinary bladder at parturition is common in male foals. Clinical signs include dysuria, stranguria, progressive abdominal distention, and depression. Some foals with ruptured bladders are able to void small volumes of urine. Ancillary tests include abdominal ultrasound, abdominocentesis, and assessment of serum and peritoneal fluid electrolytes.

Urine production

Normal urine production in young foals is large (148 ml/kg/day), urine osmolarity is low (102 ± 24 mOsm/L), and urination occurs at frequent intervals. Normal urine production in 2- to 3-day-old calves is 34 ml/kg/day and urine osmolarity is 286 to 391 mOsm/L.

Umbilicus

The umbilicus should be examined closely for patency, increased size, moistness or discharge, and tenderness. Umbilical remnant infections are an important problem in neonates. Infection generally develops during the first 2 weeks of life and can lead to umbilical abscessation, acquired patent urachus, and omphalophlebitis/arteritis. Potential complications include septicemia, septic arthritis, and osteomyelitis. Only a small part of the umbilical structures can be evaluated on physical examination, so ultrasonography is an important diagnostic tool (see main text).

Musculoskeletal System

The newborn should be examined for birth trauma, such as fractured ribs, long bones, or mandibles; brachial plexus injuries; and soft tissue trauma. The musculoskeletal system should be examined carefully, including visual inspection for flexural or angular limb deformities, palpation, and passive range of motion of all limb joints. In immature-appearing foals, radiographs of at least one carpus and one tarsus are recommended to assess the degree of ossification. Any heat, swelling, edema, or pain around the joints or physes or lameness in any neonate should be noted. *A swollen joint should be considered infected until proven otherwise.*

Nutritional myodegeneration

Skeletal muscle myopathy is an important cause of lameness in neonatal ruminants. Lambs and kids with selenium or vitamin E deficiency are often mentally bright, are reluctant to stand, walk with a stiff gait, and cry when forced to move. Evaluation of serum creatine phosphokinase, blood selenium, and plasma vitamin E concentration is useful to confirm the diagnosis.

Neurologic Examination of Neonatal Foals

Neurologic examination of neonates is similar to that described for adults (see Chapter 8 of *Large Animal Internal Medicine,* third edition). Following are some differences peculiar to young foals:

- The menace reflex is usually absent until about 2 weeks of age.
- Pupils should be responsive to light and of equal size, but foals that are excited may have dilated pupils that do not readily constrict in response to light.
- In foals younger than 1 month of age, the pupil forms a slight ventromedial angle with the horizontal axis of the palpebral fissure, in contrast to the slight dorsomedial angle in adults.
- Foals are normally hypersensitive to stimuli applied over the face and nose, responding with exaggerated, jerky head movements; they respond to noise with the same jerky movements.
- During the first few days of life, foals have a base-wide stance and a choppy, dysmetric gait.
- In lateral recumbency, newborn foals exhibit hyperreflexic spinal reflexes and have substantial resting extensor tone.
- A prominent crossed extensor reflex may accompany the flexor or withdrawal reflex until approximately 3 weeks of age.

Signs of hypoxic ischemic encephalopathy are listed in Chapter 16.

Neurologic Disorders in Neonatal Ruminants

Neurologic disease in ruminants during the perinatal period often results from birth asphyxia, congenital disease, or sepsis. Most acquired neurologic disorders in neonates are associated with disease in other organ systems (e.g., sepsis, diarrhea) and related metabolic derangements.

The Eye

The eyes should be examined for the presence of entropion, ectropion, corneal abrasions or ulcers, uveitis and hyphema (indicators of sepsis), congenital cataracts, microophthalmia, corneal dermoids, scleral injection, and scleral hemorrhage. Entropion should be corrected promptly either by injection of a small amount of penicillin subcutaneously into the lower lid or placement of one or two vertical mattress sutures in the lid.

Examination of the Postpartum Mare

When accompanying a sick newborn foal, the mare should be evaluated thoroughly and a complete foaling history obtained. The quality of the colostrum may be assessed by visual inspection (thick, sticky) or by colostrometer (specific gravity should be greater than 1.060)

Placenta

If available, the fetal membranes should be weighed and examined for integrity, abnormal thickening, discharges, villous atrophy, and other abnormalities:

- Normal placental weight for Thoroughbreds ranges from 4.5 to 6.4 kg (10 to 14 lb).
    - Placentas weighing more than 6.4 kg are potentially abnormal (edema or placentitis).
    - Placentas weighing less than 4.5 kg may be incomplete or have severe villous atrophy.
- If placentitis is suspected, fetal fluids or membranes should be cultured and sections of amnion and chorioallantois fixed in formalin for histopathologic examination.
    - The foal should be considered at high risk of being infected; broad-spectrum antibiotics are indicated, pending culture results.
    - Minimum database should include blood culture (before antibiotics are given), leukogram, and serum creatinine concentration.

18

Supportive Care of the Abnormal Newborn

(Text pp. 294-302)

Consulting Editors WENDY E. VAALA • JOHN K. HOUSE

Contributor KIMBERLY D. RAGER

GENERAL CONSIDERATIONS *(Text pp. 294-296)*

Supportive care is aimed at (1) protecting the patient from self-inflicted injury; (2) maintaining fluid, electrolyte, and metabolic homeostasis; (3) providing adequate caloric intake; and (4) preventing nosocomial infections. Basic care of recumbent foals entails the following:

- Providing soft, absorbent bedding
- Turning the foal and assisting it to stand every 2 hours
- Applying artificial tears or sterile ocular lubricant to the foal's eyes every few hours and promptly correcting entropion (see Chapter 17)
- Restoring or maintaining normal body temperature using radiant heat lamps, blankets, or heating pads and volume expansion as needed

Depending on the type and severity of the animal's condition, postural drainage, suction, oxygen therapy, or positive pressure ventilation may be indicated. If shock, severe dehydration, or metabolic derangements such as hypoglycemia are present, fluid therapy should be initiated as soon as an intravenous catheter is placed and secured.

BASIC FLUID THERAPY IN NEONATES *(Text pp. 296-298)*

In assessing the need for fluid therapy, one must consider both the degree of dehydration (sunken eyeballs, decreased skin turgor, dry mucous membranes, weakness, decreased urine output) and circulating volume (heart rate, pulse quality, capillary refill time, temperature of the limbs, blood pressure). Calculation of fluid deficits is based on the following equation:

$$\text{Fluid deficit (L)} = \%\ \text{Dehydration} \times \text{Body weight (kg)}$$

A foal or calf with moderately to severely sunken eyes is estimated to be 8% to 10% dehydrated, which translates to a fluid deficit of 3 to 4 L for a 40-kg animal.

Route of Administration

If the patient is mildly to moderately dehydrated and the gastrointestinal tract is not seriously compromised, fluid requirements can be provided via the enteral route using milk or commercial dextrose-electrolyte mixtures. However, if gut function is abnormal or if moderate-to-severe dehydration is present, the intravenous (IV) route is preferred. Intraosseous infusion is an alternative for rapid delivery of fluids in critically ill neonates when IV access is not possible (see main text).

Choice of Fluid

The optimal type of fluid for IV administration depends on the patient's electrolyte and acid-base status. In the absence of laboratory services, a balanced electrolyte solution such as lactated Ringer's is satisfactory in most cases. Saline solutions may be a more appropriate choice in foals with diarrhea, premature foals, and those receiving diuretics. Fresh or frozen plasma is often more effective than crystalloid fluids for volume expansion in seriously ill neonates.

Rate and Volume

The rate of IV fluid administration is determined by the degree of dehydration and the severity of cardiovascular compromise. Most normal foals can tolerate rapid fluid infusion, but asphyxiated, septic, or premature foals are far less tolerant of overzealous fluid administration. A general rule of thumb is to replace half the calculated deficit in the first 6 hours of fluid therapy and the rest over 12 to 24 hours. Following are some approximate fluid requirements and rates:

- Maintenance–100 ml/kg/day or 4 to 6 ml/kg/hr
- Severe diarrhea–daily fluid requirements may reach or exceed 15 to 20 L (500 ml/kg/day)
- Septic or hypovolemic shock–40 to 80 ml/kg/hr initially, until blood pressure is stable
  - If a neonate remains hypotensive despite fluid replacement, pressor agents such as dopamine and dobutamine may be indicated (see Chapter 16).

Hypoglycemia

Blood glucose levels should be checked in any depressed, weak, or seizing neonate because hypoglycemia often accompanies neonatal diseases. A continuous infusion of dextrose restores and maintains adequate blood glucose levels in most hypoglycemic neonates:

- Ten percent dextrose solution at 5 to 10 ml/kg is given fairly rapidly, followed by continuous infusion of 5% dextrose at a rate of 4 to 8 mg/kg/min (5 ml/min for a 40-kg neonate).
- Blood and urine glucose should be measured frequently during therapy.
- If hyperglycemia results, the infusion rate or concentration should be decreased (e.g., to 2 mg/kg/min) but not stopped.

Hypertonic (25% to 50%) glucose boluses should be avoided because they may aggravate preexisting central nervous system insults and frequently result in rebound hypoglycemia 30 to 40 minutes after infusion.

Acidosis

Acidosis caused by low cardiac output or decreased peripheral oxygen delivery should be treated with measures to increase tissue perfusion and oxygenation: plasma volume expansion, cardiac inotropes, and nasal oxygen insufflation. Bicarbonate therapy is not indicated for this type of acidosis and often produces disappointing results and adverse reactions. If respiratory dysfunction is present, considerable caution should be taken when using sodium bicarbonate.

Bicarbonate therapy

Bicarbonate supplementation is recommended when bicarbonate deficits are more than 10 mEq/L (serum HCO_3^- less than 15 mEq/L) or when the blood pH is less than 7.2. Bicarbonate deficits can be calculated using the following equation:

$$HCO_3^- \text{ deficit (mEq)} = 0.5 \times \text{Body weight (kg)} \times \text{Base deficit (mEq)}$$

An isotonic bicarbonate solution (1.3%) is preferred. It can be made by adding 13 g of $NaHCO_3$ to 1 L of water or 150 ml of 8.4% bicarbonate solution to 850 ml of sterile water, or 200 ml of 5% bicarbonate solution to 800 ml of sterile water. Bicarbonate solutions should be given slowly (and never combined with any calcium-containing solutions). The effect of replacement therapy should be monitored closely and the dosage adjusted accordingly. Neonates with severe diarrhea may need considerably more than the calculated deficit to maintain an adequate blood pH until the diarrhea subsides.

Hypokalemia

Hypokalemia can occur in anorexic foals, foals with diarrhea once metabolic acidosis is corrected, and those receiving diuretics. Potassium supplementation can be given using 5 to 10 g of KCl per day given orally to a colt or foal. Potassium can be safely added to IV fluids at a rate of 20 to 30 mEq/L. The rate of intravenous potassium administration should not exceed 1 mEq/kg/hr.

NUTRITIONAL SUPPORT FOR ABNORMAL FOALS *(Text pp. 298-299)*

Provision of adequate nutritional support is an essential part of critical care. If there is no medical contraindication for oral feeding and the gastrointestinal tract is functional, enteral nutrition is the preferred and most effective route of nutritional supplementation. Foals that are not nursing from the mare can be fed by bottle, bucket, or nasogastric tube. Foals less than 7 days of age should be fed every 2 hours. Mare's milk is preferred. Suitable alternatives include goat's milk and commercial mare's milk replacer.

Complications of Enteral Feeding

Complications associated with enteral feeding include colic, abdominal distention, diarrhea, constipation, flatulence, misplacement of the nasogastric tube, aerophagia, nasal and pharyngeal irritation from the tube, and aspiration pneumonia. Bowel motility can be improved in some foals with prokinetics (see Chapter 16). Diarrhea may be treated symptomatically with oral bismuth subsalicylate (1 to 2 ml/kg every 4 to 6 hours) and/or oral loperamide (0.1 to 0.2 mg/kg every 6 hours).

NUTRITIONAL SUPPORT OF THE SICK CALF *(Text p. 299)*

Maintenance nutritional requirements for a neonatal calf can be met by feeding approximately 3 L/day of whole milk. Abomasal bloat can be prevented by providing no more than 2 L per feeding and introducing solid feed at an early age. In compromised calves a smaller volume should be provided more frequently. Feeding milk replacer is discussed in Chapter 21.

PARENTERAL NUTRITION *(Text pp. 299-300)*

Indications for partial or total parenteral nutrition include chronic diarrhea, gastroduodenal ulcer disease (foals), botulism, prematurity, sepsis, and any other condition that makes the patient intolerant of enteral feedings. Parenteral nutrition is discussed further in Chapter 46.

IMMUNE SYSTEM SUPPORT IN FOALS *(Text pp. 300-301)*

Complete failure of passive transfer (FPT) is defined as serum IgG less than 200 mg/dl. *Partial FPT* is defined as serum IgG between 200 and 800 mg/dl. Foals with complete FPT should receive immunoglobulin supplementation regardless of their health status. Foals with partial FPT should receive supplementation in any circumstance that qualifies them as a high-risk neonate (see Chapter 15). Options for immunoglobulin supplementation in foals include the following:

- Colostrum (fresh or frozen)–ideally, at least 1 L good-quality colostrum within first 8 hours of life
- Oral lyophilized IgG product–in an amount to provide at least 40 g of IgG (1 g/kg body weight)

- IV plasma–at least 1 L for a 45-kg foal (20 ml/kg); more for septic foals
  - This method is recommended for foals that are too old to absorb colostrum or whose gut function is abnormal.
  - Plasma is administered at a rate of 10 ml/kg/hr; the first 100 ml should be given slowly while monitoring the foal's pulse, respiratory rate, and temperature.

Serum IgG should be measured after any type of supplementation.

RESPIRATORY SUPPORT *(Text p. 301)*

Mild hypoxemia can be improved by supporting the recumbent foal in a sternal position. Humidified oxygen should be provided via nasal insufflation at a flow rate between 2 and 10 L/min. Mechanical ventilation is necessary for persistent hypoxemia that is refractory to nasal insufflation or is accompanied by severe hypercapnia ($Paco_2$ greater than 70 mm Hg). Tracheobronchial secretion removal is enhanced by chest coupage and nebulization with mucolytic agents such as acetylcysteine or diluted bicarbonate solution.

PROPHYLACTIC ANTIBIOTIC THERAPY *(Text pp. 301-302)*

Antibiotics may be administered prophylactically to at-risk foals. Penicillin or ampicillin and an aminoglycoside, given intramuscularly or intravenously, is a good choice if the risk of infection is great. Ceftiofur (intramuscular) and trimethoprim-sulfamethoxazole (oral) are also reasonable choices. Prophylactic antibiotics should be given for 3 to 5 days or until the risk for infection has abated. Neonatal infection is discussed further in Chapter 19.

19

Neonatal Infection

(Text pp. 303-318)

Consulting Editors WENDY E. VAALA • JOHN K. HOUSE

Infection, either localized or generalized, is an important cause of morbidity and mortality in large animal neonates. Neonates that survive acute sepsis often develop localized infections, such as pneumonia, uveitis, synovitis, physitis, meningitis, hepatitis, and enteritis.

COMMON INFECTIOUS AGENTS *(Text pp. 304-305)*

Bacteria

Gram-negative bacteria are the predominant cause of infection in large animal neonates; *Escherichia coli* is by far the most common organism isolated. Other common isolates include *Actinobacillus* (foals), *Pasteurella* (calves), *Klebsiella,* and *Salmonella.* Gram-positive bacterial infections are becoming increasingly common in critically ill foals. Isolates include *Streptococcus, Staphylococcus, Enterococcus,* and *Clostridium.* Although newer antibiotics (e.g., some cephalosporins, β-lactams, fluoroquinolones) have an extended gram-negative spectrum, their gram-positive spectrum may be inadequate.

Other Microorganisms

Equine herpesvirus, equine arteritis virus, and influenza occasionally cause disease in newborn foals. Fungal infections are rare in foals, although severe and generalized candidiasis has been reported in debilitated or immunocompromised foals. Most organisms known to cause placental and fetal disease can cause disease in neonatal ruminants. However, in utero infections are far less common than postnatally acquired infections.

CLINICAL SIGNS OF NEONATAL INFECTION *(Text pp. 305-306)*

Foals

The spectrum of clinical signs associated with septicemia depends on the integrity of the foal's immune system, the duration of illness, the severity and route of infection, and the target organs.

Early signs

Initially, clinical signs are absent or vague, nonspecific, and easily attributed to other diseases:

- Lethargy, hypotonia, excessive sleepiness
- Decreased nursing frequency, followed by complete loss of suckle reflex
  - The mare's udder becomes distended and warm and may stream milk.
- Hyperemic mucous membranes with rapid capillary refill time, tachycardia, bounding peripheral pulses, warm extremities, tachypnea
  - Petechiae on the gums, sclera, inside of the pinnae, and coronary bands

Body temperature is variable; fever is an inconsistent finding in infected foals. Dehydration develops rapidly, resulting in decreased urine output and constipation. Localizing signs (see the following) may or may not be present. Prompt and aggressive intervention at this stage frequently results in a successful outcome.

Clinical course

Animals infected in utero generally begin to show signs sometime during the first 24 hours of life, whereas postnatally infected animals often appear relatively normal for at least the first 2 days of life. Bone and joint infections in neonates may not be obvious for several days to weeks, and their appearance may either follow an improvement in systemic signs of illness or not be accompanied by any signs of systemic illness.

Localizing signs

Diarrhea is the most common early localizing sign in septicemic foals. Other localizing signs include seizures, colic, respiratory distress, uveitis, subcutaneous abscess, joint distention or periarticular edema, and umbilical abscessation. Early signs of osteomyelitis or physeal infection can be subtle, consisting only of reluctance to move, stilted gait, and an inflammatory hemogram (especially increased fibrinogen).

Late sepsis

Late sepsis gives way to septic shock. Affected foals are recumbent, dehydrated, and practically moribund. Treatment of a patient in late septic shock is usually unsuccessful. Although an encouraging response to intensive therapy may be noted initially, most foals do not survive.

Neonatal Ruminants

Septicemia in neonatal ruminants commonly involves multiple organs, with the respiratory and gastrointestinal systems most often affected. Clinical signs tend to be nonspecific and include lethargy, poor suckle reflex, weakness, dehydration, tachycardia, tachypnea, and recumbency. Localizing signs include diarrhea, lameness, omphalophlebitis, neurologic and ocular symptoms, and cardiac murmurs.

Predictors in calves

Rectal temperature, heart rate, and respiratory rate are poor predictors of sepsis in calves. More useful criteria include fecal consistency, hydration status, attitude (mental awareness), and assessment of the umbilical and scleral vessels.

DIAGNOSIS OF BACTERIAL INFECTION IN FOALS *(Text pp. 306-308)*

Because of the difficulty of identifying early sepsis at a treatable stage, a sepsis scoring system (see main text) has been developed for neonatal foals that incorporates historical parameters, physical examination findings, and laboratory values. Regardless of the score, if clinical suspicion of infection is high, antibiotic therapy should be instituted and further assessment made. Following are some specific laboratory assessments that can aid diagnosis.

Hematology and Serum Biochemistry

White blood cell count

Some foals in the early stages of septicemia have a normal total white blood cell (WBC) count, but most have either an increased number of band neutrophils (more than 50 cells/μl) or toxic changes in the neutrophils. Foals dying of septicemia generally have very low WBC counts with considerable toxic changes, although a low WBC count does not necessarily predict death.

Fibrinogen

The plasma fibrinogen concentration is of particular value in detecting newborn foals that have been infected or exposed to inflammatory placental disease in utero. Fibrinogen values in these foals may be 1000 mg/dl or greater at birth (normal is 300 mg/dl or less). In the early stages of postnatally acquired infections, fibrinogen values may only be mildly increased (400 to 500 mg/dl), but with increasing chronicity fibrinogen levels may increase dramatically.

Blood glucose

Hypoglycemia (glucose less than 60 mg/dl) commonly accompanies generalized infection; values can be very low, with the foal showing few signs other than depression and weakness.

Serum IgG

Low serum IgG levels are strongly correlated with the presence of sepsis. Severe, overwhelming infections are uncommon in foals with normal IgG levels (greater than 800 mg/dl).

Other indices

Other serum chemistry abnormalities commonly associated with sepsis are metabolic acidosis (HCO_3^- less than 19 mEq/l) and azotemia (creatinine greater than 2 mg/dl). Total plasma protein concentration is highly variable and is influenced by hydration status, catabolism, and ingestion of colostral immunoglobulins. Thrombocytopenia, hypofibrinogenemia, and abnormal coagulation indices characterize disseminated intravascular coagulation (see Chapter 27).

Blood Culture

Positive blood culture is essential for a definitive diagnosis of septicemia, and it is often necessary for selection of appropriate antibiotic therapy. Blood culture is easy to perform, but it must be done with strict aseptic technique for accurate results. Both aerobic and anaerobic cultures should be requested. Other samples that can be cultured include urine, synovial fluid, cerebrospinal fluid, peritoneal fluid, feces, and transtracheal aspirate. In cases of physeal osteomyelitis, a physeal aspirate can also be cultured. If a fever spike occurs, if the WBC count changes dramatically, or if the clinical condition deteriorates, blood culture should be repeated.

TREATMENT OF BACTERIAL INFECTION *(Text pp. 308-316)*

Antibiotic Therapy

Antibiotic therapy should be started as soon as sepsis is suspected. Broad-spectrum coverage with bactericidal drugs should be initiated pending culture results. The duration of antibiotic therapy depends on the clinical status of the patient and the type of infection documented:

- Seven to ten days of therapy may be adequate for suspected but undocumented sepsis if the complete blood count and fibrinogen are normal and the patient shows no symptoms at the end of therapy.
- At least 2 weeks of treatment is suggested in blood culture-positive patients with no evidence of localized infections.
- Three to four weeks of antibiotic treatment (or more) is often required when the infection has localized, particularly in the joints or lungs.
  - Therapy is discontinued when the WBC count, fibrinogen, and radiographs are normal.

Foals

The combination of a penicillin and an aminoglycoside, such as gentamicin (6.6 mg/kg intravenously [IV] every 24 hours) or amikacin (21 mg/kg IV every 24 hours), usually provides good antimicrobial coverage. During long-term aminoglycoside therapy, efforts should be made to prevent dehydration, and urinalysis and serum creatinine should be monitored at least weekly. Other antibiotics that may be useful for empirical treatment include the following:

- Cefotaxime (20 to 30 mg/kg IV or intramuscularly [IM] three times daily), ceftriaxone, or ceftazidime
- Ceftiofur (2.2 to 6.6 mg/kg IM twice daily)
- Trimethoprim-sulfonamide combinations (15 mg/kg IV or orally [PO] twice daily)

- Chloramphenicol (25 to 50 mg/kg IV or PO four times daily)
- Ticarcillin-clavulanate (50 mg/kg IV three or four times daily)

Ampicillin, kanamycin, and tetracycline are usually of little value for treatment of gram-negative infections in neonatal foals, and up to 40% of isolates are resistant to ceftiofur, trimethoprim-sulfonamide combinations, chloramphenicol, and ticarcillin-clavulanate. Susceptibility should be documented before these antibiotics are used. Fluconazole may be effective for treatment of candidiasis (loading dose of 400 mg, followed by 200 mg every 24 hours).

Empirical therapy in neonatal ruminants

Because polymicrobial infections are common in septicemic calves, empirical therapy should have both a gram-negative and gram-positive spectrum. Antimicrobial drugs with a gram-negative spectrum include the following:

- Ceftiofur, 5 mg/kg twice daily
- Trimethoprim-sulfonamides
  - Efficacy rapidly declines as rumen function develops.
- Enrofloxacin, 2.5 to 5 mg/kg once daily
  - Prolonged administration (e.g., weeks) is not recommended.
- Aminoglycosides (should not be used in cattle because of extremely long residue times)

Antimicrobial susceptibility data for bacterial pathogens from bovine sources are given in *Large Animal Internal Medicine,* third edition.

Calf diarrhea

Antimicrobial therapy in the management of calf diarrhea is controversial because many of the causal agents are not susceptible to antibiotics. However, antimicrobial therapy is appropriate in severely debilitated calves and for treatment of specific bacterial infections (e.g., *Salmonella,* enterotoxigenic *E. coli, Clostridium perfringens*).

Respiratory disease in calves

Pneumonia in calves less than 3 days of age typically reflects aspiration of milk subsequent to inappropriate feeding practices or pharyngeal dysfunction (white muscle disease). A mixture of gram-positive, gram-negative, and anaerobic bacteria may be present, necessitating broad-spectrum antimicrobial therapy. Outbreaks of respiratory disease in calves less than 2 weeks of age may be associated with *Mycoplasma bovis* infection. Effective antibiotics include tylosin, tetracyclines, erythromycin, tilmicosin, florfenicol, aminoglycosides, and fluoroquinolones.

Septic arthritis in calves

The most common pathogens isolated from septic joints of neonatal calves are enteric organisms: *E. coli* and *Salmonella* spp. Less common isolates include *Streptococcus, Staphylococcus,* and *Arcanobacterium pyogenes.* Empirical antimicrobial therapy should be broad spectrum. Culture of synovial fluid facilitates antimicrobial selection.

Bacterial meningitis in calves

Meningitis in neonatal calves is most commonly caused by gram-negative enterics. Reasonable empirical choices include florfenicol (20 mg/kg IV) and ceftiofur (10 mg/kg twice daily).

Circulatory Support

Restoration and maintenance of effective circulating volume is a top priority in septic neonates. Guidelines are given in Chapter 18. Treatment with flunixin meglumine (1.1 mg/kg IV or 0.25 mg/kg IV every 8 hours) helps counteract the clinical and hemodynamic changes associated with endotoxemia and septic shock. Polymyxin B (6000 IU/kg, diluted in 300 to 500 ml 5% dextrose and given by slow IV infusion) is currently being used to neutralize systemic endotoxin. The dosage should *not* be increased because polymixin B can be nephrotoxic at higher dosages. Hyperimmunized plasma may also be helpful.

Immunologic Support

Administration of a colostrum supplement before 18 hours of age is indicated when an adequate supply of colostrum is not available. Multiple doses are required to deliver at least 100 g of immunoglobulin. Beyond this time, when failure of passive transfer accompanies neonatal infection, plasma is used to increase immunoglobulin levels. Between 1 and 4 L of plasma must be given IV to adequately raise IgG levels.

Supportive Therapy

Nursing care is very important in septic neonates. Provision of adequate nutrition is vital for a successful outcome (see Chapter 18). Warmth and maintenance of fluid, blood gas, and acid-base balance, as well as a clean environment, are also critical. Every sick neonate should be monitored closely for fever spikes, neutropenia, increasing lethargy, and localizing signs of infection.

MANAGEMENT OF PLACENTITIS IN MARES

Most in utero infections result from placentitis secondary to ascending bacterial infections. Prepartum clinical signs of placentitis include purulent vaginal discharge, premature udder development, and premature lactation. Transabdominal ultrasonography can be useful for evaluating the uteroplacental unit and fetal well-being (see Chapter 15). Samples of vaginal discharge should be cultured and submitted for Gram stain analysis.

Treatment

Treatment of mares with suspected placentitis includes the following:

- Systemic broad-spectrum antibiotics–trimethoprim-sulfonamide, potassium, penicillin plus gentamicin, or ceftiofur
- Flunixin meglumine
- Altrenogest (Regu-Mate; 10 to 20 ml PO every 24 hours)

If there are large areas of placental thickening, dimethyl sulfoxide (DMSO; 0.5 to 1 mg/kg IV) may decrease placental edema. In many cases, medical treatment is associated with a good outcome. However, foals born to mares suspected of having placentitis should be considered high-risk neonates.

20

Manifestations of Disease in the Neonate

(Text pp. 319-381)

Consulting Editors WENDY E. VAALA • JOHN K. HOUSE

Contributors JOHN E. MADIGAN • JONATHAN M. NAYLOR • JOHN MAAS

PREMATURITY *(Text pp. 319-324)*

Clinical Syndromes in Foals

Various terms are used to describe small or immature-appearing foals, including the following:

- Premature–foals born before 320 days' gestation
  - Common findings include small body size, short and silky hair coat, increased range of joint motion, and immature skeletal ossification.
- Unready for birth–premature foals delivered early and abruptly by induction or cesarean section or because of acute placentitis or severe systemic maternal illness
  - Features include severe flexor tendon laxity, marked joint laxity, general weakness or floppiness (including the ears), and progressive deterioration in neurologic function and homeostasis (body temperature, blood pressure, blood glucose).
- Dysmature–delayed or inappropriate fetal growth and development caused by abnormal uterine environment (e.g., placentitis, placental insufficiency, twinning, hydrops)
  - Gestational length may be shortened, normal, or prolonged.
- Intrauterine growth retardation (IUGR)–foals that are small for their gestational age
  - IUGR foals have disproportionately large heads and domed foreheads.
  - A chronic process that impedes normal growth during gestation, such as twinning or placental insufficiency, usually is involved.

Management of Premature Foals

Management of abnormal neonates is discussed in detail in Chapters 16 to 19. Following are some comments that pertain specifically to the management of premature foals.

Colostrum

It is crucial that premature foals receive ample amounts of high-quality colostrum (at least 20 ml/kg) in the first 6 hours after delivery–provided their condition is stable. In severely compromised patients, intravenous hyperimmune plasma should be provided. Small aliquots of colostrum can be administered orally once gut function seems adequate. Serum IgG should be measured at 18 to 24 hours of age to ensure successful passive transfer of immunity (IgG greater than 800 mg/dl).

Supportive care

Supportive care of premature foals should include the following:

- Antibiotic therapy
  - Many premature foals are born early as a result of in utero infection.
- Intranasal humidified oxygen and postural support (maintaining the foal in sternal recumbency or frequently turning laterally recumbent foals)
  - Positive pressure ventilation may be required if respiratory distress is severe and hypoventilation is progressive.
- A combination of parenteral and enteral nutrition
- Orthopedic support–limited exercise until tarsal/carpal ossification is near normal; heel extensions for flexor laxity; splints for incomplete ossification or angular limb deformities

WEAKNESS AND DEPRESSION *(Text pp. 324-327)*

Possible causes of weakness, with or without depression, in neonates include the following:

- Bacterial infection (see Chapter 19)
- Congenital viral infection
  - Equine herpesvirus and equine viral arteritis in foals; bluetongue virus in lambs; caprine herpesvirus in kids
  - Bovine viral diarrhea, infectious bovine rhinotracheitis, bluetongue, parainfluenza, and Akabane viruses in calves
- Prematurity (see pp. 319-321)
- Birth asphyxia (see Chapter 16)
- Birth trauma–fractured ribs, pneumothorax, hemothorax, brachia plexus injury
- Congenital malformation–cardiac, central nervous system (CNS), musculoskeletal
- Metabolic derangements–hypoglycemia, hyponatremia, hypokalemia or hyperkalemia, hypocalcemia, acidosis (respiratory or metabolic)
- Uroperitoneum with electrolyte abnormalities
- Renal failure
- Severe anemia (see p. 370)
- CNS disease–brain or spinal cord hemorrhage, ischemia/edema/necrosis, trauma, malformations, meningitis, abscessation
- Peripheral nerve or muscle disease–botulism (foals), white muscle disease, tetanus, congenital myopathy, neuropathy
- Liver disease–Tyzzer's disease (foals), ferrous fumarate toxicity (foals), hepatitis, severe hypoxic damage
- Endocrine abnormalities–hypoadrenocorticism, hypothyroidism
- Storage disorders (see Chapters 47 and 48)
- Drugs or toxins–oversedation, transplacental transfer of anesthetics and sedatives
- Gastrointestinal (GI) disease–ulceration, necrotizing enterocolitis (NEC)
- Starvation or protein-calorie malnutrition (insufficient or incorrectly prepared milk replacer)
- Hypothermia

If weakness has been present since birth, in utero bacterial or viral infections, birth asphyxia or trauma, chronic placental problems, and congenital abnormalities should top the list of suspected causes.

RESPIRATORY DISTRESS *(Text pp. 327-335)*

Diseases involving the respiratory system are common in neonates, both as primary conditions and secondary to other disease processes. Causes of respiratory distress include the following:

- Airway obstruction–choanal atresia, laryngeal edema, tracheal stenosis or collapse

- Developmental disorders–pulmonary hypoplasia, diaphragmatic hernia
- Lung parenchymal diseases–bacterial or viral pneumonia, aspiration, pulmonary edema, atelectasis, consolidation, hemorrhage, hyaline membrane disease, pneumothorax
- Nonpulmonary causes–congestive heart failure, CNS lesions, metabolic derangements (acidosis, hypoglycemia), severe anemia, hypovolemia, birth asphyxia, pleural effusion, endotoxemia (gram-negative sepsis), pain, fever or high environmental temperature

Upper Respiratory Tract Disorders

Upper respiratory tract disorders are relatively uncommon in neonates. Conditions affecting pharyngeal and laryngeal function are important because they predispose to aspiration pneumonia. Examples include iatrogenic pharyngeal and laryngeal trauma (e.g., from feeding tubes or oral medication equipment), retropharyngeal abscess, laryngeal edema and necrosis (e.g., infectious bovine rhinotracheitis in calves), and laryngeal paresis (e.g., nutritional myodegeneration, hyperkalemic periodic paralysis in foals, botulism).

Respiratory Infection

Neonatal respiratory infection most commonly takes the form of pneumonia. In most cases, pneumonia is part of a generalized septicemia. Infection with bovine respiratory syncytial virus, infectious bovine rhinotracheitis, bovine viral diarrhea, bovine coronavirus, or *Mycoplasma* spp. may also produce respiratory disease in neonatal calves. Fetal equine herpesvirus type 1 infection may cause bronchopneumonia in newborn foals. Clinical assessment and specific diagnostic tests are discussed in *Large Animal Internal Medicine,* third edition. Management of neonatal infections is discussed in Chapter 19.

Respiratory Distress Syndrome

Respiratory distress syndrome is progressive respiratory failure in a premature neonate caused by inadequate surfactant function superimposed on a structurally immature lung. It is characterized by increasingly severe respiratory distress in the first 24 to 48 hours of life. Diagnosis is based on the characteristic clinical course, negative blood cultures, and radiographic findings (interstitial infiltrates). Management involves ventilatory support and, if available, supplementary surfactant.

Meconium Aspiration Syndrome

In utero asphyxia can result in passage of meconium into the amniotic fluid. Gasping secondary to hypoxia can cause aspiration of the meconium-contaminated amniotic fluid and a variety of clinical problems (see Chapter 16). Diagnosis is based on a history of meconium-contaminated amniotic fluid and a meconium-stained newborn; clear, brownish fluid may drip from the nose. Radiographs typically show ventrocranial distribution of a pulmonary infiltrate, which is characteristic of aspiration.

Treatment

Treatment of meconium aspiration syndrome includes the following:

- Suctioning the meconium/fluid from the upper airway
- Systemic antibiotic therapy
- Ventilatory support–intranasal oxygen, coupage, good airway hygiene

DMSO (0.5 to 1 mg/kg intravenously [IV] as a 10% solution) may help by reducing pulmonary edema.

Pneumothorax

Pneumothorax is usually a consequence of positive pressure ventilation of diseased lungs, but it may occur spontaneously or as a result of birth trauma. Clinical signs include respiratory distress, shift of the cardiac point of maximum impulse, cyanosis, and hypotension. If radiography is unavailable or the patient is distressed, direct needle aspiration is both diagnostic and therapeutic. Pneumothorax may be treated conservatively if the patient is not in respiratory distress and the condition appears stable.

Disorders of Breathing Pattern

Idiopathic tachypnea

A syndrome of idiopathic tachypnea and fever has been observed in otherwise normal neonatal foals and calves. It is more common during hot, humid weather. In affected foals, body temperature typically is 102° to 108° F (39° to 42.2° C), and response to antipyretics is poor. The respiratory rate and breathing pattern resemble panting (more than 80 breaths/min).

It is extremely important to rule out pneumonia, other pulmonary abnormalities, other types of infection, metabolic acidosis, and other causes of tachypnea. Treatment is directed at lowering the body temperature (e.g., body clipping, alcohol baths, environmental cooling). If infection cannot be ruled out, antibiotic therapy should be considered. The condition usually resolves spontaneously within a few days to weeks.

Neonatal apnea and irregular breathing patterns

Periods of apnea in neonates are commonly associated with nonrespiratory factors, such as infection, CNS disorders, hypothermia, and hypoglycemia. Short-term doxapram infusion (0.02 to 0.05 mg/kg/min diluted IV, or 1 to 2.5 mg/kg/hr for a few hours) improves ventilation. Normal breathing usually resumes once the underlying problem is resolved.

Management of Respiratory Distress

Increased respiratory rate, labored respiration, and restlessness are indications for a trial of oxygen therapy. A Pao_2 less than 60 mm Hg in lateral recumbency is an objective indication for oxygen therapy. Options include the following:

- Nasal insufflation with humidified oxygen, initially delivered at 5 L/min
- Intratracheal oxygen delivery–large foals; hypoxemic neonates with rapid, shallow respiration; and foals with severe pulmonary disease unresponsive to nasal insufflation

Oxygen therapy is not effective in correcting hypoventilation, so if hypercapnia ($Paco_2$ greater than 50 mm Hg) is progressive and accompanied by increasing respiratory distress, ventilatory support (e.g., positive pressure ventilation) is usually indicated.

DISTENDED AND/OR PAINFUL ABDOMEN *(Text pp. 335-346)*

Causes of abdominal distention and pain in neonates include the following:

- Meconium impaction–primary (foals), secondary to asphyxia or sepsis
- Impending enteritis or abomasitis
- Surgical GI lesions–obstruction (e.g., hairball in calves), strangulation, malformation (atresia coli, recti, ani), intussusception, volvulus, torsion
  - Atresia coli is the most common cause of abdominal distention in neonatal calves.
- Uroperitoneum–ruptured bladder (foals), torn or necrotic urachus or ureter
- Gas or fluid accumulation in the stomach or small bowel–aerophagia, intolerance to diet, ileus
- Peritonitis–generalized infection, devitalized bowel, perforated ulcer, severe umbilical infection
- Gastric, abomasal, or duodenal ulceration
- NEC
- Other–ascites (severe liver or renal failure, severe hypoproteinemia), hemoperitoneum (ruptured umbilical vessels, spleen, or liver), congenital tumor

Uncontrollable pain and severe abdominal distention are indications for surgery, although foals with severe enteritis can present with these signs. The presence of erectile, distended loops of small intestine on radiographs is consistent with a diagnosis of obstructive disease. Intramural gas (pneumatosis intestinalis) is suggestive of NEC. With few exceptions, abdominocentesis is of limited value in neonates with acute abdominal pain.

Meconium Impaction

Meconium impaction is the most common cause of colic in newborn foals. It is rare in neonatal ruminants. Clinical signs in otherwise normal foals include repeated attempts to defecate, straining with the back arched, swishing of the tail, and restlessness. Digital examination often reveals a rectum packed with hard fecal balls. Occasionally the impaction is located more proximally (large or small colon), and radiography or ultrasonography is required for diagnosis.

Treatment

Treatment options for meconium impaction include the following:

- Most cases–gravity enema of warm water with mild soap or a commercial Fleet enema
- Refractory cases–acetylcysteine retention enema
  - Administer 6 g acetylcysteine and 20 g baking soda in 150 ml warm water, infused rectally via Foley catheter and left in the rectum for at least 15 minutes; repeat as necessary.
  - Additional therapy may include intravenous or oral fluids and oral laxatives (60 to 120 ml mineral oil with 0.5 to 1 oz psyllium, or 60 to 120 ml Milk of Magnesia).
  - Dioctyl sodium sulfosuccinate (DSS) should be avoided.

Care must be taken to avoid traumatizing the rectal mucosa. Analgesics (e.g., dipyrone, 10 to 22 mg/kg IV; flunixin meglumine, 0.25 to 1 mg/kg IV; or butorphanol, 0.01 to 0.1 mg/kg IV) may be given as necessary; xylazine should be used with caution. Surgical intervention is required in the few foals that are refractory to treatment or in uncontrollable pain.

Uroperitoneum

Uroperitoneum is a relatively common cause of abdominal distention and depression in neonatal foals, especially males. The most common cause is a ruptured urinary bladder. Clinical signs are rarely noticed before 3 days of age. The first signs may be urinary incontinence or frequent attempts to urinate with only small amounts voided. Loss of suckle, mild colic, and increasing abdominal distention are usually accompanied by worsening depression and increasing heart and respiratory rates.

Diagnosis

Diagnosis of uroperitoneum is based on clinical findings and on the following:

- Ultrasonography–large volumes of free, anechoic fluid in the abdomen and a small, irregularly shaped bladder
- Abdominocentesis–free flow of fluid that has a low cell count, low specific gravity, and a creatinine concentration at least twice that of the blood
- Serum chemistry–azotemia, hyperkalemia (may be severe enough to cause bradyarrhythmia), hyponatremia, hypochloremia, and metabolic acidosis
  - These abnormalities are not pathognomonic for uroperitoneum; foals with renal failure, urethral obstruction, white muscle disease, or enteritis may have similar changes.

Hematology and blood culture should be performed to identify primary or secondary sepsis.

Treatment

Uroperitoneum requires surgical repair. However, the patient must be stabilized before surgery:

- Aggressive fluid therapy is indicated in clinically dehydrated patients.
  - The fluids of choice in most cases are saline, dextrose, and possibly sodium bicarbonate solutions, depending on the degree of acidosis.
- Drain as much fluid as possible from the abdomen with a teat cannula or peritoneal dialysis catheter.

- Manage the hyperkalemia with continuous dextrose infusion (with or without insulin).
  - Give a continuous intravenous infusion of dextrose (4 to 8 mg/kg/min) and, if necessary, add regular insulin (0.1 to 0.2 U/kg subcutaneously [SC] or IV); monitor for hypoglycemia when giving insulin.
- Provide oxygen therapy in patients with respiratory compromise.
- Begin broad-spectrum antibiotics after samples are taken for culture.

Ileus

Abdominal distention and colic secondary to excessive gas or fluid accumulation in the GI tract are common in compromised neonates. Metabolic and infectious causes of ileus in foals include the following:

- Hypokalemia–anorexia, diarrhea, renal loss
- Hypocalcemia–prematurity, decreased dietary intake, excessive bicarbonate administration, diuretic therapy, toxemia and sepsis
- Hypoxic-ischemic bowel injury
- Bowel obstruction–meconium retention, intussusception, small intestinal volvulus
- Peritonitis
- Enterocolitis–rotavirus, *Clostridium* spp., *Salmonella* spp., dietary changes
- Endotoxemia (generalized sepsis)

Abdominal distention is a common result of overfeeding or use of certain milk replacers in calves (see Chapter 21). Discontinuing or decreasing the amount of enteral feeding and, if possible, increasing the neonate's activity usually resolve the problem.

Diagnosis

Abdominal radiographs reveal gas-distended loops of small or large intestine and may identify bowel obstruction. Sonographic examination permits evaluation of bowel wall thickness, peritoneal fluid volume and echogenicity, gut patency, intramural gas accumulation, location and degree of intestinal distention, and presence or absence of motility.

Treatment

In addition to specific therapy for the underlying condition, management of ileus includes the following:

- Nasogastric decompression
- Cessation or reduced volume and frequency of enteral feeding if gastric reflux is present
- Parenteral alimentation if enteral feeding cannot be maintained at 10% or more of body weight per day
- Enema administration to relieve distal meconium or fecal retention
- Correction of any electrolyte abnormalities
- Exercise for ambulatory foals
- Judicious use of prokinetic agents (see text)
- If indicated, percutaneous trocarization and decompression of severely distended large bowel

Inguinal Hernia

Inguinal hernias occur in colts, possibly as a result of compression during parturition. Most congenital inguinal hernias are handled conservatively with daily manual reduction and frequent observation for possible bowel strangulation. Indications for surgical intervention include rupture of the common vaginal tunic, persistent colic, severe edema of the prepuce and scrotum, and trauma to the skin overlying the hernial sac. Surgical hernias are difficult to reduce manually, and loops of intestines are often palpable in the subcutaneous tissues of the scrotum and groin.

Intussusception

Intussusceptions in foals cause varying degrees of discomfort depending on the site of obstruction and its duration. Abdominal pain can be severe but is often low grade and intermittent, accompanied by decreased fecal production. Clinical signs in calves variably include intermittent colic, absence of feces, and melena. There often is a history of diarrhea.

Diagnosis and treatment

Ultrasonography is a useful diagnostic aid; the cross-sectional view of an intussusception reveals a targetlike pattern with a thick, hypoechoic rim (severe edema of the entering and returning bowel walls of the intussusceptum). Surgical treatment is required.

Volvulus

Foals

Volvulus may involve the small or large intestine. Small intestinal volvulus is most common. Signs include abdominal distention, gastric reflux, persistent tachycardia, severe pain, and sonographic evidence of uniform, severe bowel distention with bowel wall edema (greater than 3 mm) and absence of motility. Surgical intervention is required.

Calves

Twisting of the intestinal mass around the root of the mesentery is rare but occurs more often in calves than in adult cattle. The condition is characterized by sudden onset of severe colic (e.g., kicking at the abdomen, dropping to the ground) that rapidly progresses to abdominal distention and signs of shock.

Necrotizing Enterocolitis

NEC is a syndrome of acute intestinal necrosis. Predisposing factors include prematurity, ischemic-hypoxic gut injury, intraluminal bacteria, and enteral feeding. Signs include abdominal distention and tenderness, ileus, and ascites. Generalized sepsis often accompanies NEC. Pneumatosis intestinalis develops (and is evident on abdominal radiographs and ultrasound), and the bowel often ruptures.

Abomasal Tympany in Calves

Acute abdominal distension, colic, depression, and sudden death have been reported in neonatal calves with abomasal ulcers, abomasitis, and abomasal tympany. Possible causes include dietary changes (e.g., addition of coarse roughage feeds), abomasal bezoars, copper or selenium deficiency, and various microorganisms (including *Clostridium perfringens* type A and *Campylobacter* spp.).

Clinical signs and diagnosis

Onset of clinical signs is rapid; affected calves become anorexic and depressed (and occasionally restless), and some show signs of abdominal discomfort (e.g., treading, kicking at the abdomen). Fecal output is reduced, and melena occasionally is observed. Splashing and metallic sounds are heard on succussion of the distended abdomen; passage of a stomach tube fails to relieve the distention. Initially, affected calves are likely to have a marked metabolic alkalosis; however, rapid deterioration and onset of shock is common and is accompanied by metabolic acidosis.

Treatment

Management requires rapid relief of abomasal distention by paracentesis. With the calf in dorsal recumbency, the abomasum is deflated by inserting a needle in the highest point of the distended abdominal wall between the umbilicus and xiphoid. If the calf's condition deteriorates or tympany recurs, right flank laparotomy should be performed. Dehydration and electrolyte and metabolic derangements are corrected with intravenous fluids.

Abomasal Bloat in Lambs

Abomasal bloat is a significant problem in artificially raised lambs. Predisposing factors include feeding systems that allow lambs to drink large quantities of milk replacer at infrequent intervals and housing lambs on litter. Proliferation of *Lactobacillus* spp., *Escherichia coli*, and *C. perfringens* have also been implicated. Lambs with abomasal tympany often die within hours. Early treatment with oral antibiotics is sometimes effective. Addition of 0.1% formalin to the milk replacer reduces the incidence of abomasal tympany.

Ruminal Bloat

Ruminal bloat is uncommon in calves less than 5 weeks of age. Causes include rumen putrefaction, obstruction of the cardia or esophagus, and vagal indigestion. Clinical signs include diarrhea, poor growth, rough hair coat, and recurrent bloat. Reducing the volume of milk per feeding, feeding from nipples rather than buckets, and introducing calf starter to promote rumen development help prevent the condition. Oral antibiotics (e.g., 500 mg oxytetracycline once daily for 3 to 4 days) may also help.

Gastrointestinal Ulceration

Neonatal foals

GI ulceration can occur with several neonatal diseases, including neonatal maladjustment syndrome (NMS), asphyxiation, enteritis, and septicemia. It is also observed in a significant number of clinically normal neonates. Typical signs (e.g., bruxism, excessive salivation, colic) seen in older foals are rarely observed in neonatal foals. Gastric perforation often is the first indication of the problem. Hence, antiulcer medications are often used prophylactically in compromised neonatal foals (see Chapter 30).

Neonatal calves

Abomasal ulcers are common in calves, but they rarely become symptomatic unless perforation occurs. Perforating abomasal ulcers have been associated with *C. perfringens* abomasitis, copper deficiency, dietary changes, environmental stress, mycotic infections, and abomasal bezoars. Clinical signs include abdominal distention, pain on abdominal palpation, expiratory grunt, drooling, bruxism, melena, and less commonly, chronic abdominal pain.

SEIZURES *(Text pp. 346-349)*

Seizures may be generalized or partial. Involuntary muscle activity, opisthotonos, paddling, and extensor rigidity are signs associated with generalized convulsions. With partial seizures, abnormal breathing patterns, lip smacking, chomping, rapid eye movements unassociated with sleep, small limb movements, and tremors may be the only signs indicating seizure activity.

Causes of Neonatal Seizures

Possible causes of seizure activity in large animal neonates include the following:

- Perinatal complications–hypoxic-ischemic brain injury, intracranial hemorrhage, cerebral contusion secondary to birth trauma
- Metabolic derangements–hypoglycemia, hyponatremia or hypernatremia, hypocalcemia, hypomagnesemia, metabolic acidosis
- Infection–septicemia, bacterial meningitis/encephalitis, Tyzzer's disease, botulism
- Drugs or chemical toxins–premature withdrawal of anticonvulsant medication, large amounts of theophylline, ingestion or administration of toxins, intracarotid injection
- Developmental abnormalities–hydrocephalus/hydranencephaly, storage diseases or defects in amino acid metabolism (see Chapters 47 and 48), congenital myoclonus (calves)
- Other–liver failure, idiopathic epilepsy, heat stroke

Seizure Control in Neonates

Diazepam (Valium; 5 to 20 mg for a 45-kg neonate, slowly IV) is the initial drug of choice. In some patients, one dose controls the seizures; in others, multiple doses at frequent intervals may become necessary. Longer-acting anticonvulsants are often required in these patients:

- Phenobarbital is given at an initial dose of 10 to 20 mg/kg, diluted in saline

and given IV over 15 minutes; the maintenance dosage is 10 mg/kg IV every 12 hours (oral tablets may also be used).
  ◦ Weaning from anticonvulsant therapy should be gradual.
- In foals unresponsive to diazepam and phenobarbital, phenytoin (Dilantin) is given at an initial dose of 5 to 10 mg/kg IV, followed by 1 to 5 mg/kg every 2 to 4 hours.

Neither pentobarbital nor xylazine is recommended for seizure control in foals.

Neonatal Maladjustment Syndrome in Foals

NMS is a noninfectious CNS disorder associated with gross behavioral abnormalities in newborn foals of normal gestational length. It can occur after fast, uncomplicated delivery or after dystocia and a period of asphyxia. Synonyms for these foals include barkers, wanderers, and dummies.

Clinical signs and diagnosis

The time of onset of signs varies from immediately after birth to 24 hours of age. Predominant signs may be indicative of cerebral dysfunction, spinal cord damage, or both:

- Cerebral signs–loss of suck reflex, aimless wandering, apparent central blindness, hyperexcitability or depression, extensor spasms or clonic convulsions, excessive chewing and salivation, abnormal vocalization, abnormal respiratory patterns
- Spinal cord signs–weakness (forelimbs, hindlimbs, or all limbs, depending on lesion location), ataxia, depressed spinal reflexes

Other disease processes causing similar signs must be ruled out before a diagnosis of NMS is made. Septicemia, meningitis, and metabolic disturbances, in particular, can mimic NMS.

Treatment

Initial therapy is directed at seizure control. Diazepam and phenobarbital are the most commonly used anticonvulsants. Other treatments include DMSO (1 g/kg IV, diluted to a 10% to 20% solution, once or twice daily), plasma and antibiotic therapy for foals with failure of passive transfer, antiulcer medication (see Chapter 30), and appropriate nursing care.

Meningitis

Although bacterial meningitis may occur as a primary entity, it more commonly is a result of generalized septicemia. The most common causative agents are gram-negative enteric bacteria such as *E. coli*, *Enterobacter* spp., and *Salmonella* spp. Because clinical signs of meningitis are easily confused with NMS and septicemia, diagnosis depends on cerebrospinal fluid analysis. Treatment recommendations are discussed in Chapter 33.

DIARRHEA IN NEONATAL FOALS *(Text pp. 349-352)*

Diarrhea is common in neonatal foals. Causes include the following:

- Foal heat
- Dietary intolerance–milk (lactase deficiency), milk replacers, concentrates
- Parasites–*Strongyloides westeri, Strongylus vulgaris, Cryptosporidium* spp.?
- Viral infection–rotavirus, coronavirus
- Bacterial infection–*Salmonella* spp.; *C. perfringens* types A, B, or C (NEC); *Clostridium septicum; Clostridium difficile; Campylobacter* spp.; *Bacteroides fragilis*
- Other–mechanical obstructions, foreign bodies, antibiotics, gastric ulceration, ingestion of sand or other irritants (e.g., mare's tail hairs, rope)

Neonates are especially prone to developing septicemia concurrent with diarrhea.

General Treatment Recommendations

The three main components of therapy for neonatal diarrhea are the following:

1. Fluid therapy (see Chapter 18)
   - Sodium-containing isotonic intravenous fluids are recommended in compromised neonates.

- Correct acid-base imbalance with volume expansion and bicarbonate as needed (see next section on calf diarrhea for more details).
- Unless the foal is hyperkalemic, potassium (KCl) should be added at 15 to 20 mEq/L.
- Foals that are not nursing normally may need glucose-containing fluids.
- Intravenous plasma is indicated if blood albumin is less than 2 g/dl.

2. Intestinal protectants/adsorbents (bismuth subsalicylate, kaolin, pectin, activated charcoal)
   - Preventive antiulcer therapy (see Chapter 30) may also be beneficial.
3. Antibiotic therapy as indicated
   - Administer systemic broad-spectrum antibiotics if bacteremia is suspected (see Chapter 19).
   - Oral metronidazole may be used for suspected clostridial diarrhea, together with systemic antimicrobials for concurrent gram-negative septicemia.

Nutritional support

Withholding milk can be an important part of therapy, especially with clostridial diarrhea. The foal can be muzzled for 8 to 12 hours while the mare is milked out; the foal is then provided with oral fluids via stomach tube or bottle. Most commercial electrolyte replacers provide insufficient energy and should be used for no more than 36 hours unless parenteral nutrition is provided. Milk should be gradually reintroduced.

Foal heat diarrhea

Diarrhea developing in the first 7 to 14 days of life is termed *foal heat diarrhea* because it coincides with postfoaling estrous in mares. Most cases of foal heat diarrhea are mild and require no specific therapy. Persistent diarrhea, fever, or depression with reduced nursing should be carefully evaluated and a complete blood count (CBC) and serum electrolyte measurements (including acid-base status) performed. Appropriate fluids should be administered orally or IV. In some persistent cases, intestinal protectants may be beneficial.

DIARRHEA IN NEONATAL CALVES *(Text pp. 352-366)*

Causes of neonatal calf diarrhea include rotavirus, cryptosporidia, coronavirus, enterotoxigenic *E. coli,* and in dairy calves, *Salmonella* spp. Various other agents have also been implicated (see main text). Diarrheic calves with severe systemic signs may be bacteremic or septicemic. *E. coli* and other gram-negative enteric bacteria are most often isolated in these cases. Establishing a causal diagnosis in neonatal calf diarrhea is discussed in *Large Animal Internal Medicine,* third edition.

Clinical Evaluation

Effective treatment depends on the clinical estimation of dehydration, severity of acidosis, likelihood of intercurrent infection, presence or absence of hypothermia, and metabolic derangements (hypoglycemia, hyperkalemia).

Severity of dehydration

The severity of dehydration (as a percentage of body weight) is estimated as follows:

- 6% to 8%–slight separation of eyeball and orbit; skin tent persists for 5 to 10 seconds; mucous membranes tacky
- 9% to 10%–gap of less than 0.5 cm between eyeball and orbit; skin tent persists for 11 to 15 seconds; mucous membranes tacky or dry
- 11% to 12%–gap of 0.5 to 1 cm between eyeball and orbit; skin tent persists for more than 16 seconds; mucous membranes dry

Degree of acidosis

When laboratory support is unavailable, the presence and degree of acidosis can be gauged from the calf's sucking/drinking drive, degree of weakness, and age:

- Calves 8 days old or younger with diarrhea that are standing but have a weak suck reflex typically have a base deficit of 5 to 10 mmol/L.

  - Those in sternal or lateral recumbency usually have a base deficit of 10 mmol/L or greater.
- Calves more than 8 days old with diarrhea that are standing but have a weak suck reflex typically have a base deficit of 10 mmol/L.
  - Those in sternal recumbency may have deficits of 15 mmol/L and those in lateral recumbency 20 mmol/L.

Metabolic derangements

Bradycardia (less than 90 bpm) may indicate the presence of hypothermia, hypoglycemia, or hyperkalemia. Cardiac arrhythmias are usually caused by severe hyperkalemia (K^+ greater than 8 mEq/L). The presence of bradycardia or arrhythmia indicates the need for immediate fluid therapy with bicarbonate-containing solutions.

Concurrent problems

It is important to check for intercurrent infections, such as pneumonia, umbilical infection, and joint infection. Calves that are recumbent, are less than 7 days of age, have lost their suck reflex, or have evidence of intercurrent infection are likely to be septicemic.

Fluid Therapy for Calves With Diarrhea

The total daily fluid requirement is based on the estimated severity of dehydration combined with estimates of losses through diarrhea and fluid needed to maintain essential functions:

- Replacement = % Dehydration × Body weight (kg)
- Maintenance = 50 ml/kg
- Ongoing losses from diarrhea = 1 to 4 L/day

The total requirement can be given either IV or orally. The intravenous route is best in severely depressed calves. If the oral route is used, it must be remembered that only 60% to 80% of the fluid will be absorbed. Few problems are encountered when fluid and acid-base deficits are corrected over 4 hours. The success of therapy is based on clinical signs and restoration of urination. Persistent depression is usually a sign of uncorrected acidosis or toxemia.

Bicarbonate therapy

Saline-based fluids are suitable for rehydration, but most severely depressed calves are acidotic. More consistent recovery is obtained if an alkalizing agent (e.g., lactate, acetate, gluconate, bicarbonate) is also used. Only bicarbonate is consistently effective in severely acidotic calves. Bicarbonate requirements are calculated as follows:

$$\text{Bicarbonate (mmol)} = \text{Body weight (kg)} \times \text{Base deficit (mmol/L)} \times 0.5$$

If blood gas analysis is not available, the base deficit can be calculated from serum total CO_2 or bicarbonate (base deficit = 30 mmol/L − TCO_2 or HCO_3^-) or estimated from the clinical findings. Ongoing diarrhea may require extra bicarbonate. Large amounts of bicarbonate are best given as isotonic solutions (dissolve 13 g baking soda in 1 L water).

Glucose supplementation

Most diarrheic calves are not markedly hypoglycemic, but glucose supplementation is needed to treat severe hypoglycemia (blood glucose less than 2 mmol/L or less than 36 mg/dl). Glucose is added to the intravenous fluids to a final concentration of 2.5% to 5% (see Chapter 18).

Potassium

Severe hyperkalemia is seen in some dehydrated, diarrheic calves, but it responds to rehydration and correction of acidosis. Diarrhea results in increased potassium losses, but usually there is no need to add potassium to intravenous fluids; most calves respond to saline and bicarbonate.

Oral fluid therapy

After 12 to 24 hours of intravenous fluid therapy, most calves are started on oral electrolyte solutions. This is also the route of choice for treatment of mildly affected calves. Almost all the commercial products are suitable for rehydration.

Any of the commonly used alkalinizing agents are acceptable if the calf is held off milk, but acetate-based solutions (ideally 50 to 80 mmol/L acetate) are the best choice for calves that are also receiving milk.

Milk

Milk should be withheld while the calf is depressed and not interested in sucking. In most cases, electrolyte therapy restores a calf's vigor and sucking drive within 1 to 2 days. Milk can then be reintroduced in small amounts (e.g., 1 L given two to four times daily). If the calf is not interested in drinking or gets depressed when milk is reintroduced, a high-energy oral electrolyte preparation (see main text) should be used instead.

Antibiotic Therapy in Calves With Diarrhea

Oral antibiotics can shorten the diarrheic period in enterotoxigenic *E. coli* diarrhea. Calves with *Salmonella* infections are often bacteremic, so appropriate systemic antibiotic therapy is indicated. Antibiotic resistance is high in *E. coli* and *Salmonella* spp., so culture and sensitivity testing is useful in selecting an appropriate antibiotic. Most other causes of diarrhea in calves are viral or parasitic and are not directly sensitive to antibiotics. Nevertheless, survival is often enhanced with systemic antibiotics, partly because of the benefits of controlling intercurrent infections.

Prevention of neonatal calf diarrhea is discussed in detail in *Large Animal Internal Medicine,* third edition.

LAMENESS AND RELUCTANCE TO WALK *(Text pp. 366-368)*

Infectious Lameness

Septic arthritis, septic physitis, and osteomyelitis cause lameness and reluctance to move. In most cases, they are complications of bacteremia. Sources of infection include primary bacteremia (septicemia) associated with failure of passive transfer, pneumonia, umbilical infection, enteritis, and penetrating wounds. Commonly involved organisms vary with the species:

- Foals–*E. coli, Klebsiella* spp, *Actinobacillus equuli, Salmonella* spp., *Rhodococcus equi,* and *Streptococcus* spp.
  - Gram-negative bacteria are more common in younger foals.
- Calves–streptococci and coliforms (*E. coli, Salmonella* spp.) in neonatal calves; *Arcanobacterium (Actinomyces) pyogenes* in older calves
- Lambs–streptococci, coliforms, *A. pyogenes, Erysipelothrix rhusiopathiae,* and *Fusobacterium necrophorum*

Sporadic outbreaks of polyarthritis in lambs, kids, and calves are associated with *Chlamydia* and *Mycoplasma* spp. infections.

Clinical signs

Clinical signs can be extremely variable, from sudden onset of lameness in one leg in an apparently healthy neonate with no obvious joint swelling or pain to multiple joint swelling and pain in a systemically ill neonate. Lambs and kids with septic arthritis often fail to nurse and may present with significant weight loss. Typically, polyarthritis caused by *Mycoplasma* or *Chlamydia* is associated with high fevers, conjunctivitis *(Chlamydia),* and respiratory and occasionally neurologic disease. Morbidity and mortality are high.

Diagnosis

The diagnosis is obvious in neonates with evidence of septicemia and a swollen, hot, and painful joint. However, body temperature, alertness, appetite, and peripheral leukocyte counts may be normal with localized infections. Synovial fluid analysis and radiography are important for diagnosis (see Chapter 36). The chief differential diagnosis for sudden lameness in neonates is trauma (e.g., the dam stepping on the newborn). However, any neonate less than 45 days of age with sudden onset of lameness should be considered infected until proven otherwise.

Treatment

The aims of treatment are to (1) remove the infectious agent, (2) protect and minimize cartilage damage, and (3) minimize secondary osteoarthrosis. If failure of passive transfer has occurred, an additional aim is to provide immunoglobulins through plasma transfusion (at least 2 L IV). Treatment for septicemia should begin immediately (see Chapter 19). Specific management of septic arthritis and osteomyelitis is discussed in Chapter 36.

Noninfectious Lameness

Noninfectious causes of lameness in neonates include the following:

- Nutritional myodegeneration (vitamin E/selenium deficiency; see Chapter 40)
- Rupture of the common digital extensor tendon (foals)
- Contracture of joints or tendons
- Incomplete ossification of the cuboidal bones, leading to flexural and angular deformities

UMBILICAL ABNORMALITIES *(Text pp. 368-373)*

Patent Urachus

Patent urachus is persistence after birth of the tubular connection between the bladder and umbilicus. Early severance or ligation of the umbilical cord, umbilical inflammation or infection, and excessive physical handling of the neonate have been implicated.

Clinical signs and diagnosis

Affected foals may dribble urine from the urachus during or after urination or may simply present with a constantly wet umbilical stump. Ultrasound is useful for diagnosis and for determining the involvement of the umbilical arteries or vein (omphalophlebitis; see the following). Serum IgG, CBC, and urinalysis are helpful for detecting concurrent systemic or urinary tract infection.

Treatment

Initial therapy consists of conservative management: monitoring; treatment of infection; and cauterization of the urachus with iodine, phenol, or silver nitrate sticks applied into the urachus. Persistence of urine dribbling after 2 to 3 days of cauterization, ultrasound evidence of umbilical infection, and subcutaneous swelling indicating a rent in the urachus are indications for surgery.

Omphalitis/Omphalophlebitis

Omphalitis is inflammation of umbilical structures (umbilical arteries, umbilical vein, urachus) or tissues immediately surrounding the umbilicus. Umbilical abscess or infection may remain localized or result in liver abscessation or septicemia. Organisms isolated from affected foals include *E. coli, Proteus* spp., and *Streptococcus* spp. Bacteria isolated from calves with omphalitis include *A. pyogenes, E. coli, Proteus* spp., and *Enterococcus* spp.

Clinical signs and diagnosis

In some cases, the umbilicus is swollen, painful, and draining purulent material. In other cases, the umbilicus is dry but larger in diameter than expected. Other neonates have a normal-appearing, dry navel but are severely ill from infection of the urachus, umbilical arteries, or vein. Calves with urachal abscess may show signs of dysuria or pollakiuria. Ultrasound is useful for detecting involvement of the urachus or umbilical vessels (see Chapter 17).

Treatment

Early treatment with antibiotics and supportive care (see Chapter 19) may allow resolution before development of abscessation. Established infection, which may develop within 24 hours, usually requires surgical resection of involved structures in addition to medical therapy.

ANEMIA *(Text p. 370)*

Causes of anemia in neonates include blood loss from injury, neonatal isoerythrolysis, other immune-mediated hemolytic anemias, hemoperitoneum (e.g., gastric ulcer), anemia of chronic disease (e.g., localized infections), piroplasmosis, equine infectious anemia, and iron deficiency. Blood loss causes weakness and pale mucous membranes. Hemolytic diseases produce weakness, pale or jaundiced mucous membranes, fever, and depression. Intravascular hemolysis may produce hemoglobinuria, hemoglobinemia, and hyperbilirubinemia (mostly unconjugated bilirubin). Treatment depends on the cause of anemia.

FEVER *(Text pp. 370-371)*

Fever (rectal temperature greater than 38.9° C [102° F]) is an unreliable indicator of sepsis in neonates. The chief differentials in febrile neonates are infection (viral or bacterial), seizures with muscular overactivity, massive hemolysis (e.g., neonatal isoerythrolysis), hyperthermia, and idiopathic tachypnea (see p. 334). The presence of fever in a neonate warrants rigorous diagnostic evaluation and, if infection is suspected or confirmed, aggressive treatment. Cooling is indicated for hyperthermia associated with heat stroke. Correction of the initiating cause and maintenance of fluid balance are also important.

CYANOSIS *(Text p. 371)*

Causes of cyanosis in neonates include congenital heart disease, respiratory impairment, or any circulatory condition producing a right-to-left shunt (see Chapter 5). Shock and hypothermia are important causes of peripheral cyanosis in neonates. Circulatory compromise caused by hypothermia, hypoglycemia, and shock requires aggressive fluid therapy (see the following), respiratory support, and environmental temperature correction.

OLIGURIA AND STRANGURIA *(Text pp. 371-372)*

The major causes of painful urination (stranguria) in neonatal foals are ruptured bladder and bacterial cystitis. Reduced urine production (oliguria) typically results from decreased renal perfusion; causes include cardiac anomalies, asphyxia, sepsis, diarrhea (a common cause in neonatal ruminants), and endotoxemia. Pollakiuria, dysuria, and cystitis are occasionally observed with urachal abscesses. Improving renal perfusion and urine production in oliguric neonates is outlined in Chapter 16.

SHOCK *(Text p. 372)*

Causes of shock in neonates include hypothermia, hypovolemia, cardiac insufficiency, and sepsis. Following are the basic treatment guidelines:

- If blood glucose is normal, fluid therapy should consist of lactated Ringer's solution (40 to 100 ml/kg rapidly IV).
  - If blood pressure cannot be monitored, do not exceed 2 L/hr for a 50-kg neonate.
  - Add dopamine or dobutamine infusion (2 to 5 μg/kg/min IV) if hypotension is severe.
- If hypoglycemia is present, fluids containing 5% to 10% dextrose are indicated to raise the blood glucose to 160 to 180 mg/dl.
- Bicarbonate should be given if the base deficit is more than 8 mEq/L and ventilation is adequate.
- Urine output should be monitored during fluid therapy.
- Oxygen or ventilation therapy should be provided as needed (see p. 301).

Management of septic shock is discussed in Chapter 19; fluid therapy (including glucose and bicarbonate supplementation) in neonates is outlined in Chapter 18.

ICTERUS *(Text p. 373)*

Icterus in neonates may be observed with sepsis, anorexia, liver disease, equine herpesvirus 1 infection (foals), and hemolytic anemia (notably neonatal isoerythrolysis). Liver disease in neonates may be caused by Tyzzer's disease *(Clostridium [Bacillus] piliformis* infection in foals), toxic hepatic failure (e.g., ferrous fumarate in foals), bacterial hepatitis subsequent to sepsis, or hypoxic damage. In nursing calves, lambs, and kids, *C. perfringens* type A can cause intravascular hemolysis and icterus, hemoglobinuria, and anemia.

FAILURE TO THRIVE *(Text p. 373)*

In foals, failure to thrive may be a result of twinning, prematurity, hypothyroidism, congenital heart or other organ defect, infection acquired shortly after birth that becomes chronic (e.g., pneumonia, nephritis, endocarditis, arthritis), or gastric ulcer. In calves, weak calf syndrome has been reproduced by feeding low-protein diets to prepartum cows that subsequently calved in environments in which the temperature was well below the thermoneutral zone for calves.

21

Milk Replacers

(Text pp. 382-386)

Consulting Editors A. JUDSON HEINRICHS • LORRAINE DOEPEL
RICK CORBETT

CALVES *(Text pp. 382-385)*

The goals of a milk replacer feeding program are to achieve optimum growth rates, develop a strong immune system, minimize health disorders, stimulate and optimize rumen development, and minimize the cost of feeding the preweaned calf.

General Recommendations

The composition and quality of a milk replacer influence the growth, health, and overall performance of the calf. As a general guide, milk replacers for dairy calves should contain the following levels of nutrients on a dry matter basis:

- Crude protein–18% to 24%
- Fat–10% to 22%
- Calcium–0.7%
- Phosphorus–0.6%

Guidelines for minerals and vitamins are listed in Table 21-2 of *Large Animal Internal Medicine,* third edition. Table 21-1 lists the nutritional composition of ingredients commonly used in milk replacers.

Protein Source

Replacers that use skim milk or whey proteins as the primary protein source are superior to those that use soy or other vegetable proteins. The performance and cost of products that use animal proteins (e.g., fish, plasma, hydrolyzed red blood cells) are intermediate between milk-protein replacers and soy-based replacers.

Energy Supply

During periods of extreme stress (e.g., cold temperatures in calves housed outside), the calf's energy intake should be increased by increasing the amount of replacer fed per day by 30% to 50% or by increasing the fat content of the replacer. However, overfeeding milk replacer, either the amount or concentration, reduces the dry matter intake from calf starter. This will slow rumen development and be less economical for the producer.

FOALS *(Text pp. 385-386)*

The use of milk replacer for foals becomes necessary when the mare has an inadequate milk supply or when the foal is orphaned at an early age. Milk replacers for foals should contain 18% to 22% crude protein, 12% to 16% crude fat, and 10% to 11% total solids. They should be highly digestible, easily reconstituted, and palatable.

TABLE 21-1
Composition of Ingredients Used in Milk Replacers

	Whey	Whey protein concentrate	Delactosed whey	Skim milk	Whole dried milk	Isolated soy protein	Soy protein concentrate	Soy flour	Modified wheat protein	Spray-dried blood meal	Spray-dried animal plasma
		EXPRESSED ON AN AS IS BASIS (%)					**EXPRESSED ON AN AS IS BASIS (%)**				
Dry matter	98	98	98	98	97	94	95	95	94	92	92
Protein	12	34	23	34	26	66	67	53	82	80	78
Fat	0.2	3.5	1.5	0.1	28.5	0.5	0.3	0.2	2	1.3	1.1
Lactose	74	52	55	54	34	—	—	—	—	—	—
Ash	8.5	8	16	7.9	6	4.5	7	6.3	3	5.3	8.9
Calcium	0.9	0.54	1.95	1.25	0.95	0.1	0.35	0.35	0.04	0.32	0.15
Phosphorus	0.81	0.67	1	1.05	0.75	0.76	0.18	0.73	0.4	0.24	1.7
		ESSENTIAL AMINO ACIDS (G/100 G PROTEIN)					**ESSENTIAL AMINO ACIDS (G/100 G PROTEIN)**				
Lysine	8.92	9.09	8.91	8.24	8.23	6.07	6.32	6.15	1.6	8.19	6.9
Methionine	1.92	1.94	1.91	2.65	2.62	1.11	1.32	1.26	1.85	1.01	0.7
Cysteine	2.25	2.47	2.09	1.51	1.5	1.41	1.47	1.42	2.47	0.9	1.8
Arginine	2.92	2.53	2.91	3.65	3.85	7.79	8.1	7.17	3.95	3.87	4.5
Tryptophan	2.09	2.15	2.09	1.41	1.41	1.01	1.32	1.28	0.99	1.16	1.3
Histidine	1.75	1.91	1.74	2.74	2.73	2.73	2.65	2.6	2.22	5.87	2.5
Isoleucine	6.08	5.97	8.09	6.99	7	4.85	4.65	4.62	4.44	4	2
Leucine	10.33	10.47	10.35	10.01	10	8.09	7.94	7.62	7.78	2.34	7.4
Phenylalanine	3.5	3.24	3.48	4.71	4.69	4.95	5	4.91	5.93	6.2	4.8
Threonine	7	7.29	7	4.25	4.23	3.84	4.12	4.06	2.59	3.78	4.3
Valine	5.92	5.82	5.91	5.58	6.65	5.06	5.15	4.89	4.44	7.81	5.2

General Recommendations

Orphan foals should be fed milk replacer from 1 day of age (after receiving colostrum within 24 hours of birth) until at least 4 weeks of age. General feeding recommendations are as follows:

- Age 1 to 3 days–feed 480 g/day of milk replacer powder over 12 feedings (approximately 300 ml/meal of reconstituted milk replacer)
- Age 4 to 5 days–feed 560 g/day over 8 feedings (approximately 500 ml/meal)
- Age 6 to 7 days–feed 860 g/day over 8 feedings (approximately 770 ml/meal)
- Age 8 to 10 days–feed 1100 g/day over 8 feedings (approximately 1000 ml/meal)
- Age 11 to 14 days–feed 1335 g/day over 6 feedings (approximately 1660 ml/meal)
- Age 15 to 21 days–feed 1750 g/day over 4 feedings (approximately 3225 ml/meal)
- Over 21 days–feed at least 2.5% of body weight/day over 3 to 4 feedings

LAMBS AND KIDS *(Text p. 386)*

Milk replacers for lambs are used to raise extra lambs from multiple births and orphaned lambs; they can also be used for kids. Milk replacers for lambs usually contain 21% to 24% crude protein and 24% to 30% crude fat. The lactose level should not exceed 25%; higher levels may result in abomasal bloat and diarrhea. Feeding warm milk replacer only a limited number of times during the day can also lead to abomasal bloat. Creep feed can be offered after 1 week of age. It should contain 17% to 20% crude protein, be highly digestible, and be fed fresh daily.

PART IV

Collection of Samples and Interpretations of Laboratory Tests

22

Clinical Chemistry Tests

(Text pp. 389-412)

Consulting Editor GARY P. CARLSON

Submission of samples and sources of variation in normal clinical chemistry values are discussed in *Large Animal Internal Medicine,* third edition. Normal clinical chemistry values for horses, cattle, sheep, and goats are listed in Table 22-1.

FLUID AND ELECTROLYTE BALANCE *(Text pp. 395-401)*

Sodium

Changes in serum sodium concentration reflect changes in water balance. Hyponatremia is an indicator of a relative water excess; hypernatremia is an indicator of a relative water deficit.

Hyponatremia

The more common causes of hyponatremia include the following:

- Loss of sodium-containing fluid–diarrhea, excessive sweating, blood loss, fluid drainage (e.g., high-volume gastric reflux or pleural drainage)
- Adrenal insufficiency
- Sequestration of fluid (third space problems)–peritonitis, ascites, ruptured bladder, gut torsion or volvulus
- Excessive administration of 5% dextrose to patients with renal disease
- False hyponatremia–hyperlipidemia, hyperproteinemia, hyperglycemia

Hypernatremia

Hypernatremia can occur in the initial stages of diarrhea, vomiting, or renal disease if water loss exceeds electrolyte loss. Other causes include the following:

- Pure water loss–panting, water deprivation
- Sodium excess–salt poisoning, feeding electrolytes with no access to free water

Potassium

Hypokalemia

Hypokalemia may result from depletion of the body's potassium stores or from redistribution of potassium from the extracellular to the intracellular fluid space. Reduced intake or excessive loss of potassium can occur with dietary deficiency or prolonged anorexia, vomiting, diarrhea, vagal indigestion with internal vomiting, third space problems (e.g., ileus, bowel torsion or volvulus, peritonitis), and excessive sweat loss. Hypokalemia also occurs with metabolic alkalosis.

Hyperkalemia

The more common causes of hyperkalemia include the following:

- False hyperkalemia–in vitro hemolysis or leakage from red blood cells during prolonged storage (more than 6 hours) of whole blood samples
- Hypovolemia with renal shutdown
- Metabolic acidosis
- Vigorous exercise (transient hyperkalemia)

TABLE 22-1
Clinical Chemistry: Normal Range for Large Animals

Component	Unit	Equine	Bovine	Ovine	Caprine
CHEMISTRY					
Total bilirubin	mg/dl	0.5-2.3	0-0.1	0.1-0.2	0-0.1
Direct	mg/dl	0-0.6	0	0	0
Indirect	mg/dl	0.2-2	0-0.1	0-0.12	0-0.1
Cholesterol	mg/dl	75-150	80-120	52-76	80-130
Creatinine	mg/dl	0.9-2	0.9-1.3	0.8-1.3	0.7-1
Glucose	mg/dl	89-112	33-66	56-92	53-81
Fibrinogen	mg/dl	100-400	100-600	100-500	100-400
Protein (total serum)	g/dl	5.8-7.7	6.8-8.6	6.6-8.6	6.8-8.3
Albumin	g/dl	2.3-3.6	3-4.3	2.7-3.7	3.2-3.8
Globulin	g/dl	1.7-4.7	3-4.9	2.8-5.4	3.1-4.8
Urea nitrogen	mg/dl	12-27	8-23	14-37	19-31

Data from Kaneko JJ, Harvey JW, Bruss ML, eds. *Clinical biochemistry of domestic animals,* ed 5, New York, 1997, Academic Press; and Duncan JR, Prasse KW: *Veterinary laboratory medicine,* ed 3, Ames, Iowa, 1994, Iowa State University Press; and the Veterinary Medical Teaching Hospital, University of California at Davis, 2000.

Continued

TABLE 22-1
Clinical Chemistry: Normal Range for Large Animals—cont'd

Component	Unit	Equine	Bovine	Ovine	Caprine
ENZYME					
ALP	IU/L	86-285	27-107	50-300	27-210
ASAT	IU/L	138-409	43-127	60-280	46-161
CK	IU/L	119-287	105-409	100-547	104-219
GGT	IU/L	8-22	15-39	40-94	34-65
LDH	IU/L	162-412	697-1445	238-440	123-392
LDH-1	%	6.3-18.5	39.8-63.5	45.7-63.6	29.3-51.8
LDH-2	%	8.4-20.5	19.7-34.8	0-3	0-5.4
LDH-3	%	41-65.9	11.7-18.1	16.4-29.9	24.2-39.9
LDH-4	%	9.5-20.9	0-8.8	4.3-7.3	0-5.5
LDH-5	%	1.7-16.5	0-12.4	10.5-29.1	14.1-36.8
SDH	IU/L	0-8	12-53	18-77	2-57
ELECTROLYTE					
Sodium	mEq/L	132-146	132-152	139-152	142-155
Potassium	mEq/L	2.4-4.7	3.9-5.8	3.9-5.4	3.5-6.7
Chloride	mEq/L	99-109	97-111	95-103	99-110
Calcium	mg/dl	11.2-13.6	9.7-12.4	11.5-12.8	8.9-11.7
Phosphorus	mg/dl	3.1-5.6	5.6-6.5	5-7.3	6.5
Magnesium	mg/dl	2.2-2.8	1.8-2.3	2.2-2.8	2.8-3.6
Osmolality	mOsm/kg	270-300	270-300	***	***
Anion gap	mEq/L	6-15	14-20	***	***

ACID-BASE (VENOUS BLOOD)					
pH		7.32-7.44	7.31-7.53	7.32-7.54	***
P_{CO_2}	mm Hg	38-46	35-44	37-46	***
Bicarbonate	mEq/L	20-28	17-29	20-25	***
TCO_2	mEq/L	24-32	21-32	21-28	26-30
SPECIAL					
Red cell acetylcholinesterase	IU/L	450-790	1270-2430	640	270
Ammonia	µg/dl	13-108	***	***	***
BSP (t½)	min	2-3.7	2.5-4	1.6-2.7	2.1
Serum iron	µg/dl	73-140	57-162	166-222	***
TIBC	µg/dl	200-262	63-186	***	***
Lactic acid	mmol/L	1.11-1.78	0.56-2.22	1.00-1.33	***
Ketones					
Acetone	mg/dl	***	0-10	0-10	***
Acetoacetate	mg/dl	***	0-1.1	***	***
BHB	mg/dl	***	0-10	***	***

Data from Kaneko JJ, Harvey JW, Bruss ML, eds. *Clinical biochemistry of domestic animals,* ed 5, New York, 1997, Academic Press; and Duncan JR, Prasse KW: *Veterinary laboratory medicine,* ed 3, Ames, Iowa, 1994, Iowa State University Press; and the Veterinary Medical Teaching Hospital, University of California at Davis, 2000.

ALP, Alkaline phosphatase; *ASAT,* aspartate aminotransferase; *BHB,* β-hydroxybutyrate; *BSP (t½),* bromsulphalein clearance halftime; *CK,* creatine kinase; *GGT,* γ-glutamyltransferase; *LDH,* lactate dehydrogenase; P_{CO_2}, partial pressure of carbon dioxide; *SDH,* sorbitol dehydrogenase; TCO_2, total carbon dioxide; *TIBC,* total iron-binding capacity.

- Ruptured bladder (foals)
- Hyperkalemic periodic paralysis (HYPP; primarily seen in Quarter Horses)

Chloride

Alterations in chloride concentration usually are associated with nearly proportional changes in sodium concentration. The chloride concentration tends to vary inversely with bicarbonate concentration. Thus, when disproportionate changes in chloride concentration relative to sodium occur, significant acid-base imbalances should be anticipated.

Hyperchloremia

Hyperchloremia with proportional hypernatremia is most often associated with relative water deficit (e.g., panting, water deprivation, salt poisoning). The most common cause of disproportionate hyperchloremia is hyperchloremic metabolic acidosis (e.g., renal tubular acidosis in horses).

Hypochloremia

Causes of proportional hypochloremia with hyponatremia are similar to those listed for hyponatremia. Disproportionate hypochloremia is most often associated with metabolic alkalosis. Causes include exhaustive syndrome (horses), loss of saliva in horses only, abomasal torsion, vagal indigestion with internal vomiting, and furosemide administration (horses).

Calcium

Hypocalcemia

The more common causes of hypocalcemia include the following:

- Pregnancy and lactation–parturient paresis or milk fever (cattle, sheep), lactation tetany (horses)
- Anorexia in lactating dairy cows caused by systemic diseases (e.g., ketosis, traumatic reticuloperitonitis, displaced abomasum) or acute toxemia (e.g., coliform mastitis, septicemia, pneumonia)
- Grass tetany (hypomagnesemia) in cattle
- Hypoalbuminemia (decreased total calcium; ionized calcium remains unchanged)
- Fat necrosis (cattle)
- Stress–transport (transit tetany; horses, sheep); exhaustive syndrome (horses)
- Blister beetle (cantharidin) toxicosis
- Acute renal failure (mild hypocalcemia and hyperphosphatemia)

Hypercalcemia

The more common causes of hypercalcemia include the following:

- Chronic renal failure in horses on a high-calcium diet (e.g., alfalfa hay)
    - Serum calcium is more than 14 mg/dl with modest hypophosphatemia.
- Excess vitamin D–dietary supplements or plant toxins (e.g., *Cestrum diurnum* [day-blooming jasmine] and *Solanum malacoxylon*)
- Excessive or too rapid intravenous administration of calcium

Less common causes include neoplasia (e.g., lymphosarcoma, gastric squamous cell carcinoma) and hyperparathyroidism.

Phosphorus

Imbalances of calcium and phosphorus are not always evident on analysis of serum samples. Measurement of urine creatinine clearance ratios for calcium and phosphate are more useful (see p. 411).

Hypophosphatemia

The more common causes of hypophosphatemia include inadequate dietary intake, chronic renal failure (horses), parturient paresis (low-phosphorus diets in cattle), and postparturient hemoglobinuria (lactating dairy cattle).

Hyperphosphatemia

The more common causes of hyperphosphatemia include acute renal failure, nutritional secondary hyperparathyroidism (excess phosphorus intake), and in horses, endurance exercise (transient hyperphosphatemia). Neonates normally have higher serum phosphorus values than adults (as high as 9 mg/dl).

Magnesium

Hypomagnesemia

Hypomagnesemia is reported in cattle with grass tetany and in sheep with grass staggers. Serum magnesium less than 1.8 mg/dl is considered low; values less than 1 mg/dl are likely to be associated with clinical signs. Hypomagnesemia has been reported in calves reared in confinement and fed an exclusively milk diet. It can also occur during endurance exercise in horses.

Hypermagnesemia

Hypermagnesemia occurs infrequently but may be seen with overzealous administration of Epsom salts ($MgSO_4$, orally or as an enema) and excessive intravenous administration of magnesium.

ACID-BASE IMBALANCE *(Text pp. 401-405)*

Metabolic Acidosis

Metabolic acidosis is characterized by a decrease in blood pH and bicarbonate concentration. The more common causes include the following:

- Rumen grain overload (lactic acidosis)
- Ketoacidosis–ketosis, pregnancy toxemia
- Hypovolemia with or without toxemia–acute diarrhea, strangulated bowel, peritonitis
- Uroperitoneum (ruptured bladder)
- Exercise above the anaerobic threshold (transient lactic acidosis in horses)
- Salivary loss with oral disease or esophagostomy in cattle
- Renal failure

Base deficit

The calculated base deficit provides a means of estimating the amount of bicarbonate required to correct metabolic acidosis:

$$HCO_3^- \text{ needed (mEq)} = \text{Base deficit (mEq)} \times \text{Body weight (kg)} \times 0.5$$

The base deficit is the difference between the measured bicarbonate (or total CO_2) and the normal value for that species.

Metabolic Alkalosis

Metabolic alkalosis is characterized by an increase in blood pH and bicarbonate. It occurs fairly frequently in domestic animals, particularly in association with digestive disturbances in ruminants. Causes include the following:

- Sequestration of fluid into the abomasum and forestomach (e.g., displacement, vagal indigestion or obstruction)
- Gastric reflux in horses (e.g., anterior enteritis, ileus, small bowel obstruction)
- Massive sweat loss in horses (e.g., endurance horses)
- Chloride or potassium depletion
- Extracellular fluid volume contraction without bicarbonate loss (contraction alkalosis)
- Salivary loss of chloride in horses with esophagostomy
- Diuretic usage (especially furosemide)
- Bicarbonate loading ("milk shakes") in performance horses

Respiratory Acidosis

Respiratory acidosis is characterized by a decrease in blood pH and an increase in P_{CO_2}, which develop because of reduced alveolar ventilation. The most common causes include the following:

- Acute upper respiratory obstruction–laryngeal edema
- Primary pulmonary disease–pneumonia, pleuritis, chronic obstructive lung disease
- Respiratory center depression–general anesthesia with inadequate assisted ventilation, opiates, tranquilizers, central nervous system (CNS) disease

NOTE: Exogenous bicarbonate does not correct respiratory acidosis and should not be administered to these patients.

Respiratory Alkalosis

Respiratory alkalosis is caused by hyperventilation. Causes include the following:

- Hypoxemia associated with pulmonary disease, congestive heart failure, or severe anemia
- Central stimulation of ventilation by psychogenic hyperventilation, excitement, fear, pain, gram-negative septicemia, or CNS disease

Anion Gap

The anion gap is the difference between the major cations (sodium and potassium) and the measured anions (chloride and bicarbonate). Hypoalbuminemia and hyperchloremic metabolic acidosis are the two most common causes of decreased anion gap. An increase in the anion gap usually indicates acidosis, such as lactic acidosis (anaerobic exercise, grain overload, hypovolemic shock), ketoacidosis, and uremic acidosis.

SERUM ENZYMES *(Text pp. 405-407)*

Sorbitol Dehydrogenase

Sorbitol dehydrogenase (SDH) is liver specific and a sensitive indicator of hepatocellular damage. Increases in SDH occur with severe anorexia, acute or chronic liver failure, liver abscesses, and liver damage secondary to obstructive or strangulating bowel lesions or acute toxic enteritis. This enzyme is not stable when stored at room temperature, but refrigerated samples may yield useful results even after several days of storage.

Creatine Kinase

Creatine kinase (CK) is a highly sensitive and specific indicator of muscle damage. Elevations are most commonly associated with exertional myopathies (rhabdomyolysis). Other causes include the following:

- Muscle trauma–intramuscular injections, prolonged recumbency with inability to rise (alert downer cow syndrome, muscle crush)
- Nutritional or metabolic disorders–polysaccharide storage myopathy (horses), nutritional myodegeneration (vitamin E/selenium deficiency), malignant hyperthermia
- Other–*Streptococcus equi*-associated myopathy (horses), postendurance ride multisystemic disorder, malignant edema

Vigorous exercise or prolonged shipping may result in modest elevations (up to fourfold). Hemolysis may falsely elevate CK in a sample. Persistent elevation of CK suggests active and continuing muscle damage.

Aspartate Aminotransferase

Aspartate aminotransferase (ASAT) is a nonspecific indicator of tissue damage. Elevations may be seen with muscle damage, liver disease, and in vitro hemolysis. Elevations of both CK and ASAT indicate muscle damage, whereas elevations of both SDH and ASAT indicate liver damage. Typically, extensive muscle necrosis produces much higher elevations of ASAT than does severe liver necrosis.

γ-Glutamyltransferase

The enzyme γ-glutamyltransferase (GGT) is a reliable marker of hepatobiliary disorders and cholestasis. Conditions that cause an elevation in GGT include pyrrolizidine alkaloid toxicity, chronic active hepatitis, cholangiohepatitis, cholelithiasis, aflatoxicosis, liver flukes, fatty liver syndrome in dairy cows, and hyperlipemia in periparturient pony and Miniature Horse mares. Levels of GGT are higher in neonates; burros, donkeys, and asses have GGT values 2 to 3 times higher than those in horses.

Alkaline Phosphatase

Alkaline phosphatase (ALP) is a marker of biliary obstruction and of metabolically active bone (e.g., growth, rickets, healing fractures). Elevations in ALP may be found with pyrrolizidine alkaloid toxicity, chronic active hepatitis, cholangiohepatitis, cholelithiasis, and liver fluke infestation. Because ALP is not organ specific, it is necessary to interpret elevations in relation to more organ-specific enzymes such as SDH and GGT.

Lactate Dehydrogenase

Lactate dehydrogenase (LDH) is found in relatively high concentrations in the heart, liver, muscle, kidney, erythrocytes, and leukocytes. Elevations in LDH may be seen with liver disease, extensive muscle damage (rhabdomyolysis), and some hemolytic disorders. In vitro hemolysis may falsely elevate serum LDH activity. Elevations must be interpreted in relation to more organ-specific enzymes. When available, LDH isoenzyme analysis can be helpful.

BILIRUBIN *(Text pp. 407-408)*

The total serum bilirubin concentration is of little diagnostic value in horses unless both direct (conjugated) and indirect (unconjugated) bilirubin are measured. Unconjugated, and hence total, bilirubin may be elevated with hemolytic anemia, liver failure, and in horses, fasting or anorexia. In fasted or anorectic horses, total bilirubin may be as high as 8 mg/dl. Elevation in direct-reacting bilirubin occurs with liver failure, cholelithiasis, cholangiohepatitis, and neonatal isoerythrolysis. Direct-reacting bilirubin rarely exceeds 25% of the total bilirubin in horses, and increases of this magnitude suggest biliary obstruction. In the absence of hemolytic anemia, a bilirubin value greater than 2 mg/dl indicates impaired hepatic function in ruminants.

GLUCOSE *(Text p. 408)*

Hypoglycemia

Causes of hypoglycemia include the following:

- Decreased food intake (neonates)
- Primary ketosis–pregnancy toxemia, fat cow syndrome, hyperlipemia in pregnant or lactating ponies
- Severe systemic illness–acute toxic enteritis, coliform mastitis, septicemia, colic associated with strangulated bowel, late-stage endotoxic shock
- Exhaustion after prolonged exercise in some horses
- Hepatic failure

Hyperglycemia

Hyperglycemia may be seen with excitement, transportation, or other types of stress. Other causes include severe colic in horses, later stages of Cushing's syndrome (non–insulin-responsive hyperglycemia and glycosuria), and administration of exogenous glucocorticoids or xylazine.

CREATININE *(Text pp. 408-409)*

The more common causes of elevated serum creatinine include the following:

- Prerenal azotemia–hypovolemia (e.g., acute enteritis, massive blood loss, some types of colic), congestive heart failure, dehydration after exhaustive exercise
- Renal azotemia–acute or chronic renal failure
- Postrenal azotemia–urolithiasis (renal, ureteral, or urethral calculi), ruptured bladder

Serum creatinine is not a very sensitive or early indicator of alterations in renal function, although in ruminants it is a more reliable indicator of renal failure than is blood urea nitrogen (BUN) (which can be metabolized by ruminal microflora).

BLOOD UREA NITROGEN *(Text pp. 409-410)*

BUN may be low in patients with liver failure and in normal neonates. It may be increased with any of the causes of azotemia listed earlier. Starvation or other processes that result in rapid tissue catabolism (e.g., fever, burns, corticosteroid administration) may result in modest increases in BUN.

URINALYSIS *(Text pp. 410-411)*

Urinalysis should be performed as soon after collection as possible to avoid degeneration of cellular elements, changes in pH, and bacterial overgrowth. If analysis within 30 minutes of collection is not possible, the sample should be refrigerated.

Specific Gravity

Urine specific gravity is usually measured by refractometry. The normal range for adult animals is 1.020 to 1.050. Neonates normally produce very diluted urine (specific gravity less than 1.010). Failure to produce concentrated urine (specific gravity less than 1.020 in the face of dehydration) is an indication of altered renal function. Causes include primary renal disease, diabetes insipidus, and medullary washout (severe and chronic sodium depletion).

pH

The normal range of urine pH for adult herbivores is 7 to 9. Neonatal foals tend to have a slightly acidic urine (pH less than 7). Aciduria in adults may be seen in postrace samples from racehorses, after prolonged fasting, with ketosis in ruminants, or in response to metabolic acidosis. Paradoxical aciduria is commonly seen in ruminants with hypochloremic metabolic alkalosis.

Protein

Protein normally is not detected in urine, although a false-positive reaction may be noted on urine dipsticks if the sample is strongly alkaline. Persistent and strongly positive reactions for protein in the absence of leukocytes, red cells, bacteria, or casts suggest glomerular protein loss, as occurs with glomerulonephritis or amyloidosis. The presence of bacteria and leukocytes with proteinuria suggests urinary tract infection.

Glucose

Glucose is not found in the urine of normal large animals unless the blood glucose increases above the renal threshold (100 to 140 mg/dl in ruminants, 160 to 180 mg/dl in horses). Causes of glycosuria include Cushing's syndrome, stress, other causes of catecholamine or glucocorticoid release, and in sheep, enterotoxemia (pulpy kidney). The presence of glycosuria without hyperglycemia strongly suggests renal tubular damage resulting from a toxic or ischemic insult.

Occult Blood

Both myoglobin and hemoglobin give a positive occult blood reaction on urine dipsticks. With a dark urine sample, vigorously shaking the sample produces brown foam if myoglobin is present and reddish foam if the discoloration is from hemoglobin. Hemoglobinuria caused by intravascular hemolysis generally is associated with clinical and hematologic evidence of hemolytic anemia.

Cells

Normal urine should contain 5 or fewer erythrocytes or leukocytes per high-power field. An increased number of erythrocytes indicates hematuria, which may be caused by inflammation, trauma, coagulopathy, or neoplasia. An increase in leukocytes (pyuria) indicates an inflammatory process, and when associated with bacteriuria, a septic process in the urinary tract. The presence of sheets or rafts of transitional cells suggests neoplasia.

Bacteria

Bacteria are sometimes seen in small numbers in voided urine samples. However, urinary tract infections usually are associated with significant pyuria. A catheterized sample (horse) or clean midstream catch (ruminant) should be obtained for Gram stain, culture, and sensitivity testing.

Casts

Casts are accumulations of protein and cellular material that form in the renal tubules; when present in urine, they indicate renal damage or tubular disease. Hyaline casts may be seen with glomerulonephritis, fever (with passive congestion), or severe dehydration.

Crystals

Calcium carbonate crystals are normally found in abundance in horse urine, particularly if the horse is fed alfalfa hay. Triple phosphate and calcium oxalate crystals are often found in relatively small numbers. In feedlot cattle the major crystals involved in urolithiasis are struvite ($Mg\ NH_4PO_4 \cdot 6H_2$). In the western United States, silicate stones are most common in livestock under range conditions. Carbonate and oxalate stones are common causes of urolithiasis in backyard sheep and goats fed alfalfa hay.

Urine Creatinine Clearance Ratio

Variation in the rate of urine production can lead to serious problems in the interpretation of urine electrolyte concentrations. Expression of the renal clearance as a ratio eliminates the need for quantitative urine collection. This derived value is known as the creatinine clearance ratio, or fractional excretion (FE), and is calculated by the following formula:

$$FE = [Urine(X)/Serum(X)] \times [Serum(C)/Urine(C)] \times 100$$

where X represents the electrolyte concentration and C represents the creatinine concentration.

Interpretation

Dietary salt deficiency is associated with extremely low FE of sodium and chloride; prerenal azotemia can also result in a low FE of sodium. An increase in the FE of sodium is noted with renal tubular damage and impaired sodium resorption. Calcium deficiency and phosphorus excess result in a low FE for calcium and a high FE for phosphorus.

23

Collection and Submission of Samples for Cytologic and Hematologic Studies

(Text pp. 413-414)

Consulting Editor DEBRA DEEM MORRIS

BLOOD *(Text pp. 413-414)*

Hematology

Ethylenediamine tetraacetic acid (EDTA) is the preferred anticoagulant for complete blood count; it is also suitable for platelet counts, total plasma protein, and plasma fibrinogen. If a delay is anticipated between collection and analysis, the sample should be refrigerated. Air-dried blood smears for the differential count should be prepared immediately if samples must be held longer than 2 hours.

Hemostatic Function Tests

Trisodium citrate (3.8%, mixed 1:9 with blood) is used to preserve blood for hemostatic function tests. Blood must be collected and handled with special care to prevent platelet clumping or activation of coagulation. If the sample cannot be analyzed immediately, plasma should be collected by centrifugation, harvested with a plastic pipette, and frozen. Platelet counts must be performed on a fresh sample; an estimate can be made by examining a blood smear.

BONE MARROW *(Text p. 414)*

Air-dried smears can be made directly from a bone marrow aspirate or after the sample has been anticoagulated with EDTA (e.g., collected into a syringe containing 1 to 2 drops of EDTA). Bone marrow core samples are preserved in 10% neutral buffered formalin.

LYMPH NODE ASPIRATES *(Text p. 414)*

Air-dried smears of lymph node aspirates are handled in the same way as blood smears for differential count.

24

Alterations in the Erythron

(Text pp. 415-419)

Consulting Editor DEBRA DEEM MORRIS

ANEMIA *(Text pp. 415-419)*

Anemia is functionally defined as decreased oxygen-carrying capacity of the blood. The most accurate laboratory indication is reduction of the packed cell volume (PCV), or hematocrit, below the normal range for the species (Table 24-1).

The general approach to investigating anemia is discussed in *Large Animal Internal Medicine,* third edition. Following are the clinical signs of anemia, common causes in horses and ruminants, and the possible significance of specific alterations in erythrocyte characteristics.

Clinical Signs of Anemia

The major clinical signs of anemia are tachycardia, tachypnea, reduced exercise tolerance, and depression. The PCV at which clinical signs are seen depends on the rate of development, severity of the anemia, and the physical demands placed on the animal. Anemia is accompanied by mucosal pallor, except when hemolysis results in icterus. Red urine (hemoglobinuria) indicates intravascular hemolysis, which may be accompanied by fever. Melena, hematuria, and petechial hemorrhages may indicate chronic blood loss.

Causes of Anemia

Horses

Common causes of anemia in horses include the following:

- Blood loss–parasitism (strongylosis, lice, ticks), gastric ulcers, immune-mediated thrombocytopenia, gastric squamous cell carcinoma, purpura hemorrhagica
- Hemolysis–neonatal isoerythrolysis, equine infectious anemia, red maple toxicity, equine ehrlichiosis
- Inadequate erythrocyte production–chronic inflammatory disease (e.g., abdominal abscess, pneumonia/pleuritis), purpura hemorrhagica, equine ehrlichiosis, lymphosarcoma

Less common causes of anemia in horses are listed on p. 417 of *Large Animal Internal Medicine,* third edition.

Ruminants

Common causes of anemia in ruminants include the following:

- Blood loss–parasitism (intestinal nematodes, lice, ticks), abomasal ulcer (cattle)
- Hemolysis–anaplasmosis, plant toxicity (*Brassica* spp., onions), bacillary hemoglobinuria, leptospirosis, chronic copper toxicity (sheep)
- Inadequate erythrocyte production–lymphosarcoma, liver abscess, chronic disease (e.g., bovine virus diarrhea, Johne's disease, pneumonia, abscess)

Less common causes of anemia in ruminants are listed on p. 417 of *Large Animal Internal Medicine,* third edition.

TABLE 24-1
Normal Values for Erythron Data in Ruminants and the Horse

	Cattle	Sheep	Goats	Horses
PCV (%)	24-46	27-45	22-38	32-53
Erythrocytes (× 10^6/L)	5-10	9-15	8-18	6.7-12.9
Hemoglobin (g/dl)	8-15	9-15	8-12	11-19
MCV (fl)	40-60	28-40	16-25	37-58.5
MCH (pg)	11-17	8-12	5.2-8	12.3-19.7
MCHC* (g/dl)	30-36	31-34	30-36	31-38.6
Reticulocytes	0	<0.5%	0	0
Erythrocyte diameter (m)	4-8	3.2-6	2.5-3.9	5-6
Erythrocyte fragility (% NaCl)				
Minimum (beginning hemolysis)	0.52-0.66	0.58-0.76	0.74	0.54
Maximum (complete hemolysis)	0.44-0.52	0.40-0.55	0.44	0.34
Erythrocyte sedimentation rate (mm/1 hr)	0	1-2.5	0	50-60
Erythrocyte life span (days)	160	140-150	125	140-150

PCV, Packed cell volume; *MCV,* mean corpuscular volume; *MCH,* mean corpuscular hemoglobin; *MCHC,* mean corpuscular hemoglobin concentration; *NaCl,* sodium chloride.

Evaluating Erythrocyte Characteristics

Mean corpuscular volume

A reflection of mean erythrocyte size, an increase in mean corpuscular volume (MCV) (macrocytosis) indicates a regenerative anemia. Iron deficiency results in a decreased MCV (microcytosis).

Mean corpuscular hemoglobin

An estimation of the amount of hemoglobin per erythrocyte, an increase in mean corpuscular hemoglobin (MCH) indicates either the presence of reticulocytes in the peripheral blood or hemolysis (in vivo or in vitro). Iron deficiency causes a decrease in MCH.

Mean corpuscular hemoglobin concentration

The most accurate erythrocyte index, a decrease in mean corpuscular hemoglobin concentration (MCHC) indicates reticulocytosis (erythroid regeneration) or iron deficiency. Hemolysis (in vivo or in vitro) causes an increase in MCHC.

Anisocytosis

Variation in erythrocyte size is caused by the presence of macrocytes or microcytes among normal cells. Slight to moderate anisocytosis is normal in cattle, but marked anisocytosis in ruminants is a sign of regenerative anemia. Macrocytic erythrocytes may be seen with regenerative anemia in horses, but regeneration often occurs without macrocytosis in this species. Nucleated erythrocytes and metarubricytes occasionally appear in the peripheral blood during the responsive phase of severe anemia in ruminants.

Polychromasia

Variation in erythrocyte staining is caused by the presence of bluish-staining reticulocytes. In ruminants, polychromasia is a sign of regenerative anemia. Iron deficiency results in decreased staining intensity and increased central pallor of erythrocytes (hypochromia).

Poikilocytosis

Abnormally shaped erythrocytes indicate increased erythrocyte fragility or diseases characterized by erythrocyte fragmentation. Poikilocytosis is rare in large animals, although it may accompany iron deficiency or disseminated coagulopathy.

Basophilic stippling

Basophilic stippling (tiny blue granules in Romanovsky-stained erythrocytes) is a normal feature of regenerative anemia in cattle and sheep. It may also indicate chronic lead poisoning in cattle.

Howell-Jolly bodies

Howell-Jolly bodies, basophilic nuclear remnants, are commonly seen during responsive anemias in ruminants. In healthy horses, Howell-Jolly bodies are normally found in a small number of erythrocytes.

Heinz bodies

Heinz bodies are round structures attached to one edge of the red cell, seen on new methylene blue preparations. They indicate oxidative damage to erythrocytes. Heinz body hemolytic anemia is seen in onion or *Brassica* spp. toxicity in cattle and in phenothiazine, red maple, or (rarely) onion toxicity in horses.

Autoagglutination

Aggregation of erythrocytes may be observed grossly or microscopically during immune-mediated anemia in horses and cattle, and rarely, with severe inflammatory diseases. Marked rouleaux formation, which is normal in horses, may be differentiated from agglutination by diluting the blood sample 1:4 with 0.9% saline.

Erythrocyte fragility

An increase in susceptibility of erythrocytes to hemolysis in hypotonic saline is suggestive of immune-mediated anemia, although the Coombs' test is more specific.

Direct antiglobulin (Coombs') test

A positive Coombs' test indicates the presence of antibodies on the surface of erythrocytes and may be found with idiopathic autoimmune hemolytic anemia in any species and in horses with neonatal isoerythrolysis or equine infectious anemia. However, false-negative results are common.

Erythrocytic parasites

Intraerythrocytic parasites can be found during the acute stages of anaplasmosis in cattle and babesiosis in horses and ruminants. *Anaplasma marginale* are seen as round, basophilic inclusions at the edges of red cells. *Babesia* spp. are round, bizarre, rod-shaped, or piriform (teardrop-shaped) structures. Absence of inclusions does not rule out anaplasmosis or babesiosis.

ERYTHROCYTOSIS (POLYCYTHEMIA) *(Text p. 419)*

Erythrocytosis is an increase in PCV, erythrocyte count, and hemoglobin concentration above the normal range. Erythrocytosis may be relative, caused by hemoconcentration (e.g., as seen in dehydration or shock) or splenic contraction, or absolute, caused by increased erythropoiesis.

Absolute Erythrocytosis

Primary absolute erythrocytosis (polycythemia vera) is an uncommon, idiopathic, myeloproliferative disorder. Secondary absolute erythrocytosis usually is triggered by chronic tissue hypoxia. Causes include residence at high altitude, chronic pulmonary disease, and heart defects that involve arteriovenous shunting. Rare causes of secondary erythrocytosis include hepatocellular neoplasia and a familial condition in cattle. Clinical signs of erythrocytosis are vague and include lethargy, weight loss, mucosal hyperemia, and signs of underlying disease.

25

Alterations in the Leukogram

(Text pp. 420-425)

Consulting Editor DEBRA DEEM MORRIS

PHYSIOLOGIC LEUKOCYTOSIS *(Text p. 422)*

Leukocytosis may be attributed to physiologic or pathologic causes, whereas leukopenia is always considered pathologic. Physiologic leukocytosis occurs with stress, excitation, anxiety, or exercise. The transiently elevated white blood cell (WBC) count is caused by both neutrophilia and lymphocytosis. Corticosteroids (exogenous or endogenous) cause neutrophilia and lymphopenia. Younger animals may have higher lymphocyte and total WBC counts than adults (Table 25-1).

NEUTROPHILS *(Text pp. 420-421, 422-423)*

Neutrophilia

Common causes of neutrophilia include the following:

- Physiologic (any species)–excitement, exercise, stress, exogenous corticosteroid administration
- Pathologic (any species)–chronic pneumonia, chronic peritonitis or abdominal abscess, other internal abscess, chronic salmonellosis
- Pathologic (horses)–chronic pleuritis, strangles (*Streptococcus equi* infection), thrombophlebitis, purpura hemorrhagica (vasculitis), chronic colitis
- Pathologic (ruminants)–chronic traumatic reticuloperitonitis, caseous lymphadenitis (sheep, goats), *Mycoplasma* or chlamydial polyarthritis (sheep, goats), chronic pyelonephritis, chronic metritis, liver abscess, enteritis, umbilical abscess, septic arthritis

Less common causes of neutrophilia in horses and ruminants are listed on pp. 422 and 423 of *Large Animal Internal Medicine,* third edition.

Neutrophil morphology

Evaluation of neutrophil morphology is important when interpreting a leukogram. Bacterial infections, especially those caused by gram-negative organisms, often result in toxic changes in neutrophils, including cytoplasmic foaminess, vacuolation, or basophilia; reddish-purple toxic granules; bluish cytoplasmic inclusions (Döhle bodies); and bizarre giant forms. These changes are a result of toxemia. The severity of toxemia is reflected by the number of "toxic" neutrophils and the degree of toxic changes.

Neutropenia

The usual cause of neutropenia is gram-negative septicemia or endotoxemia, especially when it is a result of gastrointestinal disease, pleuritis, metritis, or coliform mastitis. Viral diseases (e.g., equine influenza, equine herpesvirus 1),

TABLE 25-1
Normal Values for Leukogram Data (Adult Animals)

	Cattle	Sheep	Goats	Horses
White blood cells (× 10^3/μl)	4-12	4-12	4-13	5.4-14.3
Neutrophils (× 10^3/μl)	0.6-4	0.7-6	1.2-7.2	2.3-8.6
Bands (× 10^3/μl)	0-0.12	Rare	Rare	0-1
Lymphocytes (× 10^3/μl)	2.5-7.5	2-9	2-9	1.5-7.7
Monocytes (× 10^3/μl)	0.025-0.84	0-0.75	0-0.55	0-1
Eosinophils (× 10^3/μl)	0-2.4	0-1	0.05-0.65	0-1
Basophils (× 10^3/μl)	0-0.2	0-0.3	0-0.12	0-0.29
Neutrophil/lymphocyte (N/L) ratio	0.3-0.6	0.3-0.7	0.6-3.6	0.8-2.8

clostridial infections, fat cow syndrome, and toxemia- or toxin-induced bone marrow suppression are other common causes of neutropenia.

Degenerative left shift

A degenerative left shift occurs when immature neutrophils appear in the peripheral blood in greater numbers than mature neutrophils. In species other than the cow, degenerative left shift is an extremely poor prognostic sign. Neutropenia that persists for longer than 4 days is a sign of inadequate granulopoiesis, which sometimes occurs with severe toxemia, especially in cattle.

LYMPHOCYTES *(Text pp. 421-422, 423-424)*

Lymphocytosis

Pathologic lymphocytosis is uncommon. It occasionally occurs with chronic viral infections (e.g., equine infectious anemia, bovine leukosis virus [BLV]), chronic pyogenic conditions (e.g., pneumonia, liver abscess, traumatic reticuloperitonitis), and autoimmune diseases. Lymphocytic leukemia is rare in large animals, except in cattle infected with BLV (see Chapter 35).

Lymphopenia

Causes of pathologic lymphopenia include acute viral diseases (e.g., equine influenza, equine herpesvirus 1, infectious bovine rhinotracheitis), endotoxemia/septicemia, and severe bacterial infection (e.g., septic mastitis, acute pneumonia, severe peritonitis). Rickettsial diseases, malnutrition, tumors that induce corticosteroid release, and immunodeficiency may also cause lymphopenia. Persistent lymphopenia is a poor prognostic indicator.

MONOCYTES *(Text pp. 422, 424)*

Monocytosis occurs with chronic inflammation, such as granulomatous diseases and chronic bacterial infections. Stress, endotoxin release, and viremia may each cause monocytopenia.

EOSINOPHILS *(Text pp. 421, 424-425)*

Eosinophilia

Eosinophilia is uncommon in large animals but may occur with parasitic infections, allergic respiratory diseases, and dermatoses. Visceral larval migrans rarely induces peripheral eosinophilia.

Eosinopenia

Eosinopenia is difficult to evaluate because the leukograms of normal animals may contain very few eosinophils. Eosinopenia may occur secondary to increased endogenous or exogenous corticosteroids and with active inflammatory processes.

BASOPHILS *(Text pp. 421, 425)*

Basophils are rarely seen in the peripheral blood of large animal species. Stress causes a reduction in the number of basophils. Allergic dermatitis and delayed hypersensitivity reactions may be accompanied by basophilia.

26

Alterations in Blood Proteins

(Text pp. 427-433)

Consulting Editors DEBRA DEEM MORRIS • JANET K. JOHNSTON

HYPERPROTEINEMIA *(Text pp. 429-430)*

Panhyperproteinemia

Increased concentration of all blood proteins most commonly results from dehydration and is associated with an increase in packed cell volume (PCV) and a normal albumin/globulin (A/G) ratio. Total plasma protein concentrations can exceed 8 g/dl with severe dehydration.

Hyperglobulinemia

Hyperglobulinemia should be anticipated in a hyperproteinemic patient with apparently normal hydration; hyperalbuminemia occurs only with dehydration. Serum protein electrophoresis is necessary to quantitate the individual protein fractions (see main text).

Polyclonal gammopathy

The most common cause of hyperglobulinemia is a generalized increase in γ-globulins (polyclonal gammopathy), usually in response to chronic antigenic stimulation. Causes include chronic infection or abscess, chronic hepatitis, immune-mediated disorders (e.g., hemolytic anemia, thrombocytopenia, purpura hemorrhagica), amyloidosis, and neoplasia (e.g., lymphosarcoma). There usually is a concomitant decrease in albumin synthesis.

Monoclonal gammopathy

Abnormal increase of a single immunoglobulin class (monoclonal gammopathy) may be caused by multiple myeloma, lymphocytic leukemia, or other tumors of the reticuloendothelial system (e.g., lymphosarcoma). Internal parasitism, especially strongylosis, may cause a β-globulin spike, and α_2-globulins (acute-phase reactants) rapidly increase after tissue injury or inflammation. However, neither causes hyperglobulinemia in most cases.

HYPOPROTEINEMIA *(Text pp. 430-432)*

Hypoalbuminemia

Hypoalbuminemia often exists with a normal total plasma protein concentration, although a decreased A/G ratio is expected. Edema of the distal extremities, ventral body wall, and face is seen when albumin levels fall below 1.5 g/dl in horses and 1 g/dl in ruminants. Mechanisms of hypoalbuminemia include increased loss by the gut or kidney or decreased production (uncommon).

Horses

Common causes of hypoalbuminemia in horses include the following:

- Parasitism
- Renal loss–glomerulonephritis, pyelonephritis

- Gastrointestinal (GI) loss–idiopathic granulomatous enteritis, intestinal lymphosarcoma, salmonellosis, equine ehrlichial enterocolitis (Potomac horse fever), colitis X, clostridiosis, nonsteroidal antiinflammatory drug (NSAID) toxicity

Less common causes of hypoalbuminemia in horses are listed on p. 431 of *Large Animal Internal Medicine,* third edition.

Ruminants

Common causes of hypoalbuminemia in ruminants include the following:

- Protein malnutrition/starvation
- Renal loss–amyloidosis, pyelonephritis, glomerulonephritis
- GI loss–salmonellosis, Johne's disease, trichostrongyle infection

Less common causes of hypoalbuminemia in ruminants are listed on p. 431 of *Large Animal Internal Medicine,* third edition.

Panhypoproteinemia

Vigorous fluid therapy or excess water intake can cause overhydration and dilutional panhypoproteinemia. This occurs most often in animals with acute protein-losing colitis/enteritis that are receiving intravenous fluid therapy. Other causes of panhypoproteinemia include the following:

- Acute blood loss–trauma, severe epistaxis, internal vascular erosion or rupture
- GI blood or protein loss–abomasal or gastric ulceration, blood-sucking parasites (e.g., *Haemonchus* spp. in ruminants), NSAID toxicity, strangulating GI obstruction/infarction, protein-losing enteropathy (chronic granulomatous bowel disease)
- Renal blood or protein loss–vascular disorders, trauma, calculi, glomerulonephritis, pyelonephritis, neoplasia
- Coagulopathy–disseminated intravascular coagulation (DIC), immune-mediated thrombocytopenia
- Other–water intake in diarrheic animals with extensive sodium losses, severe peritonitis, congestive heart failure

Less common causes of panhypoproteinemia in horses and ruminants are listed on p. 431 of *Large Animal Internal Medicine,* third edition.

PLASMA FIBRINOGEN *(Text p. 432)*

Hyperfibrinogenemia

Hyperfibrinogenemia generally occurs with infectious, suppurative, traumatic, or neoplastic diseases. Fibrinogen normally increases in response to inflammation and then declines as the condition improves. However, the degree of hyperfibrinogenemia is not always directly correlated with disease severity. Fibrinogen is an especially useful indicator of inflammation in cattle because it is more sensitive than the leukocyte count.

Hypofibrinogenemia

Severe, diffuse liver damage (e.g., pyrrolizidine alkaloid toxicity) causes a decrease, whereas mild to moderate inflammatory liver disease can result in an increase in plasma fibrinogen. Hypofibrinogenemia is uncommon in horses with DIC. Hypofibrinogenemia may be diagnosed in error if fibrinogen is measured from samples containing clotted blood.

27

Alterations in the Clotting Profile

(Text pp. 434-439)

Consulting Editor DEBRA DEEM MORRIS

The minimum laboratory data needed to evaluate hemostasis in large animals are a platelet count, plasma fibrinogen, prothrombin time (PT), activated partial thromboplastin time (APTT), and serum fibrin/fibrinogen degradation products (FDPs). Specific clotting factor assays and other tests of hemostatic function are discussed in *Large Animal Internal Medicine,* third edition.

THROMBOCYTOPENIA *(Text pp. 434-435)*

Thrombocytopenia (platelet count less than 100,000/μl in horses and cattle; less than 250,000/μl in sheep and goats) is caused by one of three mechanisms:

- Decreased production of platelets–bone marrow infiltration with neoplastic tissue, aplastic anemia, myelofibrosis in pygmy goats
- Platelet sequestration–splenomegaly secondary to infection or venous occlusion
- Shortened platelet life span–disseminated intravascular coagulation (DIC), septicemia/endotoxemia, immune-mediated thrombocytopenia, equine infectious anemia, *Ehrlichia equi* infection, bracken fern toxicity (ruminants)

Excessive platelet consumption (shortened life span) is the most common cause of thrombocytopenia in large animals.

Clinical Manifestations

Thrombocytopenia is characterized by petechial hemorrhages on the mucous membranes, sclerae, and pinnae. Prolonged bleeding from injections or wounds and the propensity to form hematomas after minor trauma are common when the platelet count is less than 40,000/μl. Epistaxis, melena, hyphema, or hematuria may occur if the platelet count is less than 10,000/μl.

Diagnostic Approach

Other components of the hemostatic system should be evaluated because thrombocytopenia may be only part of a disseminated coagulopathy. Evaluation of a bone marrow specimen is necessary if thrombocytopenia is the only laboratory abnormality or if pancytopenia is present.

CLOTTING FACTOR ABNORMALITIES *(Text pp. 435-437)*

Clinical signs of clotting factor deficiencies relate to the tendency for spontaneous hemorrhage (e.g., epistaxis, melena, hematuria) or prolonged bleeding after trauma, diagnostic procedures, or surgery. Hematomas or hemarthrosis are common after minor trauma or even normal exercise.

Prolonged Prothrombin Time

The normal PT in horses is 7 to 9 seconds; in cattle, 22 to 55 seconds; and in goats, 9.5 to 12.5 seconds. PT becomes prolonged when fibrinogen is less than 100 mg/dl or when there is a marked deficiency of prothrombin or clotting factors V, VII, and X.

Causes

The most common mechanisms are (1) increased consumption of the relevant clotting factors, as occurs with DIC, and (2) failure of the liver to produce these factors. Reduced production occurs as a result of hepatocellular disease (e.g., pyrrolizidine alkaloid toxicity, aflatoxicosis, hepatic fibrosis) or vitamin K deficiency (e.g., moldy sweet clover hay, warfarin poisoning).

Prolonged Activated Partial Thromboplastin Time

The normal APTT in horses is 37 to 54 seconds; in cattle, 44 to 64 seconds; and in goats, 28 to 52 seconds.

Causes

The most common cause of prolonged APTT is increased consumption of clotting factors during DIC. Other possible causes are liver failure and vitamin K deficiency, as described for prolonged PT. Inherited deficiencies of factors VIII, IX, and XI and prekallikrein prolong APTT without affecting PT. When a persistently prolonged APTT is the only laboratory abnormality, hereditary clotting factor deficiency should be suspected.

ELEVATED FIBRIN/FIBRINOGEN DEGRADATION PRODUCTS *(Text p. 437)*

Measurable serum FDPs generally indicate increased fibrinolysis in response to excessive activation of coagulation (i.e., DIC). Serum FDPs may also be elevated by severe inflammation, immune-mediated thrombocytopenia, thrombophlebitis, and postoperative states that cause extensive intravascular fibrin deposition. Serum FDPs greater than 40 μg/ml most often indicate DIC; however, values less than 40 μg/ml do not exclude the diagnosis of DIC.

REDUCED PLASMA ANTITHROMBIN III *(Text pp. 437-438)*

Plasma antithrombin III (AT III) may be reduced by failure of production in the liver, excessive use (e.g., DIC), loss from the intravascular compartment (e.g., protein-losing enteropathy or nephropathy), or increased catabolism (e.g., sepsis). The major clinical sequela of AT III deficiency is a tendency to develop venous thrombosis.

PART V

Disorders of the Organ System

28

Diseases of the Cardiovascular System

(Text pp. 444-478)

Consulting Editors VIRGINIA B. REEF • SHEILA M. McGUIRK

ELECTROCARDIOGRAPHY *(Text pp. 443-445)*

The two lead systems commonly used for diagnosis of cardiac arrhythmias are the Y lead of the orthogonal lead system and the base-apex lead:

- Lead Y–attach the positive electrode over the xiphoid and the negative electrode at the front of the chest (cranially)
- Base-apex lead–attach the positive electrode to the left thorax (in the fifth intercostal space [level with the elbow] or where the apex beat is palpable), and attach the negative electrode to the skin over the right jugular furrow, one third of the way up the neck
    - ◦ With either system the ground electrode can be attached to any site remote from the heart.

The base-apex electrocardiogram (ECG) is recorded by setting the dial to one of the three standard bipolar leads (leads I, II, or III) and using the positive and negative electrodes for that lead:

- Lead I–"left arm" is the positive electrode and "right arm" is the negative electrode
- Lead II–"left leg" is positive and "right arm" is negative
- Lead III–"left leg" is positive and "left arm" is negative

The paper speed is set at 25 mm/sec, with the gain set at 1 cm/mV. Interpretation is discussed in *Large Animal Internal Medicine,* third edition.

OTHER DIAGNOSTIC TOOLS *(Text pp. 445-447)*

Other diagnostic tools and their indications include the following:

- Holter monitoring (continuous ECG recording) or radiotelemetry–intermittent or exercise-associated arrhythmias
- Echocardiography–murmurs, unexplained arrhythmias, exercise intolerance, muffled heart sounds, pericardial friction rubs or pericardial effusion, cardiovascular neoplasia, congestive heart failure (CHF), evidence of pulmonary hypertension
- Cardiac catheterization–evaluation of blood pressure waveforms, blood oxygen measurements, assessment of cardiac output and ventricular function, and angiocardiography

These modalities are described in *Large Animal Internal Medicine,* third edition.

CONGENITAL CARDIOVASCULAR DISEASE *(Text pp. 447-453)*

Congenital cardiovascular disease should be suspected in a young patient if examination reveals any of the following:

- Holosystolic or pansystolic, holodiastolic, or continuous murmur
- Murmur with a palpable thrill or wide radiation

A history of lethargy, weakness, and failure to thrive is common. If cyanosis is also present, a right-to-left cardiac shunt, obstructive pulmonary disease, or atresia/stenosis of the aorta or structures on the right side of the heart should be considered. Atrial and ventricular septal defects, patent ductus arteriosus, tetralogy or pentalogy of Fallot, and other less common cardiac defects are described in *Large Animal Internal Medicine,* third edition.

VALVULAR HEART DISEASE *(Text pp. 453-458)*

In adult animals, disorders of the heart valves are usually acquired and most commonly result in insufficiency of the affected valve. Causes include degenerative valvular changes, infection (bacterial or viral endocarditis or myocarditis), inflammation, rupture of a valve leaflet or chordae tendineae, dilation of a cardiac chamber from any cause, and rupture of the aortic root or sinus of Valsalva aneurysm. The most common bacteria isolated in cases of endocarditis are streptococci in horses and *Actinomyces pyogenes* in cattle. Bacterial endocarditis most commonly affects the tricuspid valve in cattle and the aortic valve in horses.

Clinical Findings

In most animals with valvular disease, the only abnormality is a cardiac murmur. In symptomatic animals, signs may include exercise intolerance, weight loss, and evidence of CHF, which includes tachycardia, cough, respiratory distress, jugular venous distention, subcutaneous edema, mammary vein distention in cattle, and atrial fibrillation (AF). Presenting signs vary:

- Tricuspid valve regurgitation–abnormal systolic jugular venous pulsations
- Mitral regurgitation–tachycardia, tachypnea, poor recovery after exercise, cough, and frothy fluid at the nares (pulmonary edema); lung sounds may be harsh
  - Most horses with mitral regurgitation have signs of chronic pulmonary hypertension (subtle respiratory signs, rather than acute pulmonary edema).
- Mitral valve chordae tendineae rupture–acute onset of respiratory distress with cough and expectoration of foamy fluid (pulmonary edema)
- Aortic valve lesions–"water-hammer" or bounding arterial pulse if there is significant left ventricular volume overload; ventricular premature beats and AF may also be found
- Bacterial endocarditis–tachycardia, arrhythmia, prominent heart sounds, tachypnea, cough, recurrent fever, anorexia, and weight loss
  - Evidence of disseminated sepsis (e.g., pneumonia, hematuria, pyuria) is usually present.
  - Mastitis and decreased milk production are common in cattle with bacterial endocarditis.

Auscultation

Mitral and tricuspid valve lesions primarily cause systolic murmurs. Aortic or pulmonic valve lesions typically cause a holodiastolic, decrescendo, musical murmur. The murmur is moderate to loud in intensity (greater than grade 3/6) and radiates from the point of maximum intensity (PMI) in the direction of abnormal blood flow:

- Mitral valve lesions–PMI is at left apex; usually radiates dorsally and toward the left heart base
  - Mitral valve prolapse causes a distinctive mid- to late-systolic crescendo murmur with the PMI over the mitral valve area.

  - The murmur of chordae tendineae rupture radiates widely and has a distinctive honking quality; it may be accompanied by acute onset of respiratory distress.
- Tricuspid valve lesions–PMI is on right side of chest
- Aortic or pulmonic valve lesions–PMI is at left heart base

The intensity of the murmur is not a reliable indicator of the severity of the lesion, except in horses with tricuspid regurgitation. Severely involved valves commonly have faint or no audible murmurs, especially in cattle with endocarditis.

Diagnosis

The diagnosis of valvular disease is best made with echocardiography (see main text).

Bacterial endocarditis

Laboratory findings include anemia, neutrophilia (possibly with a left shift), hyperglobulinemia, and hyperfibrinogenemia. Positive blood cultures taken during febrile episodes confirm the diagnosis when associated with echocardiographic abnormalities. However, culture results are negative in many cases. Radiographic or sonographic evidence of disseminated pneumonia may also be found in patients with right-sided lesions.

Treatment

Bacterial endocarditis

Bacterial endocarditis is treated with long-term intravenous use of bacteriocidal antimicrobials, based on blood culture and sensitivity results. Initial therapy is directed at the likelihood of a gram-positive infection. Addition of rifampin (5 mg/kg orally [PO] twice daily) can improve the short-term outlook. Aspirin (100 mg/kg/day in ruminants; 17 mg/kg every other day in horses) and low-dose heparin (30 units subcutaneously twice daily) may limit enlargement of the valvular mass.

Volume overload or CHF

Volume overload or CHF may be improved with diuretics (e.g., furosemide, 0.5 to 1 mg/kg as needed). Digoxin can be used to improve contractility with CHF:

- Intravenous dosage in horses–loading dose of 12 to 14 μg/kg, followed by a maintenance dose of either 6 to 7 μg/kg once daily or 2.2 μg/kg twice daily
- Oral dosage in horses–loading dose of 34 (elixir) to 70 (tablets) μg/kg; maintenance dose of either 17 (elixir) to 35 (tablets) μg/kg once daily or 11 μg/kg twice daily
- Cattle–loading dose of 22 μg/kg intravenously (IV), followed by a maintenance dose of 11 μg/kg IV three times daily or, preferably, intravenous infusion at a rate of 0.86 μg/kg/hr

Dehydration, acid-base imbalance, and electrolyte abnormalities should be corrected before digoxin therapy. Close monitoring of body weight, appetite, serum electrolytes, creatinine/BUN, and cardiac rhythm are essential during therapy.

Vasodilators

Horses with CHF may also benefit from vasodilator therapy. Options include hydralazine (0.5 to 1.5 mg/kg PO twice daily) and enalapril (0.5 mg/kg PO once or twice daily).

BRISKET DISEASE (COR PULMONALE) *(Text pp. 458-459)*

Cor pulmonale refers to the effect of lung dysfunction on the heart. Regardless of the cause, the underlying feature is pulmonary hypertension that leads to right-sided heart hypertrophy, dilation, and failure. The primary cause of brisket disease is hypoxic vasoconstriction from high-altitude dwelling. It is most common in calves kept at altitudes higher than 6000 feet. The disease is worsened by ingestion of locoweed (*Oxytropis* and *Astragalus* spp.). Chronic pulmonary disease, such as bronchopneumonia or lungworm infection, can also result in cor pulmonale.

Clinical Findings

The primary presenting sign often is edema of the brisket, ventral thorax, submandibular area, and occasionally limbs. Other signs can include jugular distention and/or pulsations, dyspnea and tachypnea, and tachycardia with a gallop rhythm. A cardiac murmur of tricuspid insufficiency or pulmonic valve ejection may be ausculted.

Treatment

Cor pulmonale from high altitude is potentially reversible if the animal is returned to a lower altitude. Treating any primary lung disease and administering oxygen may also help; however, once heart failure has developed, the prognosis is guarded even with appropriate treatment.

MYOCARDITIS AND CARDIOMYOPATHY *(Text pp. 460-463)*

Causes

Myocarditis is inflammation in the myocardium caused by bacterial, viral, or parasitic organisms or thromboembolic disease. Bacterial causes include *Staphylococcus aureus, Streptococcus equi, Clostridium chauvoei,* and *Mycobacterium* spp. Myocarditis can occur after bacteremia, septicemia, pericarditis, or endocarditis, regardless of the etiologic agent.

Cardiomyopathy

Cardiomyopathy is a subacute or chronic disease of the ventricular myocardium. It can result from ingestion of ionophores (monensin, lasalocid, salinomycin), gossypol, *Cassia occidentalis,* or *Phalaris* spp. Other causes include vitamin E/selenium deficiency, copper deficiency, excessive molybdenum, excessive sulfates (secondary copper deficiency), and neoplastic myocardial infiltration.

Clinical Findings

Myocarditis

Clinical manifestations are highly variable. Affected animals are often febrile or have a recent history of fever and may be tachycardic. Cardiac arrhythmias are common. Jugular distention, peripheral edema, and other signs of CHF may also be present. Horses may have myalgia, reluctance to move, or exercise intolerance.

Dilated cardiomyopathy

Most patients with dilated cardiomyopathy present with signs of heart failure. Auscultation often reveals tachycardia, gallop rhythm, muffled heart sounds, murmur of tricuspid or mitral valve insufficiency, or arrhythmia. Breath sounds are increased, tachypnea is present, and percussion of the thorax often indicates pleural or pericardial fluid. Respiratory distress is evident in some cases. Sudden death, particularly after stress or exercise, can be a feature of myocarditis or cardiomyopathy. Recumbency, collapse, and sudden death are common presenting signs in animals with ionophore toxicosis.

Diagnosis

Diagnostic tests include the following:

- Complete blood count (CBC)–neutrophilic leukocytosis may be present, but CBC may be normal
- Serum creatine kinase (CK) and lactic dehydrogenase (LDH)–may be elevated
  - Not specific for myocardial disease; elevation of cardiac troponin I or the myocardial isoenzymes LDH_1 and creatine kinase MB may be more useful
- ECG–may be evidence of conduction abnormalities in the base-apex lead

Echocardiography is useful in determining the severity of myocardial dysfunction. Samples of gastric and ruminal contents and feed should be submitted for analysis in cases of suspected ionophore toxicosis.

Treatment

Therapy for myocarditis includes treatment of the cause (if identified) and control of complications such as arrhythmias, CHF, and shock. Performance animals should be rested. Corticosteroids may be beneficial (see main text).

Digoxin

Patients with CHF may benefit from digoxin therapy, as described earlier for valvular heart disease. However, digoxin is contraindicated in patients with acute monensin toxicosis. Furosemide (0.5 to 1 mg/kg parenterally twice daily or as needed) and either hydralazine or enalapril (see p. 462) may also be useful in animals with CHF.

Quinidine

Control of arrhythmias should be attempted in animals that are hemodynamically unstable or threatened with worsening arrhythmias. Quinidine is the drug of choice for control of atrial and ventricular arrhythmias in cattle and one of the drugs of choice in horses. Quinidine is administered IV by infusion or divided bolus injections:

- Horses–1.5 to 2 mg/kg IV every 20 minutes until conversion; do not exceed a total of 6 mg/kg; alternately, administer 22 mg/kg PO every 2 hours until conversion; do not exceed a total dose of 132 mg/kg
- Cattle–48 mg/kg IV, infused over 4 hours

Concurrent administration of a balanced electrolyte solution at 3 to 4 ml/kg/hr is recommended in animals with compromised cardiovascular status.

Other antiarrhythmics

The following drugs may be used in place of quinidine in horses with ventricular arrhythmias:

- Procainamide–1 mg/kg/min IV, to a maximum of 20 mg/kg
- Lidocaine–0.1 to 0.25 mg/kg IV bolus; repeat up to a total of 0.5 mg/kg in 10 to 15 minutes
- Propafenone–2 mg/kg PO three times daily (if available in injectable form, 0.5 to 1 mg/kg in 5% dextrose, slowly IV over 5 to 8 minutes for refractory sustained ventricular tachycardia)

PERICARDITIS *(Text pp. 463-467)*

Pericarditis is inflammation of the pericardium. It results in accumulation of fluid and/or exudate in the pericardial sac. Causes include trauma (penetration of ingested foreign objects, external wounds), septicemia, extension of infection from the lungs or pleura, viral infections (e.g., equine viral arteritis, equine influenza), and neoplasia. Pericarditis is uncommon in horses. When it does occur, it is most often idiopathic (aseptic inflammatory exudate); a history of recent respiratory tract infection is common.

Clinical Findings

Fever, anorexia, depression, and weight loss may be the chief complaints. More commonly, peripheral edema, jugular distention and pulsations, tachypnea, and dyspnea are the presenting signs. Cattle may stand with the elbows abducted, have a spontaneous or induced expiratory grunt, be reluctant to move, and stand with the forequarters elevated. Horses may show signs of colic or syncopal episodes. Mucous membranes may be congested and the capillary refill time prolonged; arterial pulses are weak. Pleural effusion is common in horses with pericarditis.

Auscultation

The most consistent findings on auscultation are tachycardia, muffled heart sounds, and absence of lung sounds in the ventral thorax. In cattle, splashing sounds ("washing machine" murmur) are often heard and are attributable to accumulation of gas and fluid in the pericardium–an indication of anaerobic infection, which carries a grave prognosis. Splashing sounds are absent in horses; muffled heart sounds are the rule. However, pericardial friction rubs may be ausculted after pericardial effusion has been relieved.

Diagnosis

Changes on CBC are nonspecific and depend on the cause. Hypoalbuminemia and elevations in plasma fibrinogen and serum globulins are common. In cattle with traumatic pericarditis, fluid and gas accumulation in the pericardium and a metallic foreign body in the cranial reticulum or caudal thorax are detectable radiographically. Echocardiography is used to confirm the diagnosis (see main text).

Pericardiocentesis

Pericardial fluid is most reliably and safely obtained from the left fifth intercostal space, 2.5 to 10 cm dorsal to the olecranon and above the lateral thoracic vein. The procedure is best performed under ultrasonographic guidance. A pericardial catheter should be inserted into the pericardial space to enable repeated drainage and lavage. The following abnormalities are common in cattle with traumatic pericarditis:

- Malodorous, foamy, straw-colored or slightly blood-tinged fluid
- Elevated protein (greater than 3.5 g/dl) and white blood cell (WBC) count (greater 2500/μl, primarily neutrophils)
- Mixed population of gram-positive and gram-negative aerobic and anaerobic bacteria

In horses the protein concentration is elevated (greater than 2.5 g/dl) and the WBC count is normal or elevated (predominantly neutrophils), but aerobic and anaerobic bacterial cultures and virus isolation may be negative.

Treatment

Traumatic pericarditis in cattle

Treatment of traumatic pericarditis in cattle is unrewarding and usually is directed toward salvage or short-term survival for calving. Repeated pericardial drainage and lavage via pericardiocentesis or rib resection or pericardiectomy may be useful.

Pericarditis in horses

Moderate- to large-volume pericardial effusion should be treated aggressively with drainage and lavage of the pericardial sac and local infusion of antibiotics once or twice daily as needed (see main text). All horses with pericarditis should initially be treated with systemic broad-spectrum bacteriocidal antimicrobials. Nonsteroidal antiinflammatory drugs are useful as adjunctive therapy, as are corticosteroids (provided bacterial culture is negative and there is no cytologic evidence of sepsis).

CARDIAC TUMORS *(Text pp. 467-468)*

Cardiac neoplasia is rare in large animals. The most common primary cardiac tumor is lymphosarcoma, especially in cattle with bovine leukosis. Other tumors (e.g., squamous cell carcinomas in horses) may involve structures adjacent to the heart and extend to the heart or heart base. Nonspecific signs include anorexia, depression, weight loss, and fever. If the tumor involves the pericardium, signs of pericarditis may be seen. Myocardial involvement may result in tachycardia, arrhythmias, and murmurs (atrioventricular valve insufficiency) or signs of CHF. Ultrasonography may reveal the mass and guide biopsy for definitive diagnosis.

VASCULAR DISEASE *(Text pp. 468-471)*

Aneurysms are vascular dilations that develop from weakening of the blood vessel wall. Trauma, sepsis, parasite migration, degenerative vascular disease, atherosclerosis, and aging changes may play a role. In cattle, arteriosclerosis is often caused by excessive vitamin D_3 supplementation or ingestion of calcinogenic plants (*Solanum, Cestrum,* and *Trisetum* spp.).

Thrombosis is the formation of a clot that obstructs blood flow. Causes include trauma, venous stasis, catheterization, and hypercoagulable states. Secondary thrombosis can result from cellulitis, lymphangitis, or other sources of bacterial invasion around a vessel. Emboli are particles of other material carried in the bloodstream. They most commonly occur with bacterial endocarditis, thrombophlebitis, and parasitic arteritis.

Clinical Findings

Aneurysms

Aneurysms may be asymptomatic, but signs attributed to low blood flow (e.g., lameness, colic, edema) may be present with arterial aneurysms. Depending on the vessel, rupture may cause colic, syncope, seizures, or sudden death. With aneurysms of major cardiac vessels, there may be pain, an auscultable heart murmur, tachycardia, signs of CHF, acute onset of pulmonary edema, or sudden death when the aneurysm ruptures.

Thrombophlebitis

Thrombophlebitis is manifested by pain, swelling, redness, and thickening of the involved vein. With bilateral jugular venous thrombosis, marked swelling of the head may occur.

Aortoiliac thrombosis

In horses, thrombosis of the terminal aorta and iliac arteries often causes a vague hindlimb lameness, exercise intolerance, or poor performance. Typically, there is heavy sweating after exercise, except over the hindlimbs, which are cool. Saphenous vein filling is slow or absent, and the metatarsal and other peripheral arterial pulses of the hindlimbs are weak. Rectal examination may be normal, but abnormal findings can include weak, absent, or asymmetric iliac pulses; fremitus in the iliac arteries or terminal aorta; and thickening or aneurysmal dilation of the aorta.

Thrombosis of the cranial mesenteric artery

With verminous arteritis of the cranial mesenteric artery, a thickened, dilated cranial mesenteric artery or aorta may be palpated per rectum. The artery may be firmer than normal and have a weak pulse, with or without fremitus.

Embolism

Embolism usually is manifested by an acute episode of pain or fever and abnormal pulsation or a change in skin temperature if a peripheral artery is involved. If there is peripheral showering, superficial veins may be collapsed and muscle weakness may be present.

Diagnosis

Ultrasonography can be used to identify aneurysms or thrombosis of major arteries and peripheral vessels. In the case of catheter-associated thrombosis, positive catheter-tip culture along with positive blood culture provides evidence of septic thrombophlebitis. Ultrasound-guided aseptic aspiration of a cavitary lesion within a heterogeneous thrombus can also be performed and submitted for culture and sensitivity.

Treatment

Aneurysms

Aneurysms of major vessels carry a guarded to grave prognosis because spontaneous rupture is relatively common and there is no treatment. Once an aneurysm of a major vessel or the sinus of Valsalva is detected, the horse should be removed from athletic activities.

Catheter-induced thrombosis

The catheter should be removed if still present. Warm compresses or hydrotherapy may be helpful. Anticoagulant therapy (aspirin 100 mg/kg PO sid or heparin 30 U/kg subcutaneously twice daily) may be useful in preventing additional thrombus formation or propagation of the existing thrombus. Broad-spectrum bacteriocidal antimicrobial therapy should be instituted for suspected septic thrombophlebitis or when a cavitated thrombus is detected ultrasonographically.

ATRIAL FIBRILLATION *(Text pp. 471-474)*

AF is an arrhythmia characterized by lack of coordinated atrial electrical activity. Causes include the following:

- Atrial enlargement from myocardial disease, atrioventricular valvular regurgitation, or ventricular failure
- Myocarditis
- Autonomic nervous system imbalance (e.g., high resting vagal tone)
- Electrolyte or acid-base disturbances (metabolic alkalosis, hypocalcemia, hypokalemia, hypochloremia) such as in cattle with GI abnormalities
- Administration of anesthetic drugs, tranquilizers, or bicarbonate "milk-shakes"

Functional or benign AF can also occur from unknown causes. AF and the accompanying signs can be paroxysmal, with spontaneous conversion to sinus rhythm. Transient potassium depletion associated with furosemide administration is a common cause in horses.

Clinical Findings

Animals with AF may be asymptomatic at rest, but horses with AF usually have a history of exercise intolerance or poor performance. Other complaints may include exercise-induced epistaxis, respiratory disease, weakness, syncope, myopathy, colic, and signs of CHF. Cattle with AF usually have gastrointestinal disease (most common), foot rot, or pneumonia. Anorexia and decreased milk production are common in cattle with AF.

Auscultation

Animals with AF have an irregular cardiac rhythm with no underlying regularity and no audible fourth heart sound. The heart rate may be slow, normal, or fast. In horses the resting heart rate is rarely more than 50 beats/min unless there is underlying cardiac disease. In cattle with abdominal disease, the heart rate usually reflects the severity of the underlying disease. The arterial pulse varies in intensity, and a pulse deficit may be detected.

Diagnosis

Diagnosis is made by ECG: the RR interval is irregular and P waves are absent, replaced by fine undulations of the baseline (fibrillation or f waves). In some leads the f waves are barely visible, particularly in cattle. Echocardiography is used to determine whether cardiac disease is present. Most horses with AF have normal serum electrolytes, although the urinary fractional excretion of potassium may be low, particularly in horses that sweat excessively or routinely receive furosemide.

Treatment

Cattle with primary gastrointestinal disease often spontaneously convert to normal sinus rhythm within 5 days of resolution of the primary problem. Spontaneous conversion in horses usually occurs only in patients with small atria. Quinidine is the antiarrhythmic drug of choice for horses and cattle with AF. Pretreatment with digoxin is recommended in patients with CHF (see following discussion). In every case of AF, electrolyte and acid-base balance should be normalized before treatment. The animal should be adequately hydrated, allowed to eat and drink, or given additional oral (horses) or intravenous (cattle) fluids during therapy.

Horses

Intravenous quinidine gluconate is recommended for horses with AF of 1 month or less in duration (boluses of 0.25 to 0.5 mg/kg IV every 5 to 10 minutes to effect or up to a total of 10 mg/kg). Horses with AF of longer duration should be treated with oral quinidine sulfate:

- Record a baseline ECG before treatment.
- Give 22 mg/kg (1 g/100 lb) quinidine sulfate in water via nasogastric tube.

- After 2 hours, evaluate for adverse reactions (nasal edema, cutaneous reactions, laminitis, colic, diarrhea, ataxia); if none are found, record another ECG.
- If conversion to sinus rhythm has not occurred and the QRS duration is not more than 25% of the pretreatment value, give another dose of quinidine.
- Repeat the preceding steps every 2 hours until conversion or until a maximum of six doses have been administered.
- If at any time the QRS duration is more than 25% of pretreatment, or if a fast supraventricular arrhythmia (more than 100 beats/min) or signs of toxicity develop, discontinue every-2-hour therapy.
  - If signs do not resolve within 4 hours, discontinue quinidine therapy altogether.

If conversion has not occurred after four to six doses (88 to 132 mg/kg total), the treatment interval should be extended to every 6 hours until conversion has occurred or adverse effects are seen. Addition of digoxin (see following discussion) can be helpful if conversion has not occurred in 24 to 48 hours.

Aftercare. Continuous 24-hour ECG monitoring is recommended after conversion to check for atrial premature depolarizations. If frequent supraventricular premature extrasystoles are detected, the horse should be rested and treatment with corticosteroids considered. Exercise should not resume until the atrial premature depolarizations have resolved.

Recurrence. Recurrence of AF and side effects of quinidine therapy are more likely in horses that have had AF for more than 4 months. The recurrence rate in such cases is 60% (compared with 25% in cases of shorter duration).

Cattle

Quinidine is poorly absorbed orally in cattle, so it must be given by intravenous infusion:

- Give quinidine sulfate at 48 mg/kg in 4 L saline or lactated Ringer's solution IV at 1 L/hr.
- Administer intravenous fluids simultaneously in the opposite jugular vein.
- Monitor the patient continuously during infusion.
- Discontinue therapy after the 4-L infusion, even if conversion has not occurred.

Cattle often become depressed and develop diarrhea during quinidine infusion, but therapy can be continued. The infusion rate should be slowed if the ventricular response rate exceeds 100 beats/min. If the QRS complex is visibly prolonged or a fast (more than 120 beats/min) supraventricular arrhythmia or ventricular rhythm develops, therapy should be temporarily discontinued. Just before conversion, blepharospasm and ataxia are seen in some cattle.

Digoxin

Digoxin should be administered before initiation of quinidine therapy in patients with fast heart rates (more than 60 beats/min in horses and more than 100 beats/min in cattle). The recommended dosages and routes are given on p. 144. Only one or two doses may be needed for patients with mild tachycardia. In patients with labile heart rates or that developed supraventricular tachycardia during a previous conversion attempt, pretreatment may need to continue for up to 7 days.

VENTRICULAR TACHYCARDIA *(Text pp. 474-477)*

Ventricular tachycardia (VT) is an arrhythmia characterized by a rapid rhythm originating in the ventricle. Causes include myocarditis, myocardial necrosis or fibrosis, bacterial endocarditis (especially involving the aortic or mitral valve), autonomic nervous system imbalance (e.g., sympathetic stimulation associated with exercise), hypoxia, ischemia, electrolyte or metabolic disturbances (e.g., hypomagnesemia, hypokalemia), anesthesia, drug administration, sepsis, endotoxemia, toxic myocardial injury (e.g., monensin), or aortic root rupture. In some cases the cause is unknown. VT can be sustained or paroxysmal.

Clinical Findings

Animals with VT may be asymptomatic at rest if the rhythm is relatively slow and uniform. Patients with rapid uniform or multiform VT may present with signs of CHF. Exercise intolerance is common and may be so severe that the animal has frequent syncopal episodes. Other complaints include depression, weakness, colic, respiratory distress, cough, ventral edema, and pulmonary edema. Anorexia and decreased milk production are common in affected cows.

Cardiovascular examination

Animals with sustained VT have a rapid heart rate with either a regular (uniform) or irregular (multiform) rhythm. Heart sounds vary in intensity, with some very loud, booming sounds. Arterial pulses may be variable or uniform, with the pulse intensity being normal (slower rate) or weak (rapid rate). Pulse deficits frequently occur, and jugular pulsation is common. Signs of CHF are usually present when VT is rapid and sustained.

Diagnosis

ECG is necessary for diagnosis:

- A series of four or more ventricular premature depolarizations is diagnostic.
- The QRS complexes may be wide and bizarre, but the duration and appearance of QRS and T waves may be near normal, especially in horses.
- The morphology of the QRS complexes may be similar (uniform) or vary widely (multiform)
- The RR intervals may be regular or irregular; atrioventricular dissociation is usually present, with a slower atrial than ventricular rate; fusion beats and capture beats may be detected.

Echocardiography is used to determine whether cardiac disease is present. Marked elevations in cardiac troponin I indicate myocardial injury.

Treatment

Relatively slow, uniform VT often resolves or significantly improves just with correction of underlying electrolyte/metabolic imbalances or disease (e.g., sepsis, toxemia). Uniform VT in hemodynamically stable animals with myocarditis may resolve with rest and/or corticosteroid therapy (e.g., dexamethasone, 0.05 to 0.22 mg/kg IV or intramuscularly). A further 4 to 8 weeks of rest is indicated once VT has resolved.

Antiarrhythmic therapy

Treatment with antiarrhythmics is indicated in any animal with hemodynamically unstable or life-threatening VT: clinical signs of CHF, sustained heart rates greater than 120 beats/min in horses and greater than 140 beats/min in cattle, or multiform QRS complexes with R waves superimposed on T waves (R-on-T). These abnormalities should be treated as a cardiovascular emergency; sudden death from ventricular fibrillation is likely without antiarrhythmic therapy.

Antiarrhythmic drugs used in large animals include the following:

- Lidocaine–acts rapidly with minimal hemodynamic effects but has a short duration of action and can cause excitability and seizures in horses
  - Horses: 0.1 to 0.25 mg/kg IV bolus; repeat up to a total of 0.5 mg/kg in 10 to 15 minutes
  - Cattle: 0.5 mg/kg slowly IV; can repeat in 15 minutes
- Quinidine gluconate–very effective but slower-acting than lidocaine, has negative inotropic effects (hypotension), and can produce adverse reactions (see p. 150)
  - Give boluses of 0.25 to 0.5 mg/kg IV every 5 to 10 minutes to effect or to a total of 10 mg/kg
- Magnesium sulfate–slower-acting than lidocaine but has no adverse cardiovascular effects
  - Give 1 g/min as intravenous infusion, to effect, up to a maximum of 25 g
- Procainamide–1 mg/kg/min IV to a maximum of 20 mg/kg

- Propranolol–0.03 mg/kg IV
- Bretylium tosylate–0.5 mg/kg IV (for life-threatening VT or ventricular fibrillation)
- Propafenone–2 mg/kg PO three times daily

Many times, three or more antiarrhythmic drugs must be tried before conversion is achieved.

29

Diseases of the Respiratory System

Consulting Editors PAMELA A. WILKINS • JOHN C. BAKER • TREVOR R. AMES

Contributors ANGELINE E. WARNER • MARY ROSE PARADIS
CORINNE R. SWEENEY • FABIO DEL PIERO • BRETT DOLENTE
JANE E. AXON • PEGGY MARSH • JILL BEECH
CLIFFORD M. HONNAS • JOHN R. PASCOE • JOHN A. SMITH
NANCY E. EAST • STEVEN E. WIKSE • DAN GROOMS
ANNE M. ZAJAC • JEANNE LOFSTEDT • H. MICHAEL CHADDOCK

MANIFESTATIONS OF RESPIRATORY DISEASE
(Text pp. 479-482)

Upper Respiratory Tract

Signs of disease involving the upper respiratory tract (nares, nasal passages, paranasal sinuses, nasopharynx, larynx, and trachea) variably include the following:

- Nasal discharge (unilateral for lesions of the nares, nasal passages, and paranasal sinuses)
  - Depending on the lesion, the discharge may be mucoid, mucopurulent, purulent, or sanguineous (or frankly hemorrhagic) and may contain feed material.
  - With necrotic lesions the discharge may be malodorous.
- Tachypnea with or without dyspnea
  - Severely dyspneic animals stand with the head and neck extended and the nostrils flared and may be obviously distressed; abduction of the elbows may also be seen.
  - Open-mouth breathing is common in severely dyspneic ruminants.
- Stertorous respiration or stridor (mostly inspiratory)
- Unequal air flow from the nostrils (for unilateral lesions of the nares or nasal passages)
- Fetid breath (only with necrotic lesions)
- Cough (for lesions involving the pharynx, larynx, or trachea)
- Sneezing (most common with lesions involving the nasal passages in ruminants)
- Enlarged submandibular or retropharyngeal lymph nodes (infectious conditions)

Lower Respiratory Tract

Signs of disease involving the lungs or pleural cavity variably include the following:

- Tachypnea/hyperpnea with or without dyspnea
- Fever (infectious etiology or with severe dyspnea)
- Cough
- Nasal discharge (usually more scant than for upper airway conditions; often bilateral)

- Lethargy or depression
- Reluctance to move, evidence of thoracic pain
- Inappetence, weight loss (with or without changes in appetite)
- Exercise intolerance
- Cyanosis (if gas exchange is seriously impaired)

EVALUATION OF THE RESPIRATORY SYSTEM *(Text pp. 482-490)*

Evaluation of the respiratory system is discussed in Chapter 29 in *Large Animal Internal Medicine,* third edition. Diagnostic procedures include radiography, ultrasonography, endoscopy, tracheobronchial aspiration, bronchoalveolar lavage (BAL), intradermal skin testing, thoracocentesis, sinus trephination, guttural pouch catheterization, lung biopsy, pulmonary function testing, arterial blood gas analysis, and nuclear imaging.

Tracheobronchial Aspirate

Because of its utility for evaluating lower respiratory disorders, tracheobronchial aspiration is briefly described here:

- Sedate or otherwise restrain the patient as needed; the procedure is performed with the animal standing.
- Clip and aseptically prepare the skin over the trachea in the mid third of the neck.
- Desensitize the skin with local anesthetic and make a small vertical stab incision in the skin along the midline.
- Using the sterile technique, insert a trocar or angiocatheter needle into the trachea (between the tracheal rings), directing the needle caudally.
- Advance a 30-cm length of sterile polyethylene tubing with syringe adapter through the needle; once the tubing is in place, carefully withdraw the needle from the skin to avoid severing the tubing within the airway. If an angiocath is used, it can remain in place.
- Infuse 30 ml of sterile nonbacteriostatic saline solution into the tubing, then aspirate the fluid while gradually withdrawing the tubing; if necessary, infuse additional saline to obtain an adequate sample.
- Remove the tubing and apply a sterile dressing to the skin for 24 hours.
- Submit the sample for culture and cytologic examination.

Part I: Equine Respiratory System

BACTERIAL PNEUMONIA IN ADULT HORSES *(Text pp. 491-496)*

Pneumonia in adult horses is most often caused by *Streptococcus zooepidemicus.* Gram-negative organisms, especially *Pasteurella* spp. and, less often, *Escherichia coli, Enterobacter* spp., *Klebsiella* spp., and *Pseudomonas* spp., can complicate streptococcal pneumonia. Anaerobes, especially *Bacteroides* spp. and *Clostridium* spp., commonly complicate aerobic infections and should be considered significant when cultured.

Clinical Findings

Signs of bacterial pneumonia are indicative of lower respiratory tract disease (see p. 153). Fever may be intermittent; cough, which may or may not be spontaneous, may be productive. On auscultation, early changes include increased harshness and intensity of expiratory sounds. With more advanced pneumonia, end-inspiratory crackles and sometimes expiratory wheezes are heard. Extension of inflammation to the pleura causes rubbing sounds. The ventral thorax may be quiet, suggesting pulmonary abscess or pleural effusion.

Diagnosis

An elevated peripheral white blood cell (WBC) count with an absolute neutrophilia (with or without band forms) is often found. Hyperfibrinogenemia (500 to 1000 mg/dl) and hyperglobulinemia are common, especially with chronic pneumonia or pulmonary abscess. Thoracic radiographs are valuable for diagnosis, prognosis, and monitoring. The most common finding is opacity in the cranioventral thorax. Multiple opacities suggesting abscess are seen in some cases. The pleural space is best evaluated ultrasonographically.

Fluid analysis

When bacterial pneumonia is suspected, a tracheobronchial aspirate should be collected for aerobic and anaerobic culture, Gram stain, and cytologic examination. Antimicrobial agents should be withheld for at least 24 hours before sample collection. If pleural effusion is detected, the pleural space should also be aspirated (see p. 492), although transtracheal aspiration is often more rewarding in identifying the causal organisms.

Treatment

Therapy should be based on culture and sensitivity results from a tracheobronchial aspirate. In early cases it is reasonable to suspect *S. zooepidemicus* and treat accordingly. Appropriate choices include K- or Na-penicillin (22,000 U/kg intravenously [IV] four times daily) and procaine penicillin (22,000 U/kg intramuscularly [IM] two times daily). If mixed infections are suspected, either ampicillin (11 mg/kg IM or IV four times daily) or trimethoprim-sulfadiazine (or sulfamethoxazole) (30 mg/kg IV or orally [PO] two times daily) is a good empiric choice.

Complicated infections

Complicated infections with multiple or resistant organisms necessitate the use of antimicrobial agents specifically directed against the pathogens isolated. Appropriate choices might include the following:

- *E. coli*–ceftizoxime, amikacin, or gentamicin
- *Enterobacter* spp., *Klebsiella pneumoniae*–amikacin or ceftizoxime
- *Pseudomonas aeruginosa*–amikacin
- Most gram-negative aerobes–fluoroquinolones
- Anaerobes–metronidazole or rifampin, with appropriate therapy against aerobic isolates

Duration of therapy

Antimicrobial therapy should be continued for at least 7 days or until clinical signs resolve. If febrile episodes continue despite appropriate therapy, pleural infection or pulmonary abscess should be suspected. In every case of pneumonia, stall rest must be enforced during therapy and return to exercise should be gradual. Management of pleuropneumonia is discussed later in this chapter.

Prognosis

With an adequate duration of antibiotic therapy and rest, the prognosis in uncomplicated cases is excellent.

PNEUMONIA IN FOALS *(Text pp. 496-498)*

Pneumonia is a significant cause of morbidity and mortality in both neonatal and older foals. Bacterial pneumonia in neonatal foals is discussed in Chapters 19 and 20. Following is a discussion of pneumonia in foals between 1 and 6 months of age.

Undifferentiated Respiratory Disease

Foals 4 to 5 months of age are highly susceptible to respiratory disease. The most prominent bacterial isolate is *S. zooepidemicus.* Other gram-positive isolates include *Rhodococcus equi* (see following discussion) and *Staphylococcus epidermis.* Gram-negative organisms are found less often.

Clinical findings

Clinical findings include tachypnea, mucopurulent nasal discharge, cough, and crackles and wheezes on thoracic auscultation. High fever is not a prominent sign.

Diagnosis

The complete blood count (CBC) generally is within normal limits, although mild neutrophilia may be present. A mild to moderate bronchointerstitial pattern (without consolidation) may be seen on thoracic radiographs. Bronchial lavage fluid contains a high number of neutrophils. Gram-positive cocci with a prominent capsule can usually be seen on Gram-stained smears.

Treatment and prognosis

Appropriate antibiotic choices for initial therapy include β-lactams, such as penicillin (22,000 IU/kg IM two times daily) or ampicillin (10 to 20 mg/kg IM two times daily), and trimethoprim-sulfamethoxazole (20 to 30 mg/kg PO two times daily). A combination of both drug classes may provide better coverage than either class alone. Relapse occurs in 30% of cases, usually 1 to 5 weeks after treatment has ended. The long-term prognosis for athletic function is difficult to assess; horses that experience this type of pneumonia as foals may not perform as well as horses that do not.

R. equi Pneumonia

R. equi pneumonia is most common in foals around 2 months of age, although it can occur as early as 1 month or as late as 6 months of age. The disease is sporadic except on endemic farms.

Clinical findings

Common findings include fever (38.5° to 41° C [101.5° to 106° F]), mucopurulent nasal discharge, tachypnea, and wheezes and crackles over both lung fields on auscultation. Signs usually appear acutely, and the foal may be in respiratory distress. *R. equi* infection can also cause diarrhea, peritonitis, subcutaneous abscess, joint effusion ('reactive arthritis'), and osteomyelitis with abscess or septic arthritis.

Diagnosis

Diagnosis of *R. equi* pneumonia is based on clinical signs, radiographic evidence of pulmonary abscess, and identification (via cytologic examination or culture) of the organism in a transtracheal aspirate. *R. equi* are seen as gram-positive pleomorphic rods. Affected foals usually have leukocytosis (neutrophilia) and hyperfibrinogenemia. Serologic tests are available but are probably more useful for herd monitoring than for diagnosis. A polymerase chain reaction (PCR) test has recently been developed.

Treatment and prognosis

The antibiotic combination of choice is erythromycin estolate (25 mg/kg PO four times daily) and rifampin (10 mg/kg PO two times daily). Treatment should continue until there is no longer radiographic evidence of pneumonia, typically 6 to 8 weeks. Potential side effects of erythromycin therapy include mild diarrhea in the foal, clostridial colitis in the dam, and hyperthermia in the foal. The long-term prognosis for athletic function is guarded.

Control

Removal of manure and elimination of dusty areas are indicated to decrease the spread of the organism. Hyperimmune plasma can reduce the incidence of this disease on endemic farms when administered to foals in the first few weeks of life.

Pneumocystis carinii Infection

Pneumocystis carinii (PC) is a unicellular eukaryotic fungus. It was first recovered from Arabian foals with combined immunodeficiency syndrome but has since been recovered from other foals with no specific history of immunodeficiency. Concurrent infection with *R. equi*, enterobacteria, or *S. zooepidemicus* is common in non-Arabian foals with PC pneumonia.

Clinical outcome

Clinical presentation varies from a 3-week history of weakness, weight loss, and nasal discharge to acute respiratory distress. A severe interstitial and alveolar pattern (sometimes miliary) is seen on thoracic radiographs. The majority of reported foals died, and the diagnosis was made at necropsy. Two surviving foals responded to trimethoprim-sulfamethoxazole therapy.

Bronchointerstitial Pneumonia (Acute Respiratory Distress Syndrome)

There is a subset of foals between 1 and 7 months of age with severe respiratory distress that share some of the clinical characteristics of foals with *R. equi* or PC pneumonia but for which a consistent causative agent cannot be found. Proposed causes include endotoxemia, an inhaled or ingested toxin, viral infection (e.g., equine herpesvirus type 2 [EHV-2]), and heat shock (high ambient temperature).

Clinical findings and diagnosis

Affected foals are either found dead or present with acute onset of respiratory distress. Some foals appear normal beforehand; others are being treated for a respiratory problem. Findings include tachypnea, dyspnea, cyanosis, and hypoxemia with hypercapnia. A severe, diffuse interstitial to bronchointerstitial pulmonary pattern typically is found on thoracic radiographs.

Treatment and prognosis

Affected foals do not respond well to antibiotic treatment. Use of oxygen insufflation, bronchodilators, antiinflammatory drugs, corticosteroids, and environmental control (e.g., air-conditioned stall, alcohol bath to lower body temperature) can improve the recovery rate. The prognosis is guarded for both life and future athletic ability.

FUNGAL PNEUMONIA *(Text pp. 499-500)*

Pathogenic fungi such as *Coccidioides immitis, Histoplasma capsulatum,* and *Cryptococcus neoformans* can infect immunologically normal horses. *Aspergillus, Phycomycetes, Mucor, Rhizopus,* and *Candida* spp. tend to infect immunocompromised patients, such as those with enterocolitis, peritonitis, nephritis, endotoxemia, or septicemia. Most horses with secondary fungal pneumonia have been on antimicrobial therapy for the primary problem; many show no respiratory signs.

Diagnosis

Fungal hyphae are often present either free or in large mononuclear cells in tracheal aspirates from healthy horses. To be significant, large numbers of fungi should be accompanied by evidence of pulmonary inflammation. Percutaneous lung biopsy can confirm the diagnosis.

Aspergillosis

Clinical signs suggestive of pulmonary aspergillosis include coughing and hemoptysis. In suspect cases, careful examination of the nose and paranasal sinuses may be rewarding. Biopsy of a nasal erosion or ulcer that reveals these fungal organisms is highly predictive of concomitant or future pulmonary aspergillosis. Thoracic radiographs may reveal any infiltrative pattern, but the most common initial finding is patchy bronchopneumonia with a peripheral distribution.

Treatment

Treatment of fungal pneumonia is usually frustrating because most cases occur secondary to a severe primary disease. The drug of choice depends on the fungus involved. Specific antifungal agents include amphotericin B, ketoconazole, miconazole, 5-fluorocytosine, and iodides.

PLEUROPNEUMONIA *(Text pp. 500-504)*

Bacterial pleuropneumonia (pleuritis) is a common and often severe disorder in horses. It often is associated with a stressful event, such as long-distance transport or recent viral disease. Most affected horses have mixed infections with both aerobic and anaerobic bacteria. Common pathogens are the same as those listed for bacterial pneumonia (see p. 491).

Clinical Findings

Clinical signs include fever, anorexia, depression, cough, respiratory distress, stiff gait, weight loss, sternal or limb edema, and colic. In the acute stage, thoracic pain may be elicited by palpation over the thoracic wall. The horse may abduct its elbows and have a 'catch' to inspiration. Auscultation reveals normal lung sounds in the dorsal lung field but no sounds or only bronchial or tracheal sounds ventrally. Pleural friction rubs are present only in the acute stage; they disappear as pleural fluid accumulates. Thoracic percussion frequently confirms the presence of pleural effusion (dullness over the ventral lung field).

Diagnostic Procedures

Ultrasonography

Thoracic ultrasonography is the preferred method of diagnosis. It also allows characterization of the pleural fluid and identification of adhesions, pleural thickening, and pulmonary disease (e.g., abscess, consolidation, necrosis, atelectasis). Free gas echoes (often associated with anaerobic infection), severe fibrinous pleuritis, or loculation suggest a guarded prognosis.

Tracheobronchial aspirate

Airway specimens should be submitted for cytologic examination and culture (aerobic and anaerobic). Transtracheal aspiration (see p. 501) is preferred over transendoscopic sample collection.

Thoracocentesis

Thoracocentesis should be performed to collect pleural fluid for Gram stain, cytologic examination, and culture (aerobic and anaerobic). It should also be performed when pleural fluid accumulates rapidly, the horse is in respiratory distress, or the horse's condition deteriorates. The preferred site is the sixth or seventh intercostal space, just dorsal to the costochondral junction. Ultrasonography aids site selection. Both sides of the thorax should be tapped.

Fluid analysis. Normal pleural fluid is clear and yellow; cloudiness reflects an increased WBC count. Putrid-smelling pleural fluid is a hallmark of anaerobic infection; however, absence of odor does not exclude anaerobic infection. Pleural fluid abnormalities commonly found include the following:

- Elevated WBC count
  - Normal pleural fluid generally contains less than 10,000 cells/μl.
  - With pleuropneumonia the pleural WBC count can range from 1600 to 300,000 cells/μl.
- Elevated protein concentration (greater than 3 g/dl)

Treatment

Antimicrobial therapy

Systemic antimicrobial drugs, ideally based on culture and sensitivity results, are an essential part of treatment. Without culture results, broad-spectrum antibiotics such as a penicillin-aminoglycoside combination, trimethoprim-sulfamethoxazole, or chloramphenicol should be used. Therapy should begin with intravenous or intramuscular antimicrobials; preferably, oral antimicrobials are not administered until the horse's condition is stable and improving.

Anaerobic infections

Anaerobes are found in up to 50% of cases. Treatment of anaerobic infections is usually empiric. Options include penicillin, chloramphenicol, and metronidazole (15 mg/kg IV or PO four times daily). Metronidazole should always be given in combination with antibiotics effective against aerobes.

Pleural drainage

Drainage of pleural fluid is indicated if the fluid is thick pus or if the Gram stain is positive for bacteria and the WBC counts are elevated. Options include intermittent drainage, indwelling chest tube, pleural lavage (see following discussion), pleuroscopy and debridement, and open-chest drainage/debridement (standing or under general anesthesia). Indwelling chest tubes are indicated when continued pleural fluid accumulation makes intermittent drainage impractical. Bilateral pleural fluid accumulation requires bilateral drainage in most horses.

Pleural lavage

Pleural lavage helps dilute the fluid and remove fibrin, debris, and necrotic tissue. It is most effective in the subacute stage, before loculation develops. Warmed lactated Ringer's solution (10 L) is infused by gravity flow through a dorsally positioned tube, then allowed to drain from a ventrally positioned tube. Coughing and drainage of fluid from the nares suggest the presence of bronchopleural communication.

Other therapy

Phenylbutazone (1 to 2 g two times daily) or flunixin meglumine (500 mg one or two times daily) reduces pain and may decrease pleural fluid production, and hence may encourage the horse to eat. Corticosteroids are contraindicated. Rest and adequate nutrition are important.

Prognosis

A guarded prognosis must always be given. Prognosis for survival and return to athletic function is determined by the severity and duration of the disease and the development of complications. With early diagnosis and aggressive therapy, the prognosis for survival can be good.

STREPTOCOCCUS EQUI INFECTION (STRANGLES) *(Text pp. 504-507)*

Strangles, or *Streptococcus equi* infection, is characterized by sudden onset of fever and nasal discharge, followed by swelling and subsequent abscess of the submaxillary, submandibular, or retropharyngeal lymph nodes.

Clinical Findings

The first signs are seen 7 to 12 days after exposure and include depression, anorexia, fever, submandibular lymph node enlargement, and nasal discharge that rapidly becomes mucopurulent. Lymph node abscess usually develops 7 to 14 days after the onset of signs. The typical and favorable outcome is for abscesses to rupture onto the skin.

Complications

In most cases, recovery is uneventful once abscesses rupture and drain or are surgically lanced. However, a number of complications have been reported, including metastasis to other lymph nodes or other organs ("bastard strangles"), suppurative necrotic bronchopneumonia, guttural pouch empyema, laryngeal hemiplegia, myocarditis, and purpura hemorrhagica.

Diagnosis

Diagnosis is generally based on clinical signs. It is confirmed by isolation of *S. equi* from the nasal or lymph node discharge. Nasal swab cultures are not consistently positive for *S. equi,* so "if it looks like strangles, treat it like strangles." Asymptomatic carrier animals can be identified by culture or PCR of swabs or washes from the nasal passage or guttural pouch.

Treatment

Treatment depends on the stage of the disease. In every case, infected horses should be isolated.

Horses with early clinical signs

Development of clinical signs and lymph node abscess can be arrested with appropriate antimicrobial therapy. However, there is a high probability of relapse after cessation of therapy if the horse remains exposed to infected horses.

Horses with lymph node abscess

Therapy is directed toward enhancing maturation and drainage of the abscesses: hot packs and poultices and, if indicated, lancing; flushing of the draining abscess with 3% to 5% povidone-iodine. Antibiotic therapy is not beneficial once an abscess has formed, and it tends to prolong the disease when used at this stage. However, systemic penicillin is recommended for horses with prolonged fever, anorexia, depression, lethargy, or dyspnea. Emergency tracheotomy may be necessary in horses with severe dyspnea secondary to retropharyngeal lymph node abscess.

Horses exposed to strangles

Treatment with penicillin may prevent "seeding" of the pharyngeal lymph nodes with *S. equi* in horses exposed to strangles. Treatment should continue as long as affected horses are serving as a source of infection.

Horses with complications

Horses that develop complications from strangles must receive therapy directed at the specific problem, such as penicillin for metastatic abscess; penicillin and corticosteroids for purpura hemorrhagica; and lavage or surgical drainage for guttural pouch empyema.

Control

Recommendations for control of strangles include the following:

- Vaccination (see main text); this is ineffective in preventing disease in horses already exposed.
- Isolate all new arrivals for 2 to 3 weeks; observe for signs of disease and record rectal temperatures twice daily.
- Quarantine any suspect horse immediately.
- Disinfect all surfaces exposed to discharges from infected horses.
  - Phenolic products are recommended for facilities and equipment.
  - Iodophors and chlorhexidine are appropriate for handwashing.

Other control measures are discussed in Chapter 29 of *Large Animal Internal Medicine,* third edition.

THORACIC NEOPLASIA *(Text pp. 507-509)*

Primary tumors of the lungs or pleura are rare in horses; metastatic lesions are more common. Antemortem diagnosis of thoracic neoplasia depends on recognition of thoracic disease. Most cases involve metastatic disease, and clinical signs of the primary neoplasm often predominate. With the exception of malignant lymphoma, which may occur in young animals, thoracic neoplasia generally occurs in mature or aged horses.

Specific Neoplasms

Malignant lymphoma is the most common thoracic neoplasm in horses. Cytologic examination of pleural fluid is diagnostic in about 75% of cases. Diagnosis has also been made by biopsy of peripheral lymph nodes. Pleural mesothelioma often causes copious pleural effusion. The presence of numerous pleomorphic mesothelial cells in the pleural fluid aids antemortem diagnosis. Gastric squamous cell carcinomas commonly metastasize to the thoracic cavity. Cytologic examination of pleural fluid may allow antemortem diagnosis. Pulmonary hemangiosarcomas cause hemothorax, anemia, and dyspnea. Tentative antemortem diagnosis has been made using thoracoscopy and biopsy.

RESPIRATORY VIRUSES *(Text pp. 509-513)*

General Approach to Diagnosis and Treatment

The diagnosis of viral respiratory disease is largely presumptive based on clinical signs. Findings include fever, cough, and nasal discharge, the severity depending on the virus, the degree of challenge, and the horse's susceptibility. Fever is the initiating sign; it can be high and often is biphasic. Serous nasal discharge usually accompanies or follows the fever and may progress to become mucopurulent. Coughing is common in horses with influenza but is variable with the other viral infections.

Viral testing

On presentation it can be difficult to distinguish one viral respiratory disease from another. Viral testing is available; however, because there is currently no therapeutic benefit to knowing the specific viral agent involved, testing is not often performed. Viral testing may be indicated when multiple animals are at risk. Several methods are available:

- Virus isolation
  - Nasopharyngeal swabs and transtracheal aspirates are the best specimens.
- Serology
  - Acute and convalescent titers (taken 10 to 14 days apart) are compared; a fourfold or greater increase is considered significant.
- Detection of viral particles with fluorescent antibodies or PCR
  - PCR has been used to diagnose equine viral arteritis (EVA), influenza, and rhinopneumonitis (equine herpesvirus types 1 and 4)

An enzyme immunoassay (Directigen Flu A) for detection of influenza A in humans has been tested in horses. The test can be performed on nasopharyngeal swab samples and gives a result in 15 minutes.

Treatment

Treatment primarily involves supportive care: nonsteroidal antiinflammatory drugs (NSAIDs) and rest in an area with good ventilation and protection from foul weather. In general, a convalescent period of 3 to 4 weeks is needed for complete resolution of an uncomplicated viral respiratory infection. Rest should be enforced for at least 1 week after clinical signs have resolved. If coughing occurs when exercise resumes, rest should continue. If fever persists for more than 5 days and the nasal discharge changes from serous to mucopurulent, secondary bacterial infection should be suspected. Isolation of horses exhibiting clinical signs is important to decrease the spread of the virus.

Equine Influenza

Equine influenza has a short incubation period (1 to 3 days) and sudden onset. Disease outbreaks usually occur in horses 1 to 3 years of age. Coughing and nasal discharge either accompany the fever or appear several days later. The cough may persist up to 3 weeks. Other signs may include myalgia (or myopathy) and slight enlargement of the submandibular lymph nodes. On CBC, transient lymphopenia and eosinopenia are followed a few days later by monocytosis.

Vaccination

When chemically inactivated influenza vaccines are used, it is recommended that young horses and horses that may be heavily exposed be revaccinated every 4 to 6 months after the initial course of two injections 3 to 4 weeks apart. A less frequent schedule (every 9 to 12 months) may be adequate for older, regularly vaccinated horses. Maternal antibodies can interfere with vaccination against influenza until the foal is more than 8 months of age.

Equine Herpesvirus (Rhinopneumonitis)

The respiratory signs of EHV-1 and EHV-4 infection are clinically indistinguishable. Infection commonly occurs in the first year of life or soon after the young horse enters training. The incubation period is 3 to 7 days. CBC results may show leukopenia. Vaccines against EHV-1 and EHV-4 are available.

Equine Viral Arteritis

Manifestations of EVA range from subclinical to severe disease and death. Typically, affected animals are pyrectic for 1 to 5 days; other signs include anorexia, depression, serous nasal discharge, lacrimation, and coughing. Peripheral edema (limbs, palpebra, scrotum) and abortion have also been reported. The disease is most seroprevalent in standardbreds. Vaccination and other control measures are discussed in Chapter 29 of *Large Animal Internal Medicine,* third edition.

Other Respiratory Viruses

Other viruses that can infect the respiratory tract in horses include EHV-2, equine rhinovirus, equine adenovirus, and the newly reported Hendra virus. These viruses are briefly discussed in Chapter 29 of *Large Animal Internal Medicine,* third edition.

LUNGWORMS *(Text pp. 514-515)*

Dictyocaulus arnfieldi, equine lungworm, can cause chronic coughing in an individual horse or pony or affect several animals simultaneously. Donkeys, mules, and asses are the natural (and asymptomatic) hosts. Clinical findings are those of obstructive pulmonary disease: chronic cough, increased expiratory effort, exudate in the airways, and often audible wheezes and rales.

Diagnosis and Treatment

Presumptive diagnosis is based on clinical signs, a history of grazing with the natural hosts, and ruling out other causes of chronic coughing. The Baermann flotation technique, which can be used on feces, soil, and tissues, identifies only patent infections. It is not useful in diagnosing the more common nonpatent infections. Tracheobronchial aspirates may reveal eosinophilia without neutrophilia and sometimes larvae themselves, but eosinophilia is not pathognomonic for lungworm infection. Ivermectin is effective against immature and mature stages of the parasite.

HEMOTHORAX *(Text p. 515)*

Hemothorax may result from thoracic trauma (e.g., rib fractures), rupture of pulmonary bullae, vessel erosion by severe lung abscess or neoplasia, hemangiosarcoma involving the pleural surface, and coagulopathy. Hemothorax may be unilateral or bilateral. Diagnosis is based on clinical findings (e.g., dyspnea, tachycardia, decreased lung sounds ventrally) and thoracocentesis. Pleural fluid should be collected for cytologic examination, cell count, packed cell volume, and total protein count; it should also be cultured if infection is likely. A clotting profile and platelet count should be performed if coagulopathy is suspected.

Treatment

The underlying cause must be treated. Medical therapy, such as intranasal oxygen, analgesics, and intravenous fluids (or whole blood if blood loss is severe), may be required to stabilize cardiopulmonary function. Blood may be removed via a tube thoracostomy. In cases of hemothorax resulting from coagulopathy, drainage is not recommended unless respiratory distress occurs. Broad-spectrum antibiotics are recommended for any case of hemothorax.

PNEUMOTHORAX *(Text pp. 515-516)*

Pneumothorax is uncommon in horses. It is usually associated with trauma (e.g., puncture or laceration of the trachea or esophagus, penetrating wounds to the thorax, external wounds resulting in subcutaneous emphysema and pneumomediastinum, rib fracture with perforation of the lung).

Clinical Findings and Diagnosis

Clinical signs can include dyspnea, tachypnea, cyanosis, and evidence of trauma. Pneumothorax should be suspected when a horse with subcutaneous emphysema seems dyspneic or distressed. Auscultation and percussion reveal absence of normal lung sounds and hyperresonance in the dorsal thorax. Radiography and ultrasonography are diagnostic.

Treatment

Treatment consists of relieving the pneumothorax (if the horse is in respiratory distress) and treating the cause. Open, sucking wounds should be occluded; tracheal defects should be sutured when possible; and fractured ribs should be stabilized. Dyspneic horses should be given intranasal oxygen (15 L/min).

Relieving pneumothorax

Pneumothorax can be resolved by inserting a teat cannula or thoracostomy tube, with suction device attached, into the dorsal thoracic cavity. If pneumothorax persists or recurs, one or more chest tubes with Heimlich valves should be left in place to allow constant removal of air. The horse should be placed on broad-spectrum antibiotics.

PULMONARY EDEMA *(Text p. 516)*

Pulmonary edema rarely occurs as a primary event. When present, it is usually secondary to some other pathologic process, such as left-sided heart failure, acute renal failure, sepsis, disseminated intravascular coagulation, hypoxic acidosis, or pulmonary condition. Rapid intravenous fluid administration can also lead to pulmonary edema.

Diagnosis

Diagnosis is based on clinical findings, a history of predisposing causes, and radiography. Affected horses have a shallow, rapid respiratory pattern and may be dyspneic. Clear, slightly yellow, or pink-tinged fluid may drip from the nostrils; this finding warrants a grave prognosis. Fine crackles or wheezes may be audible on auscultation. Radiographic findings are nonspecific but include peribronchial and perivascular cuffing, increased prominence of vessels, and a hazy reticular interstitial pattern.

Treatment

Treatment consists of correcting the cause, reversing hypoxemia, decreasing plasma volume, and increasing plasma colloid osmotic pressure. Intranasal oxygen and even assisted ventilation may be needed in severe cases. Intravenous fluid therapy should be guided by the patient's needs and, if necessary, monitored by serial measurement of central venous pressure. Furosemide (1 to 2 mg/kg IV or IM) may be given as needed. Colloid solutions should be administered cautiously or in conjunction with diuretics. NSAIDs, antihistamines, and bronchodilators may be of benefit. Use of corticosteroids is controversial; if they are given, antibiotic coverage is advisable.

SMOKE INHALATION *(Text p. 517)*

Smoke inhalation injury is typically associated with exposure to fires, and there are often concurrent problems in other body systems, in particular, burns. Within the first 6 hours the patient may show signs of carbon monoxide toxicity and shock and may be depressed, disoriented, irritable, ataxic, or even moribund. As edema and necrosis in the upper airway progress, dyspnea and stridor may develop. Later stages of smoke inhalation injury include pulmonary edema (beginning 12 to 24 hours after exposure) and bronchopneumonia (which may not become apparent for up to 2 weeks after initial injury).

Treatment

Treatment depends on the stage of injury. Initially, humidified oxygen (via nasal insufflation or transtracheal catheter), nebulization, bronchodilators, diuretics, NSAIDs, and analgesics may be indicated. Upper airway obstruction may require tracheostomy. Burns and shock often require judicious use of intravenous fluids. Use of corticosteroids is controversial; prophylactic antimicrobial use is not recommended.

CHRONIC OBSTRUCTIVE PULMONARY DISEASE (CHRONIC RECURRENT AIRWAY OBSTRUCTION) *(Text pp. 517-521)*

Chronic obstructive pulmonary disease (COPD; "heaves" in its severe form) is usually associated with stabling and exposure to hay, straw, and molds. In some areas it is associated with summer pasture. Diagnosis can be difficult in horses that show signs intermittently or only when challenged.

Clinical Signs

Horses with mild COPD may breathe normally or have only slightly accentuated end-expiratory effort. Lung sounds may be normal or only slightly increased, but with deep breaths occasional wheezes may occur and the horse may cough. Coughing may be the major owner complaint. Affected horses usually show exercise intolerance. Exposure of affected horses to dust or molds can increase the expiratory effort and precipitate obvious signs of airway obstruction.

Severe COPD

Horses with severe COPD have a frequent, deep cough that may be explosive and paroxysmal. Nasal discharge, when present, may be copious, thick, and mucopurulent. The horse's nostrils may be flared, and the horse may seem anxious. Increased expiratory effort may lead to a "heave line" (hypertrophy of the external abdominal oblique). Inspiratory and expiratory wheezes may be diffuse or loudest ventrally or in the hilar area. Fine crackles may be most audible in the peripheral lung fields. Fever is rare; a severe allergic reaction can sometimes elicit a fever spike. Persistent fever should prompt suspicion of infection.

Diagnosis

Diagnosis in symptomatic horses is based on a combination of clinical signs, history, response to bronchodilators (e.g., atropine, β-adrenergic drugs), and response to environmental changes. CBC and plasma fibrinogen can be useful in differentiating between infection and COPD.

Tracheobronchial aspirates

Tracheobronchial aspirates may reveal increased mucus, Curschmann's spirals, increased numbers of neutrophils (no toxic changes), and sometimes eosinophils and damaged epithelial cells. Gram stain usually does not demonstrate a large number of bacteria. BAL is more useful, although it is unlikely to be of value in asymptomatic horses.

Treatment

Environmental management

Environmental changes are of utmost importance in managing COPD. Elimination of hay is usually more important than changes in bedding. Some horses tolerate hay as long as it is dampened; others require its complete removal from their diet. Suitable alternatives include hay cubes and alfalfa pellets. When possible, the horse should be kept outside; if not possible, the horse and its neighbors should be bedded on shavings or shredded paper. With summer pasture-associated obstructive pulmonary disease, the horse must be maintained inside.

Drug therapy

Therapeutic options include the following:

- Corticosteroids–dexamethasone IV, beclomethasone by inhalation
  - Clinically effective dosages vary among horses.
- β-Adrenergic bronchodilators–clenbuterol, pirbuterol, albuterol, given orally or by inhalation depending on the drug and formulation
  - Most inhaled β-adrenergic drugs have a short duration of action.
- Aminophylline–6 mg/kg PO two times daily initially, increasing as needed
  - Signs of toxicity (excitement tremors, sweating, tachycardia) may be seen at higher dosages.
- Atropine
  - Low dosages (e.g., 5 to 7 mg/450 kg) result in rapid improvement in symptomatic horses.
- Ipratropium–1 to 3 μg/kg by inhalation
  - Ipratropium causes bronchodilation without the undesirable effects of atropine (ileus, tachycardia, drying of secretions), but duration of action is short (4 to 6 hours).
- Cromolyn (disodium cromoglycate)–prophylactic effect by stabilizing mast cells

TUBERCULOSIS *(Text p. 522)*

Tuberculosis is extremely rare in horses, especially in the United States. The most frequent presenting complaint is chronic weight loss with weakness and lethargy. Terminally, horses with the pulmonary form are febrile and dyspneic and have a cough. Biopsy of lung lesions or culture and cytologic evaluation (acid-fast stain) of a transtracheal aspirate is needed for diagnosis. Treatment is usually not attempted (see main text).

PNEUMOCONIOSIS (SILICOSIS) *(Text pp. 522-523)*

Silicate pneumoconiosis has been reported in horses from the Monterey-Carmel peninsula of California. Clinical signs are similar to COPD and include weight loss, cough, exercise intolerance, and in some cases exercise-induced respiratory distress. Resting respiratory rates are often increased, and there is a restrictive breathing pattern. Auscultation reveals harsh breath sounds and wheezing that is exacerbated by exercise. Transtracheal aspirates primarily contain alveolar macrophages, some of which have cytoplasmic inclusions. Thoracic radiography may reveal various interstitial patterns (most severe in the caudodorsal lung fields), lymphadenopathy, pleural thickening or effusion, hyperinflation, and consolidation. Treatment is ineffective.

MYCOPLASMAL INFECTIONS *(Text p. 523)*

The importance of *Mycoplasma* spp. as respiratory pathogens in horses is debated. *Mycoplasma felis* reportedly causes pleuritis and pericarditis in horses. Clinical signs mimic those of bacterial pleuritis. Thoracocentesis should be performed for diagnostic and, if necessary, therapeutic purposes. The fluid is most often an exudate and lacks any odor. Cytologic examination reveals large numbers of neutrophils. Culture for mycoplasmas requires immediate centrifugation of the pleural fluid and placement of the supernatant in Hayflick's media. Although *Mycoplasma* spp. are sensitive to gentamicin, tetracyclines, and erythromycin, the necessity for treatment is unclear.

RETROPHARYNGEAL LYMPH NODE ABSCESS *(Text pp. 523-526)*

Retropharyngeal abscesses generally are caused by *S. equi* subsp. *equi* infection (strangles; see pp. 504-507) or are secondary to trauma. Other isolates include *S. equi* subsp. *zooepidemicus, Corynebacterium pseudotuberculosis,* and *Actinobacillus* spp.

Clinical Signs and Diagnosis

Clinical signs variably include dysphagia, painful swallowing, nasal or oral regurgitation, hypersalivation, dyspnea with or without stridor; painful throat-latch swelling, mucoid or mucopurulent nasal discharge, extension of the head and neck, fever, inappetence, depression, and weight loss. Narrowing or collapse of the pharyngeal lumen, possibly with deviation of the larynx, is evident endoscopically. Lateral radiographs of the pharynx and ultrasonography aid diagnosis. Collection of purulent material from abscessed lymph nodes assists in identification of the causal agent.

Treatment

Treatment goals are relief of respiratory distress and control of infection. Temporary tracheostomy may be needed for relief of severe dyspnea. After surgical drainage (see main text), appropriate systemic antibiotics are administered; NSAIDs may further reduce the swelling.

EXERCISE-INDUCED PULMONARY HEMORRHAGE *(Text pp. 526-529)*

Exercise-induced pulmonary hemorrhage (EIPH) is bleeding from the lung as a consequence of exercise. Most horses in race training apparently experience EIPH. The predominant clinical finding is blood in the lower airways during endoscopic examination 60 to 90 minutes after strenuous exercise. Epistaxis is seen in less than 10% of horses experiencing EIPH. Signs of impaired performance, such as slowing toward the end of a race and labored or abnormal breathing, are often reported by trainers. Astute trainers may also observe excessive swallowing after racing.

Diagnosis

In the absence of a visible source of hemorrhage rostral to the larynx, endoscopic observation of blood in the lower airways after exercise is diagnostic for EIPH. Cytologic examination of tracheal aspirates or BAL fluid is also useful: macrophages containing erythrocytes or hemosiderin indicate that the horse has previously experienced EIPH.

Treatment

Enforced rest (3 to 6 months) helps some horses, but most continue to experience EIPH when training resumes. Furosemide (0.3 to 0.6 mg/kg IV) is currently the most commonly used medication and is administered no less than 3 hours before racing in jurisdictions that approve its use. Management should include minimizing exposure to dust and infectious respiratory diseases and an adequate period of convalescence after respiratory infections. Bronchodilators, broad-spectrum antibiotics, and low-dose corticosteroids can be used to improve airway health during convalescence in horses with recurrent, performance-limiting EIPH.

PHARYNGITIS *(Text pp. 530-532)*

Pharyngitis (inflammation of the pharyngeal tissues) is a response to other diseases, particularly viral and bacterial respiratory infections, and to a lesser extent to local physical, chemical, or allergic causes. Acute and chronic forms of pharyngitis are recognized. Pharyngitis is most prevalent in horses less than 5 years of age, in which it is often termed pharyngeal lymphoid hyperplasia.

Clinical Signs and Diagnosis

Pharyngitis may be asymptomatic, but when it is severe, it can cause odynophagia, dysphagia, nasal discharge (serous, mucoid, mucopurulent, or feed contaminated), enlarged submandibular or retropharyngeal nodes, respiratory noise, pharyngeal swelling, and coughing. On endoscopic examination, hyperplasia of the lymphonodular follicles within the pharyngeal mucosa is seen. The severity is often graded from I (mild) to IV (severe).

Treatment

In many instances the signs are sufficiently mild that treatment is unnecessary. Rest from training for 4 to 8 weeks is commonly advocated in race horses. Soft feeds, especially green grass, should be offered to encourage the horse to eat. Although antimicrobial therapy is probably not indicated, it is often used to limit secondary bacterial infection. Custom preparations, usually containing an antibiotic, an antiinflammatory drug, and a hygroscopic agent (glycerin) or DMSO, are often used. The preparation is sprayed on the pharyngeal mucosa via a nasal catheter 2 to 3 times daily.

GUTTURAL POUCH DISEASES *(Text pp. 532-536)*

Guttural Pouch Tympany

Tympany of the guttural pouch occasionally occurs in foals (from birth up to 18 months of age). It is characterized by unilateral or bilateral distention of the guttural pouch with air. Affected foals have painless, soft, fluctuant swelling in the retropharyngeal space with variable signs of dysphagia and dyspnea. Mild tympany may simply cause swelling of the throat-latch region.

Diagnosis

Diagnosis is based on recognition of the characteristic swelling. Although the distention is most often unilateral, extreme distortion of a single pouch may give the impression of bilateral involvement. Radiography and endoscopy are useful for establishing the diagnosis and distinguishing bilateral from unilateral tympany.

Treatment

Guttural pouch tympany can be temporarily alleviated by percutaneous decompression or catheterization via the pharyngeal opening. Surgery is necessary for permanent resolution.

Guttural Pouch Empyema

Accumulation of purulent material in the guttural pouch (empyema) is usually unilateral and is often secondary to an infectious respiratory disease, especially *S. equi* subsp. *equi* infection (strangles). *S. equi* subsp. *zooepidemicus* is another common isolate.

Clinical signs

Clinical signs variably include intermittent purulent nasal discharge that may worsen when the horse lowers its head, lymphadenitis, parotid swelling and pain, dysphagia, and dyspnea. The nasal discharge may be unilateral or bilateral, even if only one pouch is affected. Inspissation of the purulent material results in chondroids (concretions of inspissated pus).

Diagnosis

Guttural pouch empyema should be considered in any horse with a chronic, refractory nasal discharge. Diagnostic aids include radiography, endoscopy, percutaneous centesis, and aspiration of material through the pharyngeal opening. The absence of fluid at the pharyngeal ostium does not preclude the possibility of guttural pouch empyema, especially if the material is inspissated.

Treatment

In early cases, empyema may respond to daily lavage of the affected pouch with 500 ml of saline-antibiotic solution. On initial catheterization, purulent material should be aspirated and submitted for bacterial culture and antimicrobial susceptibility testing. Although parenteral antibiotics may be of benefit, adequate drainage and local therapy are of primary importance. If response to treatment is poor or if empyema recurs, surgical drainage should be considered. Surgery is also indicated when purulent material becomes inspissated or chondroids have formed.

NOTE: Indwelling catheters and povidone-iodine solution can cause severe inflammatory changes in the guttural pouch and possibly neuritis of adjacent cranial nerves.

Guttural Pouch Mycosis

Fungal infection of the guttural pouch potentially leads to invasion of the neurovascular structures in the wall of the guttural pouch, including the internal carotid artery and cranial nerves VII, IX, X, XI, and XII. A number of fungi, most often *Aspergillus nidulans*, have been isolated from these lesions.

Clinical signs

Common signs include spontaneous epistaxis and dysphagia. Epistaxis is usually unilateral, but it can be bilateral. Episodes of epistaxis generally occur at rest and can vary from mild to severe and fatal. Dysphagia generally occurs later in the course of disease and often is permanent. Dysphagic horses cough while eating and have nasal discharge that contains food material. Other signs that may be seen include parotid pain, abnormal head posture, unilateral or bilateral nasal discharge, head shyness, abnormal respiratory noise, sweating and shivering, Horner's syndrome, visual disturbances, colic, and facial paralysis.

Diagnosis

Diagnosis involves endoscopic observation of the diphtheritic lesions in the dorsocaudal aspect of the medial compartment or elsewhere within the guttural pouch. Lesions vary in color (brown, yellow, black, or white) and in size (from discrete nodules to diffuse irregular patches). Care should be taken not to dislodge a thrombus and induce further hemorrhage.

Treatment

Surgical treatment offers the best prognosis. Options include insertion of a balloon-tipped catheter into the distal internal carotid artery followed by proximal ligation of the artery and insertion of a latex balloon or embolization coil into the artery. Medical therapy (local and parenteral antifungal treatment) is of questionable efficacy, and response to therapy is protracted.

PARANASAL SINUSITIS *(Text pp. 537-539)*

Inflammation of the paranasal sinuses (sinusitis) generally is a result of primary or secondary bacterial infection. Primary sinusitis is usually caused by *Streptococcus* spp. Maxillary sinusitis most often occurs secondary to dental disease (e.g., alveolar periostitis, patent infundibula, fractured or split teeth). Other causes of sinusitis include trauma, developmental disorders (e.g., maxillary follicular cysts), neoplasia, and fungal granulomas.

Clinical Findings

The most common presenting complaint is chronic, unilateral nasal discharge (serous, mucoid, or mucopurulent). The discharge may be intermittent or continuous. The breath may be fetid with sinusitis secondary to dental disease or tissue necrosis within the sinus. Facial distortion and reduced nasal airflow may result from expansion of material within the sinus. Percussion of the affected sinus may reveal dullness or pain, although normal resonance does not preclude the possibility of sinusitis. Other signs may include ipsilateral ocular discharge, exophthalmos, and fistula formation.

Diagnosis

Diagnostic procedures include radiography (most useful), endoscopy, percutaneous sinus centesis, and examination of the oral cavity (especially careful probing of the occlusal surfaces of the cheek teeth with a fine dental pick). Fluid obtained by sinus centesis should be examined cytologically and submitted for microbial culture and susceptibility testing. Isolation of a single organism generally indicates primary sinusitis, whereas polymicrobial infection is more compatible with sinusitis of dental origin.

Treatment

Treatment of primary sinusitis or empyema involves daily lavage of the sinus (via percutaneous centesis) with 1 L of saline to which a broad-spectrum antibiotic or antiseptic has been added. Once the results of culture and susceptibility are available, the appropriate antibiotic should also be administered systemically. If little progress is seen after 10 to 14 days or if nasal discharge recurs, sinusotomy (trephination or bone flap technique) may be required. Sinusitis that results from secondary factors (diseased teeth, granulomas, neoplasia) generally is not responsive to medical management; surgical removal of the inciting cause is required.

ETHMOID HEMATOMA *(Text pp. 539-541)*

Ethmoid hematomas are slowly expanding angiomatous masses that originate from the mucosa of the ethmoid conchae. Most affected horses are more than 8 years old. Nasal discharge with intermittent epistaxis from one or both nostrils is the most common sign. The discharge can vary from blood-tinged mucoid or mucopurulent material to a trickle of blood. Fulminant epistaxis is uncommon.

Diagnosis

Diagnosis requires endoscopy and radiography. Because ethmoid hematomas occur bilaterally in about 30% of cases, it is important to examine both the left and right ethmoidal conchae. Ethmoid hematomas vary in color from deep red or red-purple to yellow-brown, yellow-green, or bronze. Hematomas that expand dorsally into the frontal sinus may not be visible on endoscopy, but hemorrhage that originates deep to the visible portion of the ethmoidal conchae may be evident.

Treatment

The method of treatment depends on the location and size of the hematoma. Surgical ablation using curettage, cryosurgery, or laser photoablation (via sinusotomy or transnasal endoscopy) has been the preferred method. Intralesional injection of formaldehyde solution in standing, sedated horses is associated with less morbidity and similar recurrence rates. Irrespective of treatment method, the hematoma recurs in 30% to 50% of cases, from several months to years after treatment.

PART II: Ruminant Respiratory System

DISEASES OF THE NASAL CAVITY *(Text pp. 541-543)*

Mycotic Nasal Granuloma (Mycetoma)

Fungal granulomas in the nasal cavity are uncommon in ruminants. The condition is more common in warm, wet climates. The granulomas may be single or multiple, unilateral or bilateral, and located anywhere in the nasal cavity. Clinical signs include stridor, dyspnea, and mucopurulent nasal discharge, sometimes with epistaxis. Endoscopy, biopsy, and culture aid diagnosis. The lesions consist of 0.5- to 5-cm yellow, yellow-green, or red nodules or polyps.

Treatment

Treatments include surgical excision (if possible) and sodium iodide therapy. Sodium iodide (20% solution) is given at 66 mg/kg IV and repeated every 10 to 14 days until remission or until signs of iodism (lacrimation, cough, scaly skin) are seen. Because fungal granulomas can be difficult to treat and are chronically debilitating, salvage is often the most practical option.

Atopic Rhinitis and Enzootic Nasal Granuloma

Allergic rhinitis in cattle usually is caused by exposure to a plant pollen or fungal spores. Channel Island breeds and Friesians are most susceptible. Most affected animals are between 6 months and 2 years of age. A similar condition may occur in sheep.

Clinical findings

Initially the signs are seasonal, occurring in warm, moist conditions. They include sneezing, intense nasal pruritus (with snorting, head shaking, and vigorous nose rubbing), dyspnea, stertorous inspiration, and profuse bilateral nasal discharge. Lacrimation, chemosis, and blepharitis may also be present.

Chronic rhinitis may lead to granuloma formation (enzootic nasal granuloma) in which multiple firm, white nodules 1 to 2 mm in diameter or pale-pink, flat plaques are found scattered throughout the nasal cavity. The signs of chronic rhinitis are more constant, with seasonal exacerbations.

Diagnosis

Endoscopy, biopsy, cultures (viral, bacterial, fungal), antigen detection tests, and serology can be used to rule out other conditions, particularly fungal granuloma. Eosinophil counts in nasal secretions correlate with the susceptibility of the animal and activity of the disease, but no absolute level is diagnostic.

Treatment

Treatment and control entail removal of the animal from the allergen source and therapy to block the hypersensitivity reaction. Recommended drugs include antihistamines, meclofenamic acid, and corticosteroids (0.04 to 0.22 mg/kg dexamethasone IM or IV or 1 to 2.2 mg/kg prednisolone IM or IV daily). Topical corticosteroids may also be useful.

Nasal Tumors and Polyps

Tumors and polyps of the nasal cavity and sinuses are rare in ruminants. Signs common to nasal tumors include stridor, dyspnea, nasal discharge, epistaxis, foul breath, unilateral decrease in airflow, open-mouth breathing, and distortion of the facial bones. In small ruminants, other signs can include head shaking, sneezing, and exophthalmos.

Other Conditions

Nasal foreign bodies, trauma, and fractures are differential diagnoses for the conditions discussed earlier. In sheep, nasal bots are another consideration with signs referable to the nasal passages (see p. 543). Developmental anomalies, such as congenital cystic nasal turbinates in cattle, should also be considered in young animals showing upper respiratory signs.

DISEASES OF THE SINUSES *(Text pp. 543-545)*

Sinusitis

Inflammation of the paranasal sinuses is more common in cattle than in sheep and goats. Dehorning is the most common cause of frontal sinusitis, and dental disease is the most common cause of maxillary sinusitis. Other causes of sinusitis include extension of actinomycosis or nasal neoplasia, horn injuries, facial fractures, respiratory viruses, sinus cysts, lymphosarcoma, and nasal bots (sheep). *Arcanobacterium (Actinomyces) pyogenes* is the most common isolate in cattle with frontal sinusitis secondary to dehorning. *Pasteurella multocida* is the most common isolate with sinusitis not associated with dehorning.

Clinical findings

Sinusitis associated with dehorning may be acute or occur weeks or months later. The portal of entry frequently is open and discharging pus. Nonspecific signs include anorexia, lethargy, reluctance to move, and fever. In closed cases, signs may include nasal discharge, mild stridor, changes in airflow, and foul breath. The animal may hold its head at an odd angle and squint as if in pain. Percussion of the sinus may reveal a dull, full sound and elicit pain. In chronic cases, frontal bone distortion, exophthalmos, and neurologic signs may be present.

Diagnosis

Diagnosis can usually be made on the basis of clinical signs. Radiography and sinus centesis are useful when there is no recent history of dehorning or in cases of maxillary sinusitis. Sinus centesis may yield purulent material, which should be cultured and examined cytologically.

Treatment

Cattle with frontal sinusitis after dehorning should be treated by sinusotomy and drainage of the affected sinus. Trephination should be performed 3 to 4 cm from the midline, intersecting a line drawn between the caudal aspect of the orbits (see main text). The frontal sinus is compartmentalized in mature sheep and goats. Double trephination or bone flaps for exposure and curettage should be considered in these patients.

Lavage. The sinus should be lavaged daily with dilute antiseptic solutions, such as 0.1% povidone-iodine or chlorhexidine in saline, or 1:1000 potassium permanganate. Lavage is continued until infection is resolved; early cases often resolve in 10 to 14 days.

Systemic therapy. Parenteral antibiotics and NSAIDs are indicated if systemic signs are present. Penicillin (22,000 U/kg IM two times daily) is recommended in the absence of culture results. NSAID choices include aspirin (100 mg/kg PO two times daily), phenylbutazone (17.6 mg/kg PO loading dose, followed in 48 hours by 4.4 mg/kg PO once daily), and flunixin meglumine (0.5 to 1.1 mg/kg IM or IV one to three times daily).

Oestrus ovis Infestation

Infestation of the nasal cavity with the bots of *Oestrus ovis* occurs in sheep and occasionally in goats. The adult flies annoy the sheep, causing head shaking, sneezing, blowing, nose rubbing, feet stamping, and loss of grazing time. The bots, which migrate to the dorsal turbinates and sinuses, cause rhinitis with sneezing, snorting, mucopurulent (intermittently blood-tinged) nasal discharge, stridor, and reduced airflow. Chronic sinusitis is common; secondary bacterial infections may also occur. Ivermectin (200 μg/kg PO) is an effective treatment.

DISEASES OF THE PHARYNX, LARYNX, AND TRACHEA *(Text pp. 545-550)*

Pharyngeal Trauma and Abscesses

Pharyngeal trauma from iatrogenic damage, stemmy feeds, grass awns or briars, and other foreign objects may result in hematomas, foreign body granulomas, cellulitis, or abscesses. Common isolates include *A. pyogenes, Actinobacillus* spp., *Pasteurella* spp., *Bordetella* spp., *Fusobacterium necrophorum,* and *Streptococcus* spp. *Corynebacterium pseudotuberculosis* (caseous lymphadenitis) may localize in the pharyngeal nodes of goats and occasionally sheep.

Clinical signs

Signs of pharyngeal trauma vary with the severity of the resulting reaction. Prominent signs include inspiratory dyspnea and stertor, extension of the head and neck, salivation (often profuse), quidding, pain on swallowing or reluctance to swallow, regurgitation of food or saliva through the nostrils, mucopurulent or bloody nasal discharge, fetid breath, cough, bloat, and visible or palpable pharyngeal swelling. In severe cases, fever, anorexia, depression, dehydration, and ruminal stasis may be present. Aspiration pneumonia may be a secondary complication.

Diagnosis

Thorough manual examination of the oropharynx or visual examination with a speculum and light source usually confirms pharyngeal swelling and often reveals a puncture that is discharging pus. Endoscopy or radiography can be helpful in cases in which the infection is diffuse. Aspiration of material from the swelling is recommended for cytologic examination, Gram stain, and culture.

Treatment

Discrete pharyngeal abscesses are usually best drained into the pharynx with the patient standing and unsedated. The cavity is flushed with a mild antiseptic such as 0.2% povidone-iodine solution. Other options include drainage to the exterior and extirpation. Granulomas and cellulitis are treated medically. Procaine penicillin G (22,000 U/kg IM or subcutaneously [SC] two times daily), tetracyclines (11 mg/kg IM, IV, or SC one or two times daily), or sulfonamides (140 mg/kg IV loading dose, followed by 70 mg/kg IV daily) are recommended in the absence of culture results. NSAIDs (see p. 546) help relieve pain, swelling, and stertor. In severe cases, tracheostomy may be necessary.

Soft Palate Displacement and Subepiglottic Cyst

Although rare, dorsal displacement of the soft palate has been reported in cattle. Diagnosis and treatment are similar to that in horses. Subepiglottic cyst causing upper airway obstruction has also been reported in cattle. Peroral surgical removal has been described.

Necrotic Laryngitis

Necrotic laryngitis (calf diphtheria, laryngeal necrobacillosis) is infection of the laryngeal mucosa and cartilage by *F. necrophorum.* Necrotic laryngitis most often occurs in calves 3 to 18 months of age; it is common in feedlots.

Clinical signs and diagnosis

Diagnosis can usually be made on clinical signs alone. Necrotic laryngitis is characterized by acute onset of a moist, painful cough, with severe inspiratory dyspnea, stertor, and open-mouth breathing with the head and neck extended. The calf may salivate, make frequent painful swallowing movements, and sip water continually. Bilateral nasal discharge and fetid breath are common. The larynx may be palpably swollen. Anorexia, depression, fever, and hyperemic mucous membranes are present in severe cases. Untreated calves often die in 2 to 7 days.

Treatment

Sulfonamides (140 mg/kg IV loading dose, followed by 70 mg/kg daily) or procaine penicillin G (22,000 U/kg IM or SC two times daily) are the drugs of choice. Streptomycin, oxytetracycline, and tylosin (11 mg/kg IM sid or two times daily for all three drugs) are also effective. Tracheostomy may be necessary in severe cases. Supportive care is important, including shelter, adequate ventilation, easy access to feed and water, and oral or intravenous fluids if needed. NSAIDs (see p. 548) are also recommended.

Laryngeal Papillomatosis

Papillomas of the larynx are common in feedlot cattle. They cause stertorous respiration and cough. Treatment is usually not indicated.

Laryngeal Abscesses

Abscess of the arytenoid cartilages caused by *A. pyogenes* has been reported in calves and sheep. Clinical signs are indicative of upper airway obstruction. Many affected animals remain alert and afebrile and continue to eat until the terminal stages of severe dyspnea. Diagnosis is aided by endoscopy and radiography. Treatment consists of tracheostomy, antibiotics (usually penicillin at 22,000 U/kg IM or SC two times daily), and NSAIDs (see p. 548).

Tracheal Lesions

Tracheal lesions, such as stenosis, collapse, and obstruction with a foreign body or mass, are uncommon. Many patients with tracheal narrowing have normal vital signs and are alert and in good condition. However, in other cases stertorous respiration, tachypnea, dyspnea, cyanosis, fever, tachycardia, and mucosal hyperemia are observed. A "honking" cough is characteristic, especially with intrathoracic tracheal collapse. Endoscopy and radiography are the most useful diagnostic aids.

Treatment

Mild cases may respond sufficiently to confinement to be fed out for slaughter. Some small foreign objects lodged in the trachea may be retrieved endoscopically; in other cases tracheostomy is required.

Tracheal Edema Syndrome of Feedlot Cattle

Tracheal edema syndrome (tracheal stenosis, "honker cattle") is a sporadic condition that occurs in feedlot cattle. The cause is unknown. There are two forms: acute dyspnea and chronic cough.

Acute dyspnea

The acute syndrome mainly occurs in heavy cattle in the latter two thirds of the feeding period and is more common in summer. Signs include acute onset of dyspnea and loud, guttural inspiratory sounds that can be localized to the lower trachea. Dyspnea can be severe and lead to cyanosis, recumbency, and death. Broad-spectrum antibiotics and corticosteroids (dexamethasone 0.04 to 0.22 mg/kg IM or IV or prednisolone 1 to 2.2 mg/kg IM or IV daily) are recommended. Preventing stress, providing shade, and cooling with water sprays and fans are also helpful. Recovered patients tend to relapse and should be salvaged.

Chronic cough

The chronic form occurs in lighter cattle (less than 400 kg [less than 900 lb]) and is less seasonal. Affected animals may have a history of infectious bovine rhinotracheitis or pneumonia. The main sign is a persistent, hacking, nonproductive cough. The animal may be unthrifty but is otherwise normal. No effective treatment exists for this form.

BRONCHOPNEUMONIA IN RUMINANTS (RESPIRATORY DISEASE COMPLEX) *(Text pp. 551-569)*

Respiratory disease complex in ruminants consists of a single clinical entity, bronchopneumonia, but is caused by numerous combinations of infectious agents, compromised host defenses, and environmental conditions. Detailed discussions of risk factors in dairy and veal calves (enzootic calf pneumonia), feedlot calves (shipping fever), and sheep and goats can be found in Chapter 29 of *Large Animal Internal Medicine,* third edition.

Viral Agents Associated With Respiratory Disease Complex

Respiratory disease complex often involves respiratory viruses acting in combination with other infectious agents, particularly bacteria. The most important causes of viral respiratory disease in cattle are BHV-1, bovine virus diarrhea virus (BVDV), parainfluenza virus type 3 (PI-3), and bovine respiratory syncytial virus (BRSV). Bovine coronavirus may also have an important role in bovine respiratory disease complex.

BHV-1 (infectious bovine rhinotracheitis)

BHV-1 causes several disease syndromes in cattle. The respiratory form (infectious bovine rhinotracheitis, or IBR) is characterized by rhinitis and tracheitis. Clinical signs include fever, anorexia, dramatic drop in milk production, tachypnea, mild hyperexcitability, hypersalivation, coughing, nasal discharge that progresses from serous to mucopurulent, and severe hyperemia of the muzzle ("red nose"). Pustules may develop on the nasal mucosa and later form diphtheritic plaques. Conjunctivitis with excessive ocular discharge may also be present.

BVDV

A wide spectrum of disease has been associated with BVDV infection. Because of its immunosuppressive effects, it is likely that this virus is an important respiratory pathogen in cattle. A synergistic interaction among BVDV and *Mannheimia (Pasteurella) haemolytica,* BHV-1, and BRSV has been demonstrated.

Respiratory syncytial viruses

BRSV-associated disease predominantly occurs in young cattle, but the virus sporadically causes mild disease in adult cattle. In feeder-age calves, respiratory signs include high fever, depression, inappetence, tachypnea, hypersalivation, cough, and nasal and lacrimal discharges. In the later stages, dyspnea becomes pronounced. Subcutaneous emphysema and intermandibular edema are sometimes noted. Secondary bacterial pneumonia may occur. Respiratory syncytial virus has also been isolated from sheep and goats with respiratory disease.

Parainfluenza type 3

PI-3 infection can cause fever, cough, nasal and ocular discharge, tachypnea, and increased breath sounds. However, in many cases, infection is subclinical or mild. The most important role of PI-3 is in predisposing the respiratory tract to infection by other viruses and bacteria, such as *Mannheimia (Pasturella) haemolytica.* PI-3 infection is also widespread in sheep and probably in goats.

Adenoviruses

Bovine adenovirus (BAV) infection is widespread; BAV serotype 3 is most often associated with respiratory infection. Although most infections are subclinical, signs of both upper and lower respiratory tract disease and concurrent enteritis may be present. Ovine adenovirus infection is widespread in sheep and can cause respiratory and enteric disease in lambs.

Bacterial, Mycoplasmal, and Chlamydial Agents

The most common and important bacterial isolates in ruminants with pneumonia are *Mannheimia (Pasturella) haemolytica, Pasteurella multocida,* and *Haemophilus somnus.* Isolation of *A. pyogenes,* coliforms, or anaerobic bacteria often is indicative of chronic pneumonia or aspiration pneumonia and may be associated with lung abscess. *Mycoplasma* spp. are commonly isolated, usually in combination with other pathogens. *Mycoplasma ovipneumonia* can be a primary cause of mild bronchopneumonia in sheep and goats and predispose to *M. haemolytica.* Chlamydial agents are occasionally isolated. They produce only mild respiratory infections by themselves but may enhance the pathogenicity of concurrent infections.

Diagnosis of Bronchopneumonia

Diagnosis is based on clinical or necropsy findings. Identification of the infectious agents might involve virus isolation or detection of viral antigens, serology, bacterial culture, immunohistochemical staining for bacterial antigens, mycoplasma culture, and special staining or immunofluorescence techniques for chlamydia.

Treatment of Bronchopneumonia

Successful intervention with a pneumonia outbreak is based on identification and alteration of the risk factors associated with the outbreak (see main text). The basic foundation of antimicrobial therapy for bacterial bronchopneumonia is to treat early enough, treat for long enough, and treat with the appropriate antimicrobial agent. The drugs in Table 29-1 are approved by the U.S. Food and Drug Administration for treating bronchopneumonia in cattle.

Ideally, specimens for antimicrobial sensitivity testing are collected from pneumonic lung, tracheal swabs, or tracheobronchial aspirates before treatment. However, in practice, first-line antibiotics are often selected on the basis of prior performance of a drug.

Duration of therapy

Therapy should be continued for at least 48 hours after clinical signs have abated. Antibiotics are often evaluated over a standard 3-day course (longer for enzootic calf pneumonia); animals that remain febrile are classified as nonresponders. Nonresponders to first-line antibiotics may be placed on an alternate antibiotic for a set period (e.g., 4 days).

Mass medication

Mass medication with antibiotics at full therapeutic doses during a feedlot outbreak of pneumonia dramatically curtails the number of new cases and improves feed consumption. Ceftiofur HCl, enrofloxacin, florfenicol, tilmicosin, long-acting oxytetracycline, or sustained-release sulfonamides can be given to every calf, or sulfonamides can be administered in the drinking water for 5 days.

Sheep and goats

The same principles of therapy apply to bronchopneumonia in sheep and goats. Tetracycline (5 mg/kg IM two times daily for 5 or 6 days) is usually effective. Other suitable choices include sulfonamides, penicillin, and erythromycin.

Antiinflammatory therapy

Favorable responses to corticosteroid therapy (e.g., dexamethasone 5 to 25 mg IM or IV; isoflupredone acetate 10 to 20 mg IM) and antihistamines (e.g., tripelennamine 1.1 mg/kg) have been reported for outbreaks of BRSV infection. Corticosteroids should not be used indiscriminately because of the potential for immunosuppression. NSAIDs such as aspirin (100 mg/kg two times daily), flunixin meglumine (1.1 to 2.2 mg/kg, single dose or divided into two doses given every 12 hours), phenylbutazone, and ibuprofen can be beneficial when used with care. Dehydrated animals should be rehydrated before NSAIDs are administered. NSAIDs should not be overdosed or used for prolonged periods.

Antiviral therapy

Human leukocyte interferon is currently approved for prophylactic treatment of "shipping fever" associated with BHV-1 infections in certain states.

Supportive care

Sick animals should be provided shelter from rain, cold, wind, and hot sun. They should not be crowded, and the best quality feed should be provided. Mineral and vitamin deficiencies should be corrected with injectable or oral preparations. An intramuscular injection of vitamin A should be a standard part of the first day's treatment.

Prevention of Bronchopneumonia

Prevention and control, including management, vaccination, and metaphylactic antimicrobial therapy, are discussed at length in Chapter 29 of *Large Animal Internal Medicine*, third edition.

INTERSTITIAL PNEUMONIAS *(Text pp. 571-580)*

Interstitial pneumonias can be classified into four groups: (1) acute respiratory distress syndromes (ARDS), (2) hypersensitivity diseases, (3) chronic conditions

TABLE 29-1

Antimicrobials Approved by the FDA for Treatment of Bronchopneumonia of Beef Cattle

Antimicrobial	Label dosage	Route administration	Treatment interval (hr)	Withdrawal for slaughter
STANDARD PREPARATIONS				
Amoxicillin	11 mg/kg	IM, SC	12	25 days
Ampicillin	2-5 mg/kg	SC	12	6 days
Ceftiofur (sodium)	1.1 mg/kg	IM, SC	24	0 days
Ceftiofur (HCl)	1.1 mg/kg	IM, SC	24	48 hours
Enrofloxacin	2.5-5.5 mg/kg	SC	24	28 days
Erythromycin	2.2-4.4 mg/kg	IM	24	14 days
Oxytetracycline	11 mg/kg	IV, IM, SC	24	15-22 days*
Procaine penicillin G	6600 U/kg	IM, SC	24	7 days
Spectinomycin	10-15 mg/kg	SC	24	11 days
Sulfachloropyridazine	33-50 mg/kg	IV (injectable)	12	7 days
Sulfadimethoxine	200 mg/kg initial treatment	IV (injectable)	24	10 days
	130 mg/kg daily thereafter	Oral (bolus)		
Tylosin	17 mg/kg	IM	24	21 days
LONG-ACTING PREPARATIONS				
Ceftiofur HCl	2.2 mg/kg	IM, SC	48	48 hours
Enrofloxacin	7.5-12.5 mg/kg	SC	Licensed for one treatment only	28 days
Florfenicol	20 mg/kg	IM	48	28 days
	40 mg/kg	SC	Licensed for one treatment only	38 days
Oxytetracycline	20 mg/kg	IM, SC	48	28 days
Penicillin G benzathine/penicillin G procaine	8800 U/kg	IM, SC	48	30 days
Sulfadimethoxine (sustained release bolus)	137.5 mg/kg	PO	96	21 days
Tilmicosin	10 mg/kg	SC	72	28 days

*Varies with preparation

that may be sequelae of ARDS or hypersensitivity diseases, and (4) parasitic diseases. ARDS includes any respiratory condition characterized clinically by sudden onset of dyspnea (usually severe) and pathologically by any combination of the following pulmonary lesions: congestion and edema, hyaline membranes, alveolar epithelial hyperplasia, and interstitial emphysema.

Acute Bovine Pulmonary Edema and Emphysema

Acute bovine pulmonary edema and emphysema (ABPEE), or "fog fever," is an ARDS of cattle more than 2 years old that are changed from dry, sparse forage to lush, green pasture. It results from ruminal conversion of L-tryptophan to 3-methylindol, a pneumotaxic compound. The disease usually appears as a herd outbreak, but individuals may be affected to widely varying degrees. The problem is more common in the fall.

Clinical findings

Signs usually occur within 2 weeks of the pasture change. In severe cases, there is an acute onset of severe dyspnea with a loud expiratory grunt, frothing at the mouth, tachypnea, and obvious distress. Temperature and heart rate may be elevated, and subcutaneous emphysema may develop. Coughing is *not* a prominent sign. On auscultation, breath sounds are surprisingly soft; a few crackles may be heard. Up to 30% of severely affected animals may die, usually within 2 days. Those that survive typically show dramatic improvement after 3 days.

Treatment

In view of the dangers of handling affected cattle, the questionable efficacy of medical treatment, the probably irreversible nature of severe lesions, and the probability of spontaneous recovery in less severe cases, the best treatment may be no treatment. If treatment is attempted, affected cattle should be handled very cautiously. Furosemide (0.4 to 1 mg/kg IM or IV two times daily) and flunixin meglumine (0.5 to 1.1 mg/kg IM or IV sid or two times daily) may be useful.

Prevention

Prophylactic treatment with monensin or lasalocid at 200 mg/head/day PO reduces the conversion of tryptophan to 3-methylindol. Treatment must begin at least 1 day (monensin) or 6 days (lasalocid) before the pasture change and should be continued for an additional 10 days.

Acute Respiratory Distress Syndrome of Feedlot Cattle

Atypical interstitial pneumonia is an ARDS that sporadically occurs in feedlot cattle. The cause is often undetermined; dust and BRSV infection have been implicated. Signs include rapid onset of tachypnea and expiratory dyspnea with open-mouth breathing. Frothing at the mouth, cyanosis, tachycardia, and subcutaneous emphysema may also be observed. Rectal temperatures may be normal or elevated. Auscultation reveals dull areas throughout the lungs, with some crackles. Affected cattle are often found dead in the pen.

Treatment

Treatment is similar to that recommended for ABPEE. High case fatality rates may warrant immediate slaughter salvage, provided proper drug withdrawals are observed.

Moldy Sweet Potato Toxicity

This ARDS is caused by ingestion of a toxin (4-ipomeanol) produced by sweet potatoes infested with the fungus *Fusarium solani (javanicum)*. Intoxication causes acute onset of tachypnea, tachycardia, severe dyspnea with loud expiratory grunting, frothing at the mouth, and frequent deep coughing. Crackles and harsh bronchial sounds are heard on auscultation. The disease usually occurs in outbreak form. Signs typically begin within 1 day of exposure, and death may occur 2 to 5 days later. Morbidity and case fatality rates are high. Treatment has not been investigated, although the recommendations given for ABPEE may be tried.

Perilla Ketone Toxicity

Perilla ketone toxicity is an ARDS caused by ingestion of a pneumotoxin found in the leaves and seeds of *Perilla frutescens* (purple mint, Perilla mint, wild coleus, beefsteak plant), a common weed in the southeastern United States. The seed/flower stage (August to October) is especially toxic. Mature cows are most often affected. Signs include sudden onset of moderate to severe dyspnea, wheezing, frothing at the mouth, and an expiratory heave or grunt. In less severe cases the cow may pant. Poisoned cattle are frequently found dead. The recommendations for ABPEE should be followed if treatment is attempted.

Other Toxic Plants

Brassica spp. (rape, kale, turnip tops) are one of the types of pasture that can precipitate ABPEE. Morbidity and mortality rates are much higher on *Brassica* spp. pastures than on other lush forages. Pyrrolizidine alkaloids cause lung lesions in animals with chronic liver damage, although signs of liver disease usually predominate. *Crotalaria* and *Trichoderma* spp. are the most common offenders; *Senecio* spp. are a less common cause.

Toxic Gases

Ruminants may be exposed to a variety of toxic gases in their environment. The most important are ammonia, hydrogen sulfide, carbon dioxide, and methane from excreta and respiration. Treatment involves the establishment of adequate ventilation; cows should be removed from closed buildings if possible. Suggested empiric therapy includes corticosteroids (dexamethasone 0.04 mg/kg IM or IV daily), furosemide (0.5 to 1.1 mg/kg IM or IV sid to three times daily), and antibiotics to prevent secondary bacterial infections.

Hypersensitivity Pneumonitis

Hypersensitivity pneumonitis, also known as extrinsic allergic alveolitis, is an allergic respiratory disease of confined adult cattle. It is caused by inhalation of organic dusts such as moldy hay, grain, or other plant matter.

Clinical findings

The acute form is characterized by sudden onset of dullness, inappetence, hypogalactia, coughing, tachypnea, dyspnea, and transient fever. Cranioventral crackles are heard on auscultation of the lungs. The chronic form is insidious in onset and may not be detected until there is considerable fibrosis. Chronic signs include hypogalactia, weight loss, productive coughing, tachypnea, obvious hyperpnea, and widespread crackles and wheezes on auscultation.

Treatment

Treatment and control center around removal of the offending antigens if possible. Corticosteroids (e.g., dexamethasone 0.04 mg/kg IV daily) may be beneficial in acute cases.

Anaphylaxis

In ruminants the lung is the major target organ for immediate (type I) hypersensitivity reactions. Precipitating causes include vaccines, drugs, blood, *Hypoderma bovis* or *Hypoderma lineatum* larvae, insect bites, and bee stings. Severe dyspnea with frothing at the mouth and abduction of the elbows usually develops in 10 to 20 minutes. Pharyngeal and laryngeal edema cause stertor and inspiratory dyspnea. Urticaria occurs in some cases. Shivering, salivation, lacrimation, pruritus, diarrhea, fever, edema (eyes, muzzle, anus, and vulva), collapse, nystagmus, cyanosis, and discharge of froth from the nostrils may also be seen.

Treatment

Treatment should include the following:

- Epinephrine 4 to 8 mg (4 to 8 ml of 1:1000 solution) IM or SC, or 1 to 5 mg IV, for an average cow; 1 to 3 mg IM or SC for an average adult sheep or goat
- Dexamethasone (0.22 mg/kg IM or IV) or prednisolone (2.2 mg/kg IM or IV)

NSAIDs (see p. 170) and diethylcarbamazine may also be useful. Other supportive therapies include shock doses of IV fluids (40 ml/kg/hr) with sodium bicarbonate, aminophylline, furosemide, oxygen therapy, and tracheostomy if necessary.

Chronic Interstitial Pneumonias

Fibrosing alveolitis

Fibrosing alveolitis is a chronic disease of unknown and possibly multiple causes. It occurs sporadically in adult cattle in both housing and pasture conditions. The history is usually that of a chronic progressive respiratory disease. Affected cattle remain bright and alert and continue to eat until the terminal stages of cor pulmonale and heart failure. Signs include marked weight loss, consistent coughing, tachypnea, marked hyperpnea (even at rest), and dyspnea after mild exertion. Fever is not a feature. No treatment exists, and the lesions are irreversible.

Bronchiolitis obliterans

Bronchiolitis obliterans is a chronic respiratory condition of yearling or young adult cattle, characterized by a deep infrequent cough, tachypnea, hyperpnea, and exaggerated expiratory effort. Affected cattle are afebrile. The condition is speculated to be a sequela of infection with respiratory viruses, lungworm infestation, or hypersensitivity pneumonitis.

Lungworm Infestation in Cattle

Clinical infection with *Dictyocaulus viviparus* occurs in two forms: (1) primary infection, in which young stock (less than 1 year old) or previously unexposed cattle are exposed for the first time; and (2) reinfection syndrome, in which previously infected adults are subjected to massive challenge with infective larvae. This is a disease involving groups of cattle at pasture.

Clinical findings

During the prepatent phase, there is a gradual onset of coughing and tachypnea. In the patent phase, pneumonia with consolidation develops in the ventral areas of the caudal lung lobes. Signs include coughing (intermittent to marked), tachypnea, dyspnea, anorexia, and weight loss. Death is common in untreated, heavily infected animals. Recovery begins in the late patent phase. Reinfection syndrome occurs 14 to 16 days after adult cattle are placed on heavily contaminated pastures. Signs include acute hypogalactia; severe, frequent coughing; marked tachypnea; and depression. Auscultation reveals only harsh breath sounds.

Diagnosis and treatment

Larvae of *D. viviparus* are detected by the Baermann sedimentation technique (rectal fecal samples) and may also be seen in transtracheal wash fluid. No larvae are detected in reinfection syndrome. Anthelmintics approved for treatment of *D. viviparus* in the United States include levamisole, fenbendazole, oxfendazole, albendazole, ivermectin, eprinomectin, doramectin, and moxidectin (see Chapter 45).

Ascaris suum Infestation

Cattle exposed to large numbers of *Ascaris suum* eggs in areas contaminated by swine may develop interstitial pneumonia within 10 days after exposure. Recommended treatments include corticosteroids (dexamethasone 0.04 mg/kg IM or IV, or prednisolone 1 mg/kg IM or IV daily), antibiotics to control secondary bacterial infection, and anthelmintics.

Lungworm Infestation in Sheep and Goats

Lungworms in sheep and goats are most often a problem in warm climates and on irrigated pastures in hot areas. Diagnosis is by Baermann examination of fecal samples.

Dictyocaulus filaria

Mainly young animals are affected by the parasite *Dictyocaulus filaria*, but disease can occur in adults. Clinical signs include dyspnea, tachypnea, coughing, and loss of condition. Levamisole (8 mg/kg), fenbendazole (5 to 10 mg/kg), ivermectin (0.2 mg/kg PO), and moxidectin (0.2 mg/kg PO or by injection) can be used for treatment.

Muellerius capillaris

Muellerius capillaris is probably the most common of the lungworms. It is less pathogenic in sheep than in goats, in which it may cause unthriftiness, coughing, and dyspnea, and may predispose to secondary bacterial infection. Control of *M. capillaris* infections can be difficult because of inhibited larval stages. Suggested treatments in goats include fenbendazole (15 mg/kg two or three times at 35-day intervals, or 1.25 to 5 mg/kg/day, 1 week on, 1 week off, 1 week on), albendazole (10 mg/kg, or 1 mg/kg/day for 7 to 14 days), oxfendazole (7.5 to 10 mg/kg), and ivermectin (0.3 mg/kg). *M. capillaris* is largely resistant to levamisole.

Protostrongylus rufescens

Most *Protostrongylus rufescens* infestations are subclinical or produce only mild signs (nasal discharge and cough). Treatment is similar to that for *D. filaria* infestation.

PROGRESSIVE PNEUMONIAS OF SHEEP AND GOATS *(Text pp. 581-583)*

Chronic progressive pneumonias are frequently diagnosed in mature small ruminants. In sheep, ovine progressive pneumonia (OPP) and caseous lymphadenitis (CLA) are the chief causes. Chronic respiratory disease in goats is commonly associated with CLA and less frequently with caprine arthritis-encephalitis virus (see Chapter 36).

Ovine Progressive Pneumonia (Maedi-Visna)

OPP and maedi-visna are names for slow-virus diseases of sheep characterized by chronic progressive pneumonia, wasting, and indurative aseptic mastitis. OPP is usually observed in 2- to 3-year-old sheep, but adult sheep of any age can be affected. Emaciation despite a good appetite is one of the earliest symptoms. Clinical signs of OPP include exercise intolerance, tachypnea, expiratory dyspnea, and occasionally a dry cough. Pyrexia and purulent nasal discharge indicate secondary bacterial pneumonia. Death occurs within 6 to 12 months. Presumptive diagnosis of OPP can be made on the basis of clinical signs, lack of response to treatment, and serologic findings. The condition is untreatable.

Ovine Pulmonary Carcinoma

Ovine pulmonary carcinoma (OPC; sheep pulmonary adenomatosis, jaagsiekte) is a transmissible bronchioloalveolar carcinoma of sheep, possibly caused by jaagsiekte sheep retrovirus. Affected sheep usually are 2 to 4 years of age. Clinical manifestations include progressive weight loss, exercise intolerance, tachypnea, dyspnea, and occasional coughing. Abundant watery nasal discharge can often be demonstrated by raising the animal's rear limbs to lower its head. Appetite and rectal temperature are usually normal. Affected sheep die within a few weeks or months. Molecular diagnostic tests are being developed to identify affected sheep. There is no treatment.

Caseous Lymphadenitis

CLA is caused by *C. pseudotuberculosis* and is characterized by pyogranulomatous abscesses in the lymph nodes and lungs of sheep and goats. Visceral CLA with lung involvement is a common cause of severe weight loss in small ruminants. CLA is discussed further in Chapter 35.

Diagnosis

Definitive diagnosis can be reached by demonstrating abscesses in the lungs and mediastinal lymph nodes and by isolating *C. pseudotuberculosis* from a transtracheal aspirate. However, failure to isolate the organism from tracheal wash fluid does not rule out CLA as a cause of pulmonary disease. The synergistic hemolysis inhibition test can be used to diagnose early infections and aid in the diagnosis of internal abscesses. False-negative results are rare; false-positive results reportedly occur in 10% of sheep and 20% of goats.

OTHER PNEUMONIAS *(Text pp. 584-589)*

Aspiration Pneumonia

Aspiration pneumonia is caused by inhalation of large amounts of foreign material, often liquids. Signs include depression, tachypnea, dyspnea, coughing, fever, and in some cases, putrid breath. Crackles, wheezes, and occasionally pleural friction rubs can be heard on auscultation. Antibiotics combined with antiinflammatory agents (NSAIDs and corticosteroids) should be administered IV. Long-term antimicrobial therapy is required. The prognosis is guarded.

Mycotic Pneumonias

Coccidioides immitis, Aspergillus spp., *Histoplasma capsulatum, Candida albicans,* and *Mucorales* spp. occasionally cause pneumonia in ruminants. Treatment either has not been investigated or has been unsuccessful.

Other Contagious Pneumonias

Contagious bovine pleuropneumonia is a highly fatal disease of cattle caused by *Mycoplasma mycoides* subsp. *mycoides* (small-colony type). It was eradicated from the United States long ago and now occurs mainly in portions of Asia, Central Africa, Spain, and Portugal. Contagious caprine pleuropneumonia is a highly fatal disease of goats in Africa, the Middle East, and western Asia. *Mycoplasma* F38 is currently considered the cause.

Mycoplasma Pneumonia of Goats

Several species of *Mycoplasma* can cause pneumonia in goats. The large-colony type *M. mycoides* subsp. *mycoides* (Mmm) is a major cause of mortality among goat kids and does.

Clinical signs

In infected herds, kids usually appear clinically normal until 2 to 8 weeks of age, when one of three clinical syndromes occurs: (1) peracute illness characterized by high fever and death within 12 to 24 hours; (2) central nervous system syndrome with opisthotonus and death within 24 to 72 hours; and (3) an acute or subacute syndrome with high fever, multiple joint swelling and heat, and pneumonia. During an outbreak, 80% to 90% of kids die or are euthanized. Mmm infection in adult does is also life-threatening and is characterized by mastitis, polyarthritis, and pneumonia.

Diagnosis

Definitive diagnosis of Mmm infection in individuals requires isolation of the agent from milk, joint fluid, blood, urine, or tissue. Infected goat herds can readily be identified by culturing bulk tank milk. Inapparent carriers can be identified by milk culture, but false negatives are possible as the organism is shed intermittently. An enzyme-linked immunosorbent assay is available for diagnosis of Mmm.

Treatment

Tylosin or tetracyclines are commonly used treatments, but conventional antibiotic therapy is almost always unsuccessful. A small percentage of kids make a clinical recovery but often have arthritis by the time they freshen. Does that recover from mastitis become chronic carriers. Prevention and control strategies are discussed in Chapter 29 of *Large Animal Internal Medicine,* third edition.

Vena Caval Thrombosis and Metastatic Pneumonia

Metastatic or embolic pneumonia is characterized by septic embolization and multifocal abscess of the lungs. The emboli arise from septic thrombi in the caudal (and, less commonly, the cranial) vena cava. The most common cause of vena caval thrombi is liver abscess secondary to rumenitis. Less common causes include jugular phlebitis, mastitis, metritis, and foot rot. The most common isolates are *F. necrophorum, A. pyogenes,* staphylococci, streptococci, and *E. coli.*

Clinical findings

This condition is most commonly seen in feedlot cattle, but any age, breed, sex, and class of cattle may be affected. The duration of signs is variable, ranging from acute respiratory distress to a chronic history of weight loss and coughing. The classic presentation includes tachycardia, tachypnea, expiratory dyspnea and groaning, coughing, hemic murmurs and pale mucous membranes (anemia), widespread wheezes, epistaxis, and hemoptysis. The combination of respiratory signs with anemia and hemoptysis is pathognomonic. Most animals deteriorate rapidly once hemoptysis becomes evident. In chronic cases, cor pulmonale may lead to signs of right-sided heart failure, such as jugular distention and brisket edema.

Treatment

The prognosis is grave, so treatment is rarely indicated. In valuable individuals, antibiotics and supportive therapy may be tried. Penicillin is the drug of choice for the most common organisms involved; large doses (at least 22,000 U/kg IM or SC two times daily) should be given for several weeks. Supportive therapy includes furosemide (0.4 to 1.1 mg/kg IV or IM two times daily), flunixin (0.5 to 1.1 mg/kg IM or IV one to three times daily), and atropine (0.04 mg/kg SC once daily).

Tuberculosis

Mycobacterium bovis is the most common cause of tuberculosis in cattle and goats. Most infected animals do not show clinical abnormalities, yet they pose health risks to other livestock and to humans. Chronic weight loss, variable appetite, and fluctuating fevers (often accentuated after calving) may be seen. Other signs depend on the organs involved. Signs referable to the lower respiratory tract are relatively common but usually mild. The intradermal tuberculin test is routinely used to identify infected animals. This test and eradication programs are discussed in Chapter 29 of *Large Animal Internal Medicine*, third edition.

DISEASES OF THE THORACIC WALL AND CAVITY *(Text pp. 589-592)*

Pleuritis and Pleural Effusion

Pleuritis or pleural effusion is almost always secondary to such conditions as bronchopneumonia, traumatic reticulopericarditis, liver abscesses, tumors (especially lymphosarcoma), external trauma, various septicemic conditions, and hypoproteinemia. Signs of pleural inflammation and effusion in ruminants are similar to those described in horses (see pp. 501-502), although they may be overshadowed by the primary disease process.

Diagnosis

Complete blood count helps to separate infectious from noninfectious causes and distinguish relatively acute conditions (with significant left shifts) from those of a more chronic nature (with mature neutrophilia, hyperglobulinemia, and nonregenerative anemia). Pleural fluid should be collected for cytologic examination and cultured for bacteria, mycoplasma, and chlamydia. Transtracheal wash is usually indicated because of the common association with pneumonia.

Treatment

The primary problem must be treated. Pleural effusion should be drained, either intermittently (simplest) or continuously. Antibiotics are indicated in the presence of sepsis. NSAIDs (see p. 590) or narcotic analgesics (e.g., meperidine [Demerol], morphine, butorphanol) are useful to relieve pain, ease respiration, and improve appetite. Rest and good nursing care are essential.

Pneumothorax

Pneumothorax is uncommon in ruminants. Most cases result from rupture of an emphysematous bulla or from puncture of the lung by a fractured rib. Lung collapse is usually unilateral. Unless an infectious disease is responsible, affected animals are often alert and anxious, and there is a pronounced abdominal component to the breathing. Cyanosis may develop. Simultaneous auscultation and percussion may produce a "ping" over the dorsal thorax. Subcutaneous emphysema and pleuritis often accompany pneumothorax. The diagnosis is confirmed radiographically.

Treatment

If a wound is present, it should be closed and the air aspirated from the thorax. In cases of internal pneumothorax, dorsal aspiration should be attempted using a three-way stopcock on a teat cannula and a large syringe or a vacuum pump. Appropriate antibiotics are indicated.

Diaphragmatic Hernia

Diaphragmatic hernias are uncommon in ruminants. Causes include congenital, traumatic reticuloperitonitis; difficult parturition; and external trauma. Affected animals can be asymptomatic for a prolonged period. The history may include decreased milk production, weight loss, capricious appetite, difficulty in swallowing or regurgitation, abdominal pain, vomiting, and abnormal posturing of the head and neck on swallowing or regurgitation. Respiratory signs are fairly uncommon; gastrointestinal signs are more common. Radiography is the best means of confirming the diagnosis. Treatment involves surgical repair.

Pleural Mesothelioma

Pleural mesotheliomas in cattle have been reported. They result in accumulation of large amounts of pleural fluid, so signs are related to pleural effusion. If peritoneal lesions are also present (which is common), ascites occurs. Thoracocentesis yields serous, sometimes blood-tinged, or gelatinous fluid. Cytologic examination may reveal reactive mesothelial cells. There is no treatment.

30

Diseases of the Alimentary Tract

Consulting Editors MICHAEL J. MURRAY • BRADFORD P. SMITH

Contributors ANDREW T. FISCHER, JR. • JACK EASLEY
ANTHONY T. BLIKSLAGER • SAMUEL L. JONES • NATHANIEL A. WHITE II
ROBERT J. MACKAY • VANESSA L. COOK • ROBIN M. DABAREINER
GUY D. LESTER • NOAH D. COHEN • KEVIN CORLEY • GUY ST. JEAN
PAUL G.E. MICHELSEN • DAN GROOMS • JOHN C. BAKER • TREVOR R. AMES
CHARLES GUARD • FRANKLYN GARRY • GILLES FECTEAU
ROBERT WHITLOCK • JOHN MAAS • SPRING K. HALLAND

Part I: Equine Alimentary System

DIAGNOSTIC PROCEDURES *(Text pp. 593-600)*

Evaluation of the alimentary system using rectal examination, abdominocentesis, endoscopy, laparoscopy, radiography, ultrasonography, scintigraphy, biopsy, fecal examination, and absorption/digestion tests are discussed in *Large Animal Internal Medicine,* third edition.

DENTISTRY AND ORAL DISEASE *(Text pp. 600-608)*

Anatomy and function, dental examination, routine dental maintenance, and dental radiography are discussed in *Large Animal Internal Medicine,* third edition.

Clinical Signs of Dental Disease

Clinical signs of dental disease variably include abnormal behavior while eating (quidding or head tilting), reluctance to eat, loss of condition, halitosis, blood or excessive saliva in the mouth, abnormal head shaking or shyness, abnormal head carriage or signs of pain associated with position or use of the bit, oral or facial trauma, facial swelling, drainage from the mandible or maxilla, and chronic fetid nasal discharge.

Periradicular Disease (Bone Surrounding Tooth Roots)

Chronic alveolar abscess with periradicular bone erosion and drainage to the outside or into the nasal passages or paranasal sinuses is the most common form of periradicular disease.

Treatment

After radiographic assessment, treatment may involve removal of the deciduous cap that is impeding eruption of the involved cheek tooth, reshaping the neighboring cheek teeth to permit eruption, root-end resection and apical seal (root canal), or removal of the infected tooth. Antibiotic therapy is also indicated as gram-negative bacteria and anaerobes are commonly involved. Appropriate treatment choices include the following:

- Ceftiofur (2 to 4 mg/kg intramuscularly [IM] or intravenously [IV] two or

three times daily) or chloramphenicol (30 to 50 mg/kg orally [PO] four times daily for 30 days) in combination with penicillin (20,000 U/kg IV four times daily)
- Metronidazole (15 mg/kg PO three or four times daily) with penicillin only if *Bacteroides fragilis* is suspected

Management of sinusitis secondary to dental disease is discussed in Chapter 29.

Dental Decay

When oral examination reveals a black spot in a cheek tooth, deep probing and irrigation with a needle and syringe are indicated to determine the depth of the defect. Infection of the pulp secondary to infundibular decay can be managed by endodontic therapy or by tooth removal.

Periodontal Disease

Periodontal disease is progressive inflammation of the gingivae, resorption of alveolar bone, degeneration of the periodontal membrane, apical migration of the epithelial attachment, formation of periodontal pockets, and loosening of the tooth. Periodontal disease is most often associated with extreme abnormalities of wear, such as wave mouth, shear mouth, hooks, tooth loss with overgrowth of the opposing tooth, and misplaced or split teeth.

Treatment

Daily cleaning of gingival pockets with a water pick can slow disease progression. Once the disease has progressed to the point of destroying the bony attachment to the tooth, the loose tooth should be removed.

ORAL TUMORS *(Text p. 607)*

Oral tumors are rare in horses. These tumors can be divided into three basic types: odontogenic (e.g., ameloblastomas, odontomas, cementomas), osteogenic (e.g., osteosarcoma), and secondary (e.g., squamous cell carcinoma, lymphosarcoma, papilloma, melanoma). Squamous cell carcinoma is the most common oral neoplasm. These tumors are generally seen in older horses. An array of treatment options have been tried with variable results.

SALIVARY GLANDS AND DUCTS *(Text p. 608)*

Sialoliths

Sialoliths most often develop around an organic nidus (e.g., cell debris, grain husk or grass awn) in the salivary duct. Most sialoliths are hard, smooth, movable, painless, radiodense enlargements over the cheek at the level of the upper dental arcade. Abscessation with pain, hypersalivation, and fistula formation can occur. Surgical removal and primary wound closure yield good results.

Mucoceles and Ranulae

Salivary mucocele is an accumulation of salivary secretions in a single or multiloculated cavity adjacent to a ruptured duct. A ranula is a mucocele that occurs secondary to obstruction of the sublingual salivary duct. Treatment consists of creating a salivary fistula into the oral cavity or excising the mucocele and associated salivary gland.

Salivary Duct Trauma

Lacerations or iatrogenic injury to the salivary ducts can lead to salivary cutaneous fistula. These injuries should be surgically repaired by reapposing the severed duct, creating an oral opening for the duct, or resecting the salivary gland. Ablation and sclerosis of the gland can be achieved by flushing 1% formalin solution up the duct.

ESOPHAGEAL DISORDERS *(Text pp. 608-616)*

Esophageal Obstruction (Choke)

Esophageal obstruction may be primary (simple choke) or secondary to other disease processes. Most primary impactions are caused by feed (e.g., hay, apples) or bedding materials. Secondary impactions are caused by intraluminal or extraluminal abnormalities that impede food passage, such as strictures, diverticula, cysts, vascular ring anomalies, and cervical or mediastinal masses (e.g., tumors, abscesses). Complications of esophageal impaction include metabolic alkalosis; esophageal ulceration, stricture, or perforation; aspiration pneumonia; and megaesophagus.

Clinical signs

Clinical signs include anxiety, standing with the neck extended, gagging or retching, bilateral frothy nasal discharge containing saliva and food material, coughing, odynophagia, ptyalism, and dysphagia. Distention of the cervical esophagus may be evident at the site of obstruction. Other clinical signs that may be observed relate to complications stemming from the obstruction, such as dehydration, weight loss, aspiration pneumonia, and esophageal rupture.

Diagnosis

Thorough physical examination, including a complete oral examination, must be performed to rule out other causes of hypersalivation, dysphagia, and nasal discharge. Palpation of the jugular furrow may reveal a mass associated with the impaction. Crepitus or cellulitis suggests esophageal rupture. Passage of a nasogastric tube determines whether and where an obstruction is present. Although ultrasonography and radiography can be useful, definitive evaluation often requires endoscopic examination. Foreign bodies may even be retrievable via endoscopy.

Treatment

The primary goal of treatment is to relieve the obstruction:

1. Reduce esophageal spasms–options include acepromazine (0.05 mg/kg IV), xylazine (0.25 to 0.5 mg/kg IV), detomidine (0.01 to 0.02 mg/kg IV), oxytocin (0.11 to 0.22 IU/kg IM), and esophageal instillation of lidocaine (30 to 60 ml of 1% lidocaine).
2. Resolve the impaction–a nasogastric tube is used to displace the impacted material (in conjunction with external massage for cervical obstructions); it is often necessary to lavage the impaction with water via the nasogastric tube while the horse's head is lowered.

In refractory cases and when the obstruction has been present for more than 48 hours, intravenous administration of 0.9% saline containing potassium chloride (KCl; 10 to 20 mEq/L) at a rate of 50 to 100 ml/kg/day is recommended in conjunction with esophageal relaxants such as oxytocin. Some refractory cases require esophagotomy. Food and water should be withheld until the obstruction is resolved.

Aftercare

Care after resolution of the obstruction should include the following:

- Withhold food for 24 to 48 hours.
- For obstructions lasting more than 48 hours, correct dehydration, hyponatremia, hypochloremia, and hypokalemia with oral electrolyte solutions or intravenous saline with KCl (as described previously).
- Evaluate the esophagus using endoscopy (and, if indicated, ultrasonography or contrast radiography) for mucosal ulceration, esophageal rupture, masses, or strictures.
- Gradually reintroduce food.
  - After 48 hours, or once the mucosa has recovered (as assessed by endoscopy), offer soft foods (e.g., moistened pellets and bran mash).
  - Gradually reintroduce high-quality roughage over the next 7 to 21 days.
- Reevaluate every 2 to 4 weeks if mucosal injury or esophageal dilation was noted.

If aspiration pneumonia is suspected, give broad-spectrum antibiotics and metronidazole. Sucralfate (20 mg/kg PO every 6 hours) may hasten healing of esophageal ulceration. Administration of flunixin meglumine (1 mg/kg PO or IV every 12 hours) or phenylbutazone (1.1 mg/kg PO or IV every 12 hours) for 2 to 4 weeks may limit stricture formation after mucosal ulceration.

Esophagitis

Causes of esophagitis in horses include trauma (foreign bodies, nasogastric tube), infection (mural abscesses), chemical injury (medications, cantharidin), and disorders allowing reflux of gastric contents (gastric ulcer disease, motility disorders, gastric outflow obstructions, gastric paresis, intestinal ileus, impaired lower esophageal sphincter function).

Clinical signs and diagnosis

Clinical signs are nonspecific: gagging or discomfort when swallowing, hypersalivation, bruxism, partial or complete anorexia (leading to weight loss in chronic cases). Clinical signs of an underlying disease may predominate. Diagnosis requires endoscopic examination of the esophagus. The stomach should also be examined endoscopically.

Treatment

The principles of treatment for reflux esophagitis include the following:

- Control gastric acidity (see Gastric Ulceration)
- Correct any underlying disorder
- Consider using prokinetics for foals with delayed gastric emptying
  - Metoclopramide (0.02 to 0.1 mg/kg subcutaneously [SC] every 4 to 12 hours) with caution (can cause neurologic dysfunction)
  - Bethanechol (0.025 to 0.035 mg/kg SC every 4 to 24 hours or 0.035 to 0.045 mg/kg PO every 6 to 8 hours)

For esophagitis secondary to trauma or esophageal impaction, judicious use of nonsteroidal antiinflammatory drugs (NSAIDs) may be warranted. Horses with mild to moderate esophagitis should be fed frequent small meals of moistened pellets and fresh grass. Severe esophagitis may necessitate withholding food for several days.

Esophageal Hypomotility

Esophageal hypomotility results in esophageal dilation or megaesophagus. Causes include esophageal obstruction, gastric outlet or duodenal obstruction (especially in foals), reflux esophagitis, and neurologic or neuromuscular disorders. Clinical signs are similar to those of esophageal obstruction. Signs attributable to an underlying disease process may also be evident. Diagnosis requires transit studies using fluoroscopy or contrast radiography (see main text).

Treatment

Treatment should be aimed at resolving the underlying cause. Slurries of pellets should be fed from an elevated position to promote esophageal transit. Metoclopramide or bethanechol may be beneficial for increasing lower esophageal tone and gastric emptying.

Esophageal Perforation

Perforation of the esophagus may result from external trauma, excessive force with a nasogastric tube, or rupture of an esophageal lesion (e.g., impacted diverticulum). Perforation typically occurs in the cervical region. The resulting drainage of saliva and feed material within fascial planes often causes extensive tissue necrosis, cellulitis, and endotoxemia. Closed perforations may result in migration of wound discharge into the mediastinum and pleural space. Extensive subcutaneous and fascial emphysema is also a feature of esophageal perforation.

Treatment and prognosis

Treatment should involve the following:

- Conversion of closed perforations to open perforations if possible
- Extensive wound debridement and lavage

- Broad-spectrum antibiotics
- Tetanus prophylaxis
- Esophageal rest
  - Provide nourishment through a feeding tube placed in the esophagus via the wound or through a narrow nasogastric tube.
  - Oral feeding may begin once the wound has granulated and contracted to a small size.

The prognosis is poor, largely because of the extent of cellulitis, tissue necrosis, shock, and local wound complications. Wound healing takes a prolonged period. Some perforations never completely heal, forming permanent esophagocutaneous fistulae.

Esophageal Stricture

Strictures most commonly occur as sequelae to esophageal obstructions. Other causes include oral administration of corrosive medications and cervical trauma. Strictures result in partial obstruction, so clinical signs are similar to those of simple obstruction. Esophageal webs or rings can be observed endoscopically; double-contrast radiography may be required to identify mural strictures or annular stenosis.

Treatment

Strictures resulting from simple obstruction may resolve with conservative therapy (NSAIDs, antibiotics, and feeding a slurry diet), although it may take 60 days for the esophagus to heal and remodel. If there is insufficient resolution of the stricture after 60 days, methods to increase the esophageal diameter should be investigated (see main text).

Other Esophageal Disorders

Congenital esophageal disorders (stenosis, persistent right aortic arch, duplication cysts), esophageal diverticula, and esophageal neoplasia are briefly discussed in *Large Animal Internal Medicine,* third edition.

DISORDERS OF THE STOMACH *(Text pp. 617-623)*

Gastric Ulceration

Equine gastric ulcer syndrome encompasses lesions in the squamous or glandular mucosa, focal or multifocal ulceration, generalized gastritis, gastric emptying disorders, gastroesophageal reflux, and obstructive disorders. Risk factors include stress (e.g., race training, illness, pain), inappetence or disruptions in feeding or nursing, certain diets and feeding practices, and NSAID administration.

Clinical signs in foals

Clinical signs associated with gastric ulcers in foals include bruxism, dorsal recumbency, ptyalism, interrupted nursing, diarrhea, and colic. However, relatively few foals with endoscopically observed ulcers show these signs. Thus, when clinical signs are seen, severe ulceration likely exists. Chronic ulceration may result in intermittent diarrhea and colic, poor growth, rough hair coat, and a pendulous abdomen.

Clinical signs in adults

Signs associated with gastric lesions in yearlings and adult horses include colic, poor appetite, and poor bodily condition. Attitude changes, stiffness, a tucked-up abdomen, and poor performance may also be noted. However, most adult horses with gastric lesions do not demonstrate overt clinical signs. Gastric ulcers should be strongly considered in horses with recurrent colic.

Diagnosis

Diagnosis is based on the presence of age-related characteristic clinical signs, endoscopic findings (see main text), and response to treatment. In foals less than 30 days old, the presence of fecal occult blood may be indicative of gastroduodenal ulceration.

Treatment

Treatment involves addressing the underlying cause and using medications that alleviate discomfort and encourage ulcer healing (i.e., acid neutralizing or suppressive therapy). Drugs used to treat gastric and duodenal ulcers in foals and adult horses include the following:

- Proton pump inhibitors, such as omeprazole, 4 mg/kg PO once per day for 2 weeks initially
  - Ulcer healing is faster with omeprazole than with any other therapy; however, peak acid suppression is not reached until day 5 of treatment.
  - Omeprazole can prevent ulcers in horses in race training when given at 2 mg/kg PO once per day.
- Histamine type 2 (H_2) receptor antagonists for at least 3 weeks
  - Cimetidine 20 to 25 mg/kg PO every 8 hours or 6.6 mg/kg IV every 4 to 6 hours
  - Ranitidine 6.6 mg/kg PO every 8 hours or 1.5 mg/kg IV every 8 hours
  - Famotidine 3.3 mg/kg PO every 8 hours or 1 mg/kg IV every 8 hours
- Antacids such as Maalox TC (240 ml), Maalox Extra Strength (400 to 500 ml), or Mylanta II (400 to 500 ml) PO every 2 hours
- Mucosal protectants–sucralfate (10 to 20 mg/kg PO every 8 hours) or misoprostol (1.5 to 2.5 μg/kg PO every 8 hours); do not use with antacids
  - Sucralfate is most effective for ulceration in the glandular gastric mucosa.
  - Misoprostol may promote healing of glandular mucosal lesions; however, it can cause inappetence, diarrhea, and abdominal discomfort.

Clinical signs usually improve within 24 to 48 hours of initiating acid-suppressive therapy. If improvement is not observed, gastric ulceration should be considered a secondary problem. Management changes are as important as medical therapy. When possible, horses should be turned out to graze, grain should be limited, and training should cease.

Enhancing gastric emptying. Prokinetics may be indicated when gastroesophageal reflux, gastric outlet obstruction, or duodenal ulceration/inflammation is suspected. Available drugs include the following:

- Bethanechol 0.025 mg/kg SC every 4 to 6 hours, then 0.035 to 0.045 mg/kg PO every 6 to 8 hours
  - Adverse effects, although uncommon, include diarrhea, inappetence, salivation, and colic.
- Metoclopramide 0.1 to 0.25 mg/kg every 6 to 8 hours or constant intravenous infusion at 0.04 mg/kg/hr
  - Excitation can occur at the higher dosage rates.

Gastric Impaction

Gastric impaction occasionally occurs. Potential causes include certain feedstuffs (beet pulp, bran, straw, wheat, barley), impaired intestinal motility, dental disorders, and grass sickness. Impaction can be diagnosed by gastroscopy, radiography, or laparotomy. Gastric impaction can be treated medically with dioctyl sodium succinate (DSS; 4 to 8 oz of 5% solution in 4 to 6 L water via nasogastric tube) or repeated gastric lavage with water. Adjunctive treatment with bethanechol (0.02 mg/kg SC every 6 to 8 hours) may be helpful.

Gastric Rupture

Gastric rupture occurs as a sequela to gastric distention (whether from ingesta, fluid, or gas). Because of extensive peritoneal contamination, euthanasia is required.

Gastric Neoplasia

Although uncommon, squamous cell carcinoma is the most common neoplasm that affects the equine stomach. Most cases occur in older horses. The tumor can metastasize to the abdominal viscera and/or extend into the esophagus. Presenting signs include chronic weight loss, anemia, nasal reflux, and colic. Diagnosis can be made by gastroscopy, laparoscopy, contrast radiography, or peritoneal fluid analysis (with abdominal metastasis). There is no effective treatment.

Pyloric Stenosis

Pyloric stenosis can occur secondary to chronic ulceration and fibrosis or result from muscular hypertrophy (uncommon). Diagnosis is made by endoscopy (see main text). Treatment of pyloric stenosis is difficult. The objectives are to enhance gastric emptying and promote ulcer healing, as described earlier for gastric ulceration. If medical management is not effective, surgical bypass of the pylorus is indicated.

ENDOTOXEMIA *(Text pp. 633-640)*

Endotoxemia is the presence of endotoxin (gram-negative bacterial cell wall lipopolysaccharide) in the blood and the consequent clinical signs. A variety of disease conditions can precipitate endotoxemia, including gram-negative bacterial enterocolitis (e.g., salmonellosis), metritis, pleuropneumonia, wound infection, placentitis, neonatal septicemia, and damage to the gut wall (e.g., ischemic injury, enteritis, perforation, and grain overload).

Signs of Endotoxemia

Clinical signs can range from transient fever to multiple organ failure and death. Depression, restlessness, mild colic, and inappetence are typical behavioral changes. Common clinical findings include pyrexia, tachypnea, tachycardia, decreased or absent intestinal sounds, injected mucous membranes (with or without a dark "toxic" line around the gingival margins of the teeth), and prolonged capillary refill time. The inciting cause can greatly influence the clinical presentation (e.g., severe colic in horses with bowel strangulation, diarrhea in horses with salmonellosis).

Severe endotoxemia

Severe endotoxemia is manifested by signs of circulatory failure and disordered hemostasis. Affected horses usually are stuporous and totally anorectic. Other findings include dark, congested mucous membranes; rapid, weak peripheral pulses; cold extremities; sweating; muscle tremors; signs of dehydration (reduced skin turgor, dry mucous membranes, sunken eyes); drop in rectal temperature (to or below normal); oliguria or anuria; and recumbency.

Hypercoagulability

A poor prognostic sign is development of hypercoagulation syndrome, manifested as thrombosis after routine venipuncture or catheter placement, and secondary bleeding tendencies (prolonged hemorrhage from venipuncture sites and widespread mucosal petechiation). Infarction of bowel segments or lungs may cause severe clinical signs that are unresponsive to treatment.

Other signs

If moderately to severely affected animals survive for more than 24 hours, edema usually develops on the ventral abdomen and limbs. Signs of laminitis may become apparent at this stage and progress in severity despite improvement in other systemic signs of endotoxemia.

Laboratory Findings

With the exception of early and profound neutropenia (usually with a left shift and toxic changes) and hypoglycemia, laboratory findings are nonspecific and simply reflect altered tissue perfusion, organ dysfunction, and disordered hemostasis. Findings may include the following:

- Lactic acidosis, increased anion gap, hypoxemia
- Elevations in serum lactate dehydrogenase, creatine kinase, alkaline phosphatase, and bilirubin
- Azotemia and, in severe cases, proteinuria and hematuria
- Thrombocytopenia (platelet count less than 100,000/μl); hypofibrino-

genemia; increased fibrin degradation products; increased plasminogen activator inhibitor type 1; prolongation of activated partial thromboplastin, prothrombin, or thrombin time

Treatment of Endotoxemia

Circulatory support

Expansion of blood volume is the cornerstone of treatment:

- Administer balanced polyionic fluids IV (see p. 203).
  - Intravenous fluids should be supplemented with potassium (10 to 20 mmol/L). Never administer intravenous potassium faster than 1.0 mEq/kg/hr.
  - If blood pH is less than 7.2, HCO_3 is less than 15 mmol/L, or total CO_2 is less than 16 mmol/L, the base deficit should be replaced along with the initial fluid deficit.
- Compatible plasma (5 L for a 450-kg horse, 1 to 2 L for a neonate) or other colloid solutions (e.g., 6% hydroxyethyl starch [hetastarch]) may be used instead of crystalloids.
- Hypertonic saline (2 L of 7.2% NaCl for a 500-kg horse) may be used initially in horses with severe volume contraction; isotonic solutions should then be administered.
- If anuria or hypotension persists after volume expansion, infusions of dobutamine (2 to 15 μg/kg/min) and dopamine (1 to 3 μg/kg/min) should be considered.
  - Dilute 1 vial each of dobutamine and dopamine in 500 ml saline or 5% dextrose and infuse the mixture at 0.45 ml/kg/hr (200 ml/hr for a 450-kg horse).
  - Monitor heart rate and blood pressure (BP) frequently during infusion, especially in neonates.

Removal of the cause

Inflammatory effusions should be drained and appropriate antimicrobial drugs used. Intestinal problems should be corrected surgically if indicated. When endotoxemia is suspected but there is no evidence of extraintestinal gram-negative infection, antibiotics should only be given in the following circumstances: (1) foals less than 3 months old; (2) suspicion of clostridial enteritis (in which case, treat with metronidazole or vancomycin); (3) degenerative left shift or neutrophil count less than 1000/μl; or (4) evidence of dyshemostasis (e.g., jugular thrombosis or abnormal coagulogram).

NOTE: Antimicrobial therapy can temporarily worsen clinical signs. This possibility should be anticipated and minimized by timely use of NSAIDs or other antiendotoxic therapy.

Neutralization of circulating endotoxin

Options for neutralizing circulating endotoxin include the following:

- Antiserum (e.g., Endoserum) or hyperimmune plasma (e.g., Polymune J)
  - Although reports of efficacy vary, the use of 2 to 10 ml/kg hyperimmune plasma may be justified in the treatment of life-threatening endotoxemia.
- Polymyxin B 6000 U/kg (1 mg/kg) IV twice daily, given over at least 15 minutes

Inhibition of inflammatory effects

Options include the following:

- Flunixin meglumine 0.25 mg/kg IV every 6 to 8 hours
- Pentoxifylline 10 to 15 mg/kg PO twice daily
  - Concurrent use of flunixin may negate its beneficial effects.
- Heparin–should be considered in horses at high risk for laminitis (e.g., duodenitis-proximal jejunitis, grain overload) or with hypercoagulation syndrome
  - Unfractionated heparin is given at a dose of 200 to 300 IU/kg/day SC (divided twice daily) or as continuous intravenous infusion.
  - Low-molecular-weight heparin (Lovenox) is given at a dose of 50 anti-Xa IU/kg SC once per day.
  - For hypercoagulation syndrome, heparin should be given with plasma.

- Reactive oxygen species (ROS) scavengers–may be useful in limiting reperfusion injury after correction of bowel strangulation
  - Options include allopurinol (5 mg/kg IV) and DMSO (0.2 to 1 g/kg as a 10% to 20% solution IV or PO every 6 to 12 hours).

NOTE: Corticosteroids are contraindicated in the treatment of endotoxemia in adult horses.

Other treatments and preventive strategies that have been tried or are being studied are briefly discussed in *Large Animal Internal Medicine,* third edition.

MEDICAL DISORDERS OF THE SMALL INTESTINE *(Text pp. 641-648)*

Ulcerative Duodenitis

Duodenal ulceration and ulcerative duodenitis primarily affect foals and, less often, yearlings. Clinical signs are nonspecific and include fever, mild to moderate colic, mild obtundation, and diarrhea. Gastric ulceration commonly occurs secondary to duodenal ulceration and tends to be severe, often leading to reflux esophagitis. Complications of duodenal ulceration include duodenal perforation with peritonitis or adhesions, duodenal stricture with complete or partial obstruction, and ascending cholangitis, hepatitis, and pancreatitis.

Diagnosis

Duodenoscopy is the most specific means of diagnosis. Gastroscopic findings suggestive of duodenal dysfunction include excessive reflux of bile through the pylorus and ulceration at the pylorus or pyloric antrum. With severe ulceration, radiographs may reveal accumulation of fluid in the stomach and gas in the biliary ducts. Contrast studies may show delayed gastric emptying (more than 2 hours), mucosal irregularities in the duodenum, and possibly duodenal stricture.

Treatment

If duodenal ulceration is confirmed or even suspected, treatment should be aggressive. Treatment objectives are as follows:

- Decrease duodenal inflammation using corticosteroids, NSAIDs, or DMSO
  - Intravenous prednisolone (1 mg/kg once per day initially, then 0.5 mg/kg once per day) is recommended in acute cases or those in which delayed gastric emptying is suspected.
  - When oral medication can be given, prednisolone is given at 1 mg/kg PO once per day.
  - Flunixin meglumine is given at 1.5 mg/kg/day IV or IM, divided into three or four doses.
  - DMSO is given at 200 mg/kg IV as a 10% solution once or twice daily.
- Treat secondary gastric and esophageal ulceration (see Gastric Ulceration)
  - Intravenous administration of H_2 antagonists is recommended initially.
  - Once oral medication can be given, omeprazole (4 mg/kg PO once per day) should be used.
- Promote gastric emptying (see Gastric Ulceration)
- Treat related problems (e.g., peritonitis)

Foals with duodenitis should be prevented from nursing or eating feed for 1 to 3 days. During this time, parenteral feeding should be considered (see main text).

Duodenitis/Proximal Jejunitis

Duodenitis/proximal jejunitis (DPJ; anterior or proximal enteritis) is a clinical syndrome characterized by inflammation and edema of the duodenum and proximal jejunum, excessive fluid and electrolyte secretion into the small intestine, and consequently, large volumes of enterogastric reflux.

Clinical signs

Horses with DPJ present with acute onset of moderate to severe abdominal pain that often is followed by varying degrees of obtundation; copious amounts (greater than 12 L) of enterogastric reflux, which often is orange-brown with a fetid odor; and moderate small intestinal distention on rectal examination. Other findings include fever, dehydration, injected mucous membranes, prolonged capillary refill time, diminished intestinal sounds, tachycardia (more than 60 beats/min), and tachypnea.

Although abdominal pain usually abates after gastric decompression, most horses remain depressed, which is perhaps the most consistent and characteristic clinical sign of DPJ. Signs of abdominal pain recur if fluid is permitted to accumulate in the proximal intestine.

Diagnosis

Because the primary differential diagnosis is small intestinal obstruction, prompt differentiation of DPJ from obstruction is important, but on a case-by-case basis it is often difficult. Laboratory findings include the following:

- Increased packed cell volume (PCV) and total plasma protein
- Metabolic acidosis (longstanding or severe cases)
- Peritoneal fluid abnormalities–yellow and turbid (serosanguinous in severe cases); elevated protein; mild to moderate increase in white blood cell (WBC) count (more than 5000 cells/μl)

The peripheral WBC count may be normal or increased. Hyponatremia, hypochloremia, and hypokalemia can also develop. Any case in which small intestinal obstruction is suspected (distended small intestine on rectal examination, more than 2 L of nasogastric reflux) should be referred to a surgical facility.

Treatment

Treatment remains empiric, consisting of aggressive supportive therapy:

- Gastric decompression every 1 to 2 hours for as long as necessary (may be 3 to 7 days)
- Nothing by mouth until reflux abates (or decreases to less than 2 L/4 hr) and borborygmi returns
- Intravenous balanced electrolyte solutions to maintain intravascular fluid volume
  - Fluid therapy that is too aggressive can exacerbate enterogastric reflux.
  - Administration of colloid solutions may be beneficial (but costly).
- Flunixin meglumine (0.25 to 0.5 mg/kg IV every 6 hours)
- Laminitis prevention–NSAIDs, topical glyceryl trinitrate, DMSO, heparin
- Consider parenteral nutritional support (see main text)

The necessity for antimicrobial treatment is uncertain. If used, care must be taken when administering potentially nephrotoxic drugs such as aminoglycosides. Surgery should be considered in patients with prolonged (more than 7 days) nasogastric reflux, excessive fluid losses that cannot be corrected, or clinical and laboratory findings strongly suggestive of an intestinal obstruction.

Prognosis

More than 90% of horses with DPJ survive the primary intestinal insult with appropriate management. Losses (mortal or functional) are more commonly related to complications such as laminitis and intraabdominal adhesions. Other complications include peritonitis, myocardial and renal infarction, and aspiration pneumonia.

Proliferative Enteropathy

Proliferative enteropathy (PE) is a rarely diagnosed disorder of young horses (weanlings and yearlings). The hallmarks are gross thickening of the small intestine (especially the ileum and distal jejunum) with mucosal ulceration and severe hypoproteinemia. *Lawsonia intracellularis* or a similar organism may be the causal agent in some foals, but in most cases an etiologic agent cannot be identified.

Clinical signs and diagnosis

PE is a chronic, progressive disorder, so affected animals typically are not identified until the disease is advanced. Common presenting complaints include chronic weight loss, intermittent colic, diarrhea, lethargy, retarded growth, and ventral edema. Fever is found in some cases. Profound hypoproteinemia (serum protein less than 3 g/dl, albumin less than 1.5 g/dl) is a consistent laboratory finding; leukocytosis (lymphocytosis), polyclonal gammopathy, and hyperfibrinogenemia are also found in some cases. Abdominal ultrasonography may reveal a thickened small intestine.

Treatment

Treatment objectives are to reduce intestinal inflammation and, if appropriate, eliminate infection. Prednisolone (1 mg/kg PO once per day for 7 to 10 days, 0.75 mg/kg PO once per day for 7 to 10 days, then 0.5 mg/kg PO once per day for 7 to 10 days) can be effective. Erythromycin is indicated for cases of confirmed *L. intracellularis* infection. Other supportive therapy includes intravenous plasma and parenteral nutrition (in anorectic, debilitated animals).

Inflammatory Bowel Disease

Inflammatory bowel disease (IBD) is a group of intestinal disorders characterized by inflammatory cell infiltration of the bowel. It includes eosinophilic enterocolitis, lymphocytic/plasmacytic enteritis, basophilic enterocolitis, and granulomatous enterocolitis.

Clinical signs

Signs of IBD variably include progressive weight loss (typical), poor appetite, intermittent colic, diarrhea (if the large intestine is primarily involved), dermatitis, and peripheral edema. Horses with granulomatous enterocolitis typically have weight loss with a good appetite.

Diagnosis

Laboratory findings include anemia, hypoproteinemia, hypoalbuminemia, and glucose or D-xylose malabsorption. Some horses have a relative gammopathy. Ultrasonography may reveal thickening of the small intestine. Rectal mucosal biopsy is useful in some cases. Definitive diagnosis requires surgical biopsy of the intestine.

Treatment

Most reported cases of IBD have been fatal even with aggressive treatment. If treatment is attempted, corticosteroids (dexamethasone up to 0.2 mg/kg once per day) should be used.

Other Conditions

Lymphangiectasia, chyloabdomen, and neoplasia involving the small intestine are briefly discussed in *Large Animal Internal Medicine,* third edition.

SURGICAL DISORDERS OF THE SMALL INTESTINE *(Text pp. 649-653)*

Simple Obstruction

Physical obstruction of the lumen without vascular obstruction may be caused by intraluminal masses (e.g., ascarid impaction, ileal impaction) or extraluminal compression (e.g., adhesions). Signs include moderate to severe colic and loops of distended small intestine that are palpable per rectum as the condition progresses; nasogastric reflux takes some time to develop if the obstruction is in the distal small intestine. Specific conditions (ascarid impaction, ileal impaction, ileal hypertrophy, Meckel's diverticulum) are briefly discussed in *Large Animal Internal Medicine,* third edition.

Strangulating Obstruction

Strangulation obstruction is characterized by occlusion of both the intestinal lumen and its blood supply. Clinical signs are similar to those of simple obstruction. Endotoxemic shock (see p. 189) rapidly develops as the intestinal mucosa deteriorates. Consequently, the prognosis for survival is poorer than with most other types of colic. Specific conditions (e.g., epiploic foramen entrapment, pedunculated lipoma, volvulus, hernias [inguinal, umbilical, diaphragmatic], intussusceptions) are briefly discussed in *Large Animal Internal Medicine,* third edition.

Nonstrangulating Infarction

Nonstrangulating infarction occurs secondary to cranial mesenteric arteritis caused by migration of *Strongylus vulgaris.* It has become a rare surgical disorder since the introduction of broad-spectrum anthelmintics. Clinical signs are highly variable, ranging from intermittent colic to acute, severe colic. This disease should be considered in any horse with a history of inadequate anthelmintic treatment and intermittent colic that is difficult to localize. In addition to routine treatment of colic, dehydration, and endotoxemia, medical treatment may include aspirin (20 mg/kg once per day).

ACUTE DIARRHEA *(Text pp. 653-659)*

Diarrhea in adult horses almost exclusively results from a disorder of the large intestine. Disorders causing diarrhea in adult horses can be divided into two groups:

- Inflammation of the cecum and large intestine (typhlitis, colitis)
  - Acute inflammatory response (e.g., salmonellosis, clostridiosis)
  - Endoparasitism (small and large strongyle larval migration or encystation)
  - Granulomatous enteritis/inflammatory bowel disease (see p. 647)
- Noninflammatory disorders–increased intestinal hydrostatic pressure (e.g., congestive heart failure, cirrhotic liver disease), other poorly defined hypersecretory disorders

Diarrhea can result in significant losses of water, electrolytes, and buffer. In horses with colitis, evidence of endotoxemia (see p. 636) frequently accompanies, or even precedes, diarrhea. Malabsorption and protein-losing enteropathy are other features of inflammatory diarrhea. Regardless of etiology, potential complications include overwhelming endotoxemia, laminitis, septicemia with organ seeding by bacteria, immune suppression with bacterial or fungal infection, and cecal/colonic infarction.

General Approach to Diagnostic Evaluation

Diagnostic evaluation is intended to accurately assess the horse's condition and thus direct therapy toward specific requirements. In many cases the cause cannot be determined.

Complete blood count

Comparison of clinical hydration, PCV, and total plasma protein is useful in monitoring fluid and protein losses. Total WBC count, differential blood count, and morphologic evaluation are used to assess the severity of endotoxemia/septicemia. Plasma fibrinogen is used to assess the severity of inflammation.

Serum chemistry

Serum chemistry tests that should be performed include electrolytes, blood urea nitrogen (BUN) and creatinine, and assessment of acid-base status (blood pH and bicarbonate or total CO_2). Horses with acute diarrhea typically are hyponatremic, hypochloremic, and hypokalemic and may be acidotic and azotemic; hypocalcemia occurs with decreased feed intake. Serum electrolytes should be monitored daily to guide therapy.

General Approach to Treatment

Treatment of horses with acute diarrhea should include the following:

- Fluid therapy to replace water, sodium, chloride, and potassium losses (see pp. 682-692)
  - Large volumes of intravenous fluids may be required for several days.
- Intravenous plasma (3 to 10 L) for hypoproteinemic patients
- Antiendotoxin therapy (see pp. 638-639)

The use of antimicrobials is controversial. Specific antimicrobials may be indicated for documented infections, such as Potomac horse fever and clostridial enterocolitis (see the following discussion). Broad-spectrum antibiotics are justified in endotoxemic, neutropenic patients.

Salmonellosis

The horses most susceptible to acute salmonellosis are young foals, hospitalized horses receiving antimicrobials, and stressed horses. The typical presentation is acute colitis that results in profuse diarrhea (with or without colic) and signs of endotoxemia. Diarrhea is not a feature of other clinical syndromes of salmonellosis, which include fever and leukopenia, colic, and proximal enteritis.

Diagnosis

Confirmation of salmonellosis requires bacteriologic culture. Multiple (three to five) fecal cultures for *Salmonella* spp. should be performed on all horses with diarrhea; 5 to 10 g of feces (with as much solid matter as possible) should be submitted each time. Culture of a rectal mucosal biopsy specimen may be positive when fecal cultures are negative. Polymerase chain reaction (PCR) is available to detect *Salmonella* DNA in equine feces.

Treatment and prognosis

Aggressive treatment usually resolves the severe diarrhea and associated metabolic disorders within 7 to 10 days. Treatment involves intravenous administration of polyionic fluids and may include intravenous plasma and parenteral nutritional support. Antimicrobial therapy does not speed resolution, but it can decrease the spread of *Salmonella* to other organs. Fluoroquinolones may be more effective than chloramphenicol, trimethoprim-sulfa, gentamicin, or cephalosporins. Horses that have severe diarrhea and toxemia for 10 days or more are unlikely to survive, even with intensive therapy.

Potomac Horse Fever

Potomac horse fever (PHF) is caused by *Ehrlichia risticii* infection. Transmission involves a freshwater snail and trematode cercariae. The disease has been confirmed serologically in most states. Clinical signs include fever, inappetence, and a range of gastrointestinal (GI) signs from mild colic with soft stool to profuse diarrhea with signs of endotoxemia. Leukopenia and severe hypoproteinemia are common findings. Laminitis develops in 30% of cases; abortion is a reported but unusual sequela.

Diagnosis

Accurate diagnosis of PHF can be difficult because clinical signs are nonspecific and available diagnostic tests are not entirely reliable. Paired acute and convalescent blood samples should be submitted for serologic examination. A fourfold rise in titer is considered confirmatory, but failure to seroconvert does not rule out infection (see main text). Some laboratories offer PCR testing of blood samples for detection of *E. risticii* DNA.

Treatment

Treatment options include the following:

- Oxytetracycline 7 to 11 mg/kg IV twice daily for 4 days
  - Signs should resolve within 72 hours of beginning treatment.
- Doxycycline 10 mg/kg PO twice daily
  - In horses with severe GI signs, oral absorption may be adversely affected, so intravenous oxytetracycline may be the better choice.
  - Doxycycline must not be given IV.

Other therapy should include intravenous polyionic fluids and, if indicated, intravenous plasma. Relapse occurs in some horses 2 to 3 weeks after resolution and is responsive to tetracycline.

Clostridial Diarrhea

The two most important clostridial species affecting the equine intestinal tract are *Clostridium difficile* and *Clostridium perfringens*. Clostridial enterocolitis affects both foals and adult horses.

Clinical findings in foals

Clinical presentations in foals include predominantly GI signs (colic, diarrhea), neonatal septicemia, and necrotizing enterocolitis (gas- or fluid-filled intestines, thickened intestinal mucosa, intramural gas evident radiographically or ultrasonographically).

Clinical findings in adult horses

Adult horses with clostridial enterocolitis frequently present with diarrhea; in some cases colic or fever is the primary presenting problem. The spectrum of clinical signs ranges from moderate illness to severe toxemic colitis; in some cases, enteritis (ileus and gas distention of the small intestine) is the primary problem. No clinical features distinguish clostridiosis from other causes of inflammatory enterocolitis.

Diagnosis

Diagnosis of clostridial enterocolitis requires identification of toxigenic clostridia in intestinal contents or tissue. Culture requires anaerobic conditions; samples should be transported chilled (but not frozen) on ice to reach the laboratory as soon as possible. Specimens for identification of clostridial toxins or toxic genes should be handled similarly. Identification of toxin is essential for a diagnosis of clostridial enterocolitis, since many isolates are nontoxigenic.

Treatment

Treatment with metronidazole (15 mg/kg PO three or four times daily) is recommended. Vancomycin has been used with success in the few cases that proved resistant to metronidazole.

Antimicrobial-Associated Diarrhea

Acute diarrhea in horses has been associated with the use of several antibiotics, including orally administered lincomycin, trimethoprim-sulfamethoxazole, erythromycin, metronidazole, or penicillin, and parenterally administered tetracycline and ceftiofur. Antimicrobial-associated diarrhea is presumed to be secondary to disruption of normal colonic microflora and proliferation of an enteropathogen such as *Salmonella* spp., *C. perfringens,* or *C. difficile.*

CHRONIC DIARRHEA *(Text pp. 659-661)*

Chronic diarrhea may be defined as persistent diarrhea of at least 1 month's duration. The numerous causes include the following:

- Chronic inflammatory disorders
  - Infectious causes include chronic salmonellosis, parasitism (large or small strongyles), abdominal abscess, and in foals, abdominal *R. equi* infection and rotavirus.
  - Noninfectious causes include infiltrative disorders (e.g., granulomatous enteritis, lymphosarcoma), sand, NSAIDs, and gastric ulcers/delayed emptying (foals).
- Disruption in normal physiologic processes (e.g., abnormal fermentation of cellulose)

A small percentage of horses with chronic diarrhea have a primary disorder of a system other than the intestinal tract, such as congestive heart failure or hepatic disease.

Diagnostic Approach

The diagnostic approach should be based on an attempt to differentiate inflammatory from physiologic causes. The database should include the following:

- Physical examination
  - Mild to moderate dehydration and weight loss are common.
- CBC
  - Mild nonregenerative anemia is common; leukocytosis and hyperfibrinogenemia are found in some cases, but a normal CBC does not rule out an inflammatory cause.
- Peritoneal fluid analysis
  - Colonic inflammation sometimes causes an increase in protein and/or WBC count.
- Serum chemistry
  - Hyponatremia, hypokalemia, hypochloremia, azotemia, and metabolic acidosis are common.
  - Albumin and total protein are usually decreased with chronic inflamma-

tory disorders, but if hyperglobulinemia is present, the total protein may be normal or increased.
- Fecal examination for parasite ova
- Fecal culture for *Salmonella* spp., *C. difficile,* and *C. perfringens,* and assay for clostridial toxins
  - As many as 15 fecal cultures may be needed to confirm or rule out *Salmonella* infection.
  - A rectal mucosal biopsy specimen should also be cultured.

Other diagnostic tests that may be indicated include oral glucose absorption test, rectal mucosal biopsy for histopathology, and in weanlings, fecal testing (electron microscopy or enzyme-linked immunosorbent assay [ELISA]) for rotavirus. The cause of chronic diarrhea often cannot be determined. In such cases, exploratory laparotomy or laparoscopy may be warranted. Biopsy specimens from several sites in the colon, cecum, and mesenteric lymph nodes are submitted for histopathologic examination and *Salmonella* culture.

Treatment

Treatment of horses with chronic diarrhea is usually empiric because either a cause has not been determined or the cause is not amenable to treatment. Therapy may include the following:
- Larvicidal doses of fenbendazole (10 to 15 mg/kg PO daily for 5 days) for chronic parasitism
  - Prednisone (1 mg/kg PO once per day for 5 to 7 days) and aspirin (60 gr PO every other day) are recommended concurrently.
- Dietary changes (e.g., complete pelleted feed, changing roughage type)
- Removal of colonic sand by feeding psyllium
- Administration of corticosteroids for eosinophilic colitis
- Bismuth subsalicylate (1 to 4 L/day for adult horses) as nonspecific antiinflammatory therapy

Iodochlorhydroxyquin (Reaform; initially 20 mg/kg/day) is effective in some cases of chronic diarrhea caused by maldigestion of cellulose. However, diarrhea often recurs when the drug is discontinued.

SURGICAL DISORDERS OF THE LARGE INTESTINE *(Text pp. 662-665)*

Simple Obstruction

Large colon impactions are often amenable to medical therapy. Cecal impactions present much more of a dilemma because of the greater propensity for rupture. Medical management of these conditions is discussed in the following sections. Other causes of simple obstruction of the large intestine (enteroliths, sand impaction) are discussed in *Large Animal Internal Medicine,* third edition.

Large colon impaction

Impactions of the large colon with ingesta occur at sites of anatomic narrowing (pelvic flexure, right dorsal colon). The typical clinical picture is slow onset of mild colic that is well controlled with analgesics but becomes increasingly severe and refractory if the impaction is not resolved. Diagnosis is based on rectal palpation of a firm mass in the large colon. Initial medical treatment includes the following:
- Analgesics as needed
  - Options include flunixin (0.25 mg/kg IV every 6 hours, up to 1.1 mg/kg IV every 12 hours); butorphanol (0.05 mg/kg IV as needed); and xylazine (0.3 to 0.5 mg/kg IV as needed).
  - Detomidine should be used with great caution because it readily masks severe pain.
- Oral laxatives
  - Options include mineral oil (2 to 4 L/500 kg), DSS (180 to 240 ml in 4 L water) and $MgSO_4$ (1 mg/kg in 4 L water).
- Withhold feed

For impactions that persist, aggressive oral and intravenous fluid therapy (2 to 4 times maintenance) should be instituted. Surgery is indicated if the impaction remains unresolved, the horse becomes uncontrollably painful, or extensive gas distention of the colon develops.

Cecal impaction

Cecal impaction may develop as a primary condition or may arise as a complication in hospitalized horses (particularly after surgery). There are two presentations of cecal impaction:

- Impaction with dry, firm ingesta
  - Colic usually is gradual in onset (days); the cecum may rupture before colic becomes severe or signs of systemic deterioration are evident.
  - Medical treatment includes aggressive intravenous fluid therapy and judicious use of analgesics.
  - Oral laxatives are also recommended and include mineral oil (2 to 4 L/500 kg), $MgSO_4$ (1 mg/kg in 4 L water once or twice daily for up to 3 days), and psyllium (1 kg every 6 to 8 hours).
  - Surgery is indicated if the cecum is grossly distended or if medical therapy has no effect.
- Gross distention with fluid ingesta, caused by cecal dysfunction
  - Horses present with tachycardia and signs of endotoxemia (see p. 636).
  - Peritoneal fluid may be serosanguineous and have an elevated protein concentration.
  - Immediate surgery is indicated.

The diagnosis of cecal impaction is based on rectal palpation of a firm, impacted cecum or a grossly distended, fluid-filled cecum.

Nonstrangulating Obstruction of the Colon

A number of configurations of colon displacement can occur without compromise of the colonic blood supply. Clinical findings include mild to moderate colic and large colon distention on rectal palpation. If pain is recurrent, particularly if it is increasing in severity and frequency or if there is evidence of intestinal compromise (changes in abdominal fluid, systemic deterioration), the horse should be taken to surgery immediately.

Nephrosplenic entrapment

Findings on rectal palpation include gas distention of the ventral colon, displacement of the spleen toward the midline, and the presence of colon between the left kidney and spleen. When palpation is inconclusive, tentative diagnosis can be made using abdominal ultrasonography (the left kidney is obscured by gas-distended bowel). Although surgical intervention may be needed, the following nonsurgical techniques are successful in some cases:

- The horse is anesthetized and placed in right lateral recumbency; the horse is rotated into dorsal recumbency, rocked back and forth for 5 to 10 minutes, and then rolled into left lateral recumbency.
- Phenylephrine (3 to 6 μg/kg/min over 15 minutes) is administered to decrease the size of the spleen; the horse is then jogged for 30 to 45 minutes

If such manipulations are to be attempted, the clinician must be certain of the diagnosis. If the entrapment persists, the horse should be taken to surgery.

Strangulating Obstruction of the Colon

Strangulating obstructions of the colon are associated with high fatality rates. Clinical signs of large colon volvulus include rapid onset of severe, unrelenting abdominal pain that is poorly responsive to analgesics, gross distention of the colon and thus the abdomen, compromised ventilation, and visceral pooling. Affected horses may lie in dorsal recumbency. Despite severe pain and hypovolemia, the horse may be bradycardic. Rectal palpation reveals severe colonic distention, often restricting access to the abdomen beyond the pelvic brim. Immediate surgical intervention is essential.

ABNORMAL CONDITIONS OF THE DESCENDING (SMALL) COLON *(Text pp. 666-668)*

Abnormal conditions of the small colon are uncommon. American Miniature horses, Arabians, and horses more than 15 years of age appear to be at increased risk. Clinical signs and the rate of physiologic deterioration are less severe than with higher obstructions. Rectal examination and abdominocentesis are useful for determining the diagnosis and the need for surgical intervention.

Simple Obstructions

Simple obstructions of the small colon may be caused by ingesta, fecaliths, enteroliths, foreign bodies, and in neonates, meconium. Medical therapy for impaction should consist of aggressive intravenous and oral fluid therapy, laxatives and lubricants, and flunixin meglumine as necessary. The decision for surgical intervention is based on the severity of pain and abdominal distention.

Vascular Lesions

Vascular lesions involving the small colon include intramural hematoma, mesocolic tears, and rectal prolapse. Intramural hematomas may be caused by chronic mucosal ulceration or iatrogenic rectal trauma. Surgery may be indicated. Tears in the mesentery of the small colon can occur as a complication of parturition (either direct trauma or in association with rectal prolapse) and result in segmental ischemic necrosis of the small colon. Surgery is indicated.

Strangulating Obstructions

The most common cause of strangulating obstruction of the small colon is pedunculated lipoma. The incidence increases with age. Surgery is necessary.

PERITONITIS *(Text pp. 668-673)*

Peritonitis (inflammation of the peritoneum) may be classified as primary or secondary, acute or chronic, and localized or diffuse. Causes include perforating abdominal wounds, chemical irritation (bile, urine), breeding and foaling injuries, parasitism, pancreatitis, ruptured bladder or ureter, ruptured or lacerated abdominal viscus, castration, and various GI problems.

Clinical Findings

Clinical signs depend on the cause and duration. The most common presenting signs are pyrexia, anorexia, mild colic, reduced or absent borborygmi, diarrhea, tachycardia, and evidence of dehydration. The horse may stand with a guarded or splinted abdomen, be reluctant to move or defecate, and show pain on abdominal ballottement. Peracute peritonitis caused by intestinal rupture produces signs of acute, severe endotoxemia (see p. 189) and is rapidly fatal.

Rectal examination

Rectal palpation often elicits pain. Other findings may include distended bowel, abdominal masses, and enlarged mesenteric lymph nodes. However, in many cases, no abnormalities are detected. In cases of intestinal rupture, roughened peritoneal surfaces or an abnormally empty abdomen may be discerned. Examination of the urogenital tract should be performed in horses with peritonitis of unknown etiology.

Diagnosis

Abnormal laboratory values depend on the cause and duration of peritonitis. Hemoconcentration (elevated PCV and plasma total protein) is a common finding, although sequestration of protein into the abdomen may result in hypoproteinemia. Hyperfibrinogenemia (up to 1000 mg/dl) can occur after 48 hours. Horses with peritonitis of longer duration or abdominal abscess often have neutrophilia, monocytosis, and hyperglobulinemia. Ultrasonography can be useful in evaluating and obtaining abdominal fluid and identifying abdominal abscesses.

Abdominocentesis

Abdominocentesis confirms the diagnosis of peritonitis. Normal peritoneal fluid is clear, straw colored, and serous. The total nucleated cell count is less than 5000 cells/μl and the total protein is less than 2.5 g/dl (often less than 1 g/dl). The character of the fluid can provide a clue to the cause of peritonitis:

- Large quantities of colorless fluid suggest ascites or uroperitoneum.
- Serosanguineous fluid may be caused by intestinal degeneration, splenic puncture, abdominal viscera laceration, or contamination by blood from the skin.
- Green fluid results from enterocentesis or intestinal rupture, and brown fluid is associated with late-stage tissue necrosis.
- Turbid fluid indicates an increased cell count or protein concentration, and opalescence suggests chylous effusion.
- Flocculent fluid with fibrin strands indicates an exudative inflammatory process.

Peritoneal fluid values vary widely depending on the disease process. High nucleated cell counts (15,000 to 800,000 cells/μl) with more than 90% neutrophils and toxic or degenerative changes are common findings in horses with peritonitis or abdominal abscesses. (NOTE: Peritoneal fluid analyses must be interpreted carefully in horses after abdominal surgery, foaling, castration, or multiple abdominocenteses; see main text.)

Cytology and culture

Peritoneal fluid should be submitted for cytologic examination (cell morphology and Gram stain) and for aerobic and anaerobic bacterial culture and antibiotic susceptibility testing. However, failure to identify or culture bacteria from peritoneal fluid does not rule out septic peritonitis.

Treatment

Horses with peritonitis require early, aggressive therapy. Treatment involves the following:

- Patient stabilization–therapy for hypovolemia and endotoxic shock (see p. 190)
- Correction of the inciting cause (with surgery if necessary)
- Antimicrobial therapy (see following discussion)
- Flunixin meglumine (0.5 mg/kg IV every 6 hours)

Heparin (20 to 40 IU/kg SC every 8 hours) may be useful in combating infection and minimizing adhesion formation.

Antimicrobial therapy

The most common bacterial isolates include *Escherichia coli, Staphylococcus* spp., *Streptococcus* spp., and *Rhodococcus equi.* Anaerobes, especially *Bacteroides* spp., are isolated in up to 40% of cases. Broad-spectrum antimicrobial therapy, with a combination of an aminoglycoside and either a penicillin or a cephalosporin, is recommended. Suitable drugs and dosages include the following:

- Gentamicin (6.6 mg/kg IV every 24 hours) or amikacin (20 to 25 mg/kg IV every 24 hours)
- K-penicillin G (22,000 to 44,000 U/kg IV every 6 hours) or ampicillin (11 to 25 mg/kg IV every 6 to 8 hours)
- Ceftiofur (4 mg/kg IV every 8 to 12 hours)

If indicated by culture and sensitivity results, other suitable drugs include trimethoprim-sulfadiazine (30 mg/kg PO every 12 hours), chloramphenicol (25 to 50 mg/kg PO every 6 hours), and enrofloxacin (5 to 7 mg/kg PO every 24 hours; adults only). Metronidazole (15 to 25 mg/kg PO every 6 to 8 hours) is effective against most anaerobes; it can be administered intravenously or rectally in horses with ileus.

Peritoneal lavage and drainage

Peritoneal lavage and drainage should be considered for acute cases of purulent effusion and in horses not responding to medical therapy. Retrograde irrigation and drainage through a single ingress-egress catheter placed in the ventral midline is most effective (see main text).

Prognosis

The prognosis depends on the cause, severity, duration, and complications of peritonitis. With early diagnosis, correction of the inciting cause, and aggressive therapy the prognosis is fair to good for acute cases. Laminitis, diarrhea, ileus, coagulopathies, abdominal adhesions, and abscess formation adversely affect outcome.

GASTROINTESTINAL ILEUS *(Text pp. 674-678)*

Ileus is functional inhibition of propulsive bowel activity. Postoperative ileus (POI) is common after GI surgery, particularly procedures involving the small intestine. Ileus is also an important clinical feature of other disease processes, including mechanical obstruction with gas distention, gastroduodenal ulcer disease, duodenitis/proximal jejunitis, enteritis, peritonitis, cecal impaction, metabolic and electrolyte derangements (hypokalemia, hypocalcemia, uremia), and endotoxemia. In addition, certain drugs can induce ileus, including atropine, xylazine, and detomidine.

Clinical Findings

Clinical signs of POI usually develop shortly after the procedure and include abdominal pain, decreased borborygmi and fecal output, and sequestration of fluid in the small intestine, resulting in enterogastric reflux. The severity and duration of intestinal stasis is variable, lasting from minutes to days.

Rectal examination

Rectal findings in cases of persistent POI or duodenitis/proximal jejunitis often include dilated, fluid-filled loops of small intestine. Cecal distention with digesta can be palpated in horses with advanced postanesthetic cecal dysfunction (see p. 198).

Diagnosis

It is important to distinguish functional ileus from mechanical obstruction. Regardless of cause, most animals with ileus are depressed, inappetant or anorectic, and have reduced intestinal borborygmi and fecal output. Abdominal pain is typical in horses with ileus involving the proximal GI tract. The pain is caused, in part, by gastric distention and often is relieved by gastric decompression (which should also lower the heart rate).

Treatment

In addition to correcting the underlying cause, management of ileus involves the following:

- Repeated gastric decompression for ileus involving the proximal GI tract
- Fluid and electrolyte therapy to maintain adequate hydration and serum potassium, calcium, and magnesium
- Avoidance of drugs that may impair intestinal motility
- NSAID therapy (e.g., flunixin meglumine)
- Broad-spectrum antimicrobial drugs if sepsis or endotoxemia is suspected

Prokinetics

Motility-enhancing drugs, or prokinetics, have a place in the management of ileus. However, an important prerequisite is intestinal integrity; many of these drugs are less effective in the face of severe intestinal inflammation. Options include the following:

- Bethanechol–0.025 mg/kg SC or PO

- Metoclopramide–constant IV infusion at 0.04 mg/kg/hr
- Cisapride–0.1 mg/kg IM (currently available only in tablet form in the United States)
- Erythromycin–0.5 mg/kg IV, repeated as needed
- Naloxone–0.05 mg/kg IV
- Yohimbine–75 μg/kg by slow intravenous infusion
- Lidocaine–intravenous infusion at 15 to 20 mg/min over 5 to 6 hours

The relative advantages and disadvantages for each of these drugs are discussed in *Large Animal Internal Medicine,* third edition.

NONSTEROIDAL ANTIINFLAMMATORY DRUG TOXICITY *(Text pp. 679-682)*

NSAIDs have a relatively narrow therapeutic range; when administered at excessive dosages, toxicosis can occur within a few days. Some horses exhibit signs of toxicosis at recommended doses. Predisposing factors include dehydration, renal disease, hepatic disease, and sepsis. Combining two NSAIDs increases the risk of toxicity. The GI tract and kidneys are the common target organs. NSAID-induced injury can develop anywhere along the GI tract from mouth to rectum.

Clinical Signs

Clinical signs of NSAID toxicity are usually referable to the GI tract. Oral ulceration may cause difficulty with prehension or mastication. Signs of esophageal or gastroduodenal ulceration are discussed in earlier sections of this chapter. Horses with colonic ulceration may have soft stool or diarrhea (can be severe) and ventral edema secondary to enteric protein loss. Endotoxemia may result from severe intestinal mucosal damage.

Diagnosis

The diagnosis is based on a history of NSAID use, clinical signs, and laboratory findings. The most consistent laboratory abnormalities are hypoproteinemia and hypoalbuminemia, especially with ulceration in the distal intestinal tract. Some horses are also hypocalcemic. In chronic cases, anemia and occult fecal blood may be found. Several abnormalities may accompany NSAID-induced renal damage.

Diagnostic imaging

Endoscopy is useful for determining the location and extent of esophageal and gastric lesions (most common in the glandular mucosa). Ultrasonography may reveal thickening of the right dorsal colon, but the technique lacks sensitivity.

Treatment

Treatment is primarily symptomatic:

- Discontinue NSAIDs.
- Treat gastric ulceration as described on p. 681.
- Consider administering misoprostol (Cytotec).
  - To avoid side effects, start at 1.5 μg/kg PO every 8 hours for 2 to 4 days, then increase at increments of 0.5 μg/kg every 2 to 4 days until a maintenance dose of 2.5 to 3 μg/kg PO every 8 hours is reached.
- Administer crystalloid fluids for hypovolemia associated with colitis.
- Give intravenous plasma (1 to 3 L) to horses with enteropathy and signs of endotoxemia.
- Give broad-spectrum antimicrobials if signs of endotoxemia are present.
  - Parenteral is preferable to oral administration, except for metronidazole (10 to 15 mg/kg PO every 8 to 12 hours), which may also enhance mucosal healing.

Horses with strictures of the pylorus, duodenum, jejunum, or colon may require surgery.

Right dorsal colitis

Horses with right dorsal colitis should be placed on a low-bulk diet, such as a complete pelleted feed that contains both concentrate and roughage. The pelleted diet should be fed in several small meals per day. Fresh grass may be offered in small amounts if available. Feeding psyllium mucilloid (1 to 2 oz once or twice daily) may promote colonic healing.

FLUID THERAPY FOR GASTROINTESTINAL DISORDERS *(Text pp. 682-692)*

Formulating a Fluid Therapy Plan

Rational fluid therapy for GI disorders should be based on the following indices:

- Clinical estimation of the degree of dehydration (as a percentage of body weight)
  - At 5% dehydration the skin stays tented for 1 to 3 seconds; mucous membranes are moist or slightly tacky; capillary refill time is less 2 seconds; heart rate is normal; urine output is decreased.
  - At 8% dehydration the skin stays tented for 3 to 5 seconds; mucous membranes are tacky; capillary refill time may be 2 to 3 seconds; heart rate is 40 to 60 bpm; BP is decreased.
  - At 10% to 12% dehydration the skin stays tented for more than 5 seconds; mucous membranes are dry; capillary refill time is often more than 4 seconds; heart rate is more than 60 beats/min; other findings include reduced jugular filling, barely detectable peripheral pulse, and sunken eyes.
- Estimation of ongoing losses (based on the disease process)
  - Monitor the volume of nasogastric reflux removed or diarrheic feces passed.
  - Serial body weight measurements can also be useful if available.
- Available laboratory data
  - PCV greater than 50% indicates dehydration (usually at least 7% dehydration).
  - Significant plasma protein losses with GI disease can result in a low or normal total plasma protein concentration despite dehydration.
  - High urine specific gravity (greater than 1.040) indicates possible dehydration.
  - Elevated serum creatinine (up to 5 mg/dl) occurs with prolonged dehydration.

Equally important, the fluid therapy plan should be adjusted according to the patient's response.

Type of fluid

For most field situations, commercial isotonic polyionic crystalloid solutions are the safest fluids for resuscitation in dehydrated adult horses. Other options include the following:

- Hypertonic saline–2 to 4 ml/kg of 7% to 7.5% NaCl rapidly IV
  - Hypertonic saline is used to quickly restore circulating volume in shock patients, but should be used with caution in severely dehydrated patients.
  - This treatment must be followed by large volumes of isotonic polyionic crystalloids (at least 10 L for each 1 L hypertonic saline) within 2.5 hours.
- Hetastarch–10 ml/kg IV
  - When used in combination with hypertonic saline, it may be a better solution for resuscitation in dehydrated horses.
  - When using colloids such as hetastarch, plasma total protein/solids is no longer a useful guide to hydration status.
- Plasma–6 to 8 L IV for hypoproteinemic adult horses
- Oral fluids–suitable for mild dehydration in horses with adequate bowel motility
  - An isotonic solution can be made by adding 4.9 g NaCl and 4.9 g KCl per 1 L water.
  - The volume given at one time should not exceed 10 L in a 500-kg horse; at least 20 minutes should elapse before the next administration.

Administration rate

The resuscitation phase aims to rapidly restore current fluid deficits; the maintenance phase aims to prevent further fluid deficits (supply basal fluid requirements and replace ongoing fluid losses). Correction of electrolyte imbalances usually takes place during the maintenance phase. Recommended fluid rates for each phase are as follows:

- Resuscitation
  - Replace the estimated fluid deficit as rapidly as possible, but do not exceed 60 ml/kg/hr (30 L/hr for a 500-kg horse).
- Maintenance
  - The commonly recommended rate for adult horses is 3 ml/kg/hr.
  - With diarrhea, continued fluid losses may be as high as 200 ml/kg/day.

Overhydration

Clinical signs of overhydration are rare in adult horses with normal cardiac and renal function. The most important sign is pulmonary edema, manifested by dyspnea and a pink-white foamy nasal discharge. Treatment should include furosemide (0.5 to 1 mg/kg IV), intranasal oxygen, and a reduction in the rate of fluid administration.

Acid-Base and Electrolyte Disturbances

Fluids should be chosen to correct both fluid deficits and electrolyte and acid-base disturbances. In the absence of specific laboratory data, fluid therapy should probably be limited to isotonic polyionic crystalloid solutions, possibly with potassium chloride (10 to 20 mEq/L) added. Ideally, clinical response and laboratory data should be monitored frequently and treatment adjusted accordingly. Following are recommended intravenous fluid choices for specific metabolic disturbances:

- Lactic acidosis–large volumes of polyionic crystalloids (up to 60 ml/kg/hr) or hetastarch (up to 10 ml/kg/hr)
- Hyponatremia with hypochloremia–NaCl
  - Sodium should be corrected no faster than 1 mEq/L/hr.
  - If the horse is not clinically dehydrated and the hyponatremia is severe, hypertonic saline may be administered initially.
- Hyponatremia without hypochloremia–$NaHCO_3$ (as for sodium correction)
- Hypernatremia–5% dextrose or 2.5% dextrose/0.45% NaCl
  - Lower sodium no faster than 0.5 mEq/L/hr.
- Hypochloremia–0.9% (or 7.5%) NaCl to effect
- Hyperchloremia with hypernatremia–5% dextrose
  - Lower sodium no faster than 0.5 mEq/L/hr.
- Hyperchloremia without hypernatremia–5% $NaHCO_3$ slowly to effect
- Hypokalemia–KCl; 0.2 to 0.5 mEq/kg/hr; never exceed 1 mEq/kg/hr
  - In postoperative colic cases and proximal enteritis, supplement when plasma K^+ is less than 3.5 mEq/L; in patients being fed enterally, supplement when plasma K^+ is less than 3 mEq/L.
  - Add 40 mEq/L of KCl to crystalloid fluids for severe hypokalemia (K^+ less than 2.7 mEq/L) and 20 mEq/L of KCl for less severe disturbances.
  - If hypokalemia does not respond to KCl, supplement with magnesium (see following discussion).
- Hyperkalemia without clinical signs–polyionic crystalloid fluids
- Hyperkalemia with clinical signs or K^+ more than 7 mEq/L–calcium gluconate (1 ml/kg over 10 minutes), $NaHCO_3$ (1 to 2 mEq/L over 15 minutes), or 50% dextrose (2 ml/kg over 5 minutes)
- Hypocalcemia–supplement with calcium gluconate (100 to 300 ml of 23% solution) if the ionized Ca^+ is less than 4.8 mg/dl (1.2 mmol/L).
  - Calcium-containing solutions should be diluted in crystalloid fluids before administration and should not be mixed with $NaHCO_3$ or whole blood.

   - Magnesium should be supplemented in horses with refractory hypocalcemia.
- Hypercalcemia–non-calcium-containing polyionic fluids or $MgSO_4$ (2 to 8 mg/kg IV initial dose)
- Hypomagnesemia–$MgSO_4$ (as previously discussed) or MgO (8 to 32 mg/kg PO initial dose)
   - $MgSO_4$ at 2 mg/kg/min (not to exceed 50 mg/kg) is recommended for ventricular arrhythmias associated with hypomagnesemia.
- Hypermagnesemia–calcium gluconate (250 to 500 ml of 23% solution)

Inotropes, Pressors, and Vasodilators

Some horses with severe cardiovascular compromise do not respond to fluid therapy alone and may need to be treated with inotropes, pressors, or vasodilators. Indications include continued tachycardia, lactic acidosis, oliguria, and hypertension or hypotension despite appropriate fluid therapy. There are two important considerations before initiating this therapy:

1. The cause of the cardiovascular insufficiency should be addressed.
2. Minimum information required to select an appropriate drug and monitor therapy is heart rate and rhythm and measurement of arterial BP (indirectly, using a tail cuff, if direct measurement is not possible).

Treatment goals

Any of the drugs discussed here should be carefully titrated to defined endpoints:

- Inotropes and pressors–increase arterial BP sufficiently to increase urine output without inducing tachycardia or arrhythmias
   - A reasonable target is a mean BP of 65 to 75 mm Hg.
- Vasodilators–decrease mean BP to less than 120 mm Hg without inducing hypotension, tachycardia, or acidosis

It is extremely important to monitor the response to these drugs. Heart rate and rhythm, BP, acid-base balance, venous oxygen tension, and urine output should be monitored.

Drugs

Dosages and indications for the commonly used drugs are as follows:

- Dobutamine–start at 1 to 3 μg/kg/min constant intravenous infusion in isotonic saline, 5% dextrose, or lactated Ringer's solution
   - In the absence of cardiac output measurements, dobutamine should be the first drug used in hypotensive horses (mean BP of less than 65 mm Hg) that do not respond to appropriate fluid therapy.
   - The horse should be carefully monitored for tachycardia (which may indicate inadequate fluid resuscitation) arrhythmia.
- Norepinephrine–start at 0.1 μg/kg/min as constant intravenous infusion in 5% dextrose
   - Consider using this drug in hypotensive horses that do not respond to dobutamine and in those with a measured increase in cardiac output.
   - Concurrent infusion of dobutamine (5 μg/kg/min) is prudent when cardiac output is not being directly monitored.
   - It is important to carefully monitor urine output when using norepinephrine.
- Sodium nitroprusside–titrate from 0.1 μg/kg/min to 0.3 μg/kg/min constant intravenous infusion
   - Consider using this drug in severely hypertensive horses.
   - Dilute in 5% dextrose and wrap the bag in foil to protect the solution from light.
   - *It is imperative to monitor BP continuously* during the initial titration phase and frequently thereafter.

NOTE: Dopamine is not recommended for horses with GI disease.

Part II: Ruminant Alimentary System

DENTAL AND PERIODONTAL DISEASES *(Text pp. 694-696)*

Dental disease in ruminants should first be considered on a flock or herd basis. Clinical manifestations include decreased food intake, weight loss, unthriftiness, quidding, and mandibular/maxillary swellings or draining tracts. The following topics are discussed in *Large Animal Internal Medicine,* third edition: eruption times; examination of the teeth; dental attrition and erosion; periodontal disease; retention of deciduous teeth; overgrown, loose, or broken teeth; dental caries; osteodystrophia fibrosa; and tooth root abscesses.

SALIVARY GLAND DISEASES *(Text p. 697)*

Excessive Salivation

Excessive salivation (ptyalism) is a sign of many pathologic conditions, including dental disease, stomatitis, foreign objects in the mouth or pharynx, esophageal obstruction, ruminal disorders, eating spoiled silage, abomasal impaction, rabies, pseudorabies, meningoencephalitis, and various toxicities (slaframine, mercury, iodine, lead, copper, arsenic). Treatment depends on the underlying cause. NOTE: As a precaution against exposure to rabies, gloves should be worn to examine the mouth of any animal that is salivating excessively.

Other Disorders

Diagnosis and management of sialoceles, parotid gland carcinomas, and sialoadenitis in ruminants are discussed in *Large Animal Internal Medicine,* third edition.

ACTINOBACILLOSIS (WOODY TONGUE, WOODEN TONGUE) *(Text pp. 698-699)*

Actinobacillosis is a granulomatous condition caused by *Actinobacillus lignieresii,* a gram-negative rod that is a normal inhabitant of the mouth and rumen of cattle, sheep, and probably goats. The classic site of infection is the bovine tongue. Infection begins with mucosal lesions caused by plant awns (e.g., foxtails), thistles, or coarse feed. Most cases are sporadic.

Clinical Signs and Diagnosis

When the tongue is affected, the major clinical signs are inability to prehend food normally, excessive salivation, anorexia, and sometimes a visibly enlarged, protruding tongue. On palpation the tongue is firm or very hard, painful, and nodular. An ulcer filled with plant awns or stems is often present in the sulcus lingualis. Firm swelling of the submandibular area is often present. Atypical lesions may involve the lips, muzzle, lymph nodes of the head or neck, or other internal sites. In sheep, actinobacillosis typically causes hard swelling of the lips, often with fistulous tracts. Lesions are rare in goats. Definitive diagnosis requires culture.

Treatment

Iodides

The treatment of choice is sodium iodide (NaI, 70 mg/kg IV as a 10% to 20% solution), repeated at least once 7 to 10 days later. Therapy may be repeated more often (every 2 to 3 days) in refractory cases. In severe cases, organic iodides can be administered orally at 60 mg/kg daily, in addition to the intravenous iodide. If signs of iodinism develop (excessive tearing, coughing, inappetence, diarrhea, dandruff), iodine administration should be halted. Iodides can be safely given to pregnant cows, but there are anecdotal reports of iodide-induced abortion.

Other therapy

Therapy with an antimicrobial drug to which the isolate is sensitive is also recommended in severe, generalized, or refractory cases. Most strains of *A. lignieresii* are sensitive to a number of antimicrobial drugs, including ceftiofur, ampicillin, penicillin, florfenicol, aminoglycosides, sulfas, and tetracyclines, but each isolate should be tested for antimicrobial sensitivity.

ACTINOMYCOSIS (LUMPY JAW) *(Text pp. 699-700)*

Actinomycosis is a sporadic disease caused by *Actinomyces bovis,* a gram-positive, branching, filamentous bacterium that is a normal inhabitant of the ruminant mouth. The disease mainly occurs in cattle. The organism enters the tissues and bone through oral abrasions, openings, and punctures associated with dental disease, hard plant awns (e.g., foxtails), thorns, stickers, or coarse feeds. The disease mainly involves the mandible. Lesions occasionally occur in the soft tissues of the head, esophagus, forestomachs, and trachea.

Clinical Signs

Typical bovine actinomycosis causes a hard, immovable, painless bony mass on the mandible. Fistulous tracts may develop and tooth roots may be involved as the condition progresses. When teeth are affected, there may be evidence of weight loss and pain when chewing. Careful examination of the mouth is required to detect loose teeth, plant awns, or severe gingivitis and to rule out a pathologic fracture.

Diagnosis

Radiography is helpful in determining whether there is dental involvement or fracture. The lesion consists of multiple central radiolucent areas of osteomyelitis surrounded by periosteal new bone and fibrous tissue. If a fistulous tract is present, a contrast study helps determine the extent of the fistula. Before flushing, material from the core of the lesion should be aspirated or biopsied and submitted for Gram stain and culture.

Treatment

Antibiotics

Treatment options include NaI (see Actinobacillosis), isoniazid (10 mg/kg/day PO for 1 month) or, in valuable animals, penicillin (10,000 U/kg IM twice daily) or another antimicrobial to which the organism is sensitive. Treatment usually results in arrest of the lesion, but seldom does the mass regress significantly. NOTE: Isoniazid should not be used in pregnant cattle.

Other therapy

Any fistulous tracts should be vigorously curetted and flushed with povidone-iodine. If the cavity is large, it may be necessary to flush and pack with iodine-soaked gauze daily for several days (see main text). Any affected teeth should be carefully removed.

PHARYNGEAL TRAUMA/ABSCESS *(Text pp. 701-702)*

Pharyngeal trauma is relatively common in cattle and results in cellulitis, abscess, or hematoma formation. Clinical signs include anorexia, ptyalism, halitosis, extension of the head and neck, localized or diffuse pharyngeal pain, feed from the nostrils, and forestomach stasis or bloat. In severe cases there may be obvious pharyngeal swelling, fever, cough on laryngeal palpation, dyspnea, and aspiration pneumonia. Most cases resolve with broad-spectrum antimicrobial therapy for 7 to 14 days and good supportive care.

BLUETONGUE *(Text pp. 702-704)*

Bluetongue is a viral disease of wild and domestic ruminants, primarily spread by biting midges (*Culicoides* sp.). The midges, and therefore the disease, are most prevalent in summer and early fall. Clinical disease is largely restricted to sheep. Pathogenicity of local virus in endemic flocks is usually low; epizootics occur when new virus or new animals are introduced.

Clinical Signs

Clinical disease is manifested in two ways: (1) reproductive problems such as teratogenicity, abortion, and stillbirth, and (2) vasculitis involving several organ systems (bluetongue). Clinical bluetongue in sheep begins with transient high fever; edema of the face, lips, muzzle, and ears; excessive salivation; hyperemia of the oral mucosa; and profuse serous nasal discharge that becomes mucopurulent after a few days. Oral lesions progress to petechial hemorrhages, erosions, and ulcers, especially on the dental pad and commissures of the mouth. The tongue may become cyanotic (hence the name), but this is uncommon.

Other signs

Later signs of bluetongue or secondary infections include pulmonary edema, bacterial bronchopneumonia, diarrhea or dysentery, lameness and stiffness (coronitis and myopathy), sloughing of the hooves, and breaks in the wool. Severely affected sheep become depressed, are unable to rise, and die. Cardiomyopathy may result in sudden death, even during recovery.

Diagnosis

Serologic examination is commonly used to test for bluetongue infection. The competitive ELISA (C-ELISA) is the best test for detection of group antibodies. However, a positive result is not certain proof that clinical disease is caused by bluetongue virus. Virus isolation from blood obtained during the viremic, febrile stage is the most definitive means of diagnosis.

Treatment

Treatment is nonspecific: supportive and nursing care. Valuable animals should be offered soft feeds or green grass or fed gruels of alfalfa pellets via stomach tube. Water and shade must be close at hand. Sulfas or other broad-spectrum antimicrobials should be administered to prevent or treat secondary bacterial pneumonia. NSAIDs, including aspirin and flunixin, are commonly used. Control is discussed in *Large Animal Internal Medicine,* third edition.

CONTAGIOUS ECTHYMA (SORE MOUTH, ORF, CONTAGIOUS PUSTULAR DERMATITIS, SCABBY MOUTH) *(Text pp. 704-706)*

Contagious ecthyma is a common disease of sheep and goats that is transmissible to humans. The disease may be seen at any time but typically occurs in the spring in the new lamb or kid crop.

Clinical Signs

The most common presentation is a young animal with crusting, proliferative lesions of the mucocutaneous junctions of the mouth and nose and sometimes the gums. In immunologically naive older animals, lesions may also develop interdigitally and on the coronary band, tongue, conjunctivae, external genitalia, and udder or teats (especially in dams nursing affected kids). Affected animals may be reluctant to nurse, eat, walk, or be nursed, depending on the location of the lesions. The disease typically runs its course in 3 to 4 weeks.

Diagnosis

Diagnosis is usually based on finding typical lesions in a naive flock or in a naive group (young lambs or kids) in a disease-endemic flock. Definitive diagnosis usually involves virus identification from early lesions.

Treatment

The infection is usually self-limiting and of minor consequence. Young patients may need to be tube fed if the lesions are severe enough to inhibit nursing. Secondary infections, myiasis, or mastitis may be treated with topical disinfectants, antibiotics, or insecticides as appropriate. The hard crusts should not be removed because doing so may delay healing and promote scarring. NOTE: People should limit contact with and wear gloves when handling affected animals. Control is discussed in *Large Animal Internal Medicine,* third edition.

BOVINE PAPULAR STOMATITIS (PROLIFERATIVE STOMATITIS) *(Text pp. 706-707)*

Bovine papular stomatitis (BPS) is a viral disease that primarily affects young cattle. Infection is usually asymptomatic, but lesions consisting of 2- to 10-mm raised papules may be noted on the muzzle, nose, oral mucosa (particularly the hard palate), or esophagus. Most animals are afebrile and continue to eat normally. The lesions regress in 1 day to 3 weeks.

Severe bovine papular stomatitis

Outbreaks of severe disease associated with BPS have been reported. Papular and ulcerative lesions are found in the mouth, esophagus, and rumen, and they cause weight loss and diarrhea. (There are no lesions on the feet.) The mortality rate can exceed 50%. BPS has also been associated with "rat tail" syndrome of feedlot cattle, which consists of diarrhea, salivation, poor weight gain, and loss of hair from the end of the tail.

DISEASES CAUSED BY BOVINE VIRAL DIARRHEA VIRUS *(Text pp. 707-713)*

BVDV can cause a variety of clinical manifestations, ranging from subclinical infection to death. In most animals (70% to 90%), infection with BVDV is subclinical, causing mild fever, leukopenia, and development of serum-neutralizing antibodies.

Manifestations of Acute BVDV Infection

Acute bovine viral diarrhea

Acute BVD occurs in immunocompetent cattle that are not persistently infected (see following discussion) with BVDV. This syndrome usually occurs in seronegative cattle 6 months to 2 years of age. Clinical signs include fever, depression, anorexia, oculonasal discharge, oral erosions and ulceration, diarrhea, tachypnea, and in lactating cows, decreased milk production. Affected cattle are leukopenic.

Severe acute BVDV infection

An atypical form of BVDV infection has been reported in the United States and Canada. The disease has a peracute course and a high morbidity rate; mortality rates may approach 20%. Outbreaks are characterized by fever, pneumonia, and sudden death in all age groups of cattle. Reported outbreaks have been attributed to type II BVDV isolates.

Hemorrhagic syndrome

Acute BVDV infections in cattle can cause a hemorrhagic syndrome characterized by marked thrombocytopenia, dysentery, epistaxis, hemorrhages on mucosal surfaces, hyphema, bleeding from injection sites, pyrexia, leukopenia, and death. Thus far only type II BVDV has been associated with this syndrome.

Other manifestations

Acute BVDV infection has long been implicated in bovine respiratory disease complex (see Chapter 29), presumably through its immunosuppressive effects. For the same reason, acute BVDV infection also increases the animal's susceptibility to other pathogens. Acute BVDV infection can also cause venereal infections, abortion, and various congenital defects (see main text).

Persistent Infection With BVDV

Infection of a fetus with a noncytopathic BVDV isolate before the development of fetal immunocompetence may result in the birth of a calf that is immunotolerant to, and thus persistently infected (PI) with, BVDV. PI cattle are viremic and continuously shed virus, so they are the major source of BVDV transmission.

Although PI cattle may appear healthy, they are at risk of developing mucosal disease (see following discussion) and various other diseases and have a decreased survival rate compared with cattle that are not PI.

Acute mucosal disease

Mucosal disease (MD) occurs when PI cattle become infected with a cytopathic biotype of BVDV. Manifestations range from subclinical (seroconversion) to acute MD. Clinical signs of acute MD include biphasic fever, anorexia, tachycardia, polypnea, decreased milk production, and profuse, watery diarrhea (occasionally with frank blood, fibrinous casts, and a foul odor). The oral papillae may be blunted, and there may be erosions on the tongue, palate, buccal surfaces, pharynx, and in some cases, in the interdigital skin and on the teats and vulva. Erosive lesions may be diphtheritic.

Other signs may include nasal and ocular discharge, corneal opacity, ptyalism, decreased rumination, bloat, coronary band inflammation, and laminitis. Secondary bacterial infections, resulting in pneumonia, mastitis, and metritis, are common. Affected animals are often neutropenic (without a left shift) and thrombocytopenic. Cattle with MD typically become progressively dehydrated and debilitated and die within 3 to 10 days.

Chronic mucosal disease

Animals surviving acute MD develop chronic disease. Signs of chronic MD can include unthriftiness, persistently loose feces or intermittent diarrhea, chronic bloat, decreased appetite, weight loss, interdigital erosions, nonhealing erosive skin lesions, persistent nasal and ocular discharge, areas of alopecia and hyperkeratinization on the neck, and chronic lameness (laminitis, interdigital necrosis, hoof deformities). Affected animals may be persistently anemic, neutropenic, and thrombocytopenic. Cattle with chronic MD rarely survive beyond 18 months.

Diagnosis of BVDV Infection

A diagnosis of BVDV infection can be made by using serologic evaluation, virus isolation, or detection of viral antigen or RNA using PCR or another amplification method (see main text).

Virus isolation

Virus isolation is the most common method used. Serum is generally used to isolate the virus in PI cattle. Buffy coat layers or nasal swabs are more appropriate for confirming acute BVDV infection. Antemortem differentiation of PI cattle from those with acute BVDV infection requires serial isolation of virus (with samples taken at least 2 weeks apart).

Treatment

No specific treatment is available. The goals of therapy for cattle suspected of having acute BVD are supportive care and prevention of secondary bacterial infection. Broad-spectrum antimicrobial agents, fluids, electrolytes, and vitamins may be indicated. Prevention and control are discussed in detail in *Large Animal Internal Medicine,* third edition.

MALIGNANT CATARRHAL FEVER (BOVINE MALIGNANT CATARRH) *(Text pp. 714-716)*

Malignant catarrhal fever (MCF) is a highly fatal viral disease of cattle and wild ruminants. The disease is usually sporadic, although outbreaks have been reported. Treatment does not appear to be successful.

Clinical Signs

The virus causes vasculitis affecting all epithelial surfaces. Clinical signs include oral erosions, diarrhea or dysentery, severe keratoconjunctivitis, mucopurulent nasal discharge, thickened and cracked skin, encephalitis, high fever, marked lymphadenopathy, generalized weakness, dyspnea, copious ropy saliva, scabs on the muzzle, sloughing of the hooves or horns, pronounced lameness, and hematuria. When particular signs predominate, the condition may be labeled the alimentary form, encephalitic form, or skin form.

Clinical course

The course of the disease is usually 3 to 7 days. The mortality rate is high, with most affected cattle dying 1 to 3 days after developing high fever, severe diarrhea, and conjunctivitis. Peracute death without visible symptoms has also been reported. Obliterative arteriopathy is the primary lesion in surviving animals.

Diagnosis

Diagnosis is based on history of exposure (incubation period 3 to 10 weeks), clinical signs, and necropsy lesions (see main text). Serologic tests include ELISA, indirect immunofluorescence, complement fixation, and virus neutralization. Virus isolation can be attempted on nasal swabs, blood (submit at least 500 ml), and samples of spleen and lymph node. Viral antigen can also be detected by PCR.

VESICULAR STOMATITIS *(Text pp. 716-718)*

Vesicular stomatitis (VS) is a viral disease that causes sporadic (cyclic) outbreaks of disease in cattle, horses, donkeys, mules, and pigs. From 5% to 60% of cattle on a farm may be clinically affected. Vesicles that readily rupture, leaving ulcerated areas, occur in the mouth, on the teats, and on interdigital areas.

Clinical Signs

After an incubation period of 3 to 14 days (mean, 9 days), clinical signs begin with fever and painful oral lesions that cause excess salivation and reluctance to eat. Lesions on the gums and tongue may coalesce to form large, eroded areas. Teat lesions are common in dairy cattle; small ulcers in the interdigital area and on the coronary band are occasionally seen. Milk yield falls quickly. Recovery takes 2 to 21 days, depending on lesion severity and management factors, but actual healing of lesions may take as long as 60 days.

Diagnosis

The VS virus is difficult to isolate from blood, urine, feces, and oral swabs but may be isolated from tongue epithelium. Complement fixation, ELISA, and fluorescent antibody tests are available for diagnosis. State and federal regulatory veterinarians should be contacted immediately when VS is suspected.

Treatment

Mortality can be almost completely prevented if ill cattle are offered shade, fresh water, clean bedding, and soft feed. Debilitated cattle should be given broad-spectrum antibiotics to control secondary bacterial pneumonia. Cattle with teat lesions should be carefully milked last and monitored closely for mastitis. During an outbreak of VS, quarantine of premises and isolation of sick animals are required. Control is discussed in *Large Animal Internal Medicine*, third edition.

FOOT-AND-MOUTH DISEASE *(Text pp. 718-719)*

Foot-and-mouth disease (FMD) is an acute, highly contagious viral disease of cloven-hoofed livestock. Cattle and swine are the most susceptible. FMD is characterized by vesicular lesions, erosions, and ulcers in the mouth and on the muzzle, teats, interdigital area, and coronary band. FMD is exotic in the United States.

Clinical Signs and Diagnosis

FMD is clinically indistinguishable from VS except that VS also affects horses. FMD may cause fatal myocardial necrosis in young calves, and secondary bacterial pneumonia and foot infections are common. Laboratory diagnosis is made by complement fixation, virus neutralization, agar-gel precipitation, ELISA, or fluorescent antibody tests. When FMD (or VS) is suspected, state and federal authorities should be contacted immediately.

RINDERPEST (CATTLE PLAGUE) *(Text pp. 719-720)*

Rinderpest (RP) is an acute, highly contagious, and usually fatal disease of ruminants. It is exotic in the United States. Clinical signs in cattle include sudden onset of fever, depression, and anorexia; the nose is dry and mucous membranes are congested. Within days oral erosions develop, similar to those seen with VS. Purulent lacrimation and severe diarrhea (with or without dysentery) also occur with RP. The disease in sheep and goats is usually mild or subclinical.

Diagnosis

Laboratory confirmation of RP can be accomplished using virus isolation, detection of viral antigen, and serologic and histopathologic evaluation. Heparinized blood, ocular discharges, and samples of lymph node and spleen are the most reliable samples.

CHOKE AND ESOPHAGEAL DISORDERS *(Text pp. 720-722)*

Esophageal obstruction (choke) is most common in cattle because of their eating habits. Obstruction may be caused by ingestion of foreign objects or large chunks of solid feedstuffs. Rapid consumption of dry grain, particularly in pelleted form, can also cause choke in sheep. Space-occupying lesions in or near the esophagus are another possible cause of esophageal obstruction. Regardless of the cause, if the obstruction is complete, the condition is rapidly fatal because of severe bloating.

Clinical Signs

The earliest signs of complete esophageal obstruction are anxiety and ptyalorrhea (saliva dripping from the mouth because of inability to swallow), with repeated attempts to swallow. Later signs include staggering and bloat. External palpation may localize the site of obstruction in the cervical esophagus. With more slowly developing and incomplete obstructions, anorexia, dysphagia, and recurrent bloat may be observed.

Diagnosis

If there is no externally evident site of obstruction, careful attempts to pass a stomach tube usually reveal the site of the problem. Radiography with barium contrast may help identify strictures, perforations, or diverticula. Endoscopy may also aid in revealing the nature of functional or structural abnormalities.

Treatment

In cases of complete esophageal obstruction, relieving bloat is the first concern. Passage of a stomach tube may be attempted if the animal is not in respiratory distress. Otherwise, trocarization of the rumen or installation of a temporary fistula is required. Manual oral examination should precede probing attempts with a stomach tube. Suitable precautions should be taken if rabies is even remotely possible.

Cervical obstructions

Solid objects can sometimes be massaged into the pharynx by pressing along the jugular furrow. A probang with a corkscrewlike or pincerlike end can be used to grasp or engage some foreign bodies. If a mass of grain is obstructing the esophagus, external massage, probing with the stomach tube, and pumping fluid against the mass through the tube may break it up.

Intrathoracic obstructions

If the obstruction is intrathoracic and cannot be relieved with a stomach tube, a small rumen fistula can be inserted to prevent bloat and the animal can be placed in a pen without bedding, feed, or water. If the obstruction does not resolve in 24 hours, the animal can be sedated, a cuffed endotracheal tube passed to prevent aspiration, and vigorous lavage with water through a stomach tube attempted. If the obstruction still cannot be relieved, a rumenotomy may be needed.

Aftercare

Aftercare consists of providing a soft diet (e.g., well-soaked alfalfa cubes made into a mush) and administering NSAIDs. Broad-spectrum antibiotics should be given if there is suspicion of mucosal damage. Feeding through an indwelling nasogastric tube, left in place for up to 10 days, may be helpful in preventing strictures after severe esophageal trauma. Alternatively, the animal can be fed and watered through a rumen fistula.

Esophageal Dilation (Megaesophagus)

Megaesophagus is rare in ruminants. Clinical signs include regurgitation or vomiting (usually shortly after eating) and mild, recurrent bloat. Diagnosis and management are described in *Large Animal Internal Medicine,* third edition.

INDIGESTION *(Text pp. 722-745)*

Indigestion is a general term for a group of diseases characterized by dysfunction of the reticulorumen. These problems can be divided into two broad categories:

- Abnormal motor function–reticulitis/rumenitis, ruminal parakeratosis, vagal indigestion, obstruction of the cardia or reticuloomasal orifice, diaphragmatic hernia
- Abnormal microbial fermentation–inactivity of rumen microbial flora, simple indigestion, rumen acidosis, rumen alkalosis, putrefaction of rumen ingesta

Secondary indigestion is a sequela of systemic problems or disease in other organ systems. Examples include endotoxemia, fever, anorexia (from any cause), pain (especially involving abdominal viscera), hypocalcemia, and primary abomasal disease. Bloat (ruminal tympany) is a common consequence of indigestion in ruminants. It is discussed separately on p. 754.

Abnormal Reticulorumen Motor Function

Abnormal reticulorumen motor function involves diseases of the reticuloruminal wall or its innervation or those that impede passage of ingesta from the reticulorumen. Traumatic reticuloperitonitis (TRP) is probably the most important of these conditions. It is discussed separately on pp. 747-748.

Reticulitis/rumenitis

Probably the most common cause of rumenitis is acute rumen acidosis produced by grain engorgement (see p. 745). Ulceration and secondary bacterial infection of the rumen wall also occurs in oak or acorn toxicosis and with ingestion of caustic chemicals. Other causes include specific infections of the rumen wall (e.g., actinobacillosis, actinomycosis, tuberculosis) and neoplastic growths (e.g., papillomas, myxomas, fibromas, carcinomas, lymphosarcoma). Diseases that cause anorexia plus abomasal reflux predispose animals to mycotic rumenitis.

Acute and extensive lesions can cause signs similar to those of TRP: pain, inappetence, impaired forestomach function, and in some cases, death. More chronic cases may cause signs of vagal indigestion (see p. 726).

Ruminal parakeratosis

With ruminal parakeratosis, the rumen papillae are darkly colored, thickened, and clumped together. These changes predominantly occur in animals on pelleted or very finely ground rations, especially high-energy rations. Although ruminal parakeratosis may impair performance, the signs that lead to its discovery are usually those of chronic acidosis (see p. 215). In calves, parakeratosis is often associated with hairballs (trichobezoars).

Vagal indigestion

The vagal indigestion syndrome encompasses a group of motor disturbances that hinder passage of ingesta from the reticulorumen and abomasum. It is discussed separately on p. 726.

Obstruction of the cardia or reticuloomasal orifice

True mechanical obstructions of the forestomach are uncommon. The obstruction can be complete or partial and may occur at either the cardia or the reticuloomasal orifice. Causes include inflammatory and neoplastic conditions (e.g., papillomas), foreign bodies (e.g., plastic bags), and trichobezoars (in calves). Cardia obstruction leads to signs typical of esophageal obstruction. Obstruction of the reticuloomasal orifice produces signs similar to those seen with vagal indigestion (see following discussion). Rumenotomy is needed to differentiate these obstructive diseases from other problems with similar signs.

Diaphragmatic hernia

Defects in the diaphragm are uncommon in cattle. Entrapment of the reticulum may cause sudden dyspnea, tachycardia, and poor venous return, but generally, it produces signs of vagal indigestion caused by omasal transport failure (see following discussion). Signs of pain may also be present, as with TRP. Rumination is usually impaired, and vomiting of large volumes of ingesta may occur, especially after eating.

Vagal Indigestion

The pathogenesis of vagal indigestion remains to be fully clarified. Vagus nerve abnormalities are present in less than 33% of cases; inflammation involving the ruminoreticular wall is common in the remaining cases. There are four types of functional disturbance, with obstruction of ingesta flow at two sites:

1. Omasal transport failure (anterior functional stenosis)–impairs flow of ingesta through the reticuloomasal orifice. It can occur with (1) atony of the reticulorumen or (2) normal or increased rumen motility.
2. Pyloric outflow failure (posterior functional stenosis)–impairs flow through the pylorus. It occurs either (1) continuously or (2) in an intermittent, recurrent pattern.

Omasal transport failure

Failure of omasal transport with rumen hypermotility is the most common form of vagal indigestion. TRP is the most common cause. Other causes include reticuloomasal abscesses, adhesions, and peritonitis without foreign body penetration; hepatic abscesses; diffuse peritonitis; papilloma or other mass at the ruminoreticular fold, esophageal groove, or reticuloomasal orifice; inflammation of the reticular and ruminal walls; and herniation of the reticulum through a diaphragmatic defect.

Clinical findings. Accumulation of ingesta in the reticulorumen leads to gradual distention of the forestomachs and hence the left paralumbar fossa. Appetite diminishes as the rumen becomes overfilled. Continued rumen dilation leads to marked overfilling of the ventral sac, which occupies both left and right ventral quadrants. The resulting abdominal contour is often said to be shaped like a "papple" (pear-apple). Vigorous rumen contractions can be palpated in most affected animals, although some display almost complete rumen atony. Fecal volume is reduced and the feces, which has a greasy or pasty consistency, contains material with increased fiber length. Affected animals often continue to drink water, yet become mildly dehydrated.

Pyloric outflow failure

Failure of pyloric outflow causes accumulation of ingesta in the abomasum and omasum and, in advanced cases, gross distention of the reticulorumen. A common cause is persistent atony after surgical correction of abomasal volvulus. Other conditions that can impede pyloric outflow include abomasal displacement, abomasal ulceration, adhesions involving the abomasal fundus and reticulum, and advanced pregnancy (indigestion of late pregnancy).

Clinical findings. Generally, forestomach motility is not markedly affected in the early stages, and normal stratification of ingesta is maintained. Overfilling of the forestomach as a result of reflux of ingesta from the abomasum (internal vomiting) may occur, causing the chloride content of the rumen fluid to increase (normal is less than 30 mEq/L). With severe forestomach distention, motility is reduced and the rumen contents become more fluid. Marked dehydration and hypochloremic, hypokalemic metabolic alkalosis often develop. Fecal production tends to be even less than with omasal transport failure.

Abnormal Reticuloruminal Fermentation

Inactivity of rumen microflora

Inactivity of rumen microflora most commonly occurs in cattle fed poor-quality roughage (e.g., late-cut, highly lignified hay or straw). Poorly digestible feed gradually accumulates in the forestomach, often leading to distention of the reticulorumen (haybelly), which can cause moderate recurrent bloat from weak rumen contractions. Fecal passage is reduced, and feces is dry and contains undigested plant fibers. Other findings are those of nutrient deficiency. Microflora inactivity can also occur with prolonged anorexia. Rumen fill is decreased in such cases.

Simple indigestion

Simple indigestion is a common result of an abrupt ration change or ingestion of spoiled feedstuffs. The condition generally is relatively mild and self-limiting. Most affected animals are anorectic for 1 to 2 days, develop diarrhea after about 24 hours, and return to feed without treatment when rumen fermentation stabilizes. Rumen motility is reduced but usually not absent, rumen fill is not remarkably altered, and if bloat occurs it is mild.

Acute rumen acidosis

Acute rumen acidosis (grain overload, toxic indigestion) is the result of excessive consumption of readily fermentable carbohydrates (e.g., cereal grains, fruits, root crops). Excessive production of lactic acid alters the microbial flora, draws fluid into the rumen, and can directly damage the rumen mucosa. The clinical result is increased rumen fluid volume (causing rumen distention), rumen hypomotility, inappetence, dehydration, and systemic acidosis. Secondary problems can include laminitis, mycotic rumenitis, rumen wall abscessation, and dissemination of bacteria to the liver (resulting in hepatic abscess).

Severe rumen acidosis. Cattle examined a few hours after severe grain overload may still be alert but are anorectic, with a mildly distended rumen, weak rumen contractions, and mild colic. However, depression, severe dehydration, weakness, recumbency, tachycardia, tachypnea, and profuse diarrhea rapidly develop; death may ensue within 24 to 72 hours. Rectal temperature is usually normal or subnormal. Animals still capable of rising may show a staggering gait and appear blind; in fact, the pupillary light reflex may be sluggish. Recumbent animals usually lie quietly and may be stuporous.

Chronic rumen acidosis

Chronic rumen acidosis is caused by feeding excessive quantities of concentrate with low levels of well-structured fibrous roughage over a prolonged period. Affected cattle may have reduced appetite and rumen hypomotility. Lactic acid does not accumulate, but the high rate of volatile fatty acid production results in moderately acidic rumen fluid (pH 5 to 5.5). Possible consequences include ruminal parakeratosis, decreased absorption of volatile fatty acids, rumenitis with hepatic abscessation, chronic laminitis, and cerebrocortical necrosis.

Rumen alkalosis

Rumen alkalosis most commonly occurs when microbial fermentation is reduced while the animal continues to swallow saliva. Rumen fluid pH between 7.0 and 7.5 is found with prolonged anorexia, microflora inactivity caused by poorly digestible roughage, and some cases of simple indigestion. Mild rumen alkalosis (neutral pH) can also result from the generation of excessive ammonia, such as occurs with high-protein diets.

More dramatic elevations in ammonia concentration, with rumen fluid pH greater than 7.5, follow overfeeding or accidental ingestion of nonprotein nitrogen sources such as urea, biuret, and ammonium phosphate. In these animals, muscle tremors, incoordination, weakness, tachypnea, and central nervous system excitation are seen in addition to signs of forestomach dysfunction (rumen hypomotility, bloat, vomiting, abdominal pain).

Putrefaction of rumen ingesta

Putrefaction of rumen ingesta results from overgrowth of microflora (e.g., coliforms, *Proteus* spp.) that decompose feed material in a putrefactive manner. The offending microflora are supplied in fermented feeds or concentrates undergoing spoilage or in feed or water contaminated with feces. The clinical course typically is chronic. Rumen motility declines, appetite is poor, and recurrent bloat (which may be frothy) develops. The rumen fluid has a blackish-green color, putrid odor, poor protozoal and bacterial activity, and a pH of 7.0 to 8.5.

Forestomach Diseases in Calves

Reticuloruminal milk accumulation (ruminal drinking)

In preruminant calves, milk can gain access to the reticulorumen by several means: failure of esophageal groove closure (e.g., tube feeding), overfeeding of fluids beyond the capacity of the abomasum (about 2 L in a newborn calf), abomasal reflux (e.g., abomasal inflammation or ulceration), and feeding fluids that affect abomasal emptying (e.g., acidic or hypertonic fluids, severely heat-treated skim milk, nonmilk proteins).

Retention of milk in the forestomach can lead to abnormal fermentation patterns. Affected calves fail to grow normally, have a poor hair coat, and sometimes have a depraved appetite. They appear potbellied, and the rumen is distended with fluid and milk clots; rumen motility is poor, and recurrent bloat is common. Rumen fluid pH is often alkaline (although it can be acidic) and has a putrid odor. Feces is commonly pasty or fluid.

Fermentation disorders

Calves fed concentrated diets to the exclusion of forages or mixed diets with the hay pelleted or finely ground may experience ruminal parakeratosis and a form of chronic rumen acidosis that results in slowed growth and poor body condition. Affected calves often crave fibrous materials; hair coat licking is common and can lead to hairball formation in the reticulorumen.

Conversely, when calves are fed dry forage only, the indigestible fiber accumulates in the rumen, which becomes grossly distended (haybelly). The rumen contents are firm, the fluid has a neutral pH with little microbial activity or odor, rumen motility is poor, and despite the full abdomen, the calf is thin. Recurrent bloat is common in these calves.

Recurrent bloat (rumen tympany) in calves

Moderate gas distention of the rumen is a common sign of disease in calves. Usually it is the result of free-gas accumulation; frothy bloat is very uncommon in young ruminants. In most cases the calf continues to consume feed, so abnormal rumen function and development is easily overlooked. Purulent lung infections are a common cause of bloat in calves, probably as a result of intrathoracic compression of the esophagus or possibly the vagus nerves.

Clinical Signs of Indigestion

Chapter 30 in *Large Animal Internal Medicine,* third edition, contains a comprehensive discussion of physical examination findings in ruminants with indigestion. Following are the clinical signs typically associated with primary indigestion and their possible causes:

- Decreased rumen filling–fermentative indigestion or secondary indigestion (especially with persistent anorexia) in which passage of material from the rumen is not impeded

- Abdominal distention–likely causes depend on site of distention
  - Left dorsal–ruminal tympany (bloat), left abomasal displacement (mild distention)
  - Left ventral or bilateral–severe ruminal distention (or advanced pregnancy or hydrops)
  - Right side–abomasal or intestinal conditions (dilation, displacement, obstruction, ileus)
- Excessive fluid (or froth) in the rumen with loss of normal ingesta stratification–acute rumen acidosis, vagal indigestion, frothy bloat, proximal intestinal obstruction
- Excessive firm, fibrous material in the rumen–haybelly
- Firm, doughy ingesta in the ventral rumen with decreased rumen filling–prolonged rumen stasis caused by chronic disease involving anorexia
- Rumen hypermotility–early cases of frothy bloat, some cases of vagal indigestion
- Abdominal pain (present or elicited)–TRP, abomasal ulceration, reticulorumenitis
- Abnormal feces–likely causes depend on fecal abnormality
  - Decreased quantity, firm, dry, with increased fiber length–TRP, omasal transport failure, rumen inactivity with poor quality roughage, dental disease, some abomasal diseases
  - Abnormal amounts of whole cereal grains–acute or chronic rumen acidosis
  - Greasy consistency with very fine particle size–pyloric outflow failure, abomasal displacement
  - Foamy, fluid, yellowish color, acidic odor–acute rumen acidosis
  - Pasty or fluid consistency with foul odor–fermentative indigestion, enteritis
  - Decreased quantity, dry, but otherwise unremarkable–anorexia, acute indigestion
- Vomiting (rare)–vagal indigestion with rumen overdistention, reticulorumenitis, reticuloomasal orifice obstruction, diaphragmatic hernia, certain toxins (azalea, rhododendron, sneezeweed, some organophosphates)
  - Vomiting must be differentiated from esophageal disease
- Fever–TRP, reticulorumenitis

Rumen Fluid Analysis

Rumen fluid can be collected using a nasogastric tube, a specialized tube for rumen fluid collection, rumen trocarization, or centesis/aspiration. Following are the characteristics of rumen fluid from adult ruminants.

Color and consistency

Normal rumen fluid is brownish-green (may be yellowish-brown in cattle fed grain or silage). Fluid from cattle with prolonged rumen stasis or putrefaction of rumen ingesta is greenish-black. Fluid from cattle with rumen acidosis or calves with milk sequestration in the rumen is milky gray; in calves the fluid may contain milk clots. Normal rumen fluid is slightly viscous. The fluid becomes more watery when the microflora are inactive. Contamination of the sample with saliva increases the viscosity.

Odor

Normal rumen fluid is strongly aromatic. The odor is less prominent when the microflora are inactive. Abnormal odors include the acidic smell of lactic acidosis, the putrid odor of protein decomposition or spoiled milk, and the ammonia smell of urea poisoning.

pH and chloride concentration

Normal rumen fluid pH varies somewhat with the type of diet: 6 to 7 for animals on a roughage diet; 5.5 to 6.5 with a grain diet. In animals held off feed the rumen pH is more than 7 within 12 hours after a hay meal and within 24 hours after a grain meal. Rumen pH values of 7 to 7.5 are common in animals with simple indigestion and inactivity of the microflora caused by indigestible roughage. Saliva contamination of the sample falsely elevates the measured pH. The chloride concentration of normal rumen fluid is less than 30 mEq/L. Elevated rumen chloride suggests secondary indigestion caused by abomasal disease or obstruction of intestinal flow.

Sedimentation/flotation time

Sedimentation/flotation time is a simple test used to evaluate microflora activity. Immediately after fluid collection the sample is allowed to sit in a tube and the time for completion of sedimentation and flotation of solid particles is measured; normal is 4 to 8 minutes. Fluid with inactive microflora (e.g., rumen acidosis, prolonged anorexia, indigestible roughage diet) shows very rapid sedimentation and none of the material may float. When the ingesta is very frothy (e.g., frothy bloat, some cases of vagal indigestion), there may be no appreciable sedimentation or flotation.

Redox potential

The redox potential test measures the anaerobic fermentative metabolism of the bacterial population in the rumen fluid. One milliliter of 0.03% methylene blue is added to 20 ml of rumen fluid (at body temperature), and the time taken to decolorize the dye is measured. With highly active flora the initial dark blue color disappears within 3 minutes. With a hay-only diet, decolorization takes 3 to 6 minutes; with a high-grain diet, decolorization may occur in as little as 1 minute. Reduction times of 15 minutes or more are found with diets of indigestible roughage, prolonged anorexia, and rumen acidosis.

Protozoal activity and Gram stain

Evaluation of the protozoal population in normal rumen fluid reveals multiple forms and sizes, with active motion. A predominance of only small protozoa suggests a mild digestive disturbance. All protozoa are killed off at rumen pH less than 5. Gram stain of normal rumen fluid reveals a predominance of gram-negative bacteria. A predominance of gram-positive cocci and rods is seen with rumen lactic acidosis.

Treatment of Indigestion

Eliminating the underlying problem more effectively resolves indigestion than treatment directed at the clinical signs. With the exception of cardia or esophageal obstruction, the mild and recurrent free-gas bloat associated with most digestive disturbances can be handled by treating the primary problem. Inhibition of eructation caused by lesions of the cardia region can usually be confirmed and corrected (if possible) only by exploratory rumenotomy. Inflammatory lesions, including purulent lung infections, may respond to long-term administration of broad-spectrum antibiotics. Bloat is discussed separately on p. 754.

Vagal indigestion

The principles of treatment for most forms of vagal indigestion are as follows:

- Determine the likely cause (often requires exploratory laparotomy and/or rumenotomy).
- Administer appropriate therapy (e.g., antibiotics, NSAIDs, foreign body removal, relief of obstruction, ration changes, induction of parturition/cesarean section).
- Relieve forestomach distention as needed by nasogastric intubation or rumen fistula.
- Correct fluid, electrolyte, and acid-base disturbances with parenteral fluid therapy.
- Limit feed and water intake or feed a palatable, high-fiber ration (e.g., grass, long-stemmed hay).
    - Maintain hydration with intravenous fluids until reticulorumen motility is reestablished.
- Transfaunate from a healthy animal, ideally one adapted to the patient's intended diet.

  - At least 3 L of rumen fluid is needed for an adult cow; 8 to 16 L is more desirable.
- Fistulate the rumen if chronic bloat is a problem.

Response to treatment can take several weeks. Repeated development of rumen distention and continued scant fecal output, rumen hypomotility, and recurrent bloat are poor prognostic signs.

Fermentative indigestion

Treating fermentation disorders centers around restoration of a normal rumen fluid environment:

- Correct the cause (e.g., adjust the feed regimen)
- Correct rumen pH
  - Confirmed acidosis can be corrected with $Mg(OH)_2$ and $NaHCO_3$ at 1 g/kg PO initially.
  - Confirmed alkalosis can be corrected with vinegar at 2 ml/kg PO (up to 12 L).
  - These treatments are best administered via nasogastric tube in several liters of warm water.
- Correct systemic acid-base and electrolyte abnormalities (if present) with parenteral fluids
- Remove grossly abnormal rumen ingesta (e.g., spoiled milk, putrefying ingesta, excessive grain) via rumenotomy or repeated nasogastric lavage
  - From 2 to 3 days of intraruminal antibiotics may be used to kill undesirable microflora, but this must be followed with transfaunation and appropriate feeding changes.
  - Neomycin or tetracycline is indicated for rumen alkalosis or urea poisoning and chlortetracycline or erythromycin for rumen acidosis.
- Correct rumen fill (whether overdistention or emptiness)
  - Overdistention with poor quality roughage can be treated by rumenotomy or by restricting feed intake to small quantities of readily digestible feed several times per day.
  - Dissolution and passage of indigestible material can also be aided by administering mineral oil (4 L) or DSS (4 to 6 oz in 2 to 3 L water) via nasogastric tube.
  - Rumen contractions can be stimulated by mildly overfilling the rumen with warm water (20 to 30 L for an adult cow) containing 2 teaspoons/L of NaCl and KCl.
- Transfaunate repeatedly from a healthy animal (see previous discussion)
- Provide oral and parenteral mineral and vitamin supplementation (especially B vitamins) when indigestion or anorexia is chronic
  - Oral dosage of KCl (120 g [4 oz]/day) is also indicated when anorexia is prolonged.

Severe rumen acidosis

Severe grain overload requires prompt and aggressive treatment:

- Perform an emergency rumenotomy and remove the acidic rumen contents.
- Administer $Mg(OH)_2$ into the rumen and $NaHCO_3$ intravenously.
- Administer intravenous fluid therapy until the animal has recovered.
- Continue transfaunation and dietary adjustments through the recovery phase.

TRAUMATIC RETICULOPERITONITIS (HARDWARE DISEASE) *(Text pp. 747-748)*

TRP, or hardware disease, is common in cattle but rare in small ruminants. Accidental ingestion of a metal foreign object can result in penetration of the reticulum, potentially leading to localized or generalized peritonitis. In some cases only the wall of the reticulum is involved, although reticulorumen motor function may be affected (see Vagal Indigestion). The diaphragm, pericardium, heart muscle, and liver may also be involved.

Clinical Signs

Severe, acute TRP

In its most severe form, TRP is characterized by fever, anorexia, rumen hypomotility or atony, sudden decrease in milk production, and evidence of cranial abdominal pain (reluctance to move, reluctance to ventroflex or an expiratory grunt on pinching of the withers, grunt on upward pressure on the xiphoid region). Auscultation may reveal a pounding heart or muffled heart sounds bilaterally if pericarditis has developed. Other signs, such as tachycardia, reluctance to lie down, mild bloat, constipation, and abducted elbows, often abate within the first day or two.

Less severe or chronic TRP

Less severe or longstanding cases may have more subtle signs. Weight loss, rough hair coat, diarrhea, and generalized lameness, along with cranial abdominal pain that is difficult to localize, may be the only signs. If pericarditis has developed, signs of right-sided congestive heart failure (e.g., distended jugular and superficial abdominal veins) may be seen. Dyspnea may occur if left-sided heart failure is also present. Abscesses involving the liver or spleen may cause other signs of GI malfunction, particularly ruminoreticular outflow problems.

Diagnosis

The WBC count and distribution, plasma proteins, and plasma fibrinogen may be normal initially. Later, the hemogram often reflects an acute or chronic infectious process. Total plasma protein of 10 g/dl or more (primarily hyperglobulinemia) is supportive of the diagnosis. Peritoneal fluid analysis (see following discussion) may be rewarding if the peritonitis is not well localized. Pericardiocentesis (using a 5- to 10-cm spinal needle or intravenous catheter in the fifth left intercostal space, level with the point of the elbow) can also be useful. Radiography may show metallic foreign bodies in the reticulum, but surgery may be necessary to confirm their significance.

Treatment

Conservative treatment is generally attempted first and includes administration of a forestomach magnet, parenteral antibiotic therapy, and confinement in a stanchion or box stall. Many cattle recover after such therapy, with resumption of forestomach motility and appetite in 1 to 3 days. Animals not significantly improved by the third day may require a rumenotomy to remove the foreign object. Treatment of peritonitis is discussed next.

PERITONITIS *(Text pp. 748-753)*

Peritonitis is an inflammatory process that involves the serosal surfaces of the peritoneal cavity. It may result from trauma (e.g., TRP, penetrating wounds), surgery, GI ulceration, visceral rupture, internal abscess, or bowel ischemia.

Clinical Signs

Clinical signs are often nonspecific but are suggestive of GI dysfunction. Severity ranges from recurrent mild discomfort (e.g., localized abscess) to acute onset of severe toxemia and hypovolemia that is rapidly fatal (e.g., rupture of a viscus). Cattle suffering from acute, disseminated peritonitis tend to show the following signs: abdominal rigidity and tenderness, reluctance to ventroflex on withers pinch, reluctance to move, abdominal distention, scleral injection, fever, anorexia, tachycardia, dehydration, sudden hypogalactia, and rumen atony.

Diagnosis

Hematology

Depending on the severity of peritoneal contamination, abnormalities range from none to severe leukopenia with degenerative left shift, toxic neutrophils, elevated PCV, and decreased plasma proteins. Less severe cases may have neutrophilic leukocytosis and hyperfibrinogenemia.

Peritoneal fluid analysis

The right side of the abdomen, just cranial to the udder, is the preferred site for peritoneal fluid collection. Normal peritoneal fluid in cattle is clear, with specific gravity less than 1.016. The protein content is less than 3 g/dl (less than 6.3 g/dl in some studies) and the nucleated cell count is less than 10,000 cells/μl (ratio of 1:1 neutrophils to macrophages). Cytologic examination is useful in making a diagnosis of peritonitis.

Treatment

The aims of therapy are as follows:

- Stabilize the patient–correct fluid, acid-base, and electrolyte abnormalities; administer supplemental calcium and NSAIDs or short-acting corticosteroids; transfaunate.
- Correct the primary cause in a manner that does not compromise patient survival.
- Treat the infection (medically if possible).
  - Begin broad-spectrum systemic antimicrobial therapy while awaiting sensitivity results; ideally start with intravenous therapy.
  - Suitable single-antibiotic choices are tetracyclines, a third-generation cephalosporin, or a synthetic penicillin.
  - Surgery, when necessary, involves peritoneal debridement, irrigation, and drainage.

BLOAT (RUMINAL TYMPANY) *(Text pp. 754-756)*

Bloat, or ruminal tympany, is abnormal distention of the ruminant forestomach with ingesta or gas. There are three categories of bloat:

- Frothy bloat, caused by diets that lead to formation of stable froth within the rumen (e.g., lush legumes, winter wheat pasture, high-concentrate finishing rations)
- Free-gas bloat caused by high-grain rations
- Free-gas bloat caused by failure to eructate, such as esophageal obstruction, lateral recumbency, hypocalcemia, pain, general anesthesia, xylazine administration

Bloat may be fatal if the distention is extreme enough to compromise ventilation.

Clinical Signs

The degree of forestomach distention varies from that producing even filling of the left paralumbar fossa to that causing uniform, extreme abdominal enlargement. Signs of colic (kicking at the abdomen, treading, frequent lying down and rising, vocalization) may be seen. As the forestomach enlarges, breathing becomes more labored. Open-mouth breathing, cyanosis of mucous membranes, and collapse may terminate in death within minutes.

Diagnosis

Laboratory evaluation is not required for diagnosis and management in most cases of bloat. However, a sample of rumen contents should be collected when no cause is obvious. The presence or absence of froth and the pH are important features that influence therapy.

Treatment

Passage of a stomach tube generally is sufficient to relieve the discomfort of mild to moderate free-gas bloat. If no gas can be released even with manipulation of the tube, suction should be applied and the tube withdrawn and examined for froth. Unless the animal is severely dyspneic or extremely colicky, frothy bloat can be treated with surface-active agents. Poloxalene (44 mg/kg via nasogastric tube) is recommended for forage bloat and mineral oil or animal tallow for feedlot (grain) bloat.

Animals with extreme distention and severe dyspnea require immediate surgical intervention. A trocar introduced through the left paralumbar fossa relieves free-gas bloat, but an emergency rumenotomy may be necessary to evacuate frothy contents.

ABOMASAL DISPLACEMENT AND VOLVULUS
(Text pp. 756-764)

Left Displacement of the Abomasum

Left displacement of the abomasum (LDA) is the most common type of abomasal displacement. The highest incidence is seen in dairy cattle in early lactation. High-starch and low-roughage diets are often implicated. Abomasal displacements also occur in association with other common postpartum disorders, including hypocalcemia, retained placenta/metritis, and severe mastitis.

Clinical findings

Cows with LDA are inappetant or anorectic, do not chew their cud, and have decreased rumen motility, fecal output, and milk production. The feces may be drier than normal or scant and watery. Mild pain may be evident (e.g., treading, mild tachycardia). Ketonuria and acetone on the breath are commonly present. In most cases the last one or two ribs on the left are "sprung," but the paralumbar fossa is sunken. Simultaneous auscultation and percussion reveals a ping over the gas-filled abomasum (see Chapter 1). During rectal examination it may be possible to feel the abomasum to the left of the rumen or at least perceive that the rumen is displaced medially.

Diagnosis

Percutaneous needle aspiration of fluid or gas from the suspected abomasum aids diagnosis. A pH of less than 4.5 or the odor of abomasal gas (slightly acrid) confirms the presence of LDA. Mild metabolic alkalosis is common in cows with LDA; hypochloremia, hypokalemia, and hypocalcemia may also be found. Cattle examined on the farm are usually hypoglycemic with ketonuria, but after transport hyperglycemia (with or without glycosuria) may be observed.

Treatment

Treatment for LDA involves returning the abomasum to its normal position (see main text), treating the coincident electrolyte and acid-base abnormalities (often unnecessary), and providing therapy for concurrent disease conditions.

Right Displacement of the Abomasum

The clinical findings with right displacement of the abomasum (RDA) are similar to those of LDA, except that the "ping" is found on the right side (see Chapter 1). Surgery is required for correction of RDA. Because RDA can predispose the animal to abomasal volvulus and can be difficult to differentiate from early volvulus, intervention should be as prompt as possible.

Abomasal Volvulus

Abomasal volvulus causes complete outflow obstruction. Marked bilateral abdominal enlargement results from abomasal distention and rumen stasis. A large area of tympanitic resonance is detectable on the right (see Chapter 1), and splashing sounds can be heard when the abomasum is balloted behind the last rib.

Borborygmi are absent. The distended abomasum may be palpable rectally. Without intervention, cardiovascular collapse and death occur within 1 to 3 days. Colic rarely develops with abomasal volvulus.

Clinical pathology

Hypochloremic metabolic alkalosis with hypokalemia and paradoxic aciduria is often present early in the course of the disease. As the condition progresses, dehydration becomes more marked, and metabolic acidosis may supersede the alkalosis terminally. Serum chlorine less than 79 mEq/L is associated with a high mortality rate.

Treatment

Immediate surgical intervention is necessary. Fluid, electrolyte, and acid-base abnormalities must be corrected simultaneously. For early cases, large volumes (20 to 80 L) of intravenous fluids, consisting of 0.9% NaCl with 25 to 100 mEq/L of KCl added, are administered. For advanced cases with metabolic acidosis, balanced electrolyte solutions (e.g., Ringer's lactate solution) are indicated.

ABOMASAL ULCERS *(Text pp. 760-762)*

Abomasal ulcers occur in cattle of all ages. The condition is associated with stress and with high-starch diets. Concurrent diseases are often present and include the common postpartum disorders of dairy cattle (LDA/RDA, ketosis, metritis, mastitis) and lymphosarcoma.

Clinical Signs

Abomasal ulcers can be classified into four types:

1. Nonperforating–signs include mild abdominal pain, inappetence, rumen hypomotility and mild tympany, normal or reduced fecal output, and fecal occult blood
2. Nonperforating with severe blood loss–signs include inappetence or anorexia, rumen hypomotility and tympany, abdominal pain, melena, and pallor (anemia from blood loss)
   - Blood loss may be severe and acute enough to cause hemorrhagic shock.
3. Perforating with local peritonitis–clinical presentation similar to TRP
   - Abdominal pain can usually be localized to the right ventral quadrant.
   - As with TRP, acute signs usually abate over a few days.
   - In some cases, large amounts of pus accumulate within the omental bursa, resulting in a more prolonged clinical course and often causing death.
4. Perforating with diffuse peritonitis
   - Signs of septic shock develop within 24 hours and rapidly result in death.

Diagnosis

The most useful diagnostic test for abomasal ulcer disease is the fecal occult blood test. Abdominocentesis confirms diffuse peritonitis (see p. 761). Plasma fibrinogen is increased (greater than 700 mg/dl) in most cattle with peritonitis. Cattle more than 5 years of age with bleeding abomasal ulcers should be tested for bovine leukosis virus.

Treatment

Treatment is aimed at the following:

- Correcting dietary problems–replace starchy feedstuffs with good-quality hay
- Reducing stress
- Ameliorating concurrent disease problems
- Initiating specific therapy for the clinical problems caused by the ulcer
  - Intravenous or oral fluid therapy for dehydration and metabolic or acid-base disturbances

- Blood transfusion if the PCV is 14% or less; usually 4 L of whole blood once is sufficient
- Broad-spectrum antimicrobial therapy for cattle with peritonitis
- Surgery for valuable cattle with perforating ulcers

ABOMASAL IMPACTION *(Text pp. 763-764)*

Abomasal impaction most often occurs in overwintering beef cows that are fed nothing but poor-quality, coarse roughage. Other presentations or predisposing factors include feeding low-quality milk replacers to calves (that then eat their bedding or other indigestible materials); abomasal atony after correction of abomasal volvulus; and lymphosarcoma or other space-occupying lesions adjacent to the pylorus. A syndrome of abomasal dilation and mechanical transport failure causes a clinically similar condition in Suffolk sheep (see main text).

Clinical Signs

Common signs in adult cattle are reduced feed intake; scant, firm, dry feces; and poor body condition. The animal may have bilateral ventral abdominal enlargement and bulging of the left paralumbar fossa. Rumen contractions are normal or increased in frequency but often reduced in strength; later, rumen motility is often absent. The abomasum may be palpable as a firm mass following the right coastal arch. If the abomasum ruptures, signs of generalized peritonitis occur.

Diagnosis

In adult cattle, rectal examination reveals a distended rumen; the distended abomasum may also be palpable. In calves the abomasum may fill the majority of the abdomen and be doughy or firm on external palpation. Some cattle have metabolic alkalosis with chloride accumulation in the rumen, but in other cases hypochloremia and alkalosis do not develop.

Treatment

Treatment is usually unrewarding. Salvage by slaughter is often the most economic recommendation. Early cases may be resolved with easily digestible feeds, aggressive fluid therapy, and laxatives. Metoclopramide (0.3 mg/kg SC every 4 to 6 hours) may improve abomasal emptying. Installation of a nasogastric tube into the abomasum via rumenotomy and daily infusion of mineral oil (8 ml/kg), DSS (50 mg/kg), $Mg(OH)_2$ (1 g/kg), or $MgSO_4$ (2.5 g/kg) may aid in clearing the abomasum. Abomasotomy has not been successful in restoring abomasal function.

OBSTRUCTIVE INTESTINAL DISEASES *(Text pp. 764-768)*

Intestinal Atresia or Stenosis

Intestinal atresia or stenosis in neonates causes the following signs: absence of feces, progressive abdominal distention, depression, colic, and finally cardiovascular collapse. The prognosis for normal intestinal function, even after surgical correction, is poor.

Intestinal Volvulus around the Mesenteric Root

Volvulus of the small and large intestine around the mesenteric root is most common in neonates. Colic (which can be extremely violent) and abdominal distention occur acutely and rapidly progress to shock and collapse. In older cattle, tympany is restricted to the right side. Rectal examination reveals distended loops of gut and loss of normal topographic relationships. Volvulus of lesser portions of the intestinal tract causes similar signs, but onset is often slower. Colic, with accompanying tachycardia, rumen stasis, and anorexia, is present to varying degrees. Immediate surgical correction is necessary.

Intussusception

Intussusception occurs in all ruminants but is most common in neonates. Signs typically include colic initially, then chronic low-grade pain (may be absent in neonates); inappetence; dehydration; decreased fecal output; mucus and blood in dark red feces; fever; and gradual abdominal distention (often bilateral). A mass may be rectally palpable in adult cattle or through the abdominal wall in neonates; distended loops of intestine may also be found on rectal examination. If the affected bowel becomes devitalized, signs of peritonitis may develop (see p. 220). Surgical correction is required.

Cecal Dilation and Volvulus

Cecal dilation and volvulus are most common in adult dairy cattle in early lactation. Cecal dilation has a more gradual onset of signs than does volvulus.

Cecal dilation

With simple dilation, feed intake and milk production decrease and mild abdominal pain may be evident. The right paralumbar fossa is usually distended without the ribs being sprung. A large area of resonance is auscultable from the tuber coxae cranially. Manure is usually passed, but it may be scant and loose. The apex of the gas-filled cecum can be felt within or near the pelvic canal on rectal examination. Medical management with laxatives, intravenous or oral fluids, and a high-fiber diet is usually successful. Calcium therapy may also be helpful in lactating cows.

Cecal volvulus

Cecal volvulus causes abrupt onset of anorexia, agalactia, and marked abdominal pain, with tachycardia, forestomach stasis, and right abdominal distention. Manure is usually scant or absent. The apex of the cecum is usually not detectable on rectal palpation, but instead the distended body of the cecum or proximal colon impinges on the pelvic canal. Surgical intervention and fluid therapy to correct the hypokalemic, hypochloremic metabolic alkalosis are required.

Mesenteric Fat Necrosis

Mesenteric fat necrosis occurs most often in the Channel Island breeds. Many affected cattle are asymptomatic. When present, signs resemble progressive intestinal obstruction from other causes: weight loss, anorexia, diarrhea, bloody stool, abdominal enlargement, and right-sided ping with partial obstruction; fever, tachycardia, and signs of discomfort (tenesmus, treading, teeth grinding) as the obstruction becomes more severe. The condition usually is not treated.

Intestinal Incarceration

Intestinal incarceration can occur in any ruminant. Initial signs of colic followed by depression, anorexia, progressive abdominal distention, and absence of feces usually develop. Distended loops of small intestine are usually rectally palpable. Surgical intervention is required.

Ileus

Intestinal ileus can develop in any ruminant but is more common in lactating dairy cattle. Affected cows are most often presented for examination because of partial anorexia or colic. Physical examination is unremarkable, except for weak rumen contractions, right-sided abdominal enlargement (slight initially but may become marked), and absence of borborygmi. On rectal examination, distended spiral colon, cecum, or small intestine may be palpated; feces is scant or absent. The condition often resolves spontaneously; in rare instances, surgical decompression is required.

WINTER DYSENTERY IN CATTLE *(Text pp. 773-774)*

Winter dysentery is an explosive diarrheal disease of cattle that occurs in epizootic fashion within a herd, usually during the winter. The cause is unknown, but a coronavirus has been implicated.

Clinical Signs and Diagnosis

Diarrhea is accompanied by some degree of anorexia, dullness, and hypogalactia. Blood may be present in the feces of several animals in the group, typically in the first-lactation heifers. Most affected animals are afebrile. The period of illness in an individual is brief, and within a herd the outbreak usually lasts less than 2 weeks. Diagnosis is made by exclusion of other causes of epizootic diarrhea (e.g., internal parasites, moldy feed, coccidiosis, salmonellosis).

Treatment

Most animals with winter dysentery recover spontaneously in a few days. Palliative treatments, such as intestinal astringents, protectants, and adsorbents, do not seem to alter the course of disease. Provision of adequate fresh water, palatable feed, and free-choice salt is recommended.

SALMONELLOSIS *(Text pp. 775-778)*

Clinical Syndromes

Salmonellae are gram-negative enteric bacteria that can cause a variety of clinical signs in both adults and neonates. The most common signs of salmonellosis are fever and diarrhea. The diarrheic feces vary from watery to mucoid with fibrin and blood and often have a putrid odor. The systemic effects of absorbed toxins (including endotoxin) may be severe, resulting in shock.

Manifestations in calves

Bacteremia may occur rapidly, especially in neonates infected with *Salmonella dublin* or *Salmonella typhimurium*. Dyspnea, respiratory symptoms, sudden death, and occasionally diarrhea are the principal signs of *S. dublin* infection, which peaks in incidence in 6-week-old calves. Blood culture results are commonly positive. Calves infected with *S. typhimurium* are only 14 days old on average (range, 1 to 35 days) and mainly have enteric lesions. They are also often bacteremic.

Diagnosis

Definitive diagnosis requires culture of the organism from feces, blood, or tissues. *Salmonella* enteritis often causes changes in the hemogram, including hyperfibrinogenemia and either neutrophilia or neutropenia (with a left shift in severe cases). Initial dehydration may result in elevated PCV and plasma protein, but plasma protein drops as protein is lost into the bowel. Nonspecific clinical chemistry abnormalities often seen include elevated liver enzymes, hypocalcemia, and indications of prerenal azotemia.

Treatment

The keys to successful treatment of bacteremia are as follows:

- Antimicrobial drugs, based on sensitivity patterns of cultured organisms
  - Most *Salmonella* are sensitive to florfenicol and ceftiofur.
  - Resistance to penicillin, streptomycin, erythromycin, and tylosin can be anticipated.
- Fluid therapy to correct dehydration and electrolyte and acid-base disturbances
  - Sodium-containing fluids, with glucose added, are recommended.
- NSAID administration
- *S. typhimurium* antiserum (commercially available, but can cause frequent adverse reactions)

Control of salmonellosis is discussed in detail in *Large Animal Internal Medicine,* third edition.

JOHNE'S DISEASE *(Text pp. 779-782)*

Johne's disease is an insidious and chronic infection primarily of ruminants. It is caused by *Mycobacterium paratuberculosis.* The organism initially invades the ileum and then gradually spreads to regional lymph nodes and other body organs. Beef cattle have lower infection rates than dairy cattle. NOTE: Johne's disease is a reportable condition in many states.

Clinical Signs

The great majority of infected animals appear clinically normal. Only after a prolonged incubation period (2 to 10 years) do they begin to develop clinical signs, which include gradual weight loss despite a normal appetite and decreased milk production. Over several weeks, fecal consistency becomes more fluid and usually progresses to pipestream diarrhea without tenesmus, blood, or excess mucus. As the disease progresses, affected animals become increasingly lethargic and emaciated. Intermandibular edema (hypoproteinemia) typifies advanced stages of the disease. Cachexia and waterhose diarrhea characterize the terminal stages.

Diagnosis

Most animals showing clinical signs have positive fecal culture results and increased antibody titers on ELISA or agar gel immunodiffusion (AGID). Early ("silent") infection in young cattle can rarely be detected with any of the current laboratory tests. Some asymptomatic carrier adults have positive fecal cultures. The relative merits of the various diagnostic tests (AGID, ELISA, complement fixation, DNA probes, histopathology, γ-interferon tests, and fecal culture) are discussed in *Large Animal Internal Medicine,* third edition. Fecal culture remains the gold standard for routine detection of infected individuals. However, results may not be available for 12 to 16 weeks.

Treatment

No practical therapy is available for Johne's disease. In valuable cattle, remission of clinical signs may be achieved with isoniazid (22 mg/kg [10 mg/lb] PO), rifampin (22 mg/kg PO), or clofazimine (11 mg/kg [5 mg/lb] PO). The drug must be given daily; if therapy is stopped, clinical signs may reappear within a few weeks. No drug or combination has been shown to eliminate the infection or prevent shedding of *M. paratuberculosis.* Control of Johne's disease is discussed in *Large Animal Internal Medicine,* third edition.

COPPER DEFICIENCY *(Text pp. 783-786)*

Copper deficiency occurs when the diet contains an abnormally low amount of copper (primary copper deficiency) or when copper absorption or metabolism is adversely affected by high dietary levels of molybdenum, sulfates, zinc, iron, or other compounds (secondary copper deficiency).

Clinical Signs

Clinical signs of copper deficiency can include diarrhea (may be profuse), weight loss or decreased weight gain, pallor (anemia), changes in coat color or wool quality, spontaneous fractures, lameness (epiphysitis), demyelinization (enzootic ataxia of sheep and goats, swayback; see Chapter 33), and infertility. Young animals and fetuses are more susceptible than mature animals, and cattle are more susceptible than sheep.

Diagnosis

Liver biopsy for hepatic copper concentration is the preferred diagnostic sample. Hepatic copper values less than 35 μg/g (dry weight) are considered deficient. Liver biopsy can place the live patient at increased risk for black disease or bacillary hemoglobinuria, the risk of which can be decreased by prior vaccination and postbiopsy administration of penicillin. Serum or plasma copper concentrations of

0.4 μg/ml or less are considered evidence of frank deficiency. Response trials using injectable copper are also a valid means of diagnosis.

Treatment

Treatment in cattle involves subcutaneous injection of copper glycinate. Adult cattle should receive 400 mg (120 mg copper [Cu]), and calves are given 100 to 200 mg (30 to 60 mg Cu), depending on their age. One injection may be effective for up to 6 months in cases of primary copper deficiency. In cases of secondary deficiency, repeat injections may be necessary every 4 to 6 weeks. Copper glycinate often causes large swellings, granulomas, or abscesses at the injection site. Copper can also be supplemented orally (see main text). Sheep are susceptible to copper toxicity, so care is necessary when supplementing them.

COBALT DEFICIENCY *(Text pp. 786-788)*

Dietary cobalt deficiency in ruminants can cause a variety of signs, including decreased growth or weight loss, diarrhea, decreased feed efficiency, anorexia, anemia (normocytic, normochromic), pica, and lacrimation. Clinical disease is more common in growing animals. Sheep are more susceptible to cobalt deficiency than cattle. Ovine white liver disease is a recently recognized cobalt deficiency syndrome in sheep, characterized by ill thrift, weight loss, serous ocular discharge, and occasionally photosensitization.

Diagnosis

The most significant clinical chemistry analysis is tissue vitamin B_{12} concentration. Liver vitamin B_{12} values of 0.19 μg/g or less of fresh liver are indicative of cobalt deficiency. Serum vitamin B_{12} values 0.3 ng/ml or less also indicate cobalt deficiency (normal is 1 to 3 ng/ml).

Treatment

Treatment is best accomplished in the short term with vitamin B_{12} injections: 100 μg/wk or 150 μg every other week in lambs; 300 μg/wk in adult sheep; and 2000 to 3000 μg/wk in cattle.

Part III: All Large Animal Species

DISEASES CAUSED BY *C. PERFRINGENS* *(Text pp. 768-771)*

C. perfringens is a toxin-producing, spore-forming, anaerobic, gram-positive rod that causes disease in horses and ruminants. Several pathogenic biotypes have been identified. Isolation of *C. perfringens* from a necropsied animal is not sufficient basis for diagnosis, but if toxin is also demonstrated in gut contents and the history and lesions are compatible, a diagnosis of *C. perfringens* intoxication can be made. Samples for culture must come from newly dead animals. Samples of gut contents should be collected in sterile containers and cooled or frozen.

C. perfringens Type A (Yellow Lamb Disease)

Yellow lamb disease is an uncommon disease attributed to *C. perfringens* type A. Widespread hemolysis leads to anemia, weakness, hemoglobinuria, and icterus. The animals have high temperatures and usually die within 6 to 12 hours of onset. The diagnosis is always questionable because of the commensal nature of the organism and its rapid invasion after death. The finding of predominantly large gram-positive rods in impression smears from intestinal mucosa lends support to the diagnosis.

C. perfringens Type B (Lamb Dysentery)

Lamb dysentery is a highly fatal disease of young lambs in Britain and South Africa. Its clinical course and presentation are similar to those of necrotic enteritis caused by *C. perfringens* type C. Type B has not been isolated in North America.

C. perfringens Type C (Necrotic Enteritis)

Necrotic enteritis is primarily a disease of neonates and occurs in calves, lambs, foals, and piglets. It causes diarrhea that may be yellow or, in more hemorrhagic cases, brownish, with gray-red streaks of necrotic mucosa. Foals with necrotic enteritis initially show acute abdominal pain, then explosive yellow diarrhea that becomes brown and hemorrhagic. Affected animals become dehydrated, anemic, weak, and moribund despite intensive therapy. Morbidity and mortality rates are high. Once established on the premises, the disease may become endemic.

Treatment

Treatment generally is unsuccessful because of the fulminant nature of the disease. Foals can be treated with broad-spectrum antibiotics, intravenous fluids, intravenous and oral plasma, metronidazole (10 mg/kg PO twice daily), *C. perfringens* types C and D antitoxin IV, and parenteral feeding. During an outbreak, metronidazole can be given to at-risk foals, starting at 8 to 12 hours of age and continuing for 5 days. Other control measures are discussed in *Large Animal Internal Medicine,* third edition.

C. perfringens Type D (Enterotoxemia, Pulpy Kidney)

Enterotoxemia caused by *C. perfringens* type D is a disease of major importance in sheep and of lesser importance in cattle and goats. Most cases occur in animals on a highly nutritious diet.

Clinical signs and diagnosis

Sudden death of a well-fed, rapidly growing animal is the most common presentation. The disease may run its course in 30 to 90 minutes, with affected lambs showing ataxia, trembling, stiff limbs, opisthotonus, convulsions, coma, and death. Sublethal doses may result in brain damage and focal symmetric encephalomalacia. Postmortem lesions are inconsistent; the "pulpy kidney" lesion may not be seen in freshly examined specimens. Glucosuria is considered a hallmark of type D enterotoxemia.

Treatment

If initiated at first suspicion of the disease, type D antitoxin and oral antibiotics (sulfas) can have dramatic results. The diet should be adjusted during outbreaks to minimize starch intake. Lambs on rich pasture should be moved to poorer pasture or corralled and fed hay until they have been vaccinated twice. Antitoxin can be given in an outbreak, but prior vaccination is more effective (see main text).

OAK (ACORN) TOXICOSIS *(Text pp. 772-773)*

Toxicity can occur in ruminants (especially cattle) and occasionally in horses that ingest large quantities of oak buds, oak leaves, or acorns. The GI tract (including the mouth and esophagus) and kidneys are the organs most affected. Mortality rates often exceed 80%. Young cattle (less than 200 kg) often are more severely affected than adult cattle.

Clinical Signs in Cattle

The course of oak toxicosis is usually 1 to 12 days, but some cattle have protracted disease. A day or two after ingestion, animals appear anorectic and listless, have rumen hypomotility, and often have hemorrhagic diarrhea or dark diarrhea that tests positive for occult blood; feces may have a phenolic smell. Dehydration occurs rapidly, but vital signs may be remarkably normal until hypovolemia develops. As uremia progresses, scleral vessels become dark and engorged and the breath may smell of ammonia. Protracted cases most often result from renal failure, although some animals have chronic oral, esophageal, or GI ulceration and perforation.

Peracute toxicosis

With peracute toxicosis, cattle are recumbent, weak, anorectic, listless, tachycardic, and tachypneic. Rectal temperature is normal or subnormal. Marked edema is present in the perineum and vulva, and edema is obvious in the submandibular area, brisket, and ventral abdomen. Hydration appears adequate, but anuria is present. Evidence of hydrothorax, hydropericardium, and ascites may be noted. Some cattle are simply found dead.

Clinical Signs in Horses

Signs in horses are usually peracute or acute and include sudden death or colic with tenesmus, hemorrhagic diarrhea, tachycardia, hyperpnea, increased borborygmi, and injected oral mucous membranes. Acorn husks and shells may be noted in the feces. Hemoglobinuria may also occur.

Diagnosis

Cattle

In cattle with peracute or acute signs, BUN and serum creatinine are elevated. Low serum sodium, chloride, and calcium (5.1 to 6.8 mg/dl) and high serum potassium and PO_4 accompany mild metabolic acidosis with a very high anion gap (29 to 32). Elevations in neutrophil count, fibrinogen, sorbitol dehydrogenase, and γ-glutamyltransferase may also be present. If urine is being produced, isosthenuria, proteinuria, and glucosuria are often found. Abnormalities in protracted cases are more variable.

Horses

Laboratory findings in horses are similar to those in ruminants, except that marked increases in PCV occur during the acute stages. Protein, occult blood, and hemoglobin casts may be found in the urine. In addition to a history of exposure, measurement of serum or urinary phenolic (hydrolyzed tannin) content may be useful in acute cases.

Treatment

In acute stages, intravenous fluid therapy aimed at promoting diuresis and correcting acid-base and electrolyte abnormalities may be lifesaving. Calcium, sodium, and chloride deficits should be replaced and bicarbonate given if needed to correct metabolic acidosis. Furosemide (1 mg/kg IV twice daily) can be used in anuric animals. Analgesics and laxatives are used as needed in colicky horses. Antibiotics (to prevent secondary pneumonia and GI abscess), rumen transfaunation (ruminants), and ready access to grass hay and water are recommended parts of nursing care.

Prognosis

If the animal survives the acute stage and begins eating, the prognosis for recovery is good. Renal function can return to normal in 5 to 10 weeks.

RECTAL PROLAPSE *(Text pp. 788-789)*

Rectal prolapse can occur in all domestic animals. Four categories are described:

- Type I–mucosal prolapse
- Type II–complete prolapse
- Type III–complete prolapse with invagination of the small colon
- Type IV–intussusception of the rectum (or small colon in horses) through the anus

Types I and II are much more common and are more amenable to correction than types III and IV, which often cause loss of vascular integrity to the rectum or small colon and require immediate intervention.

Treatment

The first aim of therapy is identification and alleviation of the cause if possible. The animal's value and intended use and the viability of the affected tissue need to be considered when deciding between conservative and surgical options.

Types I and II

Types I and II are usually treated conservatively. Caudal epidural anesthesia may be required to reduce straining and facilitate correction. A loose purse-string suture may be placed circumferentially in the anal sphincter to prevent recurrence postreduction. The suture should be removed after 3 to 4 days. When indicated, stool softeners and enemas may be used to ease the passage of feces through the rectum. Broad-spectrum antimicrobials should be administered if there is compromise of the tissues.

Types III and IV

Types III and IV that cannot be manually reduced often require surgery. These types of rectal prolapse carry a fair to guarded prognosis.

31

Diseases of the Hepatobiliary System

Consulting Editor ERWIN G. PEARSON

Contributors NAT T. MESSER IV • JOSEPH HOYT (JOE) SNYDER
STANLEY P. SNYDER • THOMAS J. DIVERS • JOHN B. MALONE
JOHN MAAS • TERRY C. GERROS

DIAGNOSIS OF LIVER DISEASE *(Text pp. 790-795)*

Signs of Liver Disease

Many signs can be present with liver disease, but none are pathognomonic, and none are present consistently. Signs of liver disease or failure include the following: icterus (most common in horses and more common with acute hepatitis than with chronic liver disease), weight loss, ascites, change in liver size, diarrhea (most common in cattle), pruritus (uncommon), photodermatitis, hepatic encephalopathy, tenesmus and rectal prolapse (cattle), change in fecal color, hemorrhage (terminally), and pain on palpation of the liver.

Hepatic encephalopathy

Hepatic encephalopathy (HE) is a clinical syndrome, characterized by abnormal mental status, that occurs secondary to hepatic insufficiency or shunting that allows portal blood to bypass the liver. Signs are nonspecific and variably include depression or excitability, yawning (horses), excessive vocalization (ruminants), incoordination, dyspnea or inspiratory stertor (horses), aimless walking, and head pressing. Affected animals eventually become stuporous and then comatose. Blood ammonia is elevated in most cases.

Laboratory Tests of Liver Function

Liver-derived enzymes are discussed in Chapter 22; normal serum values are listed in Table 22-2. Hypoalbuminemia is uncommon in horses with liver disease; it is most likely in patients with chronic liver disease. Bromsulphalein (BSP) clearance is discussed in *Large Animal Internal Medicine,* third edition.

Bilirubin and urobilinogen

With liver damage in horses or ruminants, most of the retained bilirubin is indirect reacting (unconjugated), and the direct/total ratio usually is less than 0.3. With bile blockage or intrahepatic cholestasis the direct/total ratio may be more than 0.3 in horses and more than 0.5 in cattle. With complete biliary blockage there is no urobilinogen in the urine.

Serum bile acids

The serum concentration of bile acids is increased with hepatocyte damage, blockage of bile flow, or portosystemic shunting. In horses values greater than 14 μmol/L indicate liver damage, bile blockage, or shunting. In adult cattle the bile acid concentration in a single sample must be more than 126 μmol/L in beef cattle and more than 88 μmol/L in dairy cattle to be specific for liver disease. Levels are lower (less than 64 μmol/L) in calves younger than 6 months old.

Liver Biopsy

Liver biopsy can be useful in confirming the presence of liver disease, determining or ruling out some causes, and establishing a prognosis. In all species, adequate restraint is needed. The skin over the biopsy site is aseptically prepared and infiltrated with 2% lidocaine; a small stab wound is then made in the skin. The site of skin puncture varies among species:

- Horses–right fourteenth intercostal (IC) space, on a line between the tuber coxae and the point of the shoulder; biopsy instrument is directed slightly cranioventrally
  - Some veterinarians recommend using the twelfth or thirteenth IC space, along the same line.
- Cattle–right eleventh IC space, level with the middle of the paralumbar fossa; biopsy instrument is directed slightly cranioventrally
- Sheep and goats–ninth or tenth IC space, level with the ventral end of the last rib; biopsy instrument is directed craniomedially

Ultrasonography

Ultrasonographic examination of the liver is useful for identifying liver abscesses, choleliths, liver flukes, masses, and diffuse fibrosis. The location for best visualization varies with species:

- Horses–right or left side in the eighth to fourteenth IC spaces, ventral to the lung
- Cattle–right side in the tenth to twelfth IC spaces
- Sheep–right side in the seventh to twelfth IC spaces

Prognostic Indicators

Indicators of poor prognosis in liver disease include serum albumin less than 2.5 g/dl (horses); prothrombin time more than 30% of normal; greatly elevated γ-glutamyltransferase (GGT) and alkaline phosphatase (AP) with normal or decreased sorbitol dehydrogenase (SDH) or glutamate dehydrogenase (GLDH); marked fibrosis on histopathologic examination. Severe pyrrolizidine alkaloid toxicosis carries a particularly grave prognosis. Terminal clinical signs include hemolytic crisis (horses) and marked hepatic encephalopathy in a patient with a fibrotic liver.

ACUTE HEPATITIS IN HORSES *(Text pp. 795-796)*

Idiopathic acute hepatic disease (IAHD; Theiler's disease, serum hepatitis) is the most common cause of acute hepatitis and hepatic failure in adult horses. It is a potential complication of the use of any equine serum product in horses but is most commonly associated with the use of tetanus antitoxin (TAT).

Clinical Signs

Clinical signs of acute hepatic disease are those of acute hepatic failure, such as depression, jaundice, inappetence, pica, yawning, photoactive dermatitis, and hepatic encephalopathy. Fever is rare. Atypical signs include progressive weight loss, ventral subcutaneous edema, abnormal jugular pulses, and acute respiratory distress. Intravascular hemolysis may lead to hemoglobinuria in terminal cases. Some horses that receive TAT have clinicopathologic evidence of liver dysfunction without developing clinical signs, indicating that disease severity may vary.

Diagnosis

Diagnosis of acute hepatic disease is based on the history, clinical signs, and on findings of the following tests:

- Serum biochemistry–elevated bilirubin (unconjugated and total), bile acids, GGT, SDH, AST, lactate dehydrogenase (LDH), and AP.
- Hepatic biopsy or necropsy–widespread hepatic necrosis, most severe in the

centrilobular and midzonal areas, with the few living cells confined to the periportal areas
  - Lesions often are more advanced than the clinical course would suggest.

IAHD may occur sporadically or may affect a group of horses. Recognition of IAHD in one horse should prompt careful observation of horses on the same premises for either clinical or serum biochemical signs of IAHD.

Treatment

Therapy should be aimed at supporting liver function and controlling abnormal behavior (see pp. 820-821). Continuous intravenous administration of dextrose and balanced electrolyte solutions is recommended. If spontaneous bleeding occurs at injection sites or at sites of self-inflicted injury, plasma transfusion may be necessary to replace the deficient clotting factors. Glucocorticoids may be justified based on some evidence of an immune-mediated cause.

BLACK DISEASE *(Text pp. 796-798)*

Black disease (infectious necrotic hepatitis) is a highly and often peracutely fatal disease of grazing animals, primarily sheep. It is caused by toxins produced by *Clostridium novyi* type B. Disease occurs only when there is sufficient liver damage to provide the anaerobic environment required for growth of resident sporulated organisms. In practice the liver insult is almost always caused by larval migration of the common liver fluke, *Fasciola hepatica.*

Clinical Signs

In most cases, affected animals are simply found dead. In the unlikely instance that an affected animal is recognized before its death, the signs are nonspecific: depression, anorexia, dyspnea, and fever (declines before death).

Diagnosis

A history of sudden death, usually in an endemic area during warmer weather in a flock or herd with a poor vaccination and fluke control history, is highly suggestive. Diagnosis can often be accomplished at necropsy (see main text). Gram stain of an impression smear of the liver reveals numerous large, gram-positive rods. Further measures include identification of the organism by anaerobic culture or fluorescent antibody tests and identification of *C. novyi* type B toxins.

Treatment

C. novyi is highly sensitive to penicillin (e.g., crystalline penicillin 20,000 IU/kg intravenously [IV]) and tetracyclines (e.g., oxytetracycline 5 mg/kg IV), but toxin production is usually too far advanced for antibiotics to be of value. In the face of an outbreak, vaccination should be initiated immediately, along with mass administration of penicillin or tetracycline, preferably in a long-acting form. Prevention is discussed in *Large Animal Internal Medicine,* third edition.

BACILLARY HEMOGLOBINURIA (RED WATER) *(Text pp. 798-799)*

Bacillary hemoglobinuria (red water, icterohemoglobinuria) causes sudden death in cattle and other ruminants and, rarely, in horses. It is caused by the toxins of *Clostridium hemolyticum* (*C. novyi* type D). As with black disease, bacillary hemoglobinuria generally occurs after liver insult caused by migration of *F. hepatica* (common liver fluke) larvae.

Clinical Signs

In most cases, affected animals are found dead. In the rare instances in which the disease is recognized antemortem, general signs are similar to those described for black disease. Affected animals may also have rapid and shallow respiration, blood or blood-tinged froth at the nostrils, and rectal bleeding or bloody feces; mucous membranes are pale and icteric. Despite the name, passage of dark red, port wine-colored urine (hemoglobinuria) is rarely seen.

Diagnosis

Diagnosis is usually made at necropsy. The pathognomonic liver lesion is a large (up to 30 cm in diameter) area of coagulative necrosis. Gram-stained impression smears from the liver, or from the spleen, blood, or abdominal fluid, reveal numerous typical clostridial organisms. Laboratory confirmation depends on identification of the causative bacterium. Both fresh (refrigerated) and formalin-fixed liver tissue should be submitted.

Treatment

If there is opportunity for treatment, penicillin (at least 20,000 IU/kg, beginning with crystalline penicillin IV) is the antibiotic of choice, although tetracyclines (5 mg/kg IV twice daily or 10 mg/kg intramuscularly [IM] daily) are acceptable. Blood transfusion is advisable and should be repeated as necessary. Prevention is discussed in *Large Animal Internal Medicine,* third edition.

HEPATIC FAILURE IN FOALS *(Text pp. 799-800)*

Hepatic failure in foals can result from a variety of causes, including the following:

- Infectious–perinatal equine herpesvirus type 1 infection, leptospirosis, *Actinobacillus equuli,* Tyzzer's disease (see following discussion), other bacterial infections, septic portal vein thrombosis
- Parasitic–*Parascaris equorum* migration
- Congenital–bile duct atresia, portosystemic shunts, hepatic failure in Morgan weanlings
- Toxic–iron fumarate (see following discussion)
- Other–systemic inflammatory response syndrome and multiple organ dysfunction (an exaggerated response to sepsis), chronic neonatal isoerythrolysis, cholangitis associated with duodenal ulcer disease

Iron Fumarate Toxicity

Administration of iron fumarate before colostrum ingestion or administration may be followed in 2 to 5 days by signs of hepatic encephalopathy. Icterus is noted in most affected foals, although some foals die peracutely.

Congenital Portosystemic Shunts

Congenital portosystemic shunts are rare in horses. Clinical signs may not be noted until foals are 2 to 3 months of age and begin eating large amounts of grain or grass. Waxing and waning signs of encephalopathy are common.

Diagnosis and treatment

An elevation in plasma bile acids and ammonia with normal serum concentrations of liver-derived enzymes should arouse suspicion of a portosystemic shunt. Positive contrast portography is the diagnostic technique of choice. Successful medical management followed by shunt ligation has been described in a foal.

Tyzzer's Disease

Tyzzer's disease is an acute, rapidly fatal, focal bacterial hepatitis that affects foals between 7 and 40 days of age. The causative organism is *Clostridium piliformis.* In many cases the foal is found dead and showed no previous signs of illness. Clinical signs (e.g., fever, icterus, depression, anorexia, diarrhea, seizures), when detected, are nonspecific.

Diagnosis

Laboratory abnormalities include serum elevations of liver enzymes, bilirubin, and fibrinogen and severe hypoglycemia. The diagnosis in most cases is made at necropsy. Histopathologic examination of the liver reveals multifocal areas of necrosis in which the organism can be identified with special stains.

Treatment

Early antimicrobial therapy (large doses of intravenous penicillin and an aminoglycoside) and intravenous fluids could be helpful. However, there are no reports of successful treatment.

CHRONIC ACTIVE HEPATITIS *(Text pp. 800-801)*

Chronic active hepatitis represents a sustained inflammatory process within the liver. Several factors, including toxins, bacterial infection, and immune processes, probably are involved.

Clinical Signs

Progressive weight loss, intermittent fever, and icterus may be noted initially. Signs typical of liver failure (see pp. 790-792) may develop as liver function deteriorates. Signs of abdominal disease may be present, and some horses develop skin lesions at the coronary band or areas of necrotic, leathery skin.

Diagnosis

Serum liver enzyme activities are usually elevated, reflecting active hepatocyte damage; AP and GGT tend to be markedly elevated in the active stages. Serum bile acids and bilirubin (especially conjugated) are also increased. Definitive diagnosis is made histologically. Part of the liver biopsy specimen should be submitted for bacterial culture and sensitivity.

Treatment

Treatment of liver disease is outlined on pp. 820-821. Corticosteroids are useful in horses with lymphocytic-plasmacytic hepatic infiltrates. Dexamethasone is given at 20 to 40 mg/day for the first 4 to 7 days, then gradually reduced over the next 2 to 3 weeks. Prednisolone (400 mg/day orally [PO]) may be required for an additional 2 to 4 weeks. Antibiotics are indicated when bacterial cholangiohepatitis is suspected because of neutrophilic hepatic infiltrate or positive culture of biopsy.

PYRROLIZIDINE ALKALOID TOXICITY *(Text pp. 801-803)*

Pyrrolizidine alkaloid (PA) toxicity is a chronic, progressive, often delayed intoxication that results when animals consume plants containing PAs, such as *Senecio* spp. (e.g., tansy ragwort, groundsel), *Amsinckia* spp. (e.g., fiddleneck), and *Crotolaria* spp. (e.g., rattlebox). Cattle (especially calves) and horses are most susceptible; sheep and goats are fairly resistant.

Clinical Signs

The effects of PA toxicosis are cumulative, and because signs often are delayed, some animals may not become ill until a year or more after removal from feed sources containing the toxins.

Horses

The most common signs in horses are weight loss, icterus, and abnormal behavior (e.g., wandering, ataxia); photosensitization is occasionally seen. Subtle signs, such as poor performance, may be noted before the onset of liver failure.

Cattle

Cattle more often show diarrhea, weight loss, tenesmus, rectal prolapse, and ascites. Behavioral changes or subtle neurologic signs may also be seen in cattle, but icterus is uncommon.

Diagnosis

Although SDH and LDH are elevated initially, they may have returned to normal by the time the animal shows signs of liver failure. However, GGT, AP, and AST tend to be consistently elevated. Serum bile acids are increased; levels greater than 50 µmol/L indicate a poor prognosis in horses. Bilirubin, both direct and indirect, tends to be increased in horses in the later stages.

Liver biopsy

Liver biopsy is useful in establishing the diagnosis. The triad of fibrosis, bile duct proliferation, and megalocytosis is characteristic. However, aflatoxins may produce similar changes.

Treatment

No satisfactory treatment exists for PA toxicosis. Once obvious signs of liver failure develop, the animal usually dies within 5 to 10 days. Horses with mild clinical signs and reversible histologic lesions may survive if they retain an appetite and are not exposed to any more PA-contaminated feeds. The principles of treatment for hepatic disease should be followed (see pp. 820-821). In particular, a low-protein, high-energy diet should be fed.

OTHER HEPATOTOXINS *(Text pp. 803-805)*

Hepatotoxic plants, chemicals, and drugs are listed in Tables 31-4, 31-5, and 31-6 of *Large Animal Internal Medicine,* third edition. These toxins are also discussed in Chapter 50.

LIVER FLUKES IN RUMINANTS *(Text pp. 805-808)*

F. hepatica

Infestation with *F. hepatica,* the common liver fluke, in ruminants mimics the production effects and clinical appearance of gastrointestinal nematodiasis. In addition, migration of immature flukes through the liver predisposes the animal to black disease and bacillary hemoglobinuria (both described earlier in this chapter).

Seasonal and geographic distribution

The maximum economic effect of fluke infestation is usually seen in the late fall and winter. Explosive seasonal outbreaks of severe parasitism can occur, especially in sheep. The geographic distribution of *F. hepatica* in the United States is mainly limited to the southcentral states, Florida, and the Pacific Northwest. In tropical regions, *F. hepatica* is replaced by *Fasciola gigantica,* a similar species of somewhat greater pathogenicity.

Clinical signs

When present, clinical signs in cattle include weight loss, depression, anorexia, rough hair coat, anemia, hypoproteinemia, submandibular edema, and mild icterus (rare). Sheep and goats are more susceptible. Fatal acute disease, with ascites, abdominal hemorrhage, pallor, and icterus, can occur in association with massive entry of flukes into the bile ducts 6 to 10 weeks after infestation. Chronic infestation in sheep causes submandibular edema, ascites, and emaciation.

Diagnosis

Fecal sedimentation methods are the standard means of diagnosing liver fluke infestation (see main text). Enzyme-linked immunosorbent assays have been developed for detection of serum antibodies and coproantigen in the feces of infected animals. Supportive clinical pathology findings include anemia, hypoproteinemia, mild eosinophilia, and elevated serum liver enzymes (GGT, GLDH).

Treatment

Flukecides available in the United States that are effective against mature flukes include albendazole (10 mg/kg) and clorsulon (2 mg/kg). Clorsulon at 7 mg/kg has added efficacy against juvenile flukes more than 6 weeks old. The optimal time to treat should be based on estimated susceptibility of the fluke population (see main text). Control measures are discussed in *Large Animal Internal Medicine,* third edition.

Fascioloides magna

The large American liver fluke, *Fascioloides magna,* may infect cattle and sheep that graze common areas with deer, the natural host. Geographic distribution in the United States includes the gulf states, Great Lakes area, and the northwest. The major economic effect in cattle is condemnation of livers and other affected organs at slaughter. In sheep, infestation with only one or two flukes may be fatal. Albendazole at high dosages is moderately effective against *F. magna.*

LIVER ABSCESSES *(Text pp. 808-810)*

Hepatic abscesses can be seen in any species but are more prevalent in ruminants, especially cattle. In most cases the primary etiologic agent in cattle is *Fusobacterium necrophorum.* Rumenitis secondary to grain overload is the most common mechanism that allows *F. necrophorum* to colonize the liver. Umbilical infections can spread to the liver in young animals.

Clinical Signs

Most cases of liver abscesses in cattle are subclinical. Clinically affected animals often exhibit weight loss, decreased gain or decreased milk production, and intermittent fever and anorexia. Some animals exhibit pain when moving, lying down, or with pressure over the right caudal rib cage. Caudal vena caval thrombosis (CVCT; see Chapter 29) is a possible sequela. In horses, signs are similar to other abdominal abscesses: weight loss and intermittent colic and fever.

Diagnosis

Laboratory findings vary and usually are nonspecific but supportive of the diagnosis. Liver enzymes such as GGT and AST may be increased only if the abscess process is active. Total bilirubin is not increased unless the abscess obstructs the bile ducts, but direct bilirubin may be increased. Ultrasound examination can identify the abscess in some cases. Liver biopsy should not be performed if an abscess is suspected.

Treatment

Treatment is not usually undertaken in cattle. If antibiotic therapy is used, penicillins, oxytetracycline, and macrolides (tylosin, erythromycin) are most likely to be effective. In horses, some cases improve with long-term antibiotic therapy using penicillin or ampicillin, often in combination with rifampin or metronidazole. Surgical drainage may be possible with some abscesses (e.g., single large abscess, umbilical vein/hepatic abscess). Prevention is discussed in *Large Animal Internal Medicine,* third edition.

HEPATIC LIPIDOSIS *(Text pp. 810-816)*

Fat Cow Syndrome

Fat cow syndrome is a multifactorial condition associated with excessive mobilization of fat to the liver in well-conditioned, postparturient dairy cows. It is induced by a negative energy balance during the periparturient period and in most cases is exacerbated by concurrent diseases (e.g., metritis, retained fetal membranes, mastitis, parturient paresis, displaced abomasum).

Clinical signs

Most affected cows are either obese or very well conditioned. Presenting signs usually include depression, anorexia, weight loss, weakness (which may lead to recumbency), rumen hypomotility, and decreased milk production. Other signs vary with the concurrent disease.

Diagnosis

Most laboratory tests are poor indicators of hepatic lipidosis and are of little value in determining the severity of the disease. Liver biopsy may confirm fatty infiltration of hepatocytes (see main text).

Treatment

The most important principle in treating hepatic lipidosis is elimination of the negative energy balance and the contributing factors or diseases. Other procedures can hasten this process:

- Intravenous glucose infusion at a rate of 100 to 200 mg/kg/hr
- Protamine zinc (NPH or Lente) insulin at 200 U/1000 lb twice daily with glucose
- Short-term corticosteroid therapy (as described for treating ketosis; see Chapter 39)
- Vitamin E and selenium supplementation
- Rumen transfaunation (see Chapter 30)

Protein-Energy Malnutrition/Pregnancy Toxemia in Beef Cows

Protein-energy malnutrition and pregnancy toxemia are conditions of pregnant beef cattle on marginal diets; most cases occur in the winter. Growing, pregnant heifers are especially susceptible. Clinical signs include weight loss, weakness, depression, and in some cases, diarrhea and inability to rise. Most affected cows die 7 to 14 days after becoming recumbent.

Treatment

Treatment is often unrewarding. Alfalfa pellet gruels can be helpful if force fed. Propylene glycol (150 to 200 ml PO twice daily) can be useful as a glucose precursor. Giving intravenous fluids and treating any concurrent diseases are also important.

Pregnancy Toxemia in Ewes and Does

Pregnancy toxemia (ketosis, twin-lamb disease) occurs in ewes and does during the last 2 to 4 weeks of gestation. It is caused by negative energy balance. The incidence is greater in ewes with more than one fetus (especially if the ewe was initially overweight) and in does with three or more fetuses.

Clinical signs

Pregnancy toxemia is characterized by anorexia, weakness, depression, apparent blindness, and eventual recumbency. Neurologic signs such as tremors, star-gazing, incoordination, circling, and teeth grinding may precede terminal recumbency.

Diagnosis

Ketonuria is usually present and detected before ketonemia, but hypoglycemia is an inconsistent finding. Acidosis, hypocalcemia, and hypokalemia are common. The plasma free fatty acid concentration is usually greater than 500 μEq/L, and serum β-hydroxybutyrate is elevated (greater than 1 mmol/L). Marked neutrophilia is found in some affected animals and is particularly dramatic in does, sometimes reaching 35,000 neutrophils/μl.

Treatment

The mortality rate is high unless treatment is started early and the fetuses are removed either by inducing parturition or by cesarean section:

- Parturition can be induced with 15 to 20 mg of dexamethasone in ewes, and in does with either 10 mg of dexamethasone or 10 μg of prostaglandin $F_{2\alpha}$.
- Ketosis should be treated with intravenous glucose (250 to 500 ml of 10% to 20% glucose, followed by a slow drip of 5% to 10% glucose).
- Acidosis and hypocalcemia must be corrected if present.

Other useful therapies include rumen transfaunation, vitamin B_{12} and biotin supplementation, and oral propylene glycol (15 to 30 ml twice daily).

Hyperlipemia in Ponies

Hyperlipemia, characterized by a fatty liver and milky serum, mainly occurs in ponies and occasionally in horses. It is caused by decreased caloric intake, often secondary to other diseases, and is most common in pregnant or lactating ponies.

Clinical signs and diagnosis

Affected ponies usually are anorectic, depressed, weak, and uncoordinated; diarrhea is common. Diagnosis is based on finding opalescent plasma. Serum triglycerides are more than 500 mg/dl; free fatty acids are also increased. Bilirubin usually is elevated (from anorexia). Terminally there may be metabolic acidosis.

Treatment

It is most important to treat any primary disease and to correct the negative energy balance. Initially, slow intravenous infusion of glucose may be necessary for several days or until the lipemia clears. Heparin (100 to 250 IU/kg subcutaneously [SC] twice daily) has also been advocated. Other recommendations include the following:

- Odd days–protamine zinc insulin (PZI; 30 IU/200-kg pony IM) with glucose (100 g PO) twice daily
- Even days–PZI (15 IU/pony IM) with galactose (100 g PO) twice daily

MISCELLANEOUS LIVER DISEASES *(Text pp. 817-818)*

Congenital hyperbilirubinemias, telangiectasia, ischemia/hypoxia/congestion, fetal liver damage, hemochromatosis in Salers cattle, and hepatic neoplasia are discussed in *Large Animal Internal Medicine,* third edition.

Failure of Drug Metabolism and Excretion

A number of drugs may have delayed clearance with hepatic insufficiency, including chloramphenicol, chlorthiazide, digitalis, erythromycin, morphine, most steroids, tetracycline, and many tranquilizers and anesthetic agents.

GALLBLADDER AND BILIARY TRACT DISEASE *(Text pp. 818-820)*

Biliary tract disease is rare in large animal medicine. Intrahepatic causes of cholestasis include cholangitis, cholecystitis, choledocholithiasis, and foreign bodies. Extrahepatic causes include abscess formation, inflammatory disease near the common bile duct, and neoplasia.

Choledocholithiasis/Cholelithiasis

Cholelithiasis is the presence of gallstones in either the bile ducts or gallbladder. Choledocholithiasis describes stones found in the common bile duct; it is the most common cause of biliary obstruction and occurs most often in horses.

Clinical signs

Cholelithiasis should be suspected in horses with intermittent colic, pyrexia, and icterus. Hepatic encephalopathy, photosensitization, and weight loss are less common findings.

Diagnosis

Elevations in serum AP, AST, GGT, L-iditol 2-dehydrogenase (IDH), total bilirubin (both direct and indirect), and serum bile acids are expected. Other possible abnormalities include hyperammonemia, increased urine bilirubin, prolonged partial thromboplastin and prothrombin times, neutrophilic leukocytosis, and elevated globulins and fibrinogen.

Ultrasonography. Hepatomegaly, increased parenchymal echogenicity, and bile duct dilation are seen on ultrasonography of the liver. Choleliths may be hyperechoic or sonolucent. In horses choleliths are most likely to be seen in the cranioventral part of the right hepatic lobe, especially in the sixth to eighth intercostal spaces.

Treatment

Treatment involves relief of biliary obstruction and management of hepatitis and associated complications. Unless diffuse fibrosis is already present, surgery is indicated if there is an obstructing stone. Treatment with potentiated sulfa drugs, ampicillin, tetracycline, or chloramphenicol is recommended before surgical intervention.

Cholangitis/Cholangiohepatitis

Cholangitis or cholangiohepatitis is a common cause of bile duct obstruction in large animals. Clinical signs in horses include anorexia, subtle behavioral changes, chronic weight loss, intermittent colic, fever, and icterus.

Diagnosis

Alterations in serum liver enzymes may indicate hepatocellular damage or cholestasis or both. Other abnormalities may include conjugated hyperbilirubinemia and an inflammatory leukogram. Histopathologic examination and bacterial culture of biopsy specimens are indicated.

Treatment

Antibiotic therapy is recommended if bacterial cholangitis is suspected. Broad-spectrum aerobic drug therapy, such as a combination of ampicillin and gentamicin, trimethoprim/sulfa, ceftiofur, or enrofloxacin, is preferred for initial therapy until culture and sensitivity results are known. Anaerobic organisms may also be involved, so metronidazole can be added. Prolonged antibacterial therapy (2 weeks to 3 months) is usually required.

Biliary obstruction. Ultrasonography is important in managing suppurative cholangitis in horses because some cases are associated with biliary stones. If there are small obstructing stones or sludge, DMSO (0.5 to 1 g/kg IV daily for 3 to 5 days) and intravenous crystalloid fluids may be beneficial.

THERAPY FOR LIVER FAILURE *(Text pp. 820-821)*

Abnormal Behavior

Initial therapy should be directed toward controlling any abnormal behavior the patient may be exhibiting. Extremely agitated or convulsing animals should be sedated. Xylazine is the drug of choice for horses with maniacal behavior. Diazepam should be avoided. If blood glucose is low, 0.2 to 0.4 ml/kg of a 10% glucose solution should be given intravenously.

Hyperammonemia

Measures directed toward decreasing the blood ammonia concentration include the following:

- Nasogastric intubation with a mild laxative (e.g., mineral oil)
- Oral neomycin (10 to 30 mg/kg two to four times daily) for 1 to 2 days, either alone or in combination with lactulose (90 to 120 ml PO [adult horse] three or four times daily) or acetic acid (0.5 ml/kg PO twice daily)

Metronidazole (10 to 15 mg/kg PO twice daily) may be used, but it is not preferred because this drug is metabolized by the liver and signs of toxicity can mimic HE.

Fluid Therapy

Dehydration should be corrected with balanced electrolyte solutions (preferably without lactate) containing supplemental dextrose (20 to 50 g/L) and potassium (20 to 40 mEq/L). Potassium should also be given orally (5 to 20 g twice daily). Fresh or fresh-frozen plasma can be used if needed, but stored whole blood or hetastarch should not be used in patients with hepatic failure.

Acidosis

Acidosis may be severe in horses with hepatic failure, but attempts at correction must be made slowly. Bicarbonate therapy is recommended only when venous pH is less than 7.1 and intravenous therapy with an alkalinizing, balanced electrolyte solution has failed to improve the acidosis.

Other Therapies

Antioxidant, antiinflammatory, and antiedema therapy may be useful in some cases of acute hepatic disease and failure. Potentially useful substances include

DMSO, acetylcysteine, vitamin E, mannitol, flunixin meglumine, and pentoxifylline.

Dietary Management

Animals with hepatic disease that maintain a fair appetite often are best treated by dietary management. Energy and protein requirements (especially branched-chain amino acids in horses) should be met. Small meals fed often are ideal. Grazing of mixed grasses should be encouraged as long as the animal can be protected from sunlight. Spring-cut hay or grass should be limited, and alfalfa is best avoided in horses. Vitamin B_1, folic acid, vitamin K_1, or fresh plasma transfusion might be indicated for chronic biliary obstruction.

Example

An example of a suitable diet is 4 parts beet pulp and 1 to 2 parts cracked corn, mixed with molasses and fed four to six times daily. Milo or sorghum may be used in place of corn, and sorghum, oat, or grass hay may be substituted for beet pulp.

PANCREATIC DISEASE *(Text p. 822)*

Pancreatic disease is rare in large animals. Acute and chronic pancreatic disease have been reported in horses; only chronic pancreatic disease has been reported in cattle (typically endocrine dysfunction such as type 1 diabetes mellitus).

Acute Pancreatitis

Causes of pancreatitis include migrating parasites; bacterial and viral infections; immune-mediated damage; biliary or pancreatic duct inflammatory disease; deficiencies of vitamin E or A, selenium, or methionine; vitamin D toxicity; and possibly several commonly used drugs (see main text). Characteristic, although nonspecific, signs of acute pancreatitis in horses include moderate to severe colic, gastric reflux, and hypovolemic shock.

Diagnosis

Laboratory confirmation is difficult. Tests that may be of value include serum amylase and lipase, peritoneal fluid (PF) amylase, and fractional excretion of amylase. Serum amylase values for normal horses range from 14 to 35 IU/L; PF values range up to 14 IU/L. Elevations are difficult to interpret because they can also occur in horses with proximal enteritis, colic, and primary renal failure. In acute pancreatitis, PF amylase is higher than serum amylase.

Treatment

Treatment of acute pancreatitis is symptomatic: prevention of gastric rupture by continuous gastric decompression; control of abdominal pain; administration of large volumes of a balanced electrolyte solution; correction of hypocalcemia; and use of broad-spectrum antibiotics.

32

Diseases of the Renal System

Consulting Editors HAROLD C. SCHOTT II • DAVID C. VAN METRE
THOMAS J. DIVERS

Contributors ELIZABETH A. CARR • MONICA R. ALEMAN
LOREN G. SCHULTZ • DAVID P. GNAD • DAVID G. RENTER

Part I: Equine Renal System

ACUTE RENAL FAILURE *(Text pp. 824-829)*

Causes

Acute renal failure (ARF) in horses is usually a consequence of exposure to nephrotoxins or vasomotor nephropathy (hypoperfusion or ischemia). Vasomotor nephropathy may be more common than nephrotoxic ARF in horses.

Toxic nephropathy

Toxic causes of ARF include the following:

- Aminoglycosides–neomycin (most nephrotoxic), gentamicin, kanamycin, amikacin
  - Nephrotoxicity typically develops after several days of administration to horses with diarrhea or septicemia that are not adequately hydrated.
- Myoglobin (e.g., severe myopathy) and occasionally hemoglobin (e.g., hemolysis)
- Nonsteroidal antiinflammatory drugs (NSAIDs)–when excessive doses are given or when dehydration is not promptly corrected
- Vitamin D toxicity–administration of vitamin D or ingestion of plants containing vitamin D metabolites (e.g., day-blooming jasmine [*Cestrum diurnum*])
  - Abnormal laboratory findings include elevations in serum calcium and phosphorus.
- Heavy metals–mercury, cadmium, zinc, arsenic, lead
- Acorn poisoning (see Chapter 30)

Vasomotor nephropathy

Any condition that causes sustained, marked hypotension or release of endogenous pressor agents can initiate hemodynamically mediated (vasomotor) ARF. Risk factors include hemorrhagic shock, severe intravascular volume deficit, septic shock, and coagulopathy.

Acute glomerulopathy

Acute glomerulopathy should be considered in cases of severe ARF that cannot be attributed to vasomotor nephropathy or nephrotoxicity. Gross hematuria, proteinuria, and oliguria support the diagnosis; renal biopsy can be pursued to confirm the lesion.

Acute interstitial nephritis

Acute interstitial nephritis is a rare syndrome of ARF accompanied by rapid elevations in serum creatinine and clinical signs of uremia. The cause is unknown;

idiosyncratic drug reaction is a possibility. Treatment with corticosteroids may be of benefit in suspect cases.

Leptospirosis

ARF associated with *Leptospira interrogans* serovar *pomona* has been reported in horses. Findings include fever, inappetence, depression, azotemia, and low urine specific gravity without bacteriuria. Seroconversion or high serum titers and positive fluorescent antibody test results on urine (air-dried sample on a microscope slide) can be used to establish the diagnosis. Successful treatment has been accomplished with intravenous fluids and penicillin administration.

Clinical Findings

ARF should be suspected in the following circumstances:

- More marked depression and anorexia than would be expected with the primary disease
- Failure to produce urine within 6 to 12 hours of initiating fluid therapy

Rectal palpation may reveal enlarged, painful kidneys. Enlargement can be confirmed by renal ultrasonography. Renal ultrasonography may also reveal perirenal edema, loss of detail of the corticomedullary junction, and dilation of renal pelves.

Vasomotor nephropathy

Oliguria (often manifested as a lack of expected urination in response to fluid therapy) is an important early indicator of vasomotor ARF. When urine is eventually produced, it may be diluted (specific gravity less than 1.020) and may be discolored (hematuria or hemoglobinuria) or have microscopic evidence of hematuria.

Diagnosis

Laboratory findings in horses with ARF include the following:

- Elevated serum creatinine and blood urea nitrogen (BUN)
  - The increase in creatinine is often several times greater than that for BUN, resulting in a BUN/Cr ratio that is often less than 10:1.
- Hyponatremia, hypochloremia, and hypocalcemia
  - Hyperkalemia, hyperphosphatemia, and metabolic acidosis may also be detected in severe cases.
- Low urine specific gravity (1.020 or less) in the face of dehydration
- Gross or microscopic hematuria
  - Significant proteinuria (urine protein/creatinine ratio greater than 2:1) suggests glomerular disease.
- Increased urine enzyme activity or glucosuria
- Casts and increased numbers of erythrocytes and leukocytes in the urine sediment
- Increased fractional clearances of sodium and phosphorus (see Chapter 22)

Specific findings associated with each of these toxic agents are discussed in *Large Animal Internal Medicine,* third edition.

Renal biopsy

Glomerular injury and tubular necrosis can be confirmed by performing a renal biopsy (see main text). However, the prognosis is often more dependent on response to treatment than on biopsy results. Renal biopsy is most indicated in the evaluation of horses with ARF for which exposure to nephrotoxins or another underlying primary disease process is not apparent. NOTE: Life-threatening hemorrhage is a potential complication of renal biopsy.

Treatment

Initial treatment of ARF should focus on judicious fluid therapy to replace volume deficits and correct electrolyte and acid-base abnormalities. Most patients are not oliguric after volume replacement, so 0.9% NaCl or a balanced electrolyte solution is appropriate for fluid therapy. Specific recommendations include the following:

- Give intravenous fluids at 40 to 80 ml/kg/day to promote continued decrease in serum creatinine.

  - May need to continue at 10 to 20 ml/kg/day until creatinine has returned to normal (or steady state) and the horse is eating and drinking adequately.
  - Supplementation with NaCl (1 to 2 oz orally [PO] twice daily) promotes greater fluid intake and diuresis.
  - If diuresis induces hypokalemia, supplement with KCl (1 oz PO twice daily).
- Monitor the magnitude of azotemia and serum concentrations of Na, Cl, K, and HCO_3 daily.
  - Na and Cl are often needed in horses with polyuric ARF and can be supplied using 0.9% NaCl for fluid therapy or by oral electrolyte supplementation.
- Add 50 to 100 g/L of dextrose to intravenous fluids for anorectic horses.

Serum creatinine should be measured again within a week after fluid therapy is discontinued.

Oliguric patients

In oliguric patients, fluid and sodium replacement must be monitored carefully. Assessments include attitude, vital signs, body weight, packed cell volume (PCV) and total plasma protein, fluid input versus fluid output (see main text), and central venous pressure. The following recommendations are made for horses that remain oliguric after 12 to 24 hours of appropriate fluid therapy:

- Give furosemide at 1 mg/kg intravenously (IV) every 2 hours.
- If urine is not voided after the second dose, give mannitol (1 mg/kg IV as a 10% to 20% solution) and/or a dopamine infusion (3 to 7 μg/kg/min IV).
  - Dopamine should be administered only if blood pressure can be monitored.

If this treatment approach is unsuccessful after 72 hours, the prognosis is grave. Dialysis may be an option in selected patients (see main text).

CHRONIC RENAL FAILURE *(Text pp. 830-833)*

Chronic renal failure (CRF) is an irreversible disease process characterized by a progressive decline in glomerular filtration rate.

Causes

CRF can be divided into two broad categories:

- Primary glomerular disease–includes glomerulonephritis, nonspecific glomerulopathy, renal glomerular hypoplasia, and amyloidosis
- Primary tubulointerstitial disease–includes incomplete recovery from acute tubular necrosis, pyelonephritis, nephrolithiasis, hydronephrosis, renal dysplasia, and papillary necrosis (rare)
  - These disorders cause a pathologic condition categorized as chronic interstitial nephritis.

Because renal disease is often advanced when horses are first presented for clinical evaluation, the inciting cause may be difficult to ascertain. The pathologic diagnosis may simply be end-stage kidney disease.

Clinical Findings

Clinical signs in horses with CRF include the following:

- Weight loss–the most consistent sign
- Ventral edema–small plaque of edema often found between the forelimbs
- Moderate polyuria and polydipsia–usually present at some stage of the disease process
  - Dysuria generally is not reported unless CRF is caused by pyelonephritis.
  - Urine may be light yellow and transparent, although hematuria or pyuria is found in some horses with pyelonephritis, urinary calculi, or neoplasia.
- Accumulation of dental tartar, oral ulcers, and melena
- Stunted growth in horses with renal hypoplasia, dysplasia, or polycystic kidney disease

Laboratory Findings

A diagnosis of CRF is most commonly made in horses with azotemia and isosthenuria that present with a complaint of weight loss and/or decreased performance. However, specific clinicopathologic findings vary with appetite, diet, and the cause and severity of renal damage.

Serum chemistry

Serum chemistry findings include the following:

- Moderate to severe azotemia (creatinine usually 5 mg/dl or greater)
  - The BUN/creatinine ratio may vary, depending on protein intake, muscle mass, hydration, and degree of azotemia, but it is usually 10:1 or higher.
- Mild hyperkalemia, hyponatremia, and hypochloremia
- Hypercalcemia (greater than 20 mg/dl)–not a consistent finding and depends on dietary intake (e.g., alfalfa versus grass hay)
  - Hypophosphatemia is often found concurrently.
- Hypermagnesemia–also an inconsistent finding
- Metabolic acidosis–may be found in horses with end-stage disease
- Hypercholesterolemia and hypertriglyceridemia (hyperlipidemia)
  - Horses with advanced CRF occasionally have grossly lipemic plasma.

Hematology

Findings on complete blood count (CBC) include the following:

- Moderate anemia (PCV 20% to 30%)
- Hypoalbuminemia and hypoproteinemia in horses with glomerulonephropathy
  - Horses with advanced CRF from any cause may have mild hypoproteinemia as a result of intestinal ulceration.
  - Hyperglobulinemia may be found in horses with immune-mediated disease or chronic pyelonephritis.

Urinalysis

Findings on urinalysis may vary depending on the cause of CRF:

- The urine is relatively devoid of normal mucus and crystals, making the sample transparent.
- Urine specific gravity typically is in the isosthenuric range (1.008 to 1.014).
  - Marked proteinuria in some horses with glomerulonephropathy causes urine specific gravity values up to 1.020.
- Hematuria (gross or microscopic) may be present with pyelonephritis, calculi, or neoplasia.
- Pyuria (more than 5 white blood cells [WBCs]/high-power field) and significant bacteriuria on sediment examination may be found in horses with septic pyelonephritis.
  - These findings are inconsistent, so a urine sample should be submitted for quantitative bacterial culture in all horses with CRF.
  - More than 10,000 CFU/ml are usually found with infection, although lower numbers do not rule out septic pyelonephritis.

Assessment of urine protein concentration and urine protein/creatinine ratio can be helpful in separating glomerular disease from tubulointerstitial disease. Moderate to marked proteinuria (urine protein/creatinine ratio greater than 2:1) without hematuria provides support for glomerular disease.

Other Diagnostic Evaluations

Other evaluations that can be helpful include the following:

- Rectal examination
  - Horses with pyelonephritis and those with ureteral calculi often have enlarged ureters.
  - With CRF the kidneys are often small, with an irregular surface.
  - The right kidney usually cannot be palpated unless it is markedly enlarged.
- Ultrasonography–useful for evaluating kidney size and echogenicity
  - It may also reveal fluid distention (hydronephrosis, pyelonephritis, polycystic disease) or presence of the nephroliths.

- Cystoscopy–can be useful when hematuria or dysuria accompanies CRF
  - It also allows assessment of the ureteral orifices and urine flow from each kidney.
- Measurement of glomerular filtration rate (see main text)
- Renal biopsy–rarely indicated in horses with CRF

Treatment

Treatment is most likely to be successful if there is an acute, reversible component exacerbating the CRF. These conditions should be corrected rapidly. Therapy for stable CRF involves provision of sufficient fluids and electrolytes and nutritional support.

Fluids and electrolytes

Water should be available at all times. Salt can be provided freely as long as edema and hypertension are absent. Other recommendations are as follows:

- Monitor serum creatinine, electrolytes, and acid-base balance regularly (e.g., monthly).
- If serum Na and Cl are low, add 60 to 120 g (2 to 4 oz) of salt to the feed.
  - If edema is present, salt should be restricted, even if the patient is hyponatremic.
- If metabolic acidosis is detected (pH less than 7.35 or bicarbonate less than 20 mEq/L) and the patient is not edematous, add sodium bicarbonate (100 to 200 g/day) to the diet.

Diet

Nutritional management aimed at maintaining body condition is probably the most important aspect of supportive care in horses with CRF. Increasing carbohydrate (grain) intake and adding fat to the diet (e.g., corn oil at up to 16 oz/day) are recommended to increase caloric intake. Provision of a highly palatable diet is also important. Feeding smaller meals more frequently and varying the diet help to increase food intake. Other recommendations are as follows:

- Provide adequate amounts of dietary protein to meet or slightly exceed predicted requirements while maintaining a neutral nitrogen balance.
  - Adequacy of dietary protein intake can be assessed by evaluating the BUN/creatinine ratio.
  - Values greater than 15:1 suggest excessive protein intake, whereas values less than 10:1 may indicate protein-calorie malnutrition.
- Limit calcium intake (e.g., replace legume hay with grass hay).
- Provide supplementation with B vitamins.

Anabolic steroids may be useful for increasing appetite and limiting muscle wasting.

Other recommendations

Management changes should be kept to a minimum and any necessary changes made gradually. For patients with significant edema, diuretics may result in transient improvement. Plasma transfusions may be of temporary benefit in horses with edema and hypoalbuminemia. NSAIDs and corticosteroids are best avoided in horses with primary tubulointerstitial disease.

URINARY TRACT INFECTIONS *(Text pp. 834-836)*

Urinary tract infections (UTIs) can be divided into two categories: (1) upper urinary tract (kidneys and ureters) and (2) lower urinary tract (bladder and urethra). Urolithiasis and partial obstruction frequently accompany UTIs, either as causes or consequences of UTI.

Causes

The most common risk factors for UTI in horses are bladder paralysis, concurrent urolithiasis, and urethral damage (e.g., foaling trauma in mares, neoplasia or habronemiasis in males). The most common pathogens are *Escherichia coli, Proteus mirabilis, Klebsiella* spp., and *Enterobacter* spp.

Clinical Findings

Lower UTI

Lower UTI typically is characterized by disturbances in urine flow, such as dysuria, stranguria, pollakiuria, and incontinence. Urine scalding of the perineum (mares) or urine crystals on the sheath opening and cranial aspect of the hindlimbs (males) may develop with chronic UTI. Gross hematuria may be observed if urinary calculi are present or if the bladder or urethral mucosa has been eroded. Seldom does lower UTI cause systemic signs (e.g., fever, weight loss).

Upper UTI

Horses with upper UTI are more likely to have signs of systemic infection. Because UTI is commonly accompanied by lower UTI, dysuria may also be present.

Diagnosis

Rectal findings

Rectal examination may identify a predisposing cause for lower UTI (e.g., enlarged and atonic bladder, cystic calculi, sabulous urine sediment, bladder mass). Careful palpation of the dorsolateral aspects of the caudal abdomen (retroperitoneal space) usually reveals enlarged ureters in horses with upper UTI. With pyelonephritis, palpation may further reveal kidneys that are either enlarged or shrunken and misshapen.

Hematology and serum biochemistry

With lower UTI, results of a CBC and serum biochemical profile are usually within reference ranges. In contrast, CBC results with upper UTI often support a systemic inflammatory response. With chronic upper UTI, total protein and globulins are often increased. When upper UTI is bilateral, azotemia may also be present.

Urinalysis

On examination of the urine sediment, detection of more than 20 organisms and more than 10 WBCs/high-power field is highly supportive of UTI. Growth of more than 10^4 organisms/ml confirms the diagnosis. WBC casts in urine sediment, in association with azotemia and isosthenuria, are indicative of bilateral upper UTI, especially when accompanied by signs of systemic illness. (Note: Urine samples should be examined and processed for bacterial culture within 30 minutes after collection or they should be refrigerated.)

Other diagnostic tests

Other tests that may be of value include the following:

- Ultrasonography–useful for detecting abnormal renal size, shape, or consistency
- Endoscopy–useful for evaluating the integrity of urethral and bladder mucosa, detecting small uroliths, and assessing urine flow from each ureteral orifice
  - When unilateral pyelonephritis is suspected, each ureter can be catheterized for urine collection to document unilateral disease (see main text).

Treatment

Treatment consists of antimicrobial therapy and correction of any predisposing causes. Suitable antibiotics include trimethoprim-sulfonamide combinations, penicillins (including ampicillin), cephalosporins, tetracyclines, and chloramphenicol. Aminoglycosides should be reserved for highly resistant organisms or acute, life-threatening upper UTI caused by gram-negative organisms. Therapy should be continued for at least 7 days with lower UTIs and for 2 to 6 weeks with upper UTIs.

Monitoring the response

Urine should be cultured 2 to 4 days after beginning therapy and again 1 to 2 weeks after therapy has ended. If the UTI recurs and the same organism is isolated, a focus of upper UTI should be suspected. Recurrence of UTI with a different pathogen suggests an anatomic or functional cause of abnormal urine flow as a reason for recurrent lower or upper UTI.

URINARY INCONTINENCE *(Text pp. 836-838)*

Causes

Causes of urinary incontinence include the following:

- Urolithiasis (see pp. 841-843)
- Congenital anomalies or defects of the urinary tract (e.g., ectopic ureter)
- Trauma (e.g., breeding injury or dystocia in mares, sacral or spinal injury)
- Neoplasia
- Neurologic diseases accompanied by bladder dysfunction (e.g., equine herpesvirus myelitis, cauda equina neuritis, sorghum toxicosis)
- Decreased urethral sphincter tone (reported in mares and attributed to hypoestrogenism)
- Long-standing lumbosacral or lower back problems that make it difficult for the horse to posture to urinate

Sabulous urolithiasis

Over time, incomplete bladder emptying allows crystals normally present in the urine to accumulate in the bladder. This crystalloid sediment becomes heavy and, in some cases, quite firm and further prevents complete bladder emptying. This condition (sabulous urolithiasis) can accompany bladder paralysis of any cause but may also produce myogenic bladder dysfunction in the absence of an underlying neurologic problem.

Neurogenic incontinence

The mechanism of incontinence varies with the location of the neurologic lesion:

- Lower motor neuron (LMN)–loss of detrusor function and overflow incontinence
  - A large, easily expressed bladder is found on rectal palpation.
- Upper motor neuron (UMN)–initially characterized by increased urethral resistance, leading to increased intravesicular pressure
  - Voiding may occur as short bursts of urine passage with incomplete bladder emptying.
  - Rectal examination may reveal a turgid bladder that is either small or increased in size.

Although UMN signs are initially different from those of LMN disease, incontinence is usually not recognized until overflow incontinence develops as a result of sabulous urolithiasis and progressive loss of detrusor function. Presence of other signs associated with LMN dysfunction (e.g., loss of anal or tail tone) or UMN dysfunction (e.g., ataxia) may aid in differentiating the inciting cause of bladder paralysis.

Diagnosis

In addition to taking a complete history and performing physical and neurologic examinations, it is helpful to observe the incontinence and any attempts to urinate. Diagnostic tests to consider include the following:

- Rectal palpation
- Transrectal ultrasonography of the bladder
- Endoscopy of the lower urinary tract
- Serum biochemistry
- Urinalysis and quantitative urine culture–should be performed in all horses with incontinence because UTI is a common sequela of incontinence
- Urethral and bladder pressure profiles (see main text)
- Cerebrospinal fluid collection and analysis (if indicated)

Treatment

Antimicrobial therapy, ideally based on urine culture results, is indicated in all cases of bladder paralysis. Other treatment for incontinence varies with the underlying cause:

- Urolithiasis–removal of calculi (see following discussion) and appropriate antimicrobial therapy

- Congenital anomalies–surgical correction, if possible
- Bladder paralysis–removal of sabulous material (via lavage through a urethral catheter or via cystotomy) and temporary placement of an indwelling urinary catheter
- Urethral sphincter hypotonia in mares–estradiol cypionate (4 μg/kg intramuscularly [IM] every other day)
- Neurogenic incontinence–consider use of an autonomic drug (see main text)
    - Bethanechol (0.25 to 0.75 mg/kg subcutaneously [SC] or PO two or three times daily) for improving detrusor tone and strength of contraction
    - Phenoxybenzamine (0.7 mg/kg PO four times daily) in combination with bethanechol for UMN bladder dysfunction
    - Phenylpropanolamine (1 mg/kg PO two or three times daily) for urethral sphincter hypotonia

Treatment with autonomic drugs has largely been ineffective in controlling incontinence caused by bladder paralysis, and the long-term prognosis for recovery usually is poor.

UROLITHIASIS AND OBSTRUCTIVE DISEASE *(Text pp. 841-843)*

Renal and Ureteral Calculi

Renal and ureteral calculi can produce partial or complete obstruction of one or both sides of the upper urinary tract. Obstruction can lead to hydronephrosis. When both sides of the upper tract are affected, the condition typically progresses to CRF (see p. 245) before horses are presented for evaluation.

Diagnosis

Establishing a diagnosis of urolithiasis causing unilateral upper tract obstruction is challenging because clinical signs are mild (recurrent colic) or nonexistent and azotemia is usually absent. Ureteral stones have a propensity to lodge in the distal ureter and can sometimes be rectally palpated dorsal and lateral to the bladder neck. Careful palpation may reveal a turgid ureter and the presence of a ureterolith.

Urinalysis. Gross hematuria is uncommon unless stones have been passed into the bladder or urethra. However, urinalysis usually reveals hematuria. A quantitative urine culture should be considered part of the minimum database, especially if pyuria or bacteriuria is detected on sediment examination.

Ultrasonography. Transabdominal ultrasonography is a valuable tool for detection of nephroliths, dilation of the renal pelvis (or complete hydronephrosis), and fibrosis within the kidney. However, small nephroliths (less than 1 cm in diameter) can be missed. Transrectal ultrasonography is also useful for detection of ureteral dilation and lithiasis.

Treatment

If upper urinary tract obstruction is diagnosed before severe azotemia develops, surgery is recommended. Nephrotomy or ureterotomy may be required. When equipment is available, lithotripsy is the preferred technique for removal of ureteral stones (see main text). Before surgical intervention is pursued, both kidneys should be thoroughly evaluated for evidence of other stones; ureterolithiasis/nephrolithiasis is often bilateral.

Cystic Calculi

Cystolithiasis is the most common form of urolithiasis in horses. Intact males appear to be at greatest risk. Calculi that develop in the bladder are usually single, large spiculated stones composed of calcium carbonate crystals.

Clinical findings

The most common clinical sign is hematuria after exercise. Pollakiuria, stranguria, or incontinence may also be observed. Less commonly, dysuria may be caused by accumulation of urine sediment in the ventral aspect of the bladder (sabulous urolithiasis). Incontinence is usually present in horses with sabulous urolithiasis.

Diagnosis

Presence of a cystolith can be confirmed by rectal examination. Although rarely needed to confirm the diagnosis, ultrasonography of the entire urinary tract should be considered because calculi may be present in multiple locations. Because UTI sometimes accompanies cystolithiasis, urinalysis and quantitative urine culture are warranted during the initial evaluation.

Treatment

Treatment of cystic calculi usually consists of surgical removal (see main text) accompanied by a 7- to 10-day course of antibiotic therapy. Recommendations for reducing the incidence of recurrence include the following:

- Change from a legume to a grass hay.
- Add ammonium chloride (50 to 200 mg/kg/day PO) or ammonium sulfate (200 to 300 mg/kg/day PO) to the feed in an attempt to acidify the urine.
- Add 2 to 4 oz of salt to the feed each day to increase water consumption and urine flow.

Urethral Obstruction

Calculi, neoplasms (e.g., squamous cell carcinoma of the penis), congenital anomalies, and preputial edema and inflammation (e.g., trauma, habronemiasis) may all produce partial or complete obstruction of the urethra.

Clinical findings

Complete urethral obstruction usually causes moderate to severe signs of colic. An enlarged, turgid bladder is detected via rectal palpation. In males careful palpation of the urethra below the anus may reveal the location of an obstructing urolith or frequent contraction of the urethralis muscle. Partial urethral obstruction is usually accompanied by dysuria, incontinence, and urine scalding of the hindlimbs.

Diagnosis

Diagnosis is based on clinical signs, rectal examination findings, external examination of the penis and prepuce, and passage of a catheter or endoscope through the urethra to the bladder.

Treatment

Treatment of urethral obstruction usually involves surgery (see main text). With squamous cell carcinoma, aggressive surgical resection is warranted with larger lesions. Smaller lesions may be amenable to treatment with topical 5-fluorouracil ointment. If bladder distention is present for several days, an indwelling bladder catheter (closed system) or treatment with bethanechol (see p. 250) may help with recovery of detrusor function.

HEMATURIA *(Text pp. 843-845)*

Idiopathic Renal Hematuria

Idiopathic renal hematuria (IRH) is a syndrome characterized by sudden onset of gross, often life-threatening hematuria, which may be episodic. Hemorrhage arises from one or both kidneys. Endoscopic examination usually reveals no abnormalities of the urethra and bladder, but blood clots may be seen exiting one or both ureteral orifices.

Treatment

Treatment consists of supportive care for acute blood loss. With severe and recurrent hematuria of unilateral renal origin, nephrectomy may be indicated. However, owners must be informed that IRH may develop in the remaining kidney.

Urethral Hemorrhage

In stallions and geldings, defects or tears in the proximal urethra typically result in hematuria at the end of urination. In most cases the condition does not cause dysuria or pollakiuria. The diagnosis is made via endoscopic examination of the urethra, during which a lesion typically is seen along the dorsocaudal aspect of the urethra at the level of the ischial arch.

Treatment

Hematuria appears to resolve spontaneously in about 50% of affected horses. If hematuria persists for more than a month or if significant anemia develops, temporary subischial "incomplete" urethrotomy may be effective in geldings (see main text).

POLYURIA AND POLYDIPSIA *(Text pp. 845-847)*

Polyuria and polydipsia (PU/PD) are defined as urine output in excess of 50 ml/kg/day (greater than 25 L/day for a 500-kg horse) and water intake of more than 100 ml/kg/day (greater than 50 L/day for a 500-kg horse). It is important to remember that urine production and water consumption vary with age, diet, workload, environmental temperature, and gastrointestinal water absorption.

Causes

Causes of PU/PD in horses include the following:

- Renal failure (discussed earlier)
- Pituitary adenoma (Cushing's disease; see Chapter 39)
- Primary or "psychogenic" polydipsia (see following discussion)
- Excessive salt consumption
- Diabetes insipidus (DI) (see following discussion)
- Diabetes mellitus (see Chapter 39)
- Sepsis and/or endotoxemia
- Iatrogenic causes (e.g., sedation with α_2-agonists, corticosteroid therapy, diuretic use)

Psychogenic Polydipsia

Although rare, primary or "psychogenic" polydipsia is probably the most common cause of PU/PD in adult horses for which clients have a primary complaint of excessive urination. The polydipsia may be a stable vice; may be a response to a change in environmental conditions, stabling, or diet; or may result from medication administration. Horses with this problem generally are in good body condition and are not azotemic. The magnitude of polyuria typically is dramatic.

Diagnosis

The diagnosis is made by exclusion of renal failure, hyperadrenocorticism, and excessive salt supplementation. DI is excluded by demonstrating urinary concentrating ability after water deprivation:

- Urine specific gravity should exceed 1.025 after water deprivation of sufficient duration (12 to 24 hours) to produce a 5% loss of body weight.
- With long-standing polyuria, medullary washout (see main text) may limit the increase in urine specific gravity to 1.020 or less.
- In horses whose urine fails to concentrate after 24 hours of water deprivation, a modified water deprivation test should be tried.
  - Restrict water intake to approximately 40 ml/kg/day for 3 to 4 days.
  - By the end of this period, urine specific gravity should exceed 1.025.
- If urine specific gravity remains in the isosthenuric range (1.008 to 1.014), the polyuric horse should be carefully evaluated for CRF.

Treatment

Once it has been established that the horse is not suffering from renal disease, it is safe to restrict water intake to meet maintenance, work, and environmental requirements. Management suggestions include increasing the amount of exercise and turnout time and increasing either the frequency of feedings or the amount of roughage in the diet.

Diabetes Insipidus

There are two forms of DI:

- Neurogenic DI–inadequate secretion of antidiuretic hormone (ADH)
- Nephrogenic DI–decreased sensitivity of the collecting ducts to circulating ADH

With both forms of DI, PU/PD may be dramatic and affected animals fail to concentrate urine in the face of water deprivation (discussed earlier). With neurogenic DI, administration of synthetic ADH (60 IU IM or SC every 6 hours) results in an increase in urine specific gravity and a decrease in urine volume. Treatment is directed at managing PU/PD by restricting sodium and water intake.

NOTE: Horses with suspected DI should be monitored closely during water deprivation because affected horses may become substantially dehydrated (10% to 15%) within the first 12 hours.

RENAL TUBULAR ACIDOSIS *(Text pp. 847-848)*

With renal tubular acidosis (RTA), abnormal renal tubule function results in hyperchloremic metabolic acidosis. RTA can be categorized as primary (genetic or idiopathic) or secondary (attributed to an underlying disease process or drug administration).

Clinical Findings

Affected horses typically present with profound depression and anorexia and may have a history of poor performance, weight loss, and colic. Vital parameters generally are within normal ranges, and affected horses are not clinically dehydrated.

Diagnosis

Laboratory findings are usually within reference ranges, with the exception of electrolyte concentrations and acid-base balance. Abnormalities include the following:

- Profound metabolic acidosis (HCO_3^- less than 13 mEq/L, pH less than 7.250) and hyperchloremia (105 to 120 mEq/L)
- Compensatory decrease in P_{CO_2}
- Hypokalemia
- Mild to moderate azotemia (if the patient is dehydrated)

Urinalysis

Affected horses may have evidence of renal tubular damage on urinalysis (e.g., pigmenturia, glucosuria, abnormal sediment), and urine specific gravity may be low. Despite profound metabolic acidosis, urine pH is generally neutral or alkaline. If pursued, renal biopsy results generally support tubulointerstitial disease (chronic interstitial nephritis).

Treatment

Treatment primarily consists of intravenous and oral administration of sodium bicarbonate:

- Approximately 3000 to 9000 mEq may be required for initial correction.
  - Replace half the estimated bicarbonate deficit intravenously over 6 to 12 hours.
  - Replace the remaining deficit with a combination of intravenous and oral sodium bicarbonate (100 to 150 g PO every 12 hours).
  - Monitor serum electrolytes and acid-base balance closely.
  - Concurrent supplementation with potassium chloride (IV or PO) is usually necessary during initial correction of the acidosis.
- Oral bicarbonate administration may be required for months to maintain acid-base balance.

BLADDER RUPTURE IN ADULT HORSES *(Text pp. 848-849)*

Bladder rupture is rare in adult horses. It can occur in association with urethral obstruction, foaling, or prolonged recumbency. As azotemia develops, affected horses become depressed and inappetant. Clinical signs may not be apparent for several days, or stranguria may be observed, depending on the cause of the rupture. Abdominal distention is not as apparent.

Diagnosis

The diagnosis is based on history, rectal examination findings, laboratory results, and findings on ultrasonographic or cystoscopic examination. Postrenal azotemia develops within 24 hours after rupture and is accompanied by hyponatremia and hypochloremia. Hyperkalemia is not a consistent finding. Peritoneal fluid creatinine is at least twice that of serum creatinine.

Treatment

Surgical repair is indicated in horses with large tears in the ventral half of the bladder. In patients with small dorsal tears or incomplete tears, use of an indwelling bladder catheter (closed system) may allow the tear to heal without surgery (see main text).

URINARY SYSTEM DISEASES IN FOALS

Urinary tract disorders in foals are discussed in chapters of the main text.

Part II: Ruminant Renal System

ULCERATIVE POSTHITIS AND VULVITIS *(Text pp. 851-853)*

Ulcerative posthitis and vulvitis (enzootic balanoposthitis; pizzle or sheath rot) is an infection of the mucous membrane and surrounding skin of the prepuce or vulva in small ruminants. The causative organism is *Corynebacterium renale.*

Clinical Findings

Infection begins as a moist ulcer that is soon covered with a thin, loose, brownish, malodorous scab. If untreated, a malodorous exudate and urine accumulate within the preputial orifice. Dysuria is common; weight loss can occur in chronic cases. Fibrous adhesions may develop between the penis and prepuce, resulting in stricture and urinary tract obstruction.

Treatment

Affected animals should be isolated to limit transmission. Wool or mohair should be removed from the surrounding skin and a topical antibiotic applied. Reduction of protein or nonprotein nitrogen intake is crucial for successful treatment and may be all that is required in early cases. Systemic antibiotics (penicillin or tetracycline) are indicated for advanced cases.

UROLITHIASIS *(Text pp. 853-860)*

Urolithiasis is a metabolic disease of intact and castrated male ruminants. Calculi most commonly lodge in the urethra. Definitive diagnosis in a single animal suggests that all males in the group are at risk because of the importance of dietary and environmental factors in the pathogenesis (see main text). Clinical manifestations include acute urethral obstruction, urethral rupture, bladder rupture, chronic partial urethral obstruction, and ureterolithiasis/nephrolithiasis.

Acute Urethral Obstruction

Impacted calculi and progressive bladder distention cause stranguria and signs of abdominal pain. Anuria occurs if urethral obstruction is complete; urine may dribble from the urethral orifice in cases of partial obstruction.

Diagnosis in cattle

In cattle, calculi most frequently become lodged at the sigmoid flexure; pain or focal swelling may be appreciated over this area. Bladder distention is obvious on rectal palpation in cases of complete obstruction uncomplicated by bladder rupture.

Diagnosis in small ruminants

In sheep and goats the urethral process is the most common site of obstruction. The penis should be examined under sedation with diazepam (0.1 mg/kg IV slowly) or acepromazine (0.05 to 0.1 mg/kg IV or IM); xylazine is not recommended. Transabdominal palpation may reveal a distended bladder.

Laboratory findings

Hematologic and serum chemistry findings may be unremarkable. With time, hemoconcentration and azotemia develop; azotemia is severe in cases of hydronephrosis. Hematuria and proteinuria are consistently detected on urinalysis; crystalluria may or may not be present. Pyuria and bacteriuria are indicative of concurrent urinary tract infection.

Treatment

Steers and feeder lambs may be sent for immediate slaughter if urethral obstruction is diagnosed before the development of azotemia or urinary tract rupture. In cattle, tranquilization may be effective in relieving the obstruction in early cases.

Surgery. If the urethral process of a small ruminant is obstructed, it can be amputated with scissors or a scalpel blade. However, recurrence of obstruction is extremely common and urethral patency is usually maintained for only hours or days. Surgical options in cattle and small ruminants, as well as preoperative and postoperative considerations, are discussed in *Large Animal Internal Medicine,* third edition.

Urethral Rupture

Urethral rupture is a common complication of urethral obstruction in male cattle. Affected animals frequently are depressed and inappetant and may be febrile. Pitting edema develops in the perineum, inguinal region, prepuce, and ventral abdomen. The affected tissues become cool, dark, and nonpainful as necrosis ensues; eventually they become gangrenous and slough. A fistula may develop to allow urine to escape.

Diagnosis

Rectal examination in steers and bulls reveals a small bladder. Hematologic and serum biochemical alterations are similar to, but less severe than, those seen with bladder rupture (see following discussion). Tissue necrosis and secondary infection result in neutrophilic leukocytosis and hyperfibrinogenemia.

Rupture of the Bladder ("Water Belly")

Prolonged bladder distention secondary to urethral obstruction may result in pinpoint perforations, tears, or extensive necrosis of the bladder wall.

Clinical findings

Relief of bladder distention causes cessation of stranguria. Bilateral ventral abdominal distention develops within 1 to 2 days; ballottement may elicit a fluid wave. Dehydration, depression, weakness, and scleral injection occur secondary to uremia, and ammonia may be smelled on the patient's breath. On rectal examination the bladder is small or is not palpable. Impairment of blood coagulation may become an important clinical consideration in uremic cattle.

Diagnosis

Abdominocentesis yields a large volume of straw-colored, often blood-tinged fluid that may smell like urine (especially if warmed). A peritoneal fluid creatinine/serum creatinine ratio of 2:1 indicates uroperitoneum. Other laboratory abnormalities include the following:

- Elevated PCV and serum protein (hemoconcentration)
- Leukocytosis and hyperfibrinogenemia
- Hyponatremia, hypochloremia, and severe azotemia
    - Serum potassium tends to be normal or low in cattle, even when uroperitoneum exists for several days.
    - Hyperphosphatemia is found in some cases.

Treatment

Options for surgical repair and preoperative and postoperative considerations are discussed in *Large Animal Internal Medicine,* third edition.

Chronic Partial Urethral Obstruction

Chronic partial urethral obstruction occurs when calculi impair but do not completely obstruct urine outflow. It is uncommon. Sequelae include hypertrophy of the bladder wall, hydroureter, and hydronephrosis. Affected animals are called "dribblers" because of the characteristic slow or intermittent urine flow during voiding. Lethargy, reduced appetite, and thin body condition are evident if renal failure has developed.

Diagnosis

On rectal examination the bladder may be small and thickening of the bladder wall may be palpated. Hyponatremia, hypochloremia, hypocalcemia, hyperphosphatemia, and severe azotemia with isosthenuria are suggestive of extensive nephron damage caused by hydronephrosis.

Treatment

Options for surgical repair and preoperative and postoperative considerations are discussed in *Large Animal Internal Medicine,* third edition.

Ureterolithiasis and Nephrolithiasis

Cattle with acute ureteral obstruction may show severe colic with stretching, kyphosis, treading, collapse, and vocalization. Rectal or vaginal examination may reveal ureteral enlargement. If the left ureter is obstructed, enlargement of the left kidney may be rectally palpable.

Diagnosis and treatment

Azotemia occurs if the obstruction is bilateral. With ureteral or renal rupture, uroperitoneum or retroperitoneal accumulation of urine occur. Ultrasonography and/or radiography may help confirm the diagnosis. Ureterotomy or nephrectomy are surgical options (see main text).

Prevention of Urolithiasis

Prevention of urolithiasis or recurrence of urinary obstruction begins with analysis of the calculi and the animal's diet. Strategies for preventing specific types of calculi are discussed in *Large Animal Internal Medicine,* third edition.

URACHAL ABSCESSES/ADHESIONS *(Text p. 861)*

Urachal abscesses and adhesions are common in calves during the first few weeks of life. Diagnosis and treatment are similar to that described for foals (see Chapter 20).

BLADDER EVERSION OR PROLAPSE *(Text pp. 861-862)*

Eversion of the bladder occasionally occurs during or shortly after parturition in cows. Forceful straining pushes the bladder through the urethral orifice, exposing the bladder mucosa. Prolapse of the bladder is a rare parturient event in cattle, more commonly associated with dystocia. A full-thickness vaginal tear occurs during delivery, allowing the bladder (and possibly other viscera) to be displaced into the vagina. Prolapse exposes the serosa of the bladder.

Clinical Findings and Diagnosis

In either case a smooth, spherical mass is present within the vagina and typically protrudes from the vulva. Careful vaginal examination under epidural anesthesia is required. With bladder eversion, palpation and ultrasonography are required to identify herniation of bowel or other viscera into the everted bladder. With bladder prolapse, a flexible catheter may be passed into the urethra to remove urine from the bladder, thereby confirming the diagnosis.

Treatment

Manual reduction may not be possible if the everted bladder is edematous or if other viscera have herniated into its interior. The dorsal aspect of the urethra may be incised to widen the route through which the bladder is replaced. Laparotomy is required to assess the viability of any herniated bowel. With bladder prolapse, the bladder is emptied and replaced and the vaginal tear sutured. Antibiotic therapy is indicated in both cases.

ENZOOTIC HEMATURIA *(Text pp. 862-863)*

Enzootic hematuria is a disease of chronic or intermittent hematuria in adult cattle and sheep. It is associated with chronic ingestion of bracken fern *(Pteridium aquilinum)*. Hemorrhagic cystitis occurs initially; bladder neoplasms develop with continued ingestion. In most cases, several animals in the group are affected.

Clinical Findings

Protracted, possibly intermittent, hematuria is usually the first clinical sign; blood clots are voided on occasion. Chronic blood loss results in anemia and a decline in productivity and body condition. Icterus is not a feature of this condition. Bladder wall thickening and tumors may be rectally palpated and contribute to dysuria, pollakiuria, and rarely, urinary obstruction. Hematuria may last for months or years before severe debilitation or death occurs.

Laboratory Findings

Severe anemia is common. If bone marrow suppression is severe, there may be no evidence of a regenerative response and platelet, neutrophil, and lymphocyte counts may be depressed. Urinalysis reveals hematuria, proteinuria, and variable pyuria.

Treatment

Treatment is limited to reduction or elimination of bracken fern in the diet (either in pasture or hay). Hematuria ceases if exposure is discontinued before the onset of tumor formation.

URINARY TRACT INFECTION *(Text pp. 863-865)*

Cystitis, ureteritis, and pyelonephritis in ruminants most commonly result from ascending urinary tract infection with *C. renale* or *E. coli*. Cows are most often affected.

Clinical Findings

Cystitis

Cystitis in cows is typified by dysuria and pollakiuria with or without gross hematuria and pyuria. The cow may tread or swish its tail and retain an arched stance after urinating. Blood, purulent debris, or crystals are occasionally found on the hairs below the vulva. Rectal palpation may reveal a thickened, painful bladder.

Acute pyelonephritis

Cattle with acute pyelonephritis often have a history of abrupt reduction in appetite and milk production. Fever, depression, ruminal stasis, scleral injection, and occasional episodes of mild colic accompany signs of cystitis. With bilateral or left-sided pyelonephritis, enlargement, pain, and loss of normal lobulation of the left kidney may be evident on rectal examination.

Chronic pyelonephritis

The clinical signs of chronic pyelonephritis are vague and inconsistent. Weight loss, anorexia, and reduced milk production are common. Polyuria without gross urine abnormalities are found in some cases. Diarrhea and pale mucous membranes may also be found. Rectal findings are similar to those of the acute form, although the kidneys may not be painful or enlarged.

Diagnosis

Hematology and Biochemistry

Neutrophilic leukocytosis and hyperfibrinogenemia are present in cattle with pyelonephritis. Hyperglobulinemia may develop if the infection is established for several days. Severe, protracted proteinuria may result in hypoalbuminemia. Anemia may develop with chronic pyelonephritis. Azotemia and isosthenuria indicate bilateral involvement.

Urinalysis

Urinalysis is required for definitive diagnosis of UTI, but collection technique is important. A midstream or endstream catch is likely to provide the most accurate culture results. Tentative identification of the organism may be obtained by Gram stain. (*C. renale* is a large, pleomorphic, club-shaped, gram-positive bacillus.) UTI consistently causes hematuria, proteinuria, and bacteriuria. Leukocyte casts are definitive evidence of pyelonephritis but are not always found.

Treatment

C. renale

Penicillin is the treatment of choice for *C. renale* infection. Suitable regimens include the following:

- Procaine penicillin G (22,000 to 44,000 IU/kg IM twice daily)
- Ampicillin trihydrate (11 mg/kg IM twice daily)
- Na- or K-penicillin (22,000 to 44,000 IU/kg IV four times daily)
- Na-ampicillin (10 to 50 mg/kg IV three times daily)

Treatment should be continued for at least 3 weeks (and withdrawal times extended as appropriate). Urinalysis and urine culture should be repeated 1 week after cessation of treatment. Induction of diuresis through oral or parenteral fluid therapy may also be of value.

Note: Isolation of infected animals is recommended, and disinfection of heavily contaminated areas is advised.

E. coli

UTI with *E. coli* or other coliforms may also be successfully treated with high dosages of penicillin or ampicillin. Monitoring of appetite, attitude, rectal temperature, and urinalysis is recommended. If these indices do not improve after 96 hours of treatment, another antibiotic should be used. Suitable choices include the following:

- Trimethoprim-sulfadiazine (15 mg/kg IV once per day)
- Ceftiofur (3 mg/kg IV twice daily)

Gentamicin can also been used, but the nephrotoxicity of the drug and the prolonged slaughter withdrawal period are important considerations.

TUBULAR NECROSIS *(Text pp. 868-870)*

Causes

Tubular necrosis (TN), or tubular nephrosis, results from a variety of toxic, infectious, or hemodynamic insults to the kidneys.

Toxic causes

Toxic causes of tubular necrosis include the following:

- Metals–arsenic, mercury, cadmium, chromium, lead, zinc, copper (secondary to hemolysis)
- Medications–aminoglycosides, tetracyclines, sulfonamides (rare), ionophores, amphotericin B, polymyxin B, NSAIDs, parenteral overdose of vitamin C or D
- Plants–pigweed (*Amaranthus* spp.), Easter lily (*Lilium* spp.), oak (*Quercus* spp.), *Philodendron* spp., ponderosa pine (*Pinus* sp.), cocklebur (*Xanthium* spp.), day-blooming jasmine (*C. diurnum*), oxalate-containing plants (see main text)
- Endogenous materials–hemoglobin, myoglobin, calcium oxalate
- Miscellaneous–ethylene glycol, pentachlorophenol, mycotoxins (see main text), cholecalciferol-based rodenticides

Hemodynamic causes

Hemodynamic causes of tubular necrosis include blood loss, endotoxic shock, disseminated intravascular coagulation, and renal vein thrombosis. Depending on the nature and duration of the primary insult, the outcome ranges from reversible renal injury to renal insufficiency to ARF.

Infectious causes

Bilateral bacterial infection of the kidneys may result in acute or CRF. Renal infection may be established by ascending infection or by hematogenous spread.

Clinical Findings

The clinical signs of ARF in ruminants are nonspecific. Cattle with ARF often are presented for evaluation of poor appetite, diarrhea, or epistaxis. Depression, nasal discharge, ileus, melena, and mild free-gas bloat may also be present. The saliva may have a strong ammonia smell. Depending on the cause, anuria, oliguria, or polyuria may exist. CRF usually causes weight loss in addition to the aforementioned signs.

Diagnosis

Rectal palpation is usually unremarkable. In cases of CRF the left kidney may feel smaller than normal. Laboratory abnormalities include the following:

- Azotemia and isosthenuria
- Proteinuria, hematuria, and granular casts on urinalysis
- Hypochloremia and metabolic alkalosis–common in ruminants with ARF
    - Metabolic acidosis may be found in juvenile ruminants with tubular necrosis and concurrent diarrhea
- Hyponatremia, hypermagnesemia (with high dietary magnesium), hyperphosphatemia, hypocalcemia
- Increased fractional clearance of sodium
    - Normal values are up to 4%, depending on age, ration, and metabolic status.
    - It is prudent to compare the patient's value to that of an age-matched herd mate in a similar physiologic state and on a similar ration.

Treatment

Treatment of toxic nephrosis involves the following:

- Prevent further exposure to the toxin, or discontinue treatment with a nephrotoxic drug.
- Remove toxic material via rumenotomy, or give activated charcoal (2 to 4 g/kg PO).
- Give isotonic, sodium-containing fluids IV to induce diuresis.
    - Fluid rates 1.5 to 2 times the adult maintenance level of 60 ml/kg/day may be adequate.
    - An alternative is repeated fluid administration via stomach tube or small rumenostomy.
    - Continue fluid therapy until azotemia resolves.
    - Supplement with calcium and potassium (IV or PO) as needed.
- In oliguric or anuric patients, give furosemide (1 mg/kg IV or IM every 1 to 2 hours).
    - Mannitol (0.25 g/kg IV) or dopamine (2 to 5 μg/kg/min IV) may be required if the aforementioned measures are unsuccessful.

Supportive therapy may be necessary for 2 to 3 weeks.

LEPTOSPIROSIS *(Text pp. 870-871)*

In cattle, multiple organ systems may be involved in infection with pathogenic serovars of *Leptospira interrogans* or *Leptospira borgpetersenii*. Serovars *hardjo*, *pomona*, and *grippotyphosa* are most commonly implicated in renal infection. Serovar *hardjo* rarely causes overt renal dysfunction. Serovars *pomona* and *grippotyphosa* can cause severe hemolytic disease, interstitial nephritis, and tubular nephrosis in calves and, less commonly, adult cattle. Renal disease caused by leptospirosis appears to be uncommon in small ruminants.

Diagnosis

The microscopic agglutination test is the most widely used serologic test for diagnosis in cattle (see main text). Phase-contrast or dark-field microscopy, immunofluorescent antibody tests, and polymerase chain reaction can be performed on renal tissue, urine, or urine sediment. Urine cultures are often unrewarding.

Treatment

Treatment options in acutely infected cattle include the following:

- Oxytetracycline (10 to 15 mg/kg IM twice daily)
- Dihydrostreptomycin (12.5 mg/kg IM twice daily); not currently available for use in cattle in the United States
- Penicillin (25,000 IU/kg IM twice daily)
- Sodium ampicillin (20 mg/kg IM twice daily)

Chronic renal infection with *L. pomona* can be eliminated with a single injection of dihydrostreptomycin (25 mg/kg IM), if available. Long-acting oxytetracycline (20 mg/kg IM or SC, two doses 10 days apart) has also been recommended to treat chronic leptospiral infections and to reduce the risk of introduction of infected animals into a herd. Vaccination of newly introduced animals is also recommended.

MISCELLANEOUS DISORDERS *(Text pp. 871-872)*

Congenital Defects

Congenital defects of the urinary system (see main text) should be considered in young animals with renal disease or abnormal urination. However, diseases involving severe volume depletion, nephrotoxicity, and infectious diseases are far more common.

Other Diseases

The following uncommon or rare conditions are discussed in *Large Animal Internal Medicine,* third edition: pelvic entrapment of the bladder, amyloidosis, glomerulonephritis, hemolytic uremic syndrome, and renal neoplasia.

33

Diseases of the Nervous System

Consulting Editor MARY O. SMITH

Contributors LISLE W. GEORGE • CHRISTINE F. BERTHELEIN-BAKER
JOHN SCHLIPF • RICHARD BOWEN • WILLIAM J.A. SAVILLE
GUY LONERAGAN • DANIEL GOULD • GEORGE M. STRAIN
JOHN E. MADIGAN • BONNIE R. RUSH • THOMAS J. DIVERS
ROBERT H. WHITLOCK • BRADFORD P. SMITH • JOHN ANGELOS

CEREBROSPINAL FLUID COLLECTION *(Text pp. 873-876)*

Collection Techniques

Cerebrospinal fluid (CSF) may be collected from the lumbosacral cistern or the cisterna magna. Collection from the lumbosacral cistern is preferred if the patient is unable to tolerate anesthesia or when the lesion is located in the spinal cord.

Lumbosacral tap

A lumbosacral tap is performed with the animal sedated; the skin over the lumbosacral joint is surgically prepared and anesthetized with lidocaine. The landmarks are the dorsal spinous process of L6 cranially and S1 caudally and the tuber sacrales laterally. A spinal needle is inserted through a stab incision and advanced perpendicularly until the tip enters the lumbosacral cistern; the needle can be gently advanced to the floor of the spinal canal. A 6- to 9-inch, 18- to 20-gauge spinal needle is used for most adult horses; a 3.5-inch needle can be used in foals, small ruminants, and most cattle. NOTE: Some horses respond with violent motor activity when the cistern is penetrated.

Cisterna magna tap

A cisterna magna tap is performed with the animal under general anesthesia. The skin overlying the atlantooccipital joint is surgically prepared, the patient's head is flexed, and a 3.5-inch, 18-gauge spinal needle is inserted on the midline, 1 to 2 cm caudal to a line drawn between the cranial aspects of the wings of the atlas. The needle is inserted perpendicular to the skin and aimed toward the nose. It is slowly advanced, checking every few millimeters for CSF flow by removing the stylet.

CSF Analysis

Normal CSF is clear and colorless. Blood contamination can occur during collection (blood is unevenly mixed; sample clears as more fluid flows) or from central nervous system (CNS) trauma (blood is evenly mixed). If CNS hemorrhage occurred days previously, the fluid may have a brownish or yellow (xanthochromic) discoloration. Foamy CSF denotes a protein concentration greater than 200 mg/dl. Turbid CSF usually denotes cell counts greater than 400/µl. Normal CSF values are listed in Table 33-1 of *Large Animal Internal Medicine,* third edition.

DISEASES PRODUCING CORTICAL SIGNS *(Text pp. 876-945)*

Maedi-Visna

Visna is a chronic, progressive viral encephalitis of sheep. Nervous signs are characteristic of a diffuse encephalitis: ataxia, facial muscle twitching, proprioceptive deficits, circling, blindness, and staggering or stumbling when turning. Hyperexcitability, seizures, and coma may be seen terminally. The time between onset of signs and death may be as long as 2 years. The presence of serum antibodies is usually considered diagnostic. Antibodies and virus can also be detected in the CSF. There is no effective treatment. Respiratory signs are discussed in Chapter 29.

Caprine Arthritis-Encephalitis (Infectious Leukoencephalomyelitis)

The leukoencephalomyelitis form of caprine arthritis-encephalitis virus infection is predominantly seen in young goats. There is no effective treatment.

Clinical signs

Clinical signs include ataxia; paresis or paraplegia, hemiplegia, or tetraplegia; head tilt; nystagmus; tremors; torticollis; trismus; salivation; depression; coma; and opisthotonos. Vision and pupillary light reflexes may be reduced. Tone and spinal reflexes range from hypertonia and hyperreflexia to hypotonia and hyporeflexia, depending on the extent and location of spinal cord lesions. Specific gait disturbances also depend on lesion location. Other clinical signs variably include fever, joint swelling, vague and shifting lameness, weight loss, and tachypnea (see Chapter 36).

Diagnosis

Diagnosis is based on pathologic lesions in the CNS and joints, in conjunction with clinical and serologic findings. CSF changes are characteristic only of chronic granulomatous inflammation. Virus isolation offers little advantage over serologic examination unless the patient is a serologic nonresponder (see main text). Nucleic acid probes and polymerase chain reaction (PCR) assays have been developed.

Border Disease (Hairy Shaker Lambs)

Border disease is a congenital viral infection of sheep and goats. It is characterized in an infected flock or herd by abortion, infertility, and fetal deformities ("steel wool coat" and abnormal pigmentation; short, thickened body; shortened legs; small orbits; doming of the frontal bone; arthrogryposis). Some infected lambs have neurologic signs such as ataxia, coarse tremors, and abnormal gait.

Diagnosis

Identification of viral antigens in tissues (abomasum, pancreas, kidney, thyroid, testicles) is the most accurate method of diagnosis. Serodiagnosis of infected lambs is difficult because the lambs tend to be immunotolerant of the virus. Sheep infected as adults develop serum neutralization titers between 1:20 and 1:320.

Encephalitic Infectious Bovine Rhinotracheitis

Infection of calves with type 1 bovine herpesvirus most often results in acute upper respiratory tract disease (see Chapter 29). Occasionally, a specific strain of the virus causes meningoencephalitis. Calves younger than 6 weeks of age are most susceptible.

Clinical signs and diagnosis

Clinical signs include depression, mild nasal and ocular discharge, fever, proprioceptive deficits, head pressing, aimless circling, bellowing, salivation, odontoprisis, bruxism, paralysis of the tongue, head tilt, nystagmus, convulsions, blindness, coma, and death. Affected calves develop fulminant encephalitis within 1 to 2 days of infection and die by day 5. Virus isolation from brain tissue or nasal secretions is the most accurate method of diagnosis.

Bovine Spongiform Encephalopathy ("Mad Cow" Disease)

Bovine spongiform encephalopathy (BSE) is a slow and invariably fatal transmissible neurodegenerative disease of cattle in the United Kingdom and parts of Europe. Clinical signs are insidious in onset and begin with subtle behavioral changes that progress to extreme excitement or panic (especially during restraint), hyperesthesia, and overreaction to visual, auditory, or tactile stimuli. There is no in vivo test for BSE. Clinical suspicion can only be confirmed by microscopic examination of the brain.

Scrapie

Scrapie is a transmissible spongiform encephalopathy of sheep and goats. Clinical cases usually occur sporadically in infected flocks. Scrapie is an irreversible and fatal disease.

Clinical signs

Most affected animals are between 1 and 5 years of age. The clinical course is variable but typically slow, beginning with behavioral changes (nervousness, restlessness) and weight loss. Pruritus (and consequent skin trauma) is a common finding and increases in intensity with disease progression. Other findings can include tremors, bruxism, and ptyalism. Apathy, exercise intolerance, ataxia, seizures syncope, and depression may be present in advanced cases.

Diagnosis

Immunohistochemistry may reveal the agent (a prion) in biopsy specimens of the lymphoid tissue of tonsils or nictitating membranes, allowing diagnosis of infection in live animals. However, these tests are negative in some scrapie cases. Microscopic examination of the brain and spinal cord is the classic diagnostic method. NOTE: Scrapie is a reportable disease in the United States.

Equine Herpesvirus Type 1 Myeloencephalitis

Equine herpesvirus type 1 (EHV-1) infection typically causes respiratory disease (see Chapter 29). The virus can also cause vasculitis and subsequent ischemic necrosis of CNS tissues.

Clinical findings

Acute onset of ataxia and tetraparesis characterizes the neurologic form of EHV-1 infection. Severity can range from subtle neurologic deficits to complete recumbency. Specific neurologic signs include proprioceptive deficits (most severe in the hindlimbs), urinary incontinence, decreased tail and anal tone, and diminished perineal sensation. Cranial nerve deficits have also been reported. Other signs may include nasal discharge, limb edema, colic, ocular lesions, and anorexia. Fever is uncommon at presentation. Urine dribbling and fecal retention are common problems in affected horses.

Typically, clinical signs stabilize in 48 hours, although some patients continue to deteriorate and eventually die or are euthanized. Horses that remain standing have a much better prognosis. Most horses begin to improve during the first 5 to 7 days, although recovery may take months.

Diagnosis

Tentative diagnosis is based on characteristic neurologic signs. Typical CSF changes include increased protein and xanthochromia; however, a normal protein level does not rule out EHV-1. A fourfold or greater increase in serum neutralizing antibody titers is considered diagnostic for EHV-1 infection. A single titer of 1:256 or more is highly suggestive of recent infection. Virus isolation from the buffy coat of an EDTA-preserved blood sample or from a nasopharyngeal swab may be positive for approximately 12 days postinfection.

Pseudorabies (Mad Itch, Aujeszky's Disease)

Pseudorabies is an acute viral encephalitic disease of ruminants; horses and humans are resistant. Swine are probably the primary hosts and frequently are asymptomatic. There is no treatment.

Clinical signs

Pseudorabies has an acute or peracute course in ruminants. Affected animals may die suddenly without premonitory signs. In more slowly developing cases, the first signs are often paresthesia with pruritus and dermal abrasions. Other signs may include fever, bellowing, bloat, stamping the feet, ptyalism, chewing the tongue, ataxia, proprioceptive deficits, circling, nystagmus, and strabismus. Aggression is seen in some cases, but most affected animals are depressed. Most ruminants with pseudorabies die within 2 days of developing clinical signs.

Diagnosis

The virus can be isolated from pharyngeal or nasal secretions and can be cultured from nervous tissue, particularly spinal cord segments serving the pruritic sites.

Viral Encephalitis in Horses (EEE, WEE, VEE)

Several insect-transmitted togaviruses infect horses, birds, and humans, producing a nonsuppurative encephalitis. The most pathogenic togaviruses are eastern (EEE), Western (WEE), and Venezuelan (VEE) equine encephalitis viruses. Mortality rates for EEE range from 75% to 90%, and those for WEE range from 20% to 50%; VEE has a mortality rate between 40% and 80%.

Geographic distribution

WEE predominantly occurs in the western United States, South America, and Canada. Outbreaks occur in the western and midwestern United States; sporadic cases occur in the northeast and southeast. EEE is restricted to the eastern and southeastern United States, the West Indies, and Central and South America. The virulent form of VEE is restricted to Central and South America and the West Indies.

Clinical signs

The earliest signs are nonspecific: fever, anorexia, and stiffness. In cases of EEE and WEE, the fever is biphasic, with peaks approximately 2 and 6 days after infection. Horses with VEE tend to have persistent fever. Initially, affected horses may appear sleepy and spend a lot of time in sternal recumbency. Additional early signs include ataxia, hypermetra, proprioceptive deficits, hyperesthesia, and neck stiffness. Later signs include excitability or aggression; twitching of the muzzle or appendicular musculature; head pressing; circling; head tilt; blindness; paralysis of the pharynx, larynx, and tongue; continuous chewing movements; and frothing at the mouth or nose. Propulsive walking or somnolence may also be seen.

As the condition worsens, the horse may become comatose and exhibit psychomotor convulsions. Recumbent animals die after 3 to 5 days. Survivors show a gradual improvement in neurologic function over weeks or months. Most animals that recover from EEE have residual neurologic deficits. Survivors of WEE have fewer neurologic sequelae.

Diagnosis

CSF changes include pleocytosis (50 to 700,000 mononuclear cells/μl) and increased protein concentration (60 to 200 mg/dl). The virus may be isolated from the CSF in acute infection. A fourfold rise in antibody titer between acute and convalescent sera is used for diagnosis (see main text). The brain should be examined microscopically in horses that die.

Treatment

There is no effective treatment. Convulsions may be controlled with pentobarbital, diazepam, phenobarbital, or phenytoin (see Cerebral Trauma). Good nursing care is essential. Prevention is discussed in *Large Animal Internal Medicine,* third edition.

Borna Disease (Near Eastern Encephalitis)

Borna disease is a viral encephalitis of mammals in Europe and the Middle East. Clinical signs in horses are similar to those of other viral encephalitides. In ruminants signs include head tremors, hyperesthesia, ataxia, anorexia, propulsive walking, coma, and convulsions. The mortality rate is high. Specific antibodies can be found in the serum and CSF of most affected animals.

West Nile Virus

West Nile virus is a mosquito-borne virus that affects a broad range of animals, including horses. Birds are the principal natural host. Most infections result in subclinical or mild disease; approximately 10% of infected animals develop severe disease.

Clinical signs and diagnosis

Clinical signs typically are sudden in onset and include depression or listlessness and ataxia and paresis, particularly of the rear limbs. Some affected horses are febrile at onset. Anxiety has also been reported in affected horses. The disease progresses over 1 to 3 days to include head shaking, incessant chewing, paralysis of the lower lip or tongue, severe ataxia, ascending paralysis, and terminal recumbency. Diagnosis is based on serologic findings.

Treatment and prognosis

Treatment is limited to supportive care. The prognosis in horses showing severe clinical signs is poor. Animals with less severe disease may recover fully in 5 to 15 days.

Ovine Encephalomyelitis (Louping Ill)

Louping ill is an acute, fatal viral encephalomyelitis of sheep that occasionally infects cattle, horses, and humans. The disease is reported in Great Britain, Ireland, Norway, Turkey, and Bulgaria. There is no treatment.

Clinical signs and diagnosis

Initial clinical signs include fever, anorexia, depression, constipation, and generalized muscle tremors. Further signs include ataxia, proprioceptive deficits, head tremors, hypermetria (which causes a characteristic rabbit-hopping gait), and hyperexcitability. Later signs are indicative of cerebral cortical dysfunction. High levels of virus-specific antibody can be detected in the CSF of affected animals. The virus can be isolated from the brain or spinal cord.

Rabies

Rabies is an invariably fatal viral neurologic disease of mammals. Most cases in domestic animals result from the bite of an infected feral mammal (e.g., fox, bat, skunk, raccoon). The incubation period ranges from 3 weeks to 6 months. Regardless of the clinical manifestations, rabies is rapidly progressive and uniformly fatal. Control strategies are discussed in *Large Animal Internal Medicine,* third edition,

Clinical manifestations

Early signs are nonspecific: anorexia, depression, mild ataxia. As the disease progresses, affected animals may show repetitive muscle twitching, hyperesthesia, hypermetria, and proprioceptive deficits. Regional pruritus may cause persistent rubbing. Other clinical signs are variable. Behavioral changes range from extreme hyperexcitability, fear, or rage (furious rabies) to depression (dumb rabies) and flaccid paraparesis or tetraparesis (paralytic rabies).

Furious rabies. In cattle, furious rabies results in recumbency, coma, convulsions, bloat, tenesmus, ptyalism, pollakiuria, bellowing, hypersexuality, paraphimosis, and flaccidity of the tail and anus. Tetraplegic animals show frantic motor activity and bellow when stimulated.

Dumb rabies. Animals with dumb rabies are depressed, inappetant, and febrile. They have marked ataxia, drooped head and neck, ptosis, flaccid facial muscles, profuse salivation, yawning, repeated nibbling motions with the lips, tenesmus, and paraphimosis. Other signs include flaccidity of the tongue, tail, anus, and urinary bladder. Odontoprisis, head pressing, circling, blindness, strabismus, and nystagmus may also be seen before death.

Paralytic rabies. The first sign of paralytic rabies is ataxia or shifting-leg lameness, which rapidly progresses to paraparesis or paraplegia. Spinal reflexes and tone in the affected limbs may be decreased or absent. Most affected animals become recumbent and over several days develop encephalopathic signs (e.g., coma, seizures). This form of rabies is especially common in cattle.

Rabies in horses. Common signs in horses include recumbency, hyperesthesia, tail and anal flaccidity, ataxia, paraplegia, and fever. Less common signs include lameness, pharyngeal paralysis, and colic.

Diagnosis

The CSF may be normal or may show moderate increases in protein (60 to 200 mg/dl), mononuclear cells (5 to 30 cells/μl), and occasionally neutrophils. Definitive diagnosis is based on microscopic examination of CNS tissues. NOTE: In the United States and Canada, rabies must be reported to the state public health department.

Sporadic Bovine Encephalomyelitis

Sporadic bovine encephalomyelitis (SBE) is a chlamydial disease of cattle that comprises disseminated vasculitis and serositis. The mortality rate, which is highest in calves, is around 30%. The agent often remains endemic on a farm, and sporadic disease outbreaks occur.

Clinical signs

Initial signs include fever, anorexia, depression, and stiffness. Signs of multisystemic disease then become evident (respiratory dysfunction, hoof pain, swelling of the coronary band, polyarthritis, tenosynovitis, fibrinous peritonitis and pleuritis). As the disease progresses, meningoencephalitis causes signs that include ataxia, proprioceptive deficits, circling, head tilt, opisthotonus, hyperesthesia, stiff neck, convulsions, and coma.

Diagnosis and treatment

Detection of elementary bodies in the cells of pleural or peritoneal effusions is highly suggestive of SBE. Laboratory animal inoculation is also used for diagnosis. Oxytetracycline can be effective in early cases. The agent is also susceptible to penicillin and erythromycin.

Suppurative Meningitis

Meningitis can occur either from direct extension of infectious agents into the calvarium (e.g., compound skull fractures, dehorning, vertebral osteomyelitis) or from hematogenous spread. Specific pathogens include *Streptococcus zooepidemicus* (foals, goats), *Streptococcus suis* (foals), *Actinomyces* spp. (horses), *Cryptococcus neoformans, Pseudomonas aeruginosa* (dairy cattle, goats), and *Mycoplasma mycoides* subsp. *mycoides* (kids). Gram-negative bacteria are the dominant organisms involved in neonatal infections.

Clinical signs

The earliest clinical signs include fever, anorexia, diarrhea, neck stiffness, and hyperesthesia. Later signs variably include hyperresponsiveness to tactile stimulation, behavioral changes (from extreme depression to hyperexcitability or mania), trismus and vocalization with head and neck flexion, tetraparesis, hyperreflexia, and tendency to circle or fall to one side. Cranial nerve deficits occur inconsistently. Progression results in depression, propulsive walking, coma, and status epilepticus.

Diagnosis

Septic meningitis should be differentiated from metabolic encephalopathies by measurement of plasma sodium, glucose, and magnesium and by laboratory evaluation of hepatic function. Diagnosis of meningitis is based on CSF analysis:

- Turbid and white to amber in color; foams when shaken; clots
- Greatly elevated white blood cell (WBC) count (either predominantly neutrophilic or mononuclear)
    - More than 100 neutrophils/μl is typical of purulent meningitis.
- Elevated protein concentration (20 to 270 mg/dl); strongly positive Pándy test (for the presence of globulins)
- Low glucose concentration (often less than 50% of the blood glucose concentration)
- Bacteria commonly observed with Gram stain

Treatment

Early recognition and treatment are essential for recovery. Treatment involves the following:

- Intravenous antimicrobial therapy for 10 to 14 days

  - Third-generation cephalosporins (moxalactam, cefotaxime, ceftazidime) are good initial choices; the recommended dosage is 40 to 50 mg/kg intravenously (IV) two to four times daily.
  - Enrofloxacin and trimethoprim-sulfonamides are alternatives.
  - Penicillins and aminoglycosides penetrate the blood-brain barrier poorly.
- Supportive care–protection from self-inflicted trauma, analgesia, fluid therapy, and anticonvulsant therapy (see Cerebral Trauma)
  - Dexamethasone (0.15 mg/kg intramuscularly [IM] 15 minutes before the first dose of antibiotic and then every 6 hours for 4 days) may lessen the neurologic sequelae.

Pituitary Abscesses

Pituitary abscesses occur sporadically in ruminants but are rare in horses. A high incidence has been reported in bulls after insertion of a nose ring. *Actinomyces pyogenes* is the most common pathogen, although a variety of other organisms have been reported as primary pathogens. Because of the high mortality rate, treatment is usually not attempted.

Clinical signs and diagnosis

Clinical signs develop suddenly and progress for 7 to 10 days before the animal dies. Initial signs include ataxia, head and neck extension, base-wide stance, inappetence, depression, head pressing, and recumbency. Most affected animals have asymmetric cranial nerve deficits. Bradycardia is common. Pyogenic foci may be found at other sites, particularly around the head (e.g., sinuses, teeth, facial tissues). Exophthalmos has also been reported. Antemortem diagnosis is based on finding bradycardia, blindness, and nonresponsive pupils in conjunction with evidence of pyogenic inflammation in the CSF (see Meningitis).

Brain Abscess

The most common cause of brain abscessation in horses is *Streptococcus equi,* and in cattle it is *A. pyogenes.* The neurologic dysfunction caused by a brain abscess has a slower onset and is more asymmetric than that caused by meningitis.

Clinical findings

Early signs of cortical abscess may include ipsilateral mydriasis and contralateral vision loss. Progression causes more generalized cortical signs, including blindness, propulsive walking, circling, head tilt toward the lesion side, depression, coma, head pressing, or sudden mania. Abscesses located at the base of the brain may also result in cranial nerve deficits. In later stages, animals may become laterally recumbent and display decerebrate posture (hypertonicity, hyperreflexia, opisthotonos, coma, and convulsions).

Diagnosis and treatment

The CSF is either normal or has changes similar to those seen with meningitis. Treatment includes antibiotic therapy and supportive care. Where facilities are available, the abscess may be localized with computed tomography and, if accessible, drained via craniotomy.

Cerebral Trauma

The clinical presentation after cerebral trauma depends on the area of the brain that is damaged, the extent of the lesion, and the duration of the injury. Extreme brain swelling results in caudal displacement and herniation. Brainstem compression is characterized by cranial nerve dysfunction, severe disturbance of consciousness, and abnormal respiratory rhythm.

Blows to the poll in horses

Blows to the poll can result in basioccipital fractures, which cause asymmetric signs of vestibular disturbance, including horizontal or rotary nystagmus, ipsilateral ventrolateral strabismus, contralateral dorsomedial strabismus, head tilt, and contralateral blindness. Horses that remain ambulatory lean or circle toward the lesion side. Additional signs may include dysphagia, facial paralysis, proprioceptive deficits, recumbency (with violent struggling), depression, and coma. When the petrous temporal bone is fractured, there may be profuse bleeding from the ipsilateral nares and external ear canal.

Dehorning trauma in goats

Brain trauma from overaggressive dehorning in goats results in depression, loss of menace response, contralateral increase in extensor tonus, ipsilateral mydriasis, sluggish pupillary reflex, and loss of conscious proprioceptive responses. These signs may be delayed by several days when chemical or thermal burns are involved, and the condition may be complicated by brain abscess or bacterial meningitis.

CSF analysis

The CSF changes are characteristic:

- First 24 hours–blood in the CSF (evenly mixed); elevated protein and WBC counts
- By 48 hours–less blood in the CSF; spun fluid appears xanthochromic
  - Protein may be elevated (500 to 1000 mg/dl), but the WBC count is only marginally increased.
  - Creatine kinase is increased (10 to 100 IU/dl) for 1 to 2 days.
- Beyond 48 hours–gradual decrease in protein
  - Xanthochromia disappears by day 14.
  - Mononuclear inflammatory cells gradually increase as parts of the CNS degenerate.

NOTE: Atlantooccipital CSF collection is contraindicated if signs of increased CNS pressure (e.g., mydriasis, blindness, papilledema), uncontrolled hemorrhage from the ears or nose, or dorsal sagittal sinus fractures are observed.

Treatment principles

Successful treatment depends on early recognition and control of increased CSF pressure. Depression fractures of the frontal and parietal bones should be reduced surgically. General medical principles include respiratory support, administration of osmotic diuretics, seizure control, nutritional and fluid support, and protection from decubitus and self-inflicted damage.

Treatment of cerebrocortical edema

The following drugs and regimens have been used to manage cerebral edema in large animals:

- Methylprednisolone–30 mg/kg IV initially, then 15 mg/kg IV 2 and 6 hours later, followed by infusion at 2.5 mg/kg/hr for 48 hours
- Dexamethasone–0.1 to 0.25 mg/kg IV or IM every 4 hours for 1 to 4 days
- Mannitol–0.25 to 2 g/kg IV as a 20% solution; if response is noted, repeat every 4 to 6 hours
  - NOTE: Mannitol should not be used in animals with active CNS hemorrhage.
- Furosemide–1 mg/kg IV, IM, or subcutaneously (SC) twice daily
- Nonsteroidal antiinflammatory drugs (NSAIDs)–flunixin meglumine (1 mg/kgIV, IM, or SC twice daily), phenylbutazone (2 to 4 mg/kg IV twice daily in horses; 10 to 20 mg/kg orally [PO] initially, then 2.5 to 5 mg/kg IV on alternate days in cattle), aspirin (31.2 to 62.4 g/500 kg PO twice daily)
- DMSO–0.5 to 2.5 g/kg IV as a 10% to 20% solution twice daily

Anticonvulsant therapy

The following drugs are suggested for seizure control in large animals:

- Diazepam–0.01 to 0.2 mg/kg IV every 30 minutes as needed
- Phenobarbital–12 to 20 mg/kg IV initially (diluted in saline and given over 30 minutes), then 1 to 9 mg/kg IV three times daily or 11 mg/kg PO once per day (horses) for maintenance
  - Plasma troughs should be monitored during maintenance therapy (see main text).
- Pentobarbital–2 to 20 mg/kg IV slowly to effect; repeat every 4 hours as needed (use intravenous catheter for repeated doses), and monitor respiration carefully.
  - Seizure control in adult horses and cattle often occurs at lower dosages.
- Diphenylhydantoin (phenytoin)–1 to 5 mg/kg IV slowly (over 30 minutes)

four times daily for seizure control; 2.8 to 16.4 mg/kg PO three times daily (horses) for maintenance

- Monitor plasma troughs during maintenance therapy (see main text).

Traumatic Optic Nerve Blindness in Horses

Severe blunt trauma to the skull in young horses may result in a rapid caudal displacement of the brain and avulsion or stretching of the optic nerve. Clinical signs include blindness, loss of pupillary reflexes, and mydriasis. Ophthalmoscopic retinal changes include pallor of the optic discs, reduction in the number and caliber of retinal vessels, and linear peripapillary pigment disruptions. The condition is permanent.

Nervous Coccidiosis

Nervous coccidiosis is a neurologic syndrome of calves and yearling cattle, sheep, and goats that is associated with enteric infections by *Eimeria* spp. The condition is most common in feedlots in the northwestern United States and western Canada, especially during the winter months. The mortality rate can be high.

Clinical signs

Onset of the nervous form is usually preceded by diarrhea, tenesmus, and hematochezia. Initial CNS signs include depression, incoordination, twitching, and hyperesthesia. As the disease progresses, affected animals become recumbent and develop numerous cerebrocortical signs. Affected animals may die after 1 to 5 days of CNS signs.

Diagnosis

Fecal flotation from the patient and herd mates shows a heavy burden of coccidial oocysts. To exclude the possibility of other neurologic diseases, blood should be collected for measurement of electrolytes (calcium, magnesium, and potassium), acid-base status, glucose, and lead. If indicated, acute meningitis and salt poisoning may be ruled out by CSF analysis.

Treatment

Treatment should include calcium gluconate (2 to 4 ml/kg SC) with magnesium, and either sulfamethazine (110 mg/kg for 5 days or 1 lb/100 gallons of drinking water) or amprolium (50 mg/kg/day for 7 days). Diazepam, pentobarbital, or phenobarbital may be used for seizure control (see p. 347). Slow intravenous administration of magnesium sulfate (50 to 100 ml of a 10% solution) may also be useful as a sedative.

Sporozoan Infection in Ruminants (*Sarcocystis* Infection)

Most ruminants with *Sarcocystis* infection are asymptomatic. Clinical illness may develop when a large number of sporocysts are ingested by a nonimmune animal. Signs include fever, anorexia, weight loss, symmetric lameness, and diarrhea. Neurologic signs include ataxia, weakness, tremors, hyperexcitability, hypersalivation, recumbency, tonic-clonic seizures, leg biting, blindness, opisthotonos, and nystagmus. Affected cattle may lose the hair of the tail switch ("rat tail"); sheep may have a wool break.

Diagnosis

Background titers in normal cattle range between 1:54 and 1:486, whereas titers in infected cattle often exceed 1:10,000. During early infection there is a marked normocytic, normochromic anemia (up to 75% reduction in hemoglobin concentration). Other abnormalities may include elevations in plasma lactate dehydrogenase, alanine aminotransferase, sorbitol dehydrogenase (SDH), and blood urea nitrogen.

Treatment

Feeding monensin (100 mg/kg daily for 30 days) is prophylactic; however, the efficacy in symptomatic cattle is unknown. Treatment of infected sheep with salinomycin (1 to 2 mg/kg) has also been recommended. Amprolium at 100 mg/kg daily for 30 days may reduce the severity of *Sarcocystis* infection but may not completely eliminate clinical disease.

Neospora spp. Infection in Cattle (Protozoal Abortion)

The predominant clinical sign of *Neospora* infection in cattle is mid- to late-term abortion. Infected calves are occasionally born with neurologic dysfunction. These calves are often unable to stand and nurse and have abnormal spinal reflexes. Flexor contracture of the forelimbs, domed skull, and torticollis have also been reported. CNS signs tend to be mild initially but progress after birth. The protozoa can be seen in microscopic sections of stained tissues. Similar conditions have been described in sheep and goats.

Equine Protozoal Myeloencephalitis

Equine protozoal myeloencephalitis (EPM) is a multifocal, progressive CNS disease of horses that is primarily caused by infection with *Sarcocystis neurona.* The parasite causes inflammation and necrosis in the brain, brainstem, and spinal cord. Young Standardbred, Thoroughbred, and quarter horses are most commonly affected.

Clinical signs

Because any tissue within the CNS can be affected, neurologic signs are highly variable. Characteristic signs include asymmetric ataxia and muscle atrophy. Onset may be sudden or gradual. Other signs variably include vague, intermittent lameness; cranial nerve deficits; proprioceptive deficits; and tetraparesis. Although EPM is typified by the presence of asymmetric, multifocal neurologic abnormalities, some horses with EPM have focal or symmetric signs.

Diagnosis

Diagnosis is usually based on western blot analysis of CSF. The albumin quotient and IgG index help differentiate between intrathecal antibody production and leakage of plasma proteins across the blood-brain barrier (see main text). PCR alone is unreliable for antemortem diagnosis of EPM. Postmortem examination is still considered by many to be the gold standard.

Treatment

The standard therapy is a combination of pyrimethamine (1 mg/kg PO once per day) and sulfadiazine (20 mg/kg PO once or twice daily). One recommendation is to continue therapy at least 2 weeks beyond resolution of clinical signs or 4 weeks past a plateau in the signs. Other options include diclazuril (5 mg/kg) or toltrazuril (5 to 10 mg/kg) PO once per day for at least 28 days, and nitazoxanide (25 mg/kg once per day for 7 days, then 50 mg/kg once per day for 23 days). Although NSAIDs and DMSO are routinely used, corticosteroids should be used with caution in horses suspected of having EPM.

Prognosis

Most reports suggest an improvement rate of approximately 70% with standard therapy. However, less than 25% of horses return to their original function. The response rate may be better with diclazuril and similar drugs. The relapse rate (which is 10% to 28% with standard therapy) may also be lower with these newer drugs.

Babesia Encephalitis

Most clinical infections with *Babesia* spp. result in hemolysis and renal and liver failure. Acute encephalitis develops in a small proportion of cases. Signs include high fever, anorexia, depression, ataxia, proprioceptive deficits, mania, convulsions, and coma. CNS signs are accompanied by engorgement of scleral vessels, icterus, proteinuria, and hemoglobinuria. This condition is a reportable disease in the United States.

Polioencephalomalacia in Ruminants

Polioencephalomalacia (PEM) is malacia of the gray matter of the brain. There are several possible causes in ruminants, including excess sulfur consumption, altered thiamine metabolism, salt poisoning or water deprivation, and lead toxicity. PEM is seen in individuals and as herd outbreaks. There are two clinical manifestations of PEM: subacute and acute.

Subacute form

Clinical signs develop either within hours or over several days. Early signs include separation from the herd or flock, anorexia, staggering, apparent blindness, walking with the head held erect, slightly hypermetric gait, diarrhea, hyperesthesia, and muscle tremors (ear flicking, facial twitching). Progression results in cortical blindness, head pressing, opisthotonus, dorsomedial strabismus, miosis, repetitive chewing, profuse ptyalism, and odontoprisis. Variable nystagmus, strabismus, and head tilt may also be seen. Without appropriate treatment, signs may progress to recumbency, tonic-clonic convulsions, and death.

Acute form

Affected animals are found recumbent and comatose. Tonic-clonic seizures are common, with affected animals remaining recumbent and hypertonic between seizures.

Diagnosis

Presumptive diagnosis may be made based on history, clinical signs, or definitive diagnosis (histopathologic examination) in a herd mate. CSF changes are usually vague and include mild pleocytosis (5 to 50 WBC/μl) and increased protein (greater than 50 mg/dl). After a diagnosis of PEM, whether presumptive or definitive, attention should be focused on identifying the likely causes so that exposure of herd mates can be mitigated or limited (see main text).

Treatment

Regardless of the cause, animals with the subacute form often respond favorably to thiamine HCl (10 to 20 mg/kg IM or SC three times daily). Most patients improve within 24 hours; if there is no improvement, treatment should be continued for at least 3 days. Dexamethasone (1 to 2 mg/kg once) may be beneficial in reducing cerebral edema. Convulsions can be controlled with phenobarbital, pentobarbital, or diazepam (see p. 271). Prophylactic antimicrobial administration may be indicated in feedlot animals with PEM.

Prognosis

The majority of subacutely affected animals respond favorably to appropriate treatment. The prognosis for acutely affected animals or those with advanced subacute manifestations is grave. Survivors often are culled because of poor performance, chronic anorexia, ataxia, or blindness.

Thiamine Deficiency in Horses

Horses may develop thiamine deficiency when fed thiaminase-containing substances such as bracken fern *(Pteridium aquilinum),* horsetail *(Equisetum arvense),* and amprolium. Clinical signs include ataxia, proprioceptive deficits, heart block, bradycardia, blindness, weight loss, dysuria, cool extremities, and muscle fasciculations; seizures develop terminally. Parenterally administered thiamine is effective for treatment.

Salt Poisoning

Salt poisoning is common in livestock. It can result from overconsumption of salt-rich substances or from water deprivation.

Clinical signs

Rapid ingestion of large quantities of salt produces gastrointestinal (GI) and neurologic signs, including mucohemorrhagic diarrhea and colic, head-neck extension ("star-gazing"), blindness, aggressiveness, hyperexcitability, psychomotor seizures, vocalization, ataxia, proprioceptive deficits, head pressing, constant chewing movements, nystagmus, muscle twitching, and coma. Death results from respiratory failure. Before the onset of nervous signs, cattle with chronic salt toxicosis may appear depressed and dehydrated.

Diagnosis

Diagnosis depends on demonstration of exposure to toxic concentrations of salt (greater than 7000 ppm Na^+), a history of water deprivation, or finding serum or CSF sodium values greater than 160 mEq/L. A CSF/serum Na^+ ratio greater than 1 suggests salt poisoning. CSF sodium is consistently elevated and may exceed

200 mEq/L, but the serum sodium may be normal if the animal recently drank to repletion with ion-free water. Rumen sodium greater than 0.36% (before water repletion) is also suggestive of salt poisoning in cattle.

Treatment

Treatment is aimed at limiting the intake of ion-free (i.e., fresh) water and slowly decreasing the CNS sodium concentration while controlling cerebral edema and CNS signs:

- For calves, give hypertonic saline IV (1 to 2 L initially) and feed 2 to 4 L/day of fresh milk.
  - The need for and molar strength of repeated hypertonic saline infusions is determined by measuring plasma electrolytes twice daily (see main text).
- If neurologic signs worsen, give mannitol (0.5 to 1 g/kg IV) or dexamethasone (0.44 to 0.88 mg/kg twice daily for 2 to 3 days).
- Prevent access to water until neurologic signs abate and plasma sodium returns to normal.

Treatment is often unrewarding; most affected animals die, even with intensive medical therapy.

Vitamin A Deficiency

Vitamin A (retinol) deficiency primarily occurs in growing ruminants in feedlots. Diets that are naturally low in vitamin A include cereal grains (except corn), beet pulp, and cottonseed hulls. Other dietary or management conditions that favor vitamin A deficiency include grazing on dry pastures, exclusive feeding of cereal grains that have been stored at high temperature and humidity, and prolonged feeding of mineral oil to prevent frothy bloat.

Clinical signs

Clinical signs are related to increased intracranial pressure, secondary infections, parasitism, and other nutritional deficiencies. Neurologic signs are age dependent; signs in include anorexia, ill thrift, blindness, diarrhea, and pneumonia; signs in adults include star-gazing, blindness, diarrhea, anasarca, nystagmus, strabismus, exophthalmos, loss of pupillary light reflexes, and tonic-clonic convulsions.

Ophthalmoscopic findings. The pupils are dilated and unresponsive; the border of the optic disc becomes indistinct dorsally (giving the appearance of an inverted heart); the retinal vessels become tortuous or appear occluded as they course over the disk; and the disc becomes faded. These characteristic findings (particularly absent pupillary light reflexes) help distinguish vitamin A deficiency from PEM and salt poisoning.

Diagnosis

Measurement of vitamin A and carotene in the plasma and feed is the most direct method of diagnosis (see main text). CSF changes include mononuclear cell pleocytosis (40 to 50 cells/μl) and increased protein (140 mg/dl).

Treatment

Affected cattle should receive 440 IU/kg of vitamin A parenterally, then 6000 IU/kg PO every 50 to 60 days until the diet has been enriched. Cattle with acute encephalopathy and simple papilledema may respond favorably after a short period of supplementation. Cattle with severe retinal degeneration do not regain their vision.

Hydrocephalus/Hydranencephaly in Cattle

Hydrocephalus/hydranencephaly is relatively common in cattle. Normotensive hydrocephalus (hydranencephaly) and hypertensive hydrocephalus are reported. Most cases of hydranencephaly in ruminants are caused by in utero infection with bluetongue; bovine viral diarrhea (BVD); Akabane, Cache Valley, or Aino virus; or border disease. Hypertensive hydrocephalus may be congenital or acquired. Causes of acquired hydrocephalus include cerebral abscesses, *Coenuris cerebralis* infestation, pachymeningitis, lymphosarcoma, and vitamin A deficiency.

Clinical signs

Congenitally hydrocephalic animals frequently are born dead or are weak and die shortly after birth, showing various CNS signs. Occasionally, there is doming of the calvarium or protrusion of a cystic structure through the open fontanelle. In viral-induced cases of hydranencephaly, skeletal deformities may also be observed. Patients with hydrocephalus caused by compressive lesions may display unilateral or bilateral signs of increased intracranial pressure, such as head tilt (toward the lesion side), ipsilateral mydriasis, and contralateral menace deficit.

Diagnosis

Diagnosis in calves and lambs is commonly based on the presence of characteristic clinical signs and domed skull. Whenever hydranencephaly is suspected, blood should be collected for virus isolation, serology, and quantitative immunoglobulin determination (see main text).

Ammoniated Forage Toxicosis (Cow Bonkers)

Overapplication of anhydrous ammonia to forages may result in toxicosis, particularly in nursing calves. Affected animals are hyperesthetic and ataxic. At rest the animal assumes a sawhorse stance, but when excited it becomes hyperactive, appears to be blind, and circles compulsively. Other signs include vocalization and dysphonia. Periods of frenzy may result in recumbency and convulsions. Afterward the animal rests quietly, with occasional muscle tremors. The concentration of ammonia in the CSF and blood may be increased. Affected calves may benefit from treatment with acepromazine (0.045 mg/kg IV) and thiamine (1.14 mg/kg IM).

Lead Poisoning

Lead poisoning in ruminants is characterized by acute encephalopathy; in horses it manifests as polyneuritis. Common sources include lead arsenate defoliants, batteries, motor oil, linoleum, roofing felt, paint, machinery grease, caulking compounds, and foliage near lead smelters.

Clinical signs in ruminants

Initially, affected cattle stand alone and are depressed; hyperesthesia, muscle fasciculations, and rapid twitching of the eyelids or other facial muscles may develop. These signs progress to ataxia, proprioceptive deficits, blindness, head pressing, odontoprisis, coma, and convulsions. Despite the blindness, pupillary reflexes are usually normal. Some animals display episodic running, hyperesthesia, and bellowing; there may be frothy saliva at the lips. Bloat and diarrhea may be observed if other substances were ingested with the lead.

Clinical signs in horses

Signs of lead poisoning in horses include weight loss (can be severe), incoordination, laryngeal/pharyngeal paralysis, dysphonia, proprioceptive deficits, loss of anal tone, facial paralysis, and difficulty masticating. Aspiration pneumonia is common; fine muscle tremors occur intermittently. Psychomotor seizures precede death.

Diagnosis

Diagnosis is based on finding increased lead concentrations in blood and tissues. Normal ranges vary considerably among laboratories. Consideration of the reference ranges obtained with similar methodology is essential when interpreting blood lead values (see main text). Environmental sources of lead can be detected by measuring lead in soil or pasture.

Hematologic and CSF changes. Most lead-poisoned livestock have a normal hemogram. If present, lead-related changes are indicative of hemolytic anemia with an inappropriately large bone marrow response. Specific findings include Howell-Jolly bodies, metarubricytes, and basophilic stippling. These changes are not pathognomonic but are suggestive in horses. Increases in CSF protein (50 to 100 mg/dl) and WBCs (5 to 50 cells/μl) may be found.

Chronic poisoning. Livestock that are chronically poisoned with small amounts of lead may have a normal blood lead concentration but a high lead concentration in bone. Poisoning can be diagnosed by giving calcium disodium EDTA (75 mg/kg IV) and measuring the urine lead concentration, which may rise fortyfold within a few hours (see main text). Measurements of free erythrocyte porphyrins and erythrocyte α-aminolevulinic acid are preferred for diagnosis of chronic lead poisoning (see main text).

Treatment

Therapy should include removal of the lead from the digestive tract, chelation therapy, fluid and nutritional support, and anticonvulsant therapy as needed (see p. 268). Two chelation regimens with calcium disodium EDTA have been reported:

- Slow intravenous infusion at 73 mg/kg daily for 5 days; treatment is discontinued for 2 days and then reinstituted for 5 days
  - Therapy is guided by posttreatment blood lead analysis and renal function tests.
- Intravenous injection at 110 mg/kg every 12 hours for 2 days; treatment is discontinued for 2 days and then reinstituted for 2 more days

Oral supplementation with zinc is recommended after EDTA therapy. Thiamine (2 to 5 mg/kg daily) is an effective adjunct in cases of acute lead poisoning in cattle. In ruminants ingested lead is best removed from the digestive tract via rumenotomy; magnesium sulfate is administered concurrently. Oral administration of chelators is contraindicated.

Gasoline and Petroleum Distillate Toxicosis

Ingestion of natural gas condensate or petroleum distillate by livestock causes depression, ataxia, diarrhea, recumbency, coma or semicoma, absent menace response, decreased palpebral reflex, and hypotonia. Affected animals appear to be anesthetized. Some animals die suddenly. Feces and rumen contents have a strong odor of petroleum or gasoline, and gas chromatography reveals peaks of aromatic hydrocarbons. Rumenotomy should be considered in early cases. Treatment is usually futile when the animal is recumbent and unresponsive.

Ethylene Glycol (Antifreeze) Toxicosis

Antifreeze poisoning primarily occurs in ruminants. Clinical signs, which develop within 3 to 4 days of ingestion, include blindness, progressive hindlimb ataxia, salivation, depression, nystagmus, tonic-clonic seizures, and status epilepticus. Pupillary reflexes are usually intact.

Diagnosis and treatment

Laboratory findings include azotemia, hypophosphatemia, hypocalcemia, acidosis, hyperosmolality, and increased γ-glutamyltransferase (GGT); hemolytic anemia and hemoglobinuria are occasionally seen. Ethylene glycol can be detected in the rumen for at least 4 days after ingestion. Treatment with 20% ethanol (50 ml/hr) is recommended but is unsuccessful in advanced cases. Oral administration of activated charcoal may be worthwhile.

Flatpea Poisoning

Signs of flatpea (*Lathyrus* spp.) intoxication include depression, muscle tremors, spasmodic torticollis, and dark brown urine. Affected animals become recumbent and are reluctant to rise. When stimulated to move, they display circling, head pressing, odontoprisis, and seizures. Normal behavior and gait may resume in interictal periods. Blood ammonia concentrations are elevated. Treatment is empiric: vinegar (1 to 2 L PO), diazepam, and removal from the forage.

Leukoencephalomalacia (Moldy Corn Disease, Blind Staggers)

Leukoencephalomalacia is a highly fatal disease of horses caused by ingestion of corn contaminated with the fungus *Fusarium moniliforme.* Outbreaks of multifocal neurologic disease and hepatic disease occur in groups of horses exposed to tainted feedstuffs.

Clinical signs

Clinical signs develop suddenly and include somnolence, flaccidity of the facial and pharyngeal muscles, muscle fasciculations over the neck and withers, ataxia, proprioceptive deficits, head pressing, mania, facial desensitization, blindness, seizures, and tendency to circle or lean to one side. Most animals die while convulsing.

Diagnosis

Antemortem diagnosis relies on recognition of cerebral cortical disease and exposure to moldy corn. Serum liver enzymes (aspartate aminotransferase, GGT, SDH) and bilirubin levels may be elevated. The major pathologic feature is liquefactive necrosis of one or both cerebral hemispheres.

Treatment

There is no specific treatment. Antiinflammatory medications (DMSO, flunixin), antibiotic therapy, thiamine (5 g IV every 12 hours), and supportive care have been effective in a few cases. However, survivors usually have permanent neurologic dysfunction.

Blue-Green Algae Toxicosis

Ingestion of stagnant pond water containing toxic species of blue-green algae may cause peracute intoxication in livestock. Development of toxic stands of blue-green algae requires specific environmental conditions, such as water pH greater than 6, organic pollution, and warm temperatures. Release of the toxin produces a rotting fish odor.

Clinical signs

Death can occur within minutes after ingestion of toxic water, so dead animals may be found near the pond. In more chronic cases, affected animals show ataxia, depression, anorexia, hemorrhagic diarrhea, icterus, and photosensitization (secondary to hepatic necrosis). Death occurs within 2 to 72 hours. Treatment is generally unsuccessful.

Diagnosis

Diagnosis is based on an association between livestock deaths and ingestion of pond water, identification of toxic algae in the water, the presence of hepatic disease in chronically affected animals, and the ability to rule out other causes of sudden death. Rumen contents should be divided, with half placed in 10% neutral buffered formalin for microscopic analysis and the other half refrigerated and submitted for mouse bioassay or chromatographic identification of the toxin.

Intracarotid Drug Injection

Inadvertent intracarotid injection with hypertonic or caustic drugs causes cortical necrosis. This problem is more common in horses than in cattle. Onset of clinical signs is peracute: during injection the animal recoils backward and falls over. Some horses strike, rear violently, or run wildly; others simply fall and become comatose. Severely affected animals may die; surviving animals may have residual neurologic deficits. Violent horses should be placed in a padded stall, sedated with diazepam, and treated with dexamethasone (0.88 to 2.2 mg/kg). Administration of mannitol or other osmotic diuretics should be avoided.

Coenuriasis

Coenuriasis is caused by CNS invasion with *Coenuris cerebralis*, the intermediate stage of the canine tapeworm *Taenia multiceps*. Ruminants and horses are susceptible. The clinical presentation is that of a space-occupying cranial lesion; signs progress to lateral recumbency and coma. In advanced cases the calvarium over the parasitic cyst enlarges and softens.

Diagnosis and treatment

Diagnosis is based on the history (endemic area) and supportive clinical and radiographic findings (see main text). Praziquantel (Droncit, 100 mg/kg daily for 5 days) is effective in sheep. Administration of an NSAID and dexamethasone may enhance posttreatment survival rates. Surgical cyst removal has been reported.

Brain Tumors

Clinical signs with most brain tumors are the result of brainstem compression. Signs include hypermetric gait, ataxia, depression, facial paresis or paralysis, facial anesthesia or analgesia, head tilt, strabismus, nystagmus, and unilateral loss of menace response. Migration of facial tumors into the cranial vault through the cranial nerve foramina may also result in facial swelling, exophthalmos, Horner's syndrome, or asymmetric nasal air flow.

Cholesteatomas in Horses

Cholesteatomas are common lesions in the brains of older horses. Signs of cerebral dysfunction (e.g., seizures) develop only when the masses grow sufficiently large to obstruct CSF flow or compress the brain directly. Antemortem diagnosis can be made by computed tomography. There is no specific treatment.

Epilepsy

Epilepsy is a condition of recurrent seizures not attributable to a neurologic or metabolic disorder. A seizure may be generalized or partial (focal). Seizures may be preceded by a prodromal aura and followed by postictal depression of variable duration (minutes to days).

Signalment

Seizure disorders have been described in various cattle breeds (e.g., Romagnola, Swedish Red, Brown Swiss, Hereford, Angus, Brahman), and in Arabians, some pony breeds, and Paso Finos. A condition known as *benign epilepsy* is seen in foals of many breeds, especially Arabians. Unlike true epilepsy, it is usually outgrown. Idiopathic epilepsy in mares associated with elevated estrogen levels has been reported. NOTE: Seizures in very young or aged animals are frequently not of epileptic origin.

Management

Following are some guidelines for managing epilepsy:

- Measure plasma Na, K, Mg, and Ca in all animals with seizures of unknown origin.
- Control generalized seizures or status epilepticus with anticonvulsants.
  - Begin anticonvulsant drugs at the lowest possible dose (see p. 268) and increase the dose every 1 to 3 days until the seizures are controlled.
  - If the seizures cannot be controlled without causing depression or ataxia, add a second anticonvulsant, gradually increasing the dose until the seizures cease.
  - Monitor the trough blood concentration of all anticonvulsants used (see main text).
  - Withdrawal of anticonvulsant therapy should be made gradually over 4 weeks.
- Also treat ruminants with seizures with thiamine (see Polioencephalomalacia).
- Consider ovariectomy in mares with estrus-related seizures.

Horses with epilepsy should not be ridden or used for sporting purposes.

Narcolepsy and Cataplexy

Narcolepsy is characterized by episodes of excessive daytime sleepiness, weakness, and rapid-eye-movement sleep. Between attacks the animal appears normal. Cataplexy, a sudden episode of voluntary muscle paralysis, can range from weakness of facial, neck, and forelimb muscles to atonic, areflexic paralysis of all nonrespiratory muscles. Episodes last seconds to minutes. Imipramine (0.5 mg/kg) may counteract excessive sleepiness.

Head Shaking in Horses

Head shaking is a well-recognized problem in horses. Head shaking may be vertical, horizontal, or both, and is frequently accompanied by agitation. Onset often occurs in the spring or early summer, and signs usually begin shortly after the start of exercise. Possible causes include middle ear disorders, ear mites, larval harvest mite infestation, cranial nerve abnormalities, ocular disease, guttural pouch mycosis, dental abnormalities, allergic vasomotor rhinitis, a photoperiod mechanism leading to optic-trigeminal summation (photic head shaking), and neuropathic pain involving the trigeminal nerve.

Diagnostic approach and treatment

Evaluation should include a complete physical examination; ophthalmic, otoscopic, neurologic, and dental examinations; endoscopic examination of the nasal passages, pharynx, and guttural pouches; radiography of the skull; and a complete blood count and serum chemistry panel. In the absence of any abnormal findings, treatment with cyproheptadine (0.3 mg/kg PO twice daily) results in improvement in some cases.

Miscellaneous Conditions

The following conditions are briefly discussed in *Large Animal Internal Medicine,* third edition: Murrurundi disease, humpyback disease, *Morbillivirus* encephalomyelitis, mycotic encephalitis, *Cowdria (Rickettsia) ruminantium* infection (heartwater), cerebral theileriosis, cerebral trypanosomiasis, Nardoo fern poisoning, *Helichrysum argyrosphaerum* poisoning, nitrofurazone toxicosis, ceroid lipofuschinosis (Batten's disease), and citrullinemia.

DISEASES INVOLVING BRAINSTEM AND CRANIAL NERVE DYSFUNCTION *(Text pp. 946-957)*

Listeriosis

Listeriosis is an acute meningoencephalitis caused by *Listeria monocytogenes.* It is common in ruminants but rare in horses. Contaminated forage is a common source of infection. Clinical forms include abortion, neonatal septicemia, ophthalmitis, diarrhea and septicemia in ewes, and neurologic disease. Neurologic listeriosis may present as a multifocal brainstem disorder, diffuse meningoencephalitis, or spinal cord myelitis. The condition usually affects individual animals, but outbreaks can occur.

Clinical Signs

Common signs include fever, anorexia, depression, proprioceptive deficits, head pressing, compulsive walking or circling, and cranial nerve deficits. The fever often disappears after 3 to 5 days. Disease progression is associated with decreased consciousness, coma, and convulsions. Lambs may develop spinal myelitis without brainstem disease. Signs include paraparesis, tetraparesis, paraplegia, or tetraplegia; proprioceptive deficits; and recumbency. Sensorium and appetite are normal in some lambs but markedly depressed in others.

Diagnosis

Signs of multifocal brainstem disease with fever in a ruminant are suggestive of listeriosis; *Haemophilus somnus* infection (cattle) and aberrant parasite migration are important differentials. CSF analysis is helpful in diagnosing listeriosis (protein greater than 40 mg/dl, WBC count greater than 12 mononuclear cells/μl), but changes do not correlate well with disease severity or prognosis. Confirmation is based on identification of multifocal microabscesses in the brainstem and isolation of *L. monocytogenes* from infected brain tissue. The agent is rarely isolated from CSF.

Treatment

L. monocytogenes is susceptible to most commonly used antimicrobials. Recommended treatment involves either oxytetracycline (10 mg/kg twice daily) or penicillin G (40,000 IU/kg IM three or four times daily for 7 days, then 22,000 IU/kg daily for 14 to 21 days). When using penicillin, intravenous therapy with potassium penicillin G (44,000 IU/kg three or four times daily) may be used for the first 3 to 5 days. Good nursing care is important. However, animals that are recumbent, comatose, or convulsive rarely survive despite intensive antibiotic and supportive therapy.

Thromboembolic Meningoencephalitis

Thromboembolic meningoencephalitis (TEME) is a fulminant neurologic disease of cattle caused by *H. somnus* septicemia. It is most common in feedlot cattle in the winter.

Clinical Signs

Signs occur peracutely, although they may be preceded for 1 to 2 weeks by a dry, harsh cough and dyspnea. Death often occurs within 36 hours after the onset of neurologic signs, which begin with fever, anorexia, depression, ataxia, and proprioceptive deficits. Cerebellar and caudal brainstem lesions cause head tilt, nystagmus, strabismus, blindness, muscle tremors, opisthotonos, coma, and convulsions. Other findings may include harsh bronchovesicular sounds and pleural friction rubs, lameness and joint swelling, and retinal hemorrhages, hyphema, and hypopyon.

Diagnosis

Cattle with acute TEME have antibody titers greater than 1:400 (greater than 1:1024 in convalescing cattle). CSF changes are characteristic of CNS hemorrhage (see p. 261). In untreated cases the organism may be isolated from pleural fluid, tracheal aspirates, urine, blood, and preputial washings; isolation from CSF is usually unsuccessful. Specimens should be inoculated directly onto growth media as soon as they are collected. Kidney and brain tissues are the best to submit for postmortem isolation.

Treatment

H. somnus is susceptible to many antimicrobials, including tetracyclines, penicillin, aminoglycosides, and ampicillin. Oxytetracycline (10 mg/kg IV twice daily for 3 days or 20 mg/kg of the long-acting formulation every 48 hours for three treatments) is most cost effective. It should be followed by daily treatment with penicillin (10,000 to 20,000 IU/kg) until recovery is complete.

Bacterial Otitis Media-Interna in Ruminants

Otitis media-interna is common in cattle and sheep. It usually occurs as a sequela to severe respiratory infections. In calves the tympanum is often ruptured, and clear, yellow proteinaceous fluid is discharged through the external ear canal. Sheep with *Pseudomonas* otitis may develop necrotizing dermatitis of the ear canal.

Signs of otitis interna

Extension of the infection into the labyrinths can result in vestibular signs, such as head tilt (toward the lesion side), constant horizontal nystagmus (fast phase away from the lesion side), and a tendency to stumble or fall toward the lesion side. Head shaking may precede the vestibular signs (and may cause an aural hematoma). Most patients with otitis media also develop facial nerve dysfunction. Some sheep develop signs of cortical or brainstem disease, including unilateral blindness and contralateral mydriasis.

Treatment

Treatment with oxytetracycline (6 mg/kg IM or IV every 24 hours, or 20 mg/kg IM of a long-acting formulation every 48 hours) or penicillin (40,000 IU/kg IM or IV) may be effective if continued for several weeks. Other drugs that may be beneficial include lincomycin, spectinomycin, ampicillin, gentamicin, and enrofloxacin.

Ear Mite Infestations

Severe ear mite infestations can perforate the tympanum and result in vestibular disease. Infestation can been resolved with rotenone drops (daily for 5 to 10 days), fenthion (Spotton, 0.2 ml) drops, or ivermectin (0.2 mg/kg SC).

Peripheral Vestibular Disease in Horses

Vestibular disease in horses has several possible causes, including extension of bacterial infection from the guttural pouch, polyneuritis equi, viral or bacterial labyrinthitis, and skull fractures. Staphylococci, streptococci, and *Aspergillus* spp. have been isolated from cases of suppurative otitis in horses.

Clinical signs

The horse may seem uncomfortable and shake its head or rub the affected ear for 2 to 3 weeks before the onset of vestibular signs. Neurologic signs appear suddenly. Horses with mild disease develop ataxia, head tilt, facial paralysis, nystagmus (rapid phase away from the lesion side), and ventrolateral strabismus (ipsilateral). Affected horses circle or lean against the stall wall for support. There is often a mild proprioceptive deficit that is worse on the affected side. Horses with severe calvarium fractures fall and become recumbent, lying on the lesion side.

Peripheral versus central lesions. Horses with peripheral vestibular lesions remain appetent and alert. Horses with vestibular disease accompanied by petrous temporal bone fractures and meningitis tend to be depressed, febrile, and inappetant. Those that develop septic meningitis show rapid deterioration of mental status, rigidity or flailing of the limbs with mild stimulation, neck stiffness, hyperesthesia, fever, otorrhea, and dysphagia.

Diagnosis and treatment

Evaluation should include skull radiographs and endoscopic examination of the guttural pouch. High dosages of penicillin (20,000 to 40,000 IU/kg IV four times daily) are recommended for peripheral vestibular disease. If penicillin-resistant bacteria are suspected, third-generation cephalosporins or trimethoprim-sulfonamide combinations can be used. NSAIDs and corticosteroids (in the acute stages) may be helpful. Good nursing care is important.

Nigropallidal Encephalomalacia (Yellow Star Thistle Poisoning)

Nigropallidal encephalomalacia occurs in horses that ingest large quantities of yellow star thistle *(Centaurea solstitialis)* or Russian knapweed *(Centaurea repens).* Signs appear suddenly after chronic ingestion and include weight loss, depression, ataxia, proprioceptive deficits, yawning, lowered head, protruding tongue, tremor of the tongue and lips, and facial hypertonicity when feed is offered. Retraction of the lips and a fixed grimace with the mouth held half open are characteristic. Prehension, mastication, and deglutition are uncoordinated. The signs stabilize after several days, but affected animals usually do not recover.

Ruptured Rectus Capitis Ventralis Muscles

Traumatic avulsion of the rectus capitis ventralis muscle can occur when horses flip over backward and hyperextend the neck and head. Tearing of the tendinous insertion damages cranial nerves IX to XI. Clinical signs include epistaxis (mild and transitory), laryngeal hemiplegia, dysphagia, and pharyngeal paralysis. Radiography can be helpful in establishing the diagnosis (see main text). The neurologic signs usually resolve in time.

Horner's Syndrome

Horner's syndrome results from interruption of ocular sympathetic pathways. Specific causes include guttural pouch mycosis, traumatic lesions of the basisphenoid area, cervical trauma, space-occupying lesions in the cranial thorax, periorbital abscesses or tumors, esophageal rupture, and ligation of the carotid artery. Horner's syndrome has also occurred after intravenous injection with xylazine, vitamin E/selenium, or phenylbutazone.

Clinical signs

Clinical signs in horses variably include miosis, enophthalmos, ptosis, regional hyperthermia, excessive sweating on the ipsilateral side of the face, congested nasal mucosae, inspiratory stridor, and dermatitis (from chronic sweating). The palpebral reflex and menace response are normal. Sweating on the neck may also be seen if there is damage to the cervical sympathetic nerves. Clinical signs in cattle are similar except that there is lack of sweating on the planum nasale on the affected side. In sheep and goats, clinical signs are limited to mild ptosis.

Diagnosis

Thorough physical examination should include palpation of the jugular furrows and auscultation and percussion of the thorax. The pharynx, and in horses the guttural pouches, should be examined endoscopically. The cervical vertebrae and, if indicated, the thorax should be radiographed. The site of denervation can usually be localized by physical examination and instillation of epinephrine (0.1 ml of 1:1000 solution) into the eye. Mydriasis occurs within 20 minutes with postganglionic lesions, but takes 30 to 50 minutes with preganglionic lesions.

Treatment

Treatment depends on the underlying cause. Except for Horner's syndrome following intravenous injection of xylazine, neurologic signs are often irreversible even if the primary cause is eliminated.

Guttural Pouch Mycosis—Neurologic Sequelae

Guttural pouch mycosis is discussed in Chapter 29. When present, neurologic signs are related to dysfunction of cranial nerves IX to XII. Signs variably include head shaking, dysphagia, head shyness, laryngeal hemiplegia, protrusion of the tongue, abnormal head posture (extended or low), facial sweating, shivering, Horner's syndrome, facial paralysis, brachiocephalicus and trapezius muscle atrophy, and signs of vestibular disease.

Miscellaneous Conditions

The following breed-specific conditions are discussed in *Large Animal Internal Medicine,* third edition: space-occupying cranial nerve lesions in Groningse Blaarkop calves and heritable exophthalmos and strabismus in Jersey, Holstein, Brown Swiss, and shorthorn cattle.

CEREBELLAR DISEASES *(Text pp. 957-960)*

Cerebellar Hypoplasia in Calves

Infection with the BVD virus between 90 and 170 days of gestation can result in abortion, stillbirth, hydranencephaly, or cerebellar hypoplasia. BVD virus infection is discussed further in Chapter 30.

Clinical signs

Signs of cerebellar dysfunction are usually present at birth and include trunkal ataxia, falling backward, opisthotonos, base-wide stance, coarse intentional head tremors, hypermetria, hyperreflexia, and nystagmus or strabismus. Severely affected animals may be unable to stand. Affected calves may have a deficient menace response and appear blind; retinal degeneration and corneal opacity are sometimes seen with congenital BVD. Neurologic signs rarely improve.

Diagnosis

Diagnosis is based on clinical signs and identification of BVD antibodies in precolostral blood. The virus can be cultured from the blood of some affected calves. (Bluetongue virus occasionally causes cerebellar lesions in calves and lambs.)

Cerebellar Abiotrophy

Cerebellar abiotrophy has been reported in Holstein, Angus, and Limousin heifers and in Arabian foals. Signs may be present at birth, but in most cases they appear in the first 3 to 9 months (calves) or 2 to 4 months (foals). Signs in calves are similar to those listed earlier for cerebellar hypoplasia except that vision is preserved. In foals signs range from subtle ataxia to complete, diffuse cerebellar dysfunction. The signs may remain static (calves, foals), slowly progress for a time and then plateau (foals), or slowly progress until the animal becomes recumbent and unable to rise (calves). There is no effective treatment.

Miscellaneous Conditions

Other breed-specific cerebellar conditions in cattle include hereditary hypermetria in shorthorn calves, cerebellar malformation in Ayrshire calves, bovine familial convulsions and ataxia in Angus cattle, familial ataxia in Hereford calves, and micrognathia and cerebellar hypoplasia in Angus calves. These conditions are discussed in *Large Animal Internal Medicine,* third edition.

STORAGE DISEASES AND INBORN ERRORS OF METABOLISM *(Text pp. 960-966)*

The following storage diseases cause neurologic signs in certain livestock breeds:
- α-Mannosidosis–Angus, Murray gray, Simmental, Galloway, and Holstein cattle
- β-Mannosidosis–Anglo-Nubian goats and Salers calves
- Generalized glycogenosis–Holstein cattle and Suffolk sheep
- Bovine generalized glycogenosis–shorthorn and Brahman cattle
- Globoid cell leukodystrophy–polled Dorset sheep
- Neuronal lipodystrophy–sheep and Angus and Beefmaster calves
- Shaker calf syndrome–newborn horned Hereford calves
- Maple syrup urine disease–newborn Hereford and polled shorthorn calves
- Hereditary neuraxial edema–newborn Hereford and Hereford-Friesian crossbred calves
- Inherited myoclonus–Peruvian Paso foals
- Congenital encephalomyelopathy–quarter horse foals

These conditions are discussed in *Large Animal Internal Medicine,* third edition.

Locoweed Poisoning

Chronic ingestion of *Astragalus* or *Oxytropus* spp. (locoweed) causes an acquired neurovisceral storage disease. Horses are most susceptible, but cattle, sheep, and goats can also be affected.

Clinical signs in horses

Signs include ataxia, proprioceptive deficits, and depression with alternating periods of frenzied or maniacal activity. At rest affected horses show intentional head tremor, flaccidity of the nose and lips, repetitive movements with the lips and tongue, and dysphagia. High-stepping, stringhalt-like gaits are seen in some horses. The signs worsen markedly when affected horses are handled or transported. Tranquilization usually is ineffective for controlling the hyperexcitability.

Clinical signs in ruminants

Signs in adult cattle include proprioceptive deficits; hypermetria; weakness; depression; dull, staring eyes; and loss of herding instinct. Poisoned sheep have a star-gazing attitude, appear blind, and are nervous and stiff; normal flocking behavior is absent. Ptyalism may also occur.

Diagnosis and treatment

Cytoplasmic vacuolation in the lymphocytes on stained blood smears is diagnostic in animals with clinical signs and a history of exposure. There is no effective long-term treatment. Some authors recommend tranylcypromine (60 mg PO), protriptyline (60 mg PO), or reserpine (3.125 g/500 kg). Cattle with mild signs recover completely within 60 days of removal from the pasture. Horses that survive retain the altered behavior.

GRASS STAGGERS *(Text pp. 966-971)*

Ryegrass Staggers and Similar Conditions

Ataxia and tremors (grass staggers) can occur in livestock that ingest toxic stands of perennial ryegrass *(Lolium perenne),* annual ryegrass *(Lolium rigidium),* Bermuda grass *(Cynodon dactylon),* Dallis grass (either pasture or hay) infected with the ergot fungus *Claviceps paspali,* or moldy corn stalks infested with *Penicillium cyclopium.* Affected animals appear normal at rest but tremble when excited; the gait is stiff and hypermetric. Other signs include intentional head tremor, trunkal sway, and base-wide stance.

Features specific to each intoxication are as follows:
- Ryegrass staggers–affects horses, cattle, and sheep
  - Clinical signs may occur within 48 hours or several weeks after animals are introduced to toxic pastures.
  - If the animals are removed from toxic pastures when signs are first seen, mortality is low, but several months may elapse before the signs resolve completely.

- Bermuda grass staggers–cattle are most susceptible, followed by sheep, goats, and horses
  - Signs may appear as early as 36 hours after consuming toxic forage (either pasture or hay).
  - Most animals recover between 2 days and 2 months after removal from the pasture.
- Dallis grass staggers–horses susceptible, but most common in cattle
  - Toxic stands of Dallis grass can be recognized by the presence of numerous small, reddish-brown or black sclerotia on the seedhead.
  - Animals recover spontaneously within 1 to 3 months of removal from the pasture.
- *Penicillium cyclopium* (tremorgen) intoxication–affects ruminants
  - Diagnosis is based on clinical signs, demonstration of the mycotoxin in the feed, and identification of the fungal elements in the feces.
  - Affected animals recover completely when removed from the forage.

Canary Grass *(Phalaris)* Staggers

Canary grass stagger occurs in cattle or sheep grazing canary grass (*Phalaris* spp.). There are two clinical forms: acute death from cardiovascular collapse (which occurs within the first 72 hours of exposure) and a more chronic nervous form.

Clinical signs

The nervous form occurs after exposure of at least 2 weeks' duration; clinical signs may be delayed for as long as 4 months after removal from the grass. Signs include hyperexcitability, fine muscle fasciculations (particularly of the masseter muscles), licking of the lips, wrinkling of the facial muscles, repetitive chewing, inability to swallow, flaring of the nostrils, ptyalism, nystagmus, intentional head tremor, ear and tail twitching, base-wide stance, reduced menace response, and deficient pupillary reflexes. The gait is stiff, with both rear limbs moving in unison ("rabbit hopping").

Diagnosis and management

For confirmation of the diagnosis, the amount of tryptamine alkaloids in suspect grasses can be measured (see main text). If toxic pastures must be used, administration of cobalt (28 mg per sheep weekly) is protective. Animals usually recover within 8 days after removal from offending pastures, but signs can persist for up to 1 month and relapse can occur for up to 5 months.

NOTE: *Phalaris* spp. may also contain potentially toxic concentrations of nitrate or cyanide. In any outbreak of suspected *Phalaris* toxicosis when acute deaths are encountered, cyanide and nitrate poisoning should be considered.

DISEASES PRODUCING SPINAL CORD OR PERIPHERAL NERVE SIGNS *(Text pp. 971-999)*

Cervical Stenotic Myelopathy (Wobbler Syndrome)

Cervical stenotic myelopathy (CSM) is a common cause of symmetric ataxia in young horses (6 months to 3 years). The condition involves spinal cord compression by malformed cervical vertebrae. CSM appears to be a manifestation of developmental orthopedic disease. Thoroughbreds are particularly predisposed; males are affected more often than females. Neurologic deficits typically progress for a short time, then stabilize.

Clinical evaluation

Neurologic examination is performed to assess the symmetry and severity of weakness, ataxia, and spasticity. The deficits are accentuated by circling, elevation of the head, and maneuvering over obstacles and inclines. At rest affected horses may have a base-wide stance and demonstrate delayed responses to proprioceptive positioning. The neck muscles may appear atrophied, and the articular processes of C5 and C6 may be prominent.

Diagnosis

Diagnosis is based on clinical and radiographic findings. CSF is usually unremarkable; mild xanthochromia or a mild increase in protein content may be seen. Myelography is required for definitive diagnosis, identification of the location of affected sites, and classification of compressive lesions as dynamic or static. Radiographic findings, myelography techniques, and diagnostic criteria are described in detail in *Large Animal Internal Medicine,* third edition.

Treatment

Conservative management consists of antiinflammatory therapy (glucocorticoids, DMSO, NSAIDs), exercise restriction, and dietary modification (see main text). Surgical intervention comprises either dorsal laminectomy or cervical vertebral interbody fusion.

Equine Degenerative Myeloencephalopathy

Equine degenerative myeloencephalopathy (EDM) is a symmetric, noncompressive disease of the spinal cord and brainstem in young horses. Dietary deficiency of vitamin E and genetic factors have been implicated. Most affected horses are 6 to 8 months of age at onset.

Clinical signs and diagnosis

The disease is characterized by symmetric ataxia, which usually is of equal severity in the forelimbs and rear limbs. Other signs include deficits of the cervical and the cervicoauricular reflexes (see Chapter 8) and laryngeal paresis/paralysis. Radiographic evaluation of the cervical spine and CSF protein and WBC counts in horses with EDM are normal. Plasma vitamin E may be below the reference range (300 to 1050 μg/dl) in some, but not all, unsupplemented affected horses.

Treatment and prognosis

Vitamin E should be supplemented orally at a rate of 6000 IU/day, mixed in 60 ml of corn oil and added to the feed. EDM is usually chronically progressive; the signs may stabilize for an indefinite period, but they are irreversible.

Equine Motor Neuron Disease

Equine motor neuron disease (EMND) is a sporadic, acquired neurodegenerative disease of adult horses. The disease occurs secondary to chronic vitamin E deficiency. The diet of affected animals is deficient in green foodstuffs (e.g., pasture), often consisting of pelleted or sweet feed and grass hay without any source of vitamin E supplementation.

Clinical signs

Clinical signs vary with the stage and duration of the disorder:

- Subacute form–acute onset of trembling, fasciculations, lying down more than normal, frequent shifting of weight in the rear legs, abnormal sweating, and weight loss
  - Head carriage may be abnormally low.
  - Appetite and gait usually are not noticeably affected.
- Chronic form–trembling and fasciculations subside
  - The horse stabilizes but with varying degrees of muscle atrophy (may be severe).
  - The tail head may be held in an abnormally high resting position.

Diagnosis

The diagnosis is based on epidemiologic information, clinical signs, measurement of plasma vitamin E (less than 1 μg/ml) and muscle enzymes (mildly elevated), and surgical biopsy of the sacrocaudalis dorsalis muscle or spinal accessory nerve (see main text).

Treatment and prognosis

Oral vitamin E supplementation at a dosage of 5000 to 7000 IU/day may result in improvement, although full recovery is unlikely. Sudden death has been reported in some horses that appeared to have recovered after treatment.

Spinal Fractures, Luxations, and Spinal Cord Trauma

Vertebral fractures are a common cause of spinal cord injury in large animals. The clinical presentation depends on the site of the lesion, the severity of spinal cord compression, and the involvement of specific anatomic tracts (see Chapter 8).

Vertebral fractures are painful, so patients usually show some distress in the early stages.

Diagnosis

Plain radiographs are the most definitive method of diagnosis. Acute CSF changes include diffuse blood contamination, high RBC count and protein concentration, and normal or high WBC count. CSF changes more than 24 hours after injury include xanthochromia, normal or slightly increased red blood cell and WBC counts, and increased protein concentration.

Treatment

Treatment of acute injuries might involve the following:

- Antiinflammatory therapy–DMSO (0.25 to 1 g/kg IV as a 40% solution in 5% dextrose) and dexamethasone (0.1 to 0.2 mg/kg four times daily for 2 to 4 days)
- Analgesia–NSAIDs or narcotic analgesics (e.g., morphine 0.2 to 0.4 mg/kg)
  - Morphine can also be given epidurally (0.1 mg/kg in 10 to 20 ml saline).
  - Analgesics and tranquilizers should be used with caution in ambulatory patients.
- Fracture stabilization (if possible)
  - Water flotation tanks and slings may be appropriate for stabilization in selected cases.
  - Cervical fractures and luxations in small ruminants may be stabilized by incorporation of the head, neck, and cranial thorax in a fiberglass cast.
  - Surgical stabilization may be an option in certain cases.
- Nursing care–evacuation of bladder and rectum as needed

Most recoveries from spinal cord contusion occur spontaneously and are not appreciably influenced by drug therapy.

Spinal Abscesses

Most spinal cord abscesses originate from vertebral body osteomyelitis. The bone is usually infected hematogenously. The more common infectious agents in ruminants are *Corynebacterium pseudotuberculosis, A. pyogenes, Pasteurella hemolytica, Staphylococcus aureus,* and *Fusobacterium necrophorum.* Common agents in foals include *Salmonella* spp., *Actinobacillus equuli, Escherichia coli,* β-hemolytic streptococci, *Rhodococcus equi,* and *Klebsiella pneumoniae.*

Clinical signs

If the infection remains localized in the vertebral body or if extensive bone infection results in vertebral fracture, the signs are consistent with occlusion of the spinal canal. If the infection erodes through the dura mater, the animal develops signs of septic meningitis (see p. 266). Other signs of spinal abscess include heat, pain, swelling, and crepitus over the affected area and signs of bacteremia.

Diagnosis

Plain radiographs are the best method of diagnosis. A random pattern of lucency and increased bone density characteristic of osteomyelitis is seen in the affected vertebrae. Nuclear scintigraphy can be useful when the bone lesions are not well defined radiographically. Myelography may be used to identify the site of the spinal cord compression.

Hematology. A CBC may indicate chronic inflammation (hyperfibrinogenemia, neutrophilia with left shift, monocytosis, and nonresponsive anemia). Plasma globulin levels are increased in adults but may be increased or decreased in neonates.

CSF analysis. In most cases the abscess does not infiltrate the pachymeninges, so the CSF is either normal or shows only mildly increased protein content (60 to 120 mg/dl) and xanthochromia. CSF changes with meningitis are described on p. 266.

Treatment

If a spinal abscess is recognized early, prolonged antimicrobial therapy generally is effective. When culture (blood, urine, feces, CSF) is inconclusive, a broad-spectrum antimicrobial should be selected. Potassium penicillin G (10,000 IU/kg

IV three or four times daily) with either amikacin (7.5 to 10 mg/kg IM four times daily) or gentamicin (1 mg/kg IM three times daily) is a suitable combination. These drugs are given for 1 to 2 weeks and followed by 2 to 3 months of treatment with trimethoprim-sulfonamide (horses) or procaine penicillin G (cattle). NSAIDs may be administered for pain relief. Surgical drainage of the abscess and curettage of the necrotic bone may be options in selected cases.

Spinal Tumors

With the exception of lymphosarcoma, spinal tumors in domestic animals are rare. A diagnosis of tumorous spinal invasion should be considered when there is progressive neurologic disease that is characterized by flaccid tail and anus, dysuria, urine scalding, distended bladder, perineal analgesia or anesthesia, or paraparesis. CSF analysis can be useful if the tumor is located within the lumbosacral cistern. In other cases the CSF is normal or shows signs of mild hemorrhage. There is no effective treatment.

Cerebrospinal Nematodiasis

Migration of parasitic larvae through the CNS can produce acute neurologic signs. Parasitic agents in horses include *Micronema deletrix, Hypoderma lineatum* and *Hypoderma bovis* (warble flies), *Strongylus vulgaris, Draschia megastoma,* hydatid cysts, and *Setaria* spp. In cattle the condition is principally produced by *Setaria* spp. and *H. bovis.* Small ruminants that share pastures with white-tailed deer may become infected with *Parelaphostrongylus tenuis.*

Clinical signs

The parasites may attack any region of the CNS, but most clinical cases are the result of lesions in the brainstem or spinal cord. Clinical signs variably include paraparesis, tetraparesis, paraplegia, or tetraplegia; asymmetric proprioceptive deficits; hyperreflexia or areflexia; regional anesthesia; neurogenic atrophy; and cranial nerve deficits. *H. bovis* infestation may be apparent by the skin lesions caused by burrowing larvae.

Diagnosis

Parasitic myeloencephalopathy must be considered in all cases of acute asymmetric disease of the spinal cord, cerebellum, or brainstem. Antemortem diagnosis can be difficult. Identification of eosinophils in the CSF is helpful but is not found in every case.

Treatment

Although severe reactions are often associated with death of the parasites in the CNS, administration of parasiticides is recommended. Both corticosteroids (e.g., dexamethasone 0.1 to 0.25 mg/kg) and NSAIDs should be given on the day before treatment and for at least 5 days thereafter. Recommended anthelmintic regimens include the following:

- *S. vulgaris*–thiabendazole (440 mg/kg) or mebendazole (30 mg/kg) daily for 2 days
- *H. bovis*–crufomate (75 mg/kg as Ruelene 13.5%), trichlorfon (40 mg/kg PO), famphur (13.2%; 1 fl oz/90 kg, not to exceed 4 oz for cattle), or ronnel (100 mg/kg PO)
  - Ivermectin may also be effective.
- *P. tenuis*–levamisole (7 mg/kg PO once), diethylcarbamazine (40 to 100 mg/kg twice 72 hours apart), or thiabendazole (250 to 440 mg/kg daily for 2 days)
- *Setaria* spp.–diethylcarbamazine (80 to 100 mg/kg once)

Occipitoatlantoaxial Malformation

Occipitoatlantoaxial malformation, a disease that occurs in horses and ruminants, involves a spectrum of cervical spinal abnormalities. Lesions include loss or flattening of the occipital condyles, asymmetric flattening of the articular surfaces of the axis, and shortened dens. The condition is heritable in Arabians.

Clinical findings

Clinical signs are highly variable and range from normal neurologic function to brainstem compression, sudden death, or stillbirth. Typically, tetraparesis/tetraplegia is seen at or shortly after birth. The signs are symmetric in most cases and include proprioceptive deficits, hyperreflexia, and hypertonia. Some patients are reluctant to move the neck and head; clicking, creaking, or crepitation may be perceived over the cervical spine when the head is moved. Animals with asymmetric bone lesions often show torticollis, whereas patients with symmetric lesions hold their heads in extension.

Diagnosis and treatment

The bone lesions are readily apparent radiographically. Surgical fusion of the atlantoaxial joints, with or without laminectomy, may be appropriate in certain cases.

Spastic Paresis (Elso Heel)

Spastic paresis is characterized by marked asymmetric spasticity and hypertonia of the rear limbs. It has been reported in several cattle breeds and in pygmy goats. Spastic paresis is seen in young animals (onset at 3 weeks to 1 year of age) and occurs at all times when the animal stands. The excessive extensor motor activity results in inability to flex the hock during limb protraction. The spasticity is progressive. Surgical techniques have been described (see main text). Lithium gluconate (4 g/100 kg IM daily for 10 to 30 days) reportedly is efficacious in the early stages.

Coyotillo Poisoning

Ingestion of the fruit of the coyotillo plant *(Karwinskia humboldtiana)* produces a stiff gait, hypotonia, and either hyperreflexia or areflexia. The condition occurs in the southwestern United States. Goats are most susceptible.

Acquired Torticollis

Torticollis is deviation of the head and neck. Causes of acquired torticollis include fracture or subluxation of the cervical vertebrae, basilar skull fractures, dystrophic muscle degeneration, unilateral muscular contracture from injections, lupinosis, traumatic rupture of the cervical muscles, hydranencephaly, asymmetric neurodegeneration, and congenital vertebral deformity. If the spinal cord is intact, there are no neurologic deficits.

Tetanus

Tetanus is a highly fatal disease characterized by generalized muscle rigidity. It is caused by exotoxins produced by *Clostridium tetani.* All species of livestock are susceptible, although cattle are more resistant than horses and small ruminants. In horses, puncture wounds are the most common route of infection. Dairy cattle are most often infected via the uterus. The organisms may proliferate in the forestomachs of cattle in sufficient numbers to induce disease.

Clinical signs

In most susceptible animals the incubation period is 2 to 4 weeks. The earliest signs may be colic (horses) or bloat (ruminants) and vague stiffness or lameness in the infected limb. By 24 hours after onset, generalized spasticity is usually evident, with a stiff gait and extended head. The limbs are held in a characteristic "sawhorse" posture. There is excessive facial muscle tone, causing the lips to be retracted, the ears pulled slightly down and caudal, and the jaws clamped tightly shut (lockjaw). Muscle spasms can be elicited by auditory, ocular, or tactile stimulation. In horses and sometimes in ruminants, retraction of the eye and flashing of the third eyelid across the cornea occurs after stimulation. Aspiration pneumonia may develop as a result of dysphagia.

Clinical course. Severely affected animals become recumbent and lie on their side with the head and legs in full extension. Survivors begin to show improvement after 2 weeks, but signs may persist for as long as 1 month, and lameness may be permanent.

Diagnosis

There are no reliable tests for confirmation of the diagnosis, although attempts should be made to culture *C. tetani* from the suspected site of entry. A history of previous vaccination does not exclude the possibility of tetanus.

Treatment

Treatment guidelines are as follows:

- Provide muscle relaxation.
  - Options include acetylpromazine (0.05 to 0.1 mg/kg), acetylpromazine (0.06 mg/kg) with 5% sodium pentobarbital (2 to 4 ml/50 kg), diazepam (0.01 to 0.4 mg/kg IV), and mephenesin (10 to 20 mg/kg).
  - Place an intravenous catheter to minimize stimulation during treatment.
  - Keep the patient in a quiet, darkened stall and pack its ears with cotton.
- Provide good footing and deep bedding.
- Eliminate the infection–surgically debride the affected area and infiltrate with penicillin G.
  - Also give either potassium penicillin (22,000 IU/kg IV three or four times daily) or procaine penicillin (22,000 IU/kg IM twice daily).
- Neutralize any unbound toxin–infiltrate the tissue around the wound with tetanus antitoxin.
  - Some reports suggest that intracisternal administration of tetanus antitoxin (50,000 IU) can stabilize clinical signs (see main text).
- Maintain hydration and nutritional status–elevate food and water containers, give intravenous fluids and electrolytes as needed, and consider feeding via nasogastric tube or rumenostomy.
- Establish active immunity–immunize with tetanus toxoid at the start of treatment and give a second dose 1 to 2 months later.

Animals that survive for more than 7 days have a fair to good chance for complete recovery. Prevention is discussed in *Large Animal Internal Medicine,* third edition.

Triaryl Phosphate Poisoning (Chronic Organophosphate Poisoning)

Ingestion of industrial lubricants containing triaryl phosphates causes slowly progressive incoordination and paralysis. A similar condition occurs in some families of sheep after treatment with organophosphorous anthelmintics.

Clinical signs

Onset of slowly progressive neurologic signs begins 10 days to a few months after exposure. Signs include rough hair coat, bloat, dyspnea, muscle weakness, and hindlimb incoordination, which may progress to a dog-sitting posture. The tail, bladder, and rectum often are paralyzed, with consequent incontinence, constipation, and perineal scalding. Most animals retain a normal appetite and sensorium. The condition is irreversible.

Diagnosis

Red blood cell cholinesterase is low or undetectable at clinical onset but may return to normal by the time profound paralysis develops. Confirmation is usually based on histopathologic findings in peripheral nervous tissues.

Miscellaneous Conditions

The following uncommon, breed-specific, and exotic conditions are discussed in *Large Animal Internal Medicine,* third edition: ankylosing spondylitis in Holstein bulls, fibrocartilaginous embolization in lambs, systemic neuroaxonal dystrophy in Suffolk sheep, weaver syndrome (bovine progressive degenerative myeloencephalopathy) in Brown Swiss and Angler cattle, progressive spinal myelinopathy in Murray Grey cattle, bovine spinal muscular atrophy in Brown Swiss cattle, spinal dysmyelination in Brown Swiss–Braunvieh calves, progressive ataxia in Charolais calves, inherited periodic spasticity (crampy syndrome, stretches, barn cramps) in cattle, doddler syndrome (hereditary lethal spasms) in Jersey cattle, congenital vertebral anomalies (e.g., spina bifida, hemivertebrae, Arnold-Chiari syndrome), myelodysplasias (e.g., syringomyelia, spinal dysraphism, hydromyelia), and cycad palm poisoning (*Zamia* paralysis).

MOTOR UNIT AND CAUDA EQUINA DISEASES
(Text pp. 999-1013)

Electromyography and Nerve Conduction Testing

Electrodiagnostic techniques such as electromyography (EMG) and peripheral nerve conduction testing are useful when signs of generalized weakness, muscle atrophy, tremors, or obscure lameness are present. These tests are described in *Large Animal Internal Medicine,* third edition.

Botulism: General Comments

Botulism is caused by the neurotoxin of *Clostridium botulinum.* Botulism can occur in three ways: (1) ingestion of preformed toxin (the most common form in cattle and adult horses); (2) ingestion of spores, leading to toxicoinfectious botulism ("shaker foal" syndrome); and (3) wound contamination with botulism spores. Horses are much more susceptible to botulism than cattle. In North America, horses are most commonly affected by the type B toxin, which is associated with forages such as hay.

Diagnostic Approach

Typically, botulism is a diagnosis of exclusion. Laboratory support for the diagnosis requires one of the following:

- Demonstration of botulinum toxin in the patient's serum, GI contents, or wound
- Demonstration of *C. botulinum* spores in the GI contents or feed materials
- Detection of an antibody response to *C. botulinum* in recovering patients

A tentative diagnosis may be based on the presence of botulinum spores and toxin in feedstuffs recently consumed by animals showing clinical signs compatible with botulism (gradual progression of muscle weakness leading to recumbency, with dysphagia and tongue weakness). Because initial signs of botulism vary somewhat among species and with age, foals, adult horses, and cattle are discussed separately.

Botulism in Foals

Botulism is most common in foals 2 to 5 weeks of age, although it can occur at any age. Treatment is described in the section on Botulism in Adult Horses.

Clinical signs

Early signs include lying down more than normal and generalized weakness and muscle tremors ("shaker foal") when forced to stand. Affected foals are well nourished, are bright and alert, and (initially) have normal vital signs. Other findings include dribbling milk from the mouth when nursing, weak tongue (the tongue is easy to pull from the mouth and is retracted slowly once released), mild mydriasis, weak eyelid tone, and ileus and constipation. Progressive symmetric myasthenia with absence of fever and other signs of systemic disease leading to recumbency is the predominant clinical sign in foals.

Clinical course

As the disease progresses, aspiration pneumonia and, terminally, respiratory failure cause elevations in heart and respiratory rates. A small proportion of foals stabilize at a certain level of neuromuscular weakness, then gradually recover over 10 to 14 days with intensive nursing care.

Botulism in Adult Horses

Clinical signs

Early signs of botulism in adult horses that may be detected by an astute owner include weakness, decreased ability to swallow hay and water, slight depression, decreased exercise intolerance, and slowness to eat. Colic is the initial clinical sign in some cases. Moderately affected horses walk with a shuffling gait (sometimes with toe dragging) and show evidence of muscle weakness. Decreased eyelid and tail tone may be detected; moderate mydriasis that persists for several days is an early sign.

One of the most sensitive early indicators of botulism is decreased tongue strength and delayed retraction when the horse's tongue is gently pulled from the horse's mouth. Another is assessment of the horse's ability to consume grain and the time it takes to consume an 8-oz cup of grain (normally less than 2 minutes). Dropping grain mixed with saliva while eating is characteristic. Decreased tongue strength and dysphagia typically occur before the onset of obvious muscle weakness.

Clinical course

As the disease progresses, the dysphagia becomes more complete and the myasthenia (often with muscle tremors) more obvious, leading to recumbency and difficulty rising. Death occurs as a result of respiratory paralysis (or euthanasia). Mildly affected horses may have only transient dysphagia and recover with minimal treatment. Large doses of toxin result in peracute, rapidly progressive illness. These horses may become recumbent within 8 to 12 hours of the first detectable signs. Once an adult horse with botulism is recumbent and unable to rise, the prognosis is grave.

Treatment

Botulism in horses is usually fatal unless affected animals are promptly treated with antitoxin (specific or multivalent botulinum antiserum). The recommended dose is 200 ml (30,000 IU antitoxin) for a foal and 500 ml (70,000 IU) for an adult horse. Only one dose of antitoxin is needed. However, because the antitoxin has no effect on bound toxin, once signs have progressed to recumbency, the prognosis for survival is greatly reduced, even with the antitoxin.

Nursing care is an important part of therapy. It should include the following:

- Stall confinement; frequent turning for recumbent patients
- Broad-spectrum antibiotic therapy for complications such as aspiration pneumonia
  - Avoid using aminoglycosides.
- Fluid therapy and supportive alimentation (feeding via nasogastric tube)
  - Give mare's milk or a suitable substitute to nursing foals.
  - Give a slurry of alfalfa meal (e.g., 4 lb in up to 12 L water twice daily) to adult horses.
  - Monitor hydration daily by assessing PCV and total plasma protein.
- Mineral oil via nasogastric tube to prevent impaction colic
- Bladder catheterization as needed
- Gastric ulcer therapy for foals (see Chapter 30)

Dysphagic horses that are able to stand gradually regain the ability to swallow over 3 to 7 days. The more complete the dysphagia, the slower the recovery. Return to full strength often takes more than a month. Recumbent foals are usually able to stand after 7 to 10 days of intensive nursing care. Very few adult horses that become recumbent and unable to rise recover without meticulous nursing care.

Botulism in Cattle

Most cases of botulism in cattle occur as a herd outbreak. Multiple animals with progressive weakness and clinical signs similar to milk fever typifies botulism in cattle. Careful investigation usually identifies a source of botulinum toxin (e.g., small-grain silage stored in plastic, feed containing an animal carcass).

Clinical signs

Affected cattle are anorectic, depressed, lethargic, hypogalactic, and may develop paresis that leads to recumbency. Rumen contractions are decreased in strength and frequency, and the feces is firm. The pupils tend to be dilated and poorly responsive to light. Tongue weakness (assessed by grasping the animal's tongue and gently pulling it from the mouth) is characteristic. Affected cattle may drool small amounts of saliva and often become dehydrated because of their inability to swallow. Muscle tremors and truncal ataxia, even to the point of dribbling urine, may be apparent before the animal becomes recumbent.

Clinical course

Cattle that absorb a moderate amount of toxin typically exhibit signs of weakness 24 to 48 hours before becoming recumbent. They are unable to rise for 2 to 3 days before death from respiratory failure, dehydration, or complications of recumbency. Large doses of toxin may lead to clinical signs within 12 to 24 hours of ingestion (uncommon). Smaller doses may not yield clinical signs for 7 to 10 days. In a typical herd outbreak, many cattle have subclinical signs (weak tongue, decreased jaw tone, possibly mild dysphagia) and never become recumbent.

Neuritis of the Cauda Equina

Neuritis of the cauda equina, a disease of adult horses, involves inflammatory changes in various nerve roots, particularly those of the cauda equina and cranial nerves. The cause is unknown, although an autoimmune mechanism is suspected. Instability of the caudal spine caused by luxations or fractures, equine herpesvirus myelitis, and sorghum intoxication can each cause similar signs.

Clinical signs

Initially affected horses show hyperesthesia, particularly around the tail head, and they rub and chew at this area. The condition can progress to hypoesthesia or anesthesia of the affected areas. In the chronic form, gradually progressive paresis of the tail, bladder, rectum, and anal sphincter develops, which may terminate in paralysis. Fecal retention or incontinence is sometimes a feature. Urinary incontinence occurs in many affected horses; the bladder is atonic, distended, and easily expressed manually. In severe cases, overflow incontinence develops, with consequent urine scalding and urinary tract infections. In cases in which nerve roots of the lumbosacral spinal cord are involved, there is hindlimb weakness and ataxia, possibly with muscle atrophy.

Cranial nerve involvement. Signs of cranial neuritis depend on the nerves affected and the severity of the disease. The motor branch of the trigeminal nerve is most commonly involved, resulting in temporal and masseter muscle atrophy with drooling and dysphagia.

Diagnosis

CSF changes include mononuclear and neutrophilic pleocytosis (sometimes greater than 100 cells/μl) and moderately to markedly increased protein. Denervation of affected muscles is found on EMG. Detection of circulating antibodies to P2 myelin protein may be a useful test.

Treatment

Treatment with corticosteroids early in the course of the disease may be helpful, although no therapy has consistently been shown to be effective. General supportive care should be given, including fluid therapy when necessary, and manual evacuation of the bladder and rectum. Gradual deterioration usually culminates in euthanasia.

Sorghum Toxicity

A syndrome of ataxia and cystitis in horses, cattle, and sheep has been linked to ingestion of *Sorghum* spp. The first sign is usually hindlimb ataxia, commonly followed by urinary incontinence. The perineal muscles are relaxed, and urine dribbles from a flaccid, distended bladder. In stallions and geldings the penis is relaxed. Tail paresis may also be present in horses and cattle. Cystitis secondary to urine retention may be severe and can lead to pyelonephritis.

Diagnosis and treatment

No diagnostic test is available, and there is no specific treatment. Withdrawal of *Sorghum* spp. from the diet results in gradual improvement over weeks or months, although recovery may not be complete. Treatment of bacterial cystitis is discussed in Chapter 32.

Stringhalt

Stringhalt is a disorder that produces characteristic hyperflexion of one or both hocks in affected horses. It occurs in both sporadic and epidemic forms. Affected horses appear normal at rest but have involuntary hyperflexion of the hock when moving. The disorder may be unilateral or bilateral and can vary in severity from a slight exaggeration of normal movement to a motion wherein the rear foot strikes the belly. The signs generally worsen on turning or backing.

Sporadic form

Traumatic injury, particularly to the dorsoproximal metatarsus, appears to be the cause in some sporadic cases. Clinical signs usually are unilateral, and spontaneous recovery is rare. Surgical therapy (tenotomy or tenectomy of the lateral digital extensor tendon) has been the treatment of choice. Conservative treatment using gradually increasing exercise and intraarticular corticosteroids is effective in some cases.

Epidemic form

Plant toxicity may be the cause of the epidemic form of stringhalt. Outbreaks in the western United States have been associated with ingestion of *Hypochoeris radicata.* Most cases manifest with bilateral signs, and most horses eventually recover without treatment. Because a toxic etiology is suspected, it is recommended that the horses be removed from the pasture. Administration of phenytoin (10 to 15 mg/kg PO once or twice daily) results in clinical improvement in many cases.

Tick Paralysis

An ascending lower motor neuron paralysis can occur in livestock infested with certain ticks (*Dermacentor* spp. in the United States, *Ixodes holocyclus* in Australia). Clinical signs are of progressive generalized paresis that terminates in recumbency and death from respiratory failure in as little as 24 hours. Animals infested with *Dermacentor* spp. recover if the ticks are removed before the patient is moribund. *Ixodes*-induced paralysis is often fatal despite tick removal.

Grass Sickness

Grass sickness is a disorder of unknown etiology that occurs in horses, ponies, and donkeys in Great Britain and northern Europe (and possibly Colombia). The major clinical finding is a decrease in or cessation of gut motility. The course of the disease varies from peracute, with sudden death, to chronic, with some animals surviving for many months.

PERIPHERAL NERVE DISORDERS *(Text pp. 1013-1018)*

Most peripheral nerve disorders in large animals are traumatically induced; injections, abscesses, tumors, and parasitic invasion are uncommon causes. Signs of damage to specific peripheral nerves include the following:

- Suprascapular nerve–slight outward bowing of the scapulohumeral joint during weight bearing; eventual neurogenic atrophy of the supraspinatus and infraspinatus muscles
- Brachial plexus–complete flaccidity of the forelimb and inability to bear weight; absent triceps and biceps reflexes; and desensitization of the entire forelimb
- Radial nerve–limb position varies depending on location of lesion
  - Proximal radial nerve paralysis (at elbow level) is characterized by a dropped elbow, flexion of all distal limb joints, and inability to protract or bear weight on the leg.
  - More distal lesions result in flexion of the carpus, fetlock, and pastern joints; the animal can bear weight on the limb if the carpus and distal limb are supported in extension.
  - Chronic radial nerve dysfunction results in atrophy of the forelimb

extensor muscles; sensory deficits tend to be vague and vary among patients.

- Femoral nerve–inability to extend and fix stifle, constant flexion of distal joints result in collapse of limb during weight bearing
  - There is analgesia/anesthesia of the medial thigh as far distal as the hock.
  - Chronic lesions result in atrophy of the quadriceps femoris and caudal part of the gluteal muscles.
- Sciatic nerve–at rest limb hangs behind animal; stifle dropped and extended; digit is constantly knuckled
  - If the limb is positioned properly, the animal usually can bear weight for a limited period.
  - There is analgesia/anesthesia of the entire limb distal to the stifle (except the medial thigh).
  - Chronic denervation results in atrophy of the caudal thigh muscles and all muscles distal to the stifle.
- Peroneal nerve–hyperextension of the hock and flexion of the fetlock and pastern; desensitization over the craniolateral aspect of the limb from stifle to hoof
- Tibial nerve–hock is overflexed and pulled higher than normal when limb is protracted
  - At rest the pelvis is asymmetric (the affected side is lower).
  - There is anesthesia/analgesia of the caudomedial aspect of the leg.
  - Chronic loss of function results in atrophy of the gastrocnemius and digital flexor muscles.
- Obturator nerve–severe abduction or splaying of hindlimbs when on a slippery surface
  - In severe cases the patient is sternally recumbent, with the hindlimbs extending laterally.

Treatment of Peripheral Nerve Dysfunction

Medical management of peripheral nerve injuries consists of the following:

- Reduction of neural inflammation–dexamethasone (0.05 mg/kg) daily for the first 3 to 5 days after injury; phenylbutazone; cold therapy (first 24 hours after injury)
- Relief of musculoskeletal pain–NSAIDs or narcotic analgesics (e.g., Demerol 1 to 2 mg/kg or morphine 0.07 to 0.14 mg/kg)
- Prevention of secondary complications (e.g., mastitis, fractures, joint damage)
  - Use a dry dirt stall with deep bedding; turn recumbent animals 6 to 8 times daily.
  - In patients with obturator paralysis, prevent splaying with a hobble rope around the distal metatarsi that limits the maximum distance between the limbs to 14 to 20 inches.
  - Calcium gluconate can be given empirically to down cows (500 ml SC daily), as may potassium chloride (100 g in 20 L water by stomach tube daily).
- Prevention of malnutrition and dehydration

Down Cows (Alert Downers)

Such conditions as hypocalcemia, hypophosphatemia, musculoskeletal injuries, pelvic swelling from dystocia (calving paralysis, obturator paralysis), and spinal cord compression may result in an alert downer: a cow that is unable to rise but is alert and will eat and drink. Secondary muscle or nerve damage associated with recumbency is often a complicating factor. A warm water flotation system has been developed for rehabilitating alert downer cows (see main text).

34

Mammary Gland Health and Disorders

Consulting Editors JEFF W. TYLER • JAMES S. CULLOR

BOVINE MASTITIS *(Text pp. 1019-1032)*

Mastitis is the most common disease in adult dairy cows. Contagious mastitis has the infected quarter as its primary reservoir, and bacteria are spread to healthy quarters or to other cows by contaminated milking equipment, human hands, or other means. The most common agents are *Streptococcus agalactiae, Corynebacterium bovis, Staphylococcus aureus,* and *Mycoplasma* spp. Environmental mastitis follows bacterial invasion of the mammary gland from the environment. Common agents include coliforms (*Escherichia coli, Klebsiella* spp., *Enterobacter* spp.), *Pseudomonas* spp., *Serratia* spp., *Proteus* spp., and *Streptococcus uberis.*

Clinical Categories

Inflammation of the mammary gland can be classified as either subclinical or clinical. Clinical mastitis is characterized by grossly abnormal milk (ranging from a few milk clots to serum with clumps of fibrin) and evidence of mammary gland inflammation (e.g., redness, heat, swelling, pain). Clinical categories can be divided into acute, gangrenous, and chronic mastitis.

Subclinical mastitis

Subclinical mastitis occurs when the mammary gland is infected and the number of leukocytes (somatic cells) is increased but the milk appears grossly normal and there are no visible signs of mammary inflammation. It is detected by routine tests such as the California Mastitis Test, somatic cell counts (SCCs), and routine culture. The most common isolates are *S. agalactiae* and *S. aureus.* In time, most subclinical infections result in mammary fibrosis (a firmer, larger gland) and decreased milk production.

Acute mastitis

Acute mastitis is characterized by a swollen (edematous or firm), painful gland and an abnormal hindlimb gait. Systemic signs (e.g., anorexia, depression, fever) may be mild or severe. Toxic patients may have hypocalcemia that is unresponsive to calcium administration and a clinical presentation that resembles milk fever. Mammary secretions in cases of acute mastitis may contain flakes or clots of milk and can be watery, serous, or purulent.

Acute gangrenous mastitis

Gangrenous mastitis is uncommon. It is characterized by signs of toxemia and gangrenous destruction of the affected gland. One to four quarters may be involved. Initially, the affected gland is red, swollen, and warm, but within a few hours the teat becomes cold and the secretions watery and sanguineous. The gland soon exhibits a sharply delineated area of blue discoloration that proceeds to slough over the next 10 to 14 days. Secondary bacterial infection, necrosis, and continued sloughing of most of the glandular tissue in that quarter ensues. The most common pathogens are *S. aureus* and *Clostridium perfringens.*

Chronic mastitis

Cows with chronic mastitis show no clinical signs until the condition is exacerbated and signs of acute mastitis become evident. SCCs typically are chronically elevated, and the milk periodically contains flakes, clots, or shreds of fibrin. Over time, fibrosis results in reduced milk production. The bacteria most commonly isolated are coliforms, *S. agalactiae,* and *S. aureus.*

Diagnosis of Mammary Gland Infection

Routine milk culturing should be initiated when one or more of the following occurs:

- The bulk tank SCC is more than 250,000.
- Dairy Herd Improvement Association SCCs reveal that more than 15% of lactating cows in the herd have a linear score greater than 4.5.
- New clinical cases comprise more than 2% of the herd per month.
- Acutely ill cows comprise more than 1% of the herd per year.

Clinical cases should undergo bacterial culture on samples collected separately from each quarter. Culture of all cows in the herd is indicated when a pathogen is known to be a problem in the herd. The object is to identify infected cows for segregation and treatment, so composite samples (a sample from each quarter collected in one tube) generally suffice. Monthly culturing of bulk tank milk is also an important screening tool (see main text).

Sample collection

Following are some guidelines for proper sample collection:

- Collect samples just before milking.
- Thoroughly wash the udder and teats, dry with a paper towel, and swab the teat end with 70% alcohol.
- Strip each teat two or three times before collecting a milk sample.
- Sample each quarter individually (unless collecting composite samples for herd screening).
- Keep the samples refrigerated until plated.

A comprehensive discussion on microbiologic techniques (including sample handling, plating, and interpretation) is contained in *Large Animal Internal Medicine,* third edition.

Mastitis Therapy

The goals of therapy are to (1) prevent death in peracute cases, (2) restore normal milk composition and production, (3) eliminate sources of infection, and (4) prevent new infections in the dry period. Both parenteral and intramammary antibiotics should be administered if systemic signs are present. Intramammary therapy is then continued once systemic signs have abated. Antimicrobial selection and management of specific infections are briefly discussed below; detailed discussions can be found in *Large Animal Internal Medicine,* third edition.

Antimicrobial selection

In general the choice of antimicrobial agent is dictated by antibiotic sensitivity, drug distribution, and government regulations regarding antibiotic residues (see text). The following antibiotics have been approved for use in bovine mastitis in the United States:

- Prescription–pirlimycin, hetacillin, cloxacillin, amoxicillin, novobiocin, and sulfamethazine (not approved for lactating cows)
- Over-the-counter–penicillin G, dihydrostreptomycin, cephapirin, erythromycin, and novobiocin

Staphylococcal mastitis

Staphylococcal mastitis must be considered a herd problem. Treatment of clinical cases is of little value because the efficacy of current antimicrobial therapy for lactating cows is limited.

Streptococcal mastitis

Streptococcal mastitis is primarily caused by *S. agalactiae.* Intramammary administration of penicillin G (100,000 U/quarter) is highly effective against this pathogen.

Coliform mastitis

Spontaneous recovery without treatment is the usual course with coliform mastitis. However, some patients become severely toxic, and treatment must be initiated early for a successful outcome. Frequent milking (stripping every 2 hours) is important. Administration of oxytocin (20 IU) may enhance stripping of the affected gland and removal of inflammatory mediators. Patients exhibiting toxic shock require circulatory support in addition to antimicrobial therapy. Suggested treatments include intravenous fluids and electrolytes, hypertonic saline, corticosteroids, and nonsteroidal antiinflammatory drugs (e.g., flunixin meglumine).

Mycoplasma mastitis

Mycoplasma spp. are susceptible in vitro to many antimicrobial agents, including tetracyclines, kanamycin, neomycin, gentamicin, and novobiocin, but intramammary infusion does not alter the clinical course. Thus treatment has little benefit and may only delay slaughter or sale of milk.

Control

The National Mastitis Council recommends a five-point control program: (1) milking machine maintenance, (2) teat dipping, (3) early treatment of clinical cases, (4) dry cow therapy, and (5) culling of cows with chronic mastitis. Dairy cows should also be vaccinated against gram-negative mastitis using an R-mutant bacterin. These and other control measures are discussed in *Large Animal Internal Medicine,* third edition.

EQUINE MASTITIS *(Text p. 1032)*

Mastitis in mares can occur at any stage of lactation, but most cases develop within a few weeks after weaning. The most consistent signs are mammary swelling, heat, pain, and ventral edema; some mares are also depressed and inappetant. Mild lameness in the hindlimb nearest the inflamed gland is occasionally seen. Lameness and swelling may be severe when draining lymph nodes become involved; these nodes may abscess when infected with *Corynebacterium pseudotuberculosis.*

Diagnosis

Culture and antimicrobial susceptibility tests should be performed in each case. Strict hygiene is essential when collecting milk samples for culture. *Streptococcus zooepidemicus* is the most common isolate. Others include *Streptococcus equi, Streptococcus equisimilis, S. agalactiae, Streptococcus viridans, Actinobacillus* spp. (including *Actinobacillus suis*), *Pasteurella ureae, Enterobacter aerogenes, Corynebacterium pseudotuberculosis, Staphylococcus* spp., *Pseudomonas aeruginosa, Klebsiella pneumoniae,* and *E. coli.*

Treatment

Trimethoprim-sulfonamide (5 mg/kg of trimethoprim orally twice daily) or a combination of penicillin (20,000 IU/kg intramuscularly [IM] twice daily) and gentamicin (2 mg/kg intravenously or IM three times daily) are suitable antibacterial choices while awaiting culture results. Supportive care that includes frequent milking, and hot packs or hydrotherapy may also be of benefit. Bovine intramammary infusion products can be used, but no efficacy data are available for mares.

SMALL RUMINANT MASTITIS *(Text p. 1032)*

Sheep

The bacteria most commonly isolated from ewes' milk are *S. aureus,* coagulase-negative staphylococci, *Streptococcus* spp., *C. bovis, Pasteurella hemolytica,* and *E. coli.* Acute mastitis with life-threatening toxemia and possibly gangrenous destruction of the mammary gland is most often caused by *S. aureus* or *P. hemolytica.* Lameness is often the first sign of mastitis in ewes. Routine udder palpation is a typical component of flock management. Ewes with evidence of scarring or fibrosis of the udder are culled.

Dairy Goats

Coagulase-negative staphylococci and *S. aureus* are the most common mammary pathogens in dairy goats. Following are recommendations for managing specific types of mastitis in does.

S. aureus

S. aureus can cause subclinical or clinical mastitis (including acute gangrenous mastitis). Unlike in cows, this organism often causes large nodular abscesses within the affected gland in goats. *S. aureus* is difficult to eliminate from the mammary gland. Segregating or culling infected does is strongly recommended.

Coagulase-negative staphylococci

Coagulase-negative staphylococci have been isolated in pure cultures from subclinical, acute, and chronic caprine mastitis cases and are sensitive in vitro to procaine penicillin.

Mycoplasma mycoides subsp. *mycoides*

Mycoplasma mycoides subsp. *mycoides* has been associated with mastitis, decreased milk production, systemic illness, and peracute death in kids and adult goats. Transmission via colostrum or milk can cause pneumonia and arthritis in kids. Current antimicrobial agents are not effective in vivo against this pathogen. Herd culture and culling programs are recommended.

Mycoplasma putrefaciens

Though not as prevalent as *M. mycoides, Mycoplasma putrefaciens* is a major cause of sudden agalactia in dairy goats. It is highly contagious but self-limiting and does not cause systemic illness. Normal levels of lactation may return within 90 days.

Streptococcus spp.

Clinical cases of mastitis caused by *Streptococcus* spp. present with fever and a warm, firm, enlarged, agalactic mammary gland. Subcutaneous administration of penicillin (10,000 IU/kg twice daily for 5 to 7 days) or intramammary infusion of a bovine product (at half dose) may be effective in eliminating the pathogen.

Hard Udder or Hard Bag

In addition to signs of systemic illness, caprine arthritis-encephalitis and ovine progressive pneumonia viruses can cause fibrosis of the mammary gland and agalactia (hard udder or hard bag). These infections are discussed elsewhere in the text.

MAMMARY GLAND EDEMA *(Text pp. 1033)*

Physiologic udder edema is common in mares and in prepartum dairy cattle, especially high-producing cows and first-calf heifers. Its primary importance is in its clinical similarity to pathologic edema associated with mammary infection. Unless the edema is serious, treatment is unnecessary. Prolonged massage and hydrotherapy of the mammary gland can be of benefit. In mares, hand walking, salt deprivation, and diuretics are also beneficial.

BLOODY MILK *(Text pp. 1033-1034)*

Contamination of mammary secretions with blood predominantly results from trauma; it may also occur subsequent to prepartum udder edema and rupture of small mammary vessels. Milk discoloration varies in degree and typically disappears within 1 week of parturition; shorter clinical courses are common. The streak canal often becomes blocked with frank blood clots, necessitating frequent hand stripping. Antibiotic treatment is neither efficacious nor indicated.

35

Diseases of the Hematopoietic and Hemolymphatic Systems

Consulting Editor GARY P. CARLSON

Contributors DEBRA DEEM MORRIS • GUY H. PALMER • STUART LINCOLN
JERRY L. ZAUGG • LISLE W. GEORGE • MARK C. THURMOND
JOHN E. MADIGAN • ARLENA B. PIPKIN • MONICA R. ALEMAN
SHARON J. SPIER

BLOOD LOSS *(Text pp. 1039-1042)*

Acute Blood Loss

Massive acute blood loss induces hypovolemic shock: tachycardia, tachypnea, cold extremities, pallor, muscle weakness, and eventual death from cardiovascular collapse. Hemoperitoneum may cause signs of colic, and hemothorax is generally attended by dyspnea. The packed cell volume (PCV) and total plasma protein show little change in the first 12 to 24 hours after acute blood loss.

Treatment principles

Initial treatment should be aimed at stopping the hemorrhage with pressure wraps or ligation as appropriate. However, it may be inadvisable to attempt to control internal hemorrhage if the patient is a poor anesthetic risk. Hypovolemic shock should be treated with sodium-containing crystalloid solutions (40 to 80 ml/kg intravenously [IV]). Hypertonic saline (7.2% NaCl at 4-6 ml/kg IV) can be useful in patients with severe hemorrhagic shock.

Blood transfusion

Whole blood transfusion should be considered when the PCV is less than 20% in an animal with acute blood loss or when the PCV decreases to 12% or less over 24 to 48 hours. Ideally, compatibility testing should be performed before transfusion (see main text). However, the first transfusion in a horse or ruminant that has not been previously transfused or sensitized by immunization or pregnancy is usually well tolerated. Guidelines for transfusion are as follows:

- Usually 6 to 8 L of whole blood is sufficient for adult horses and cattle.
- Give 0.1 ml/kg blood over 5 to 10 minutes and monitor for adverse effects (tachypnea, dyspnea, restlessness, defecation, tachycardia, piloerection, muscle fasciculations, collapse).
- If no adverse effects are seen, resume transfusion at up to 20 ml/kg/hr.

Transfusion should be slowed or stopped if any adverse effects are noted. Severe reactions should be treated with epinephrine (0.01 to 0.02 ml/kg of 1:1000). Patients with only mild signs may respond to a slowed transfusion rate or administration of corticosteroids or flunixin meglumine. However, the safest approach is to discontinue transfusion and administer isotonic crystalloid solutions.

Chronic Blood Loss

Several diseases can result in chronic blood loss that is insidious until clinical signs of anemia develop (usually at a PCV of less than 15%). Causes include bleeding gastrointestinal lesions (e.g., parasitism, ulceration), certain renal diseases, hemostatic dysfunction, and bloodsucking external parasites. Chronic severe blood loss may result in iron deficiency anemia. The aim of treatment is to address the primary cause of blood loss; treatment of the anemia itself is rarely indicated.

INHERITED COAGULATION DISORDERS *(Text p. 1042)*

Inherited deficiencies of specific clotting factors have been described in horses and in Holstein cattle. Clinical signs, when present, reflect the tendency for hemorrhage from large vessels, such as subcutaneous hematomas; hemarthrosis; epistaxis; melena; hematuria; and prolonged bleeding after trauma, diagnostic procedures, or surgery. Petechial hemorrhage is not a feature. Definitive diagnosis is based on specific quantitative assays of intrinsic clotting factors (see main text). Treatment involves replacement of clotting factors using fresh plasma.

VASCULITIS *(Text pp. 1042-1043)*

Vasculitis (inflammation and necrosis of blood vessel walls) is generally a secondary manifestation of a primary infectious, toxic, or neoplastic disorder. Clinical manifestations include the following:

- Areas of dermal or subcutaneous edema, which may progress to skin infarction, necrosis, and exudation
- Hyperemia, petechial and ecchymotic hemorrhages, or ulceration of mucous membranes

Vasculitis can affect any organ system, so lameness, colic, dyspnea, or ataxia may also be noted. Secondary problems often include cellulitis, thrombophlebitis, laminitis, and pneumonia.

General Approach to Diagnosis

Laboratory findings vary with the underlying disease, length of illness, organ involvement, and complications. The platelet count generally is normal. Definitive diagnosis requires histopathologic evaluation of full-thickness punch biopsy specimens (6 mm or larger in diameter) from affected areas. Biopsy specimens should be preserved in 10% formalin and in Michel's transport medium.

Purpura Hemorrhagica in Horses

Purpura hemorrhagica represents an allergic reaction that follows respiratory tract infection, most often with *Streptococcus equi.* Typically, respiratory infection precedes clinical signs of purpura by 2 to 4 weeks. Clinical signs include well-demarcated areas of edema, usually on the head, ventral abdomen, or extremities, with petechial or ecchymotic mucosal hemorrhages. The edema is often sensitive, and affected horses are depressed and reluctant to move.

Treatment

Treatment of purpura hemorrhagica and other vasculitis syndromes is directed at the following:

- Removing the antigenic stimulus–discontinue any medications being given when signs first developed; investigate an underlying infectious cause.
  - Horses with a streptococcal infection should receive procaine penicillin (22,000 U/kg intramuscularly [IM] twice daily) or potassium penicillin G (same dose IV four times daily) for at least 2 weeks.
- Reducing the immune response–give dexamethasone (0.05 to 0.2 mg/kg IV or IM each morning) initially, then continue with prednisolone (0.5 to 1 mg/kg IM twice daily).
  - Once the edema begins to resolve, gradually reduce the dosage of corticosteroids (over 7 to 21 days) as long as signs do not recur.
  - Continue antimicrobial coverage while administering corticosteroids.

- Reducing vessel wall inflammation with nonsteroidal antiinflammatory drug (NSAID) administration.
- Supportive care–provide hydrotherapy and pressure wraps.

Skin sloughing, laminitis, cellulitis, pneumonia, and diarrhea are common complications.

Equine Viral Arteritis

Clinical cases of equine viral arteritis (EVA) are characterized by fever, anorexia, serous ocular and nasal discharge, and edema of the limbs, ventral abdomen, and conjunctivae. Signs develop 1 to 10 days after infection. Late-pregnant mares may abort 3 to 8 weeks later. Diagnosis is based on isolation of the virus or seroconversion. Affected horses usually recover within 4 weeks with supportive care, but a persistent viral carrier/shedder state can occur.

Other Conditions

Two other conditions in which vasculitis is a feature are equine infectious anemia (EIA) and equine granulocytic ehrlichiosis (*Ehrlichia equi* infection). These diseases are discussed on p. 1043.

THROMBOCYTOPENIA *(Text pp. 1043-1045)*

Thrombocytopenia is defined as a platelet count less than 100,000/μl. Mechanisms are briefly discussed and clinical findings are described in Chapter 27.

Persistent, life-threatening hemorrhage caused by thrombocytopenia may be treated with a transfusion of compatible fresh whole blood or, preferably, platelet-rich plasma.

Immune-Mediated Thrombocytopenia

Immune-mediated thrombocytopenia (IMTP) may be primary (idiopathic) or secondary to the administration of drugs (e.g., penicillin, heparin, quinidine, thiazides, digoxin, sulfas, erythromycin), infections (e.g., EIA), neoplasia (e.g., lymphosarcoma), or other immunologic disorders (e.g., autoimmune hemolytic anemia, alloimmune thrombocytopenia in neonates).

Clinical signs

Clinical signs include mucosal hemorrhages and the propensity to bleed from small vessels. Horses with idiopathic IMTP are usually bright and afebrile, without overt hemorrhage despite very low platelet counts. Clinical signs in neonates with alloimmune thrombocytopenia include depression, loss of suckle, bleeding tendency, blood loss, and rapidly developing anemia.

Diagnosis

Laboratory findings include the following:

- Severe thrombocytopenia (less than 40,000/μl)
- Prolonged bleeding time and abnormal clot retraction, but normal thrombin time (TT), prothrombin time (PT), activated partial thromboplastin time (APTT), and plasma fibrinogen
  - Fibrin degradation products (FDPs) may be mildly increased.

Anemia and hypoproteinemia develop if there is ongoing blood loss. In most cases, megakaryocytic hyperplasia is evident on examination of bone marrow aspirates or biopsy specimens. NOTE: Thrombocytopenia in a horse with obvious primary disease should prompt a thorough hemostatic workup to rule out disseminated intravascular coagulation (DIC) (see following discussion).

Treatment

Treatment of any unexplained case of thrombocytopenia involves the following:

- Discontinue all current medications or replace medically necessary drugs with the substitute that is chemically most dissimilar.
  - Patients with drug-induced IMTP usually respond within 14 days of drug withdrawal.
- Administer corticosteroids–dexamethasone (0.05 to 0.2 mg/kg IV or IM

once per day) generally results in an elevation in the platelet count within 4 to 7 days.
- Once the platelet count is greater than 100,000/μl, the dose can be reduced by 10% to 20% per day while monitoring the platelet count.
- Corticosteroids can usually be discontinued after 10 to 21 days, provided the platelet count has been normal for at least 5 days.

Alternative treatments are discussed in *Large Animal Internal Medicine,* third edition. Chronic refractory IMTP suggests an underlying disease.

COAGULATION DISORDERS *(Text pp. 1045-1063)*

Disseminated Intravascular Coagulation

DIC is the most common type of hemostatic dysfunction in large animals. It is characterized by widespread fibrin deposition in the microcirculation (and subsequent ischemic damage) and hemorrhagic diathesis caused by the consumption of procoagulants and hyperactivity of fibrinolysis.

Causes

DIC is never a primary disease. Inciting causes include localized or systemic septic processes, neoplasia, gastrointestinal disorders, renal disease, and hemolytic anemia. DIC is particularly prevalent in horses with acute gastrointestinal disorders that cause colic.

Clinical findings

Clinical manifestations range from diffuse thrombosis to severe hemorrhagic diathesis. DIC usually occurs in a compensated form, so overt hemorrhage is rare. Microvascular thrombosis and subsequent ischemia can lead to renal failure, gastrointestinal hemorrhage (and melena in ruminants), acute laminitis (horses), and thrombosis of major peripheral veins (horses). Other signs depend on the primary disease process.

Diagnosis

Numerous hemostatic tests may be abnormal during DIC; however, no one test consistently or specifically provides a definitive diagnosis. Clinical signs and specific situations suggest the possibility of DIC, and laboratory tests are used only to provide support. The combination of thrombocytopenia with mild to moderate prolongation of the PT or APTT strongly suggests DIC. Serum FDPs are often elevated, but they are usually normal in early or compensated DIC. Repeated hemostatic testing is advised when there is a strong suspicion of DIC.

NOTE: Hemostatic function tests are unreliable unless blood samples are collected and handled properly. These tests are discussed in Chapter 27.

Treatment

Therapy for DIC is highly controversial; the only uncontested modalities are those directed toward treatment of the primary disorder and general supportive measures to combat shock and maintain tissue perfusion (e.g., intravenous fluids, flunixin meglumine [0.25 mg/kg IV three times daily]). If significant life-threatening hemorrhage occurs (which is rare), fresh plasma should be administered at 15 to 30 ml/kg IV. The efficacy of heparin for DIC in horses is unproved. If heparin therapy is considered, there must be adequate plasma antithrombin III (AT III) available; plasma administration may be necessary. Corticosteroids may worsen DIC.

Warfarin Toxicosis

Horses may develop a hemorrhagic diathesis after warfarin administration or ingestion of coumarin rodenticides. Clinical findings include hematomas, ecchymoses of mucous membranes, epistaxis, and hematuria. Lack of petechial hemorrhages helps rule out DIC. The diagnosis is based on a history of exposure, signs of large-vessel hemorrhagic diathesis, and prolonged PT (and sometimes APTT) with no other clotting abnormalities.

Treatment

Warfarin therapy should be stopped. Vitamin K_1 (0.5 to 1 mg/kg subcutaneously [SC] every 6 hours) must be given until the PT returns to normal and is stable. Significant hemorrhage can be controlled by administration of fresh plasma. If the anemia is life-threatening, whole blood transfusion should be considered. NOTE: Vitamin K_3 must not be used because it is highly nephrotoxic in horses.

Sweet Clover Toxicosis

Sweet clover (*Melilotus* spp.) toxicosis is caused by ingestion of dicumarol in moldy sweet clover hay or silage. This disease can occur in any species but is most common in cattle in the northern plains states. Signs are first noticed 2 to 7 days after the moldy hay is fed. Early signs include epistaxis and melena; subcutaneous hematomas and periarticular swellings develop as the disease progresses. Accidental and surgical wounds cause severe hemorrhage.

Diagnosis

Laboratory findings are similar to those described for warfarin toxicosis. The platelet count remains normal, which differentiates this syndrome from DIC and bracken fern toxicosis. Chemical analysis for dicumarol in suspected feed or in the blood or liver of affected animals aids diagnosis; however, the disease cannot be excluded if dicumarol is not detected.

Treatment

Treatment involves discontinuing the use of contaminated feed and administering vitamin K_1 (1.1 to 3.3 mg/kg IM). A response should be observed within 24 hours. Animals with severe anemia resulting from blood loss or those with ongoing hemorrhage should be treated with plasma or fresh whole blood.

HEMOLYTIC ANEMIA *(Text pp. 1048-1063)*

Hemolytic disorders are characterized by an increased rate of red blood cell (RBC) destruction. Clinical manifestations vary with the degree of anemia, the rate of RBC destruction, and the underlying disease process.

Common Clinical Findings

Clinical signs

Common signs with severe anemia include fatigue, depression, anorexia, pallor, tachycardia, and tachypnea. Icterus is characteristic, but intense icterus is noted only after massive RBC destruction and often is transient. Fever is commonly encountered with infectious causes and during periods of active RBC destruction. Neurologic abnormalities (e.g., bizarre behavior, mania), collapse, and death may occur when severely anemic animals are handled.

Clinical pathology

Hematologic manifestations vary with the rate of RBC destruction, the time course, and the underlying disease process. The anemia may be modest or severe. Ruminants usually show evidence of enhanced erythropoiesis (e.g., anisocytosis, polychromasia, reticulocytosis, nucleated RBCs) after a few days. In all species, responsive anemias often are accompanied by neutrophilia and a regenerative left shift. The bone marrow usually shows an erythropoietic response with a decreased myeloid/erythroid (M/E) ratio. An increase in serum bilirubin (primarily indirect) is a reflection of active RBC destruction.

Anaplasmosis

Anaplasmosis is an infectious, transmissible disease of ruminants. It is primarily caused by *Anaplasma marginale* (cattle) and *Anaplasma ovis* (sheep, goats) and is characterized by progressive anemia. In the United States, bovine anaplasmosis is endemic in the southeast and much of the west.

Clinical signs in cattle

Disease is often mild in calves younger than 9 months of age (and asymptomatic in young calves), and is increasingly severe in older cattle. Fever is often the first sign in adult cattle, but it subsides within 12 to 24 hours. Anorexia, dramatic decrease in milk production (dairy cattle), suppression of rumination, constipation, dryness of the muzzle, pallor, and lethargy are often noted subsequently.

Some cattle become aggressive. The convalescent period is protracted (3 to 4 weeks); icterus and weight loss are common at this stage.

Clinical signs in small ruminants

A. ovis infection is often asymptomatic. The anemia occasionally becomes severe enough to cause signs similar to those of *A. marginale* infection in cattle.

Diagnosis

Acute bovine anaplasmosis is characterized by anemia, which can be precipitous. During the decline in PCV, *A. marginale* morula can be detected within RBCs on Wright-stained, new methylene blue-stained, or Giemsa-stained blood smears. Evidence of erythrocyte regeneration is present after a few days. The icterus index is variable. Serologic tests are useful in detecting persistently infected asymptomatic animals (see main text).

Treatment

Oxytetracycline (11 mg/kg IV once per day for 3 to 5 days or 20 mg/kg of a long-acting formulation IM once or twice at 72-hour intervals) is effective for acute anaplasmosis. If the PCV is 12% or less, whole blood transfusion (4 to 8 L for adult cattle) may be necessary. Care must be taken not to overstress severely anemic animals. To achieve complete clearance, long-acting oxytetracycline must be administered at 20 mg/kg every 3 days for four treatments. Prevention is discussed in *Large Animal Internal Medicine,* third edition.

Babesiosis in Cattle

Babesiosis (redwater, tick fever) is a tick-borne intraerythrocytic disease caused by protozoa of the genera *Babesia* and *Theileria.*

Clinical signs

Findings include fever (can be high), depression, icterus, anorexia, tachycardia, tachypnea, anemia, hemoglobinemia, hemoglobinuria, abortion, and death. The anemia may develop rapidly. Cerebral babesiosis, characterized by hyperexcitability, convulsions, opisthotonos, coma, and death, may be observed, especially with *Babesia bovis.* Most cases with cerebral involvement are fatal. Many cattle that survive acute babesiosis recover but become chronic carriers. Other survivors often experience episodes of recrudescence, eventually succumbing to the disease.

Diagnosis

Clinical signs in cattle in enzootic areas may be sufficient for a presumptive diagnosis. Positive diagnosis requires identification of the organisms within RBCs on Giemsa-stained thin blood smears (acute infections), positive serologic tests, inoculation of splenectomized calves with blood, or identification using DNA or RNA probes.

Treatment

The most commonly used babesiacides are diminazine diaceturate (Berenil or Ganeseg, 3 to 5 mg/kg), phenamidine diisethionate (Lomdine, 8 to 13 mg/kg), imidocarb dipropionate (Imizol, 1 to 3 mg/kg), and amicarbalide diisethionate (Diampron, 5 to 10 mg/kg). Acute cases with PCVs greater than 12% usually respond well to treatment, but the prognosis is poor if hemoglobinuria or cerebral signs are present. Supportive therapy (e.g., blood transfusions, fluids, hematinics, prophylactic antibiotics) are important; however, wild, excitable cattle may best be left alone. Prevention is discussed in *Large Animal Internal Medicine,* third edition.

Babesiosis in Horses

Babesiosis, or piroplasmosis, in horses is caused by *Babesia caballi* or *Theileria equi* (formerly *Babesia equi*). Once infected, survivors remain chronic carriers. Equine piroplasmosis is widely distributed throughout the tropics and subtropics and to a lesser extent in temperature regions; however, it is not a problem in the United States.

Clinical signs

Clinical findings, following an incubation period of 5 to 28 days, include fever (can be high), anemia, jaundice, hemoglobinuria, and death. Other nonspecific signs include depression, anorexia, incoordination, lacrimation, mucous nasal discharge, eyelid edema, and recumbency. *T. equi* is the more pathogenic of the two species and is more likely to cause hemoglobinuria and death. Hemoglobinuria is rare in animals infected with *Babesia caballi,* but the urine is often dark yellow in color; *B. caballi* causes a more persistent fever and anemia.

Diagnosis

Diagnosis is based on clinical signs and detection of parasite-infected RBCs in Giemsa-stained blood smears. (A unique characteristic of *T. equi* is that the parasites divide into four cells to form a Maltese cross.) Serologic tests may be positive within 14 days after exposure. A polymerase chain reaction (PCR) test is also available for diagnosis of both infections.

Treatment

If diagnosed early and treated promptly, recovery is the rule. *B. caballi* and *T. equi* both respond to the same babesiacidal drugs used to treat bovine babesiosis; however, *T. equi* is more refractory to treatment than *B. caballi.* The drug of choice for eliminating the carrier state is imidocarb (2.2 mg/kg twice every 24 hours for *B. caballi;* 4 mg/kg four times every 72 hours for *T. equi*). The higher dosages of imidocarb often produce transient colic.

Leptospirosis

Leptospira infection sometimes causes an acute hemolytic syndrome in calves and lambs. Clinical findings include fever, depression, icterus, anemia (can be severe), and petechial hemorrhages. The diagnosis is made by demonstration of the organism in the urine and an increase in serum antibody titer. Leptospirosis is discussed further in Chapters 32, 37, and 41.

Bacillary Hemoglobinuria

Bacillary hemoglobinuria is an acute hemolytic disorder caused by *Clostridium novyi* type D. It is discussed in Chapter 31.

Equine Infectious Anemia

EIA is a viral disease of horses, donkeys, and mules that is characterized by episodes of hemolytic anemia. There is no effective treatment or vaccine, and infected animals remain carriers for life. Control measures are discussed in *Large Animal Internal Medicine,* third edition.

Clinical signs

The acute form follows initial exposure to the virus; signs (which may be mild) include fever, depression, and petechial hemorrhages. Horses occasionally develop fulminant infection that results in death. The subacute or chronic stage presents with more classic signs of EIA: recurrent episodes of fever, depression, anemia, icterus, lymphadenopathy, petechiae, edema, and weight loss. The frequency of episodes and the severity of the signs decrease over time, such that chronically infected horses may manifest few clinical or hematologic indications of the disease.

Diagnosis

During febrile episodes, moderate to severe hemolytic anemia and thrombocytopenia are noted; Coombs' test may be positive. Mild lymphocytosis and monocytosis are often associated with active disease. The complete blood count in chronic carriers often is normal, except for marginally low RBC indices. The diagnosis is based on serologic examination using either enzyme-linked immunosorbent assay or agar gel immunodiffusion (AGID) (Coggins' test). Note: EIA is a reportable disease.

Autoimmune Hemolytic Anemia

Autoimmune hemolytic anemia is associated with the production of antibodies directed against the patient's own RBCs. The condition rarely occurs as a primary disorder. Most often it is secondary to disease processes, such as purpura hemorrhagica, lymphosarcoma, other neoplasms, protein-losing enteropathy, and chronic bacterial infection, or to drug administration (e.g., procaine penicillin in horses).

Clinical signs

Presenting signs vary with the degree of anemia and the primary disease. Animals with marked anemia (PCV less than 15%) manifest signs typical of those seen with other severe hemolytic anemias.

Diagnosis

The hemolytic process often is rapid and persistent, leading to pronounced anemia (PCV less than 10%). Hematologic features are those expected with a responsive hemolytic anemia. Erythrophagocytosis and autoagglutination may be noted on blood smears. Moderate neutrophilic leukocytosis is common; thrombocytopenia occurs in some individuals.

Coombs' test. Diagnosis is usually based on direct Coombs' test (see main text). However, Coombs' test is not positive in every case, so the diagnosis may depend on ruling out other causes of hemolytic anemia and on the response to therapy. NOTE: Prior treatment with corticosteroids could lead to a false-negative Coombs' test.

Treatment

Guidelines for treatment are as follows:

- Address the primary problem–discontinue the medication or change to another class of drug in cases that may be drug-induced.
- Immunosuppressive therapy–administer dexamethasone (30 to 40 mg/day for a 450-kg horse) for 3 to 5 days; gradually decrease over the next 7 to 14 days, depending on response to therapy.
  - Once the hemolysis is under control, change to prednisolone (400 to 500 mg/day orally [PO]).
- Supportive care–provide a quiet, restful environment and good nutrition, including vitamin supplementation.
  - Hematinics are generally of little benefit.
  - Blood transfusion should not be considered unless the anemia is life-threatening and the immune response can be controlled with corticosteroids.

Immune-mediated hemolytic anemias that are secondary to other diseases can be managed successfully only if the primary problem is amenable to treatment.

Heinz Body Hemolytic Anemia

Acute hemolytic anemia can develop after exposure to a variety of oxidizing agents, including phenothiazine drugs, methylene blue, acetylphenyl hydrazine, wild or domestic onions, plants in the *Brassica* family (e.g., rape, kale), and wilted or dried red maple *(Acer rubrum)* leaves. Dietary situations that can lead to Heinz body anemia include chronic copper toxicity (in sheep on low-molybdenum diets), ingestion of ryegrass *(Secale cereale),* and selenium deficiency.

Clinical findings

Clinical signs vary with species, toxin, amount ingested, time course, and complicating factors such as hemoglobin nephrosis and acute renal failure. Weakness, depression, anorexia, and exercise intolerance are the usual presenting complaints. Mucous membranes generally are pale and may be icteric (can be marked); brownish discoloration (methemoglobinemia) may be noted in horses with red maple toxicosis. Heart and respiratory rates are elevated. Urine output may be reduced, and the urine may be dark (as a result of increased hemoglobin, methemoglobin, or bilirubin). The mortality rate with red maple toxicosis is high (60% to 65%).

Diagnosis

The anemia usually is profound. In the early stages a high percentage of erythrocytes have Heinz body inclusions (ovoid or serrated refractile granules near or protruding from the cell margin). They are best visualized with stains such as crystal violet or new methylene blue applied to unfixed blood smears. After the first 3 or 4 days, there is usually hematologic evidence of an active erythrogenic response in all species except the horse.

Serum biochemistry. Serum bilirubin (particularly indirect reacting) is elevated. Total plasma proteins usually remain within normal limits, and Coombs' test is negative. Red maple poisoning results in modest elevations of liver-derived serum enzymes. Hemoglobinemia and hemoglobinuria may occur and can lead to renal failure.

Treatment

Treatment involves removal of the source of the toxin and provision of supportive care. Blood transfusion can be beneficial in severely anemic patients. Intravenous fluids are indicated in animals with hemoglobinuria or azotemia. Vitamin C therapy has little impact on survival in horses with red maple toxicosis.

Postparturient Hemoglobinuria

A syndrome of intravascular hemolysis, hemoglobinuria, and anemia (often severe) sporadically occurs in high-producing, multiparous dairy cows in the first month postpartum. Hypophosphatemia is implicated. Depression, inappetence, hypogalactia, and icterus are noted. Blood transfusion and intravenous fluids are indicated in valuable cows with life-threatening anemia. Administration of sodium acid phosphate (60 g/300 ml of water IV) should be followed by oral phosphorus supplementation.

Copper Toxicosis

An acute, highly fatal hemolytic crisis occurs in growing lambs, and occasionally in calves, and is associated with the sudden release of hepatic copper stores after a long period of excessive copper intake.

Clinical signs and diagnosis

Clinical findings include depression, anorexia, weakness, hemoglobinemia, hemoglobinuria, and anemia; high death losses can occur within 1 to 2 days. Icterus and evidence of active erythropoiesis may be noted in surviving animals. During the acute hemolytic crisis the blood copper concentration is significantly increased.

Treatment

Therapy includes intravenous fluids, oxygen insufflation, and blood transfusion (if the PCV is less than 8%). Chelation therapy with D-penicillamine (Cuprimine, 52 mg/kg daily for 6 days) and daily oral administration of ammonium molybdate (100 mg/sheep) and anhydrous sodium sulfate (1 g/sheep) may help mobilize excessive hepatic copper. Ammonium tetrathiomolybdate (50 to 100 mg/sheep PO twice weekly) shows some promise (see main text).

Miscellaneous Conditions

The following conditions are uncommon or exotic causes of hemolytic anemia: haemobartonellosis and eperythrozoonosis in ruminants, theileriasis in ruminants, trypanosomiasis, L-tryptophan-indole intoxication in horses, water intoxication (salt poisoning) in calves, hemolytic syndrome in horses with terminal liver failure, and congenital erythropoietic porphyria in cattle. These conditions are discussed in *Large Animal Internal Medicine,* third edition.

DEPRESSION ANEMIA *(Text pp. 1063-1065)*

Anemia caused by depression of erythropoiesis is the most common form of anemia in domestic animals. Depression anemia can be caused by (1) deficiency of iron, copper, cobalt, vitamin B_{12}, or folic acid; (2) chronic inflammatory diseases or neoplasia; or (3) processes that damage or displace bone marrow elements (e.g., aplastic anemia, bracken fern poisoning).

General Approach to Diagnosis

Depression anemia is often mild to moderate in severity and generally is only slowly progressive. With the exception of chronic iron or copper deficiency, depression anemia tends to be normocytic and normochromic. Bone marrow evaluation is a useful diagnostic tool in animals with nutritional deficiencies or when bone marrow damage or dyscrasia is suspected.

Iron Deficiency Anemia

Iron deficiency is most commonly associated with chronic blood loss (see p. 1040). Iron depletion is first indicated by decreased marrow iron, evident by staining bone marrow aspirate with Prussian blue. As blood loss continues and iron deficiency progresses, serum iron decreases (normal is 100 μg/dl), whereas the iron-binding capacity may increase (normal is 300 μg/dl). It is only late in this process that microcytic, hypochromic erythrocytes are found. Treatment is contingent on resolution of the process responsible for the chronic blood loss.

Copper Deficiency

Copper deficiency can occur as a primary problem in milk-fed animals or in pastured animals in copper-deficient areas. More commonly, copper deficiency occurs secondary to other trace mineral imbalances, such as molybdenum excess. Clinical signs are most prominent in young animals and may include decreased growth rate, rough and depigmented hair, diarrhea, osteoporosis with spontaneous fractures, anemia, and, in lambs, enzootic ataxia (see Chapter 33).

Diagnosis and treatment

The anemia is usually microcytic and hypochromic. Copper deficiency can be documented by measuring serum copper (as ceruloplasmin); erythrocyte superoxide dismutase; or the copper content of hair, liver, or kidney. Copper can be supplied as a dietary supplement or as an injectable copper glycinate preparation (see Chapter 30).

Bracken Fern Toxicosis

Bracken fern toxicosis in cattle causes bone marrow depression and subsequent pancytopenia. Toxic effects are cumulative and clinical signs occur suddenly 2 to 8 weeks after cattle gain access to the plant. Signs include fever, melena, epistaxis, hematuria, mucosal petechiae, hyphema, and bleeding from the eyes and vagina. Death may follow in 1 to 3 days.

Diagnosis and treatment

Hematologic examination reveals a platelet count less than 40,000/μl and profound leukopenia with essentially no neutrophils. Antibiotic therapy and blood/platelet transfusion may be appropriate, but severely affected cattle (platelet count less than 50,000/μl and leukocyte count less than 2000/μl) usually die.

Other Conditions

The following causes of depression anemia are discussed in *Large Animal Internal Medicine,* third edition: vitamin B_{12} and folic acid deficiency, anemia of inflammatory disease, anemia secondary to organ dysfunction, bone marrow hypoplasia, and aplastic anemia.

ERYTHROCYTOSIS (POLYCYTHEMIA) *(Text pp. 1066-1067)*

Absolute erythrocytosis is caused by increased erythropoiesis that creates a circulating erythrocyte mass above normal for the species. Relative erythrocytosis caused by hemoconcentration, endotoxemia, or splenic contraction (horses) is much more common.

Absolute Erythrocytosis

Absolute erythrocytosis is usually secondary to chronic diseases that produce tissue hypoxia, such as residence at high altitude, congenital heart defects with right-to-left shunting, and some forms of chronic pulmonary disease. In these instances the erythrocytosis is physiologically appropriate. In contrast, excessive erythropoietin production associated with certain renal, hepatic, or endocrine disorders causes erythrocytosis that is physiologically inappropriate.

Clinical findings and diagnosis

Absolute erythrocytosis causes characteristic "muddy" hyperemia of the mucous membranes, lethargy, and weight loss. Thrombotic complications, such as laminitis and renal failure, may also be seen. Diagnosis is based on persistently elevated PCV, hemoglobin, and RBC count, without clinical evidence of shock or dehydration, and unresponsiveness to intravenous fluid therapy. Appropriate erythrocytosis is confirmed by measuring arterial Po_2 and documenting hypoxemia. Inappropriate erythrocytosis is characterized by a normal Pao_2.

Treatment

Treatment is difficult because the underlying cause often cannot be corrected. Phlebotomy is indicated to keep the PCV less than 60% for appropriate erythrocytosis and less than 50% for inappropriate erythrocytosis.

BOVINE LYMPHOSARCOMA *(Text pp. 1067-1070)*

Lymphosarcoma occurs sporadically in calves and young cattle. The most common form of bovine lymphosarcoma appears endemically in cattle older than 2 years of age and is associated with bovine leukemia virus (BLV) infection. There is no treatment. Control is discussed in *Large Animal Internal Medicine,* third edition.

Clinical Signs

Affected cattle often present with a history of weight loss, abrupt drop in milk production, lymphadenopathy (most often prescapular, femoral, and supramammary), exophthalmos, and inappetence/anorexia. Other signs may include diarrhea, ataxia, paresis, ketosis, and infertility. Physical examination often reveals evidence of organ system failure or secondary infection. Subclinical lymphosarcoma may be diagnosed in cows submitted for routine reproductive examination.

Diagnosis

Rectal palpation

Rectal palpation is the most useful diagnostic procedure in cases lacking peripheral node enlargement or exophthalmos. Tumor masses palpated in the abdomen typically are multiple and range in size from only slightly enlarged lymph nodes to lesions of 50 cm in diameter. The internal iliac nodes are involved in most cattle with abdominal tumors.

Hematology

The hemogram is often unremarkable. Microcytic, hypochromic anemia may be present in cattle with gastrointestinal hemorrhage. Lymphocytosis is not usually associated with lymphosarcoma, although a large number of bizarre, immature-appearing lymphocytes are seen in some cases. Fibrinogen levels are inconsistent, but measurement may be helpful in differentiating lymphosarcoma from abscess.

Cytology and biopsy

Cytologic examination is not a reliable diagnostic tool with lymphosarcoma, although it can be helpful. Histopathologic examination of biopsy specimens from tumors or nodes is more useful. Tissue should be sent for biopsy; this should be done by surgically removing as much of the node (or mass) as possible.

Serology

Almost all adult cattle with lymphosarcoma are BLV positive, so serologic examination can be useful in establishing the diagnosis. In fact, the presence of antibodies to BLV is considered a prerequisite for a diagnosis of lymphosarcoma, except in periparturient cows. However, less than 2% of BLV-infected cattle have lymphosarcoma, so serology is merely supportive of clinical suspicions.

LYMPHOMA IN HORSES *(Text pp. 1071-1072)*

Lymphoma (formerly lymphosarcoma) is one of the most common neoplasms in horses. Clinical signs depend on lesion location and the organ systems involved. Four forms of equine lymphoma are described (see following discussion). With all but the cutaneous form, the prognosis is poor.

Approach to Diagnosis

Diagnosis depends on demonstration of neoplastic cells by cytologic evaluation of bone marrow or pleural or peritoneal fluid or by histologic examination of biopsy specimens from enlarged lymph nodes, tumor masses, or infiltrated tissues.

Hematology and serum chemistry

A modest neutrophilic leukocytosis with an elevated fibrinogen is often seen, and many patients have a polyclonal gammopathy and hypoalbuminemia. Anemia is common and is frequently associated with an immune-mediated hemolytic process. In most cases the lymphocyte count is normal or decreased. Frank leukemia is rare, but atypical lymphocytes may be noted on blood smears in 20% to 30% of cases, particularly late in the disease. Hypercalcemia has been reported in a number of cases.

Generalized or Multicentric Form

The most common form of equine lymphoma is generalized or multicentric. Affected horses often present with severe depression, emaciation, generalized lymphadenopathy, and ventral edema. Additional signs are associated with specific internal organ involvement. Although rare, leukemia is seen most often with this form of lymphoma.

Intestinal or Alimentary Form

Intestinal or alimentary lymphoma is most common in horses younger than 5 years of age. Affected horses are often very thin and may have a history of mild recurrent colic or recurrent fever. Altered stool character may also be noted. Peripheral lymph nodes generally are not enlarged, but intestinal lymphadenopathy may be noted on rectal palpation. The oral glucose absorption test may indicate malabsorption, and a test for fecal occult blood may be positive.

Mediastinal or Thymic Form

Mediastinal or thymic lymphoma is associated with respiratory signs, pleural effusion, edema of the ventral thorax, and regional lymphadenopathy (thoracic inlet and retropharyngeal area). Temperature and pulse and respiratory rates are often elevated. Cytologic examination of pleural fluid is often diagnostic.

Cutaneous Form

One of the most common forms of lymphoma in horses is cutaneous. However, it is questioned whether this form truly represents a malignant neoplastic process. Lesions are confined to the skin and regional lymph nodes, and they tend to wax and wane.

Clinical signs

Multiple subcutaneous nodules ranging from less than 1 cm to more than 20 cm in diameter develop regionally or over most of the body. The nodules may appear suddenly, and frequently regress, only to reappear. They tend to gradually increase in size but may remain static for years. Local lymph nodes may become involved, but generalized lymphadenopathy and internal organ involvement seldom occur. The hemogram in most cases is normal.

Treatment and prognosis

This form of lymphoma is responsive to corticosteroids. Lesions often regress almost completely over 1 to 2 weeks in response to dexamethasone (20 mg daily). However, unless gradually tapering doses are continued for long periods, the lesions tend to recur, often in a more vigorous and rapidly expanding form. Affected horses may live and function well for many years.

MYELOPROLIFERATIVE DISEASE *(Text pp. 1072-1073)*

Myelogenous neoplasia occurs rarely in horses, and most often in those less than 5 years of age. It should be considered in animals with signs of depression, recurrent fever, and petechial hemorrhages that have hematologic evidence of thrombocytopenia, neutropenia, and nonregenerative anemia. Diagnosis is based on bone marrow evaluation (see main text). There is no effective treatment.

GRANULOCYTOTROPIC EHRLICHIAL INFECTIONS *(Text pp. 1073-1074)*

Ehrlichia phagocytophila

Ehrlichia phagocytophila causes tick-borne fever in ruminants in Europe. Infection in sheep is characterized by an initial febrile phase in which the animal appears dull and listless, loses body weight, and develops thrombocytopenia and leukopenia. The illness resolves after 1 to 12 days; relapse occasionally occurs if the infection was untreated. The disease predisposes the animal to bacterial, fungal, and viral infections. Tick-borne fever is treated with tetracyclines.

Equine Granulocytic Ehrlichiosis

Equine ehrlichiosis is a tick-borne disease caused by the rickettsia *E. equi.* Clinical signs include fever, depression, anorexia, limb edema, mucosal petechiae, ataxia, and reluctance to move. Seasonal incidence parallels tick exposure. The incubation period is 10 to 20 days.

Diagnosis

Presumptive diagnosis is based on a history of tick exposure, clinical signs, and hematologic findings (anemia, leukopenia, and thrombocytopenia). Diagnosis involves identification of the characteristic cytoplasmic inclusions (pleomorphic, blue-gray bodies with a spoke-wheel appearance) in neutrophils and eosinophils on a Giemsa- or Wright-stained blood smear (early cases); seroconversion; or a positive PCR test. Subclinical infection (positive titer) is common in endemic areas.

Treatment

The disease is usually self-limiting; recovery typically occurs in 10 days with supportive care. Treatment with oxytetracycline (7 mg/kg IV once per day for 5 to 7 days) can shorten the clinical course. In rare cases, horses treated for fewer than 7 days relapse within the following 30 days.

ANTHRAX *(Text pp. 1074-1076)*

Anthrax is an acute, contagious, and usually fatal septicemia caused by *Bacillus anthracis,* a spore-forming, aerobic bacillus that is a normal inhabitant of alkaline soil in many parts of the country. Anthrax affects a wide range of mammalian species, including humans. Cattle and sheep are most commonly affected. Anthrax typically occurs during the warm, dry months. Epizootics tend to follow periods of change, such as heavy rainfall or flooding after drought.

Clinical Signs

The incubation period is usually 3 to 7 days but can range from 1 to 14 days. Clinical signs vary, but the most common sign is sudden death.

Ruminants

Clinical signs in ruminants include marked pyrexia, rumen stasis, anorexia, hematuria, bloody diarrhea, abrupt decrease in milk production, and possibly blood-tinged or yellow milk. A period of aggression is usually followed by depression, muscle tremors, respiratory distress, and convulsions. Death usually occurs in 1 to 3 days. Nonautolyzed carcasses typically exude bloody discharges from body orifices and show marked splenic swelling. Chronic anthrax is characterized by localized edematous swellings on the shoulders, ventral neck, and thorax.

Horses

Clinical signs in horses include marked pyrexia, colic, enteritis, dyspnea, and edematous swellings on the ventral neck, thorax, and abdomen. Death usually occurs in 2 to 4 days.

Diagnosis

Anthrax should be considered when any animal dies after having been observed in good health during the preceding 24 hours. Antemortem identification of *B. anthracis* is often unrewarding.

Postmortem diagnosis

Necropsy should not be performed on a carcass suspected of having anthrax unless it is performed in an area that can be easily and thoroughly disinfected. A diagnosis of anthrax can be confirmed without a complete necropsy if appropriate tests are performed. Blood should be collected from a superficial vessel (ear or jugular vein) and transported to the laboratory via sealed syringe, sterile swab, or blood smear. An intact eyeball or section of spleen sealed in a leak-proof bag can also be used for bacterial isolation.

Cytology. The simplest and quickest method of diagnosis is by examining a blood smear. Using Giemsa stain, the bacilli appear in single or short chains with purplish-pink capsules. With Gram stain, young bacteria appear gram positive, but older organisms may appear gram negative.

Treatment

If anthrax is suspected, immediate segregation of infected animals is advised. *B. anthracis* is highly susceptible to a wide range of antimicrobials, including penicillin, streptomycin, and tetracycline. The first dose should be given intravenously; intramuscular administration can then be continued for at least 5 days. Prevention and control are discussed in *Large Animal Internal Medicine,* third edition.

LYME DISEASE *(Text pp. 1076-1077)*

Lyme disease (borreliosis) is caused by the spirochete *Borrelia burgdorferi.* The organism is transmitted by ticks. Clinical syndromes in horses and ruminants are not well characterized, but include inflammatory arthritis, uveitis, and possibly brain involvement.

Diagnosis and Treatment

Animals from endemic areas have serologic evidence of exposure, but most seropositive animals do not show clinical signs of disease. Definitive diagnosis is difficult; it is sometimes possible to culture the organism from blood, urine, or cerebrospinal fluid. The organism is sensitive to tetracyclines and moderately sensitive to penicillin; amoxicillin, ceftriaxone, and imipenem are also effective.

TULAREMIA *(Text p. 1078)*

Tularemia is an infectious disease caused by *Pasteurella (Francisella) tularensis,* a non-spore-forming, gram-negative rod. Transmission to livestock occurs chiefly through ticks, fleas, deerflies, and other biting insects. Sheep are the most commonly affected livestock species; massive epidemics with high mortality rates have been reported.

Clinical Signs and Diagnosis

The disease causes an acute septicemia, with localization and development of granulomatous lesions in the viscera, particularly the liver and spleen. Signs are nonspecific and include fever, anorexia, and depression and in some cases cough, tachypnea, and diarrhea. Stiffness and limb edema may also be seen. The course of disease is usually 2 to 14 days. Diagnosis is based on culture of the organism from blood or affected tissues.

Treatment

Treatment early in the course of infection is effective. Aminoglycosides, tetracyclines, and cephalosporins are each good choices until susceptibility results are available. Removal of ticks from affected animals and herd mates is important.

CORYNEBACTERIUM PSEUDOTUBERCULOSIS INFECTIONS *(Text pp. 1078-1083)*

Corynebacterium pseudotuberculosis is a gram-positive, intracellular, facultative anaerobe that survives well in the environment. It causes external and internal caseous lymphadenitis (CLA) in sheep and goats; cutaneous excoriated granulomas and mammary, visceral, or mixed infections in cattle; and ulcerative lymphangitis and external and internal abscesses in horses.

Clinical Forms in Sheep and Goats

There are two forms of CLA in sheep and goats: external and internal abscesses. External abscess is the most common form.

External abscesses

External abscess is characterized by suppuration and necrosis of the large superficial lymph nodes (mandibular, parotid, prefemoral, prescapular). The abscess exudate is thick or inspissated and may appear white in sheep and greenish in goats. Because CLA represents a major herd health problem, culturing of the abscess to determine the causative agent is important.

Internal abscesses

Internal abscesses may be found in the lungs, kidneys, and mediastinal, bronchial, mesenteric, or lumbar lymph nodes. Chronic weight loss is the most common presenting complaint. Other signs are related to the organ or tissues affected.

Clinical Forms in Cattle

The most common clinical form in cattle is cutaneous excoriated granuloma. Other forms are mammary (mastitis), visceral (most often involving the lung), and mixed infections. With the cutaneous form, ulcerative granulomatous lesions up to 20 cm in diameter exuding thick, greenish pus or bloody serum are most often found on lateral areas of the body (e.g., face, neck, thorax, flanks). The lesions do not appear to cause significant illness or decreased milk production, and they heal spontaneously in 2 to 4 weeks.

Clinical Forms in Horses

Three forms of *C. pseudotuberculosis* infection have been described in horses: ulcerative lymphangitis (least common), external abscesses (most common), and internal abscesses.

Ulcerative lymphangitis

Ulcerative lymphangitis is a severe cellulitis of one or more limbs, accompanied by multiple small sores or abscesses and fever, lameness, inappetence/anorexia, and lethargy. Infection often becomes chronic, resulting in chronic lameness, weight loss, and debility. Many cases are attributed to unhygienic conditions.

"Pigeon fever"

"Pigeon fever" infection is characterized by ventral midline, inguinal, or pectoral abscesses. The abscesses can become very large, particularly in the pectoral and inguinal areas. They have a thick capsule and may be deep in the tissue, making maturation slow and drainage difficult. Moderate fever, inappetence, and weight loss may be present during abscess maturation.

Diagnosis

Diagnosis is based on culture of material aspirated or drained from the abscesses. The synergistic hemolysis inhibition test can be used for serologic identification of infected animals. In sheep and goats this test can be used to monitor the prevalence of CLA in a herd or flock and the status of incoming animals. In horses the test is most often used to determine exposure in animals suspected of having deep tissue or internal abscesses.

Treatment

External abscesses

The usual recommendations for treating abscesses (allowing maturation of the abscess before lancing, and ensuring adequate drainage and lavage) should be followed. In most horses the abscesses resolve without further complication after lancing and lavage. A small percentage of horses have recurrent abscesses; an even smaller percentage develop internal abscesses. In small ruminants, drainage does not always result in permanent resolution. In valuable animals the abscesses can be carefully removed intact under regional or general anesthesia.

Internal abscesses and ulcerative lymphangitis

Long-term (6 to 12 weeks) antibiotic therapy may be the only option with internal abscesses and ulcerative lymphangitis. The most commonly used drugs are procaine penicillin (20,000 U/kg IM twice daily), potassium penicillin (40,000 U/kg IV four times daily), and trimethoprim-sulfamethoxazole (15 mg/kg PO twice daily). Erythromycin (4 to 15 mg/kg twice daily IM or IV in ruminants, PO or IV in horses) is also an excellent choice. Rifampin (2.5 to 5 mg/kg PO twice daily) has shown promise, but it should always be administered with penicillin, erythromycin, or trimethoprim-sulfamethoxazole.

36

Diseases of the Bones, Joints, and Connective Tissue

Consulting Editor SUSAN M. STOVER

Contributors HAROLD F. HINTZ • ANDREW T. FISCHER, JR. • JOHN MAAS
JEFFREY P. WATKINS • NANCY E. EAST • JAMES A. ORSINI
MELINDA H. MACDONALD • KEVIN HAUSSLER • K.C. KENT LLOYD
BRADFORD P. SMITH • PATRICIA A. HOGAN • CLIFFORD M. HONNAS
MICHAEL A. LIVESAY • ROBERT L. LINFORD • ERIC W. DAVIS
ANITA J. EDMONDSON • DENNIS M. MEAGHER • STEVEN C. ZICKER
PAMELA WAGNER VON MATTHIESSEN • ANDRIS J. KANEPS
CAROL L. GILLIS • LAURIE A. McDUFFEE

PHYSITIS (EPIPHYSITIS) *(Text pp. 1085-1086)*

Physitis is a disturbance of endochondral ossification that affects the physes of young animals. Horses are more often affected than ruminants. Suggested factors in horses include genetic capacity for rapid growth, conformation, excessive intake of a high-energy diet, calcium malnutrition, trace mineral imbalances (e.g., copper, zinc), and overexercise.

Clinical Signs and Diagnosis

Most cases occur between 4 and 8 months of age, although physitis can develop in horses up to 2 years of age. The most common clinical finding is symmetric enlargement of the distal physes of the radius, tibia, or third metacarpal and metatarsal bones or the proximal physis of the first phalanx. Radiographic findings include a widened, irregular zone of cartilage with a squashed lipping appearance.

Treatment

The first step in treating physitis is to evaluate the ration. Dietary recommendations include a reduction of soluble carbohydrate (grain) intake and provision of adequate amounts of calcium and phosphorus. Nonsteroidal antiinflammatory drugs (NSAIDs) may be indicated to diminish the pain and prevent flexural deformities.

OSTEOCHONDROSIS *(Text pp. 1086-1088)*

Osteochondrosis is a developmental disease characterized by a defect in endochondral ossification, which leads to a dissecting cartilage flap (osteochondrosis dissecans [OCD]), subchondral bone cyst, or physitis. It is recognized more often in horses than in ruminants.

Clinical Signs

OCD may be diagnosed in weanlings or adult horses, but it is most commonly recognized when horses are first placed in training. Onset of clinical signs may be insidious or acute. The severity of lameness varies from nonexistent to severe, but most cases have joint effusion. OCD can occur in any joint; the most commonly affected are the tarsocrural, femoropatellar, and fetlock joints. Subchondral bone cysts occur while animals are growing, but clinical signs often are absent until the horse starts training. Joint effusion is not as common as with OCD.

Diagnosis

Lameness of any type is best evaluated by careful physical examination, gait evaluation, regional anesthesia, and radiography. The contralateral joint should always be radiographed because of the frequently bilateral nature of osteochondrosis. Radiographic features are described in *Large Animal Internal Medicine,* third edition.

Treatment

There are two options for treatment of osteochondrosis: conservative (e.g., extended periods of rest, dietary management) and surgical (e.g., arthroscopic removal of osteochondral fragments, debridement). Subchondral bone cysts in the medial femoral condyle that do not respond to conservative therapy within 3 to 6 months should be treated surgically. Cysts in the proximal interphalangeal joint are usually treated by arthrodesis.

RICKETS IN RUMINANTS *(Text pp. 1088-1089)*

Rickets (osteodystrophy) is a disease of young, growing animals that is characterized by defective mineralization of developing bones. It primarily affects rapidly growing animals and is most commonly associated with phosphorus or vitamin D deficiency, although calcium deficiency can result in rickets. Animals that receive little or no direct sunlight (e.g., winter grazing, confinement) or vitamin D supplements are at increased risk.

Clinical Signs

Clinical signs include stiffness, reluctance to move, lameness, joint enlargement, arching of the back, enlargement of the costochondral junctions, and bowing of the long bones. Tooth eruption is delayed and irregular, and the teeth are mottled and poorly calcified. Patients are often inappetant and have decreased growth, weight gain, and feed efficiency.

Diagnosis

Diagnosis is based on an accurate and complete dietary history and on clinical signs. Important radiographic findings include cortical thinning, bowing of the long bones, and enlargement and widening of the physeal plates.

Clinical pathology

Serum alkaline phosphatase activity is greater than in normal growing animals. Serum calcium and phosphorus concentrations are often normal, although hypophosphatemia can be expected with phosphorus deficiency. With inadequate dietary calcium or vitamin D, hypocalcemia is usually seen only in the terminal stages.

Treatment

The first step is to provide adequate dietary calcium and phosphorus. Suitable supplements include dicalcium phosphate, bone meal, and limestone with monoammonium phosphate. Vitamin D (10,000 to 30,000 IU/kg intramuscularly [IM]) is administered if indicated.

ANGULAR LIMB DEFORMITIES *(Text pp. 1089-1094)*

Angular limb deformities (ALDs) are deviations of the limb in the frontal plane. Valgus denotes lateral deviation of the limb distal to the origin of the deformity; varus denotes medial deviation. ALDs are either congenital or acquired. In general, they are caused by laxity of periarticular supporting structures, incomplete ossification of carpal or tarsal bones, or asynchronous physeal growth. ALDs occur most often and are of most clinical significance in foals.

Evaluation

Important historical information includes age, onset and progression of the deformity, and intended use of the foal. Physical examination should include careful palpation to determine whether the deformity can be temporarily corrected by manipulation of the limb. Deformities resulting from laxity of periarticular supporting structures can be corrected manually, whereas deformities resulting from asynchronous growth or from cuboidal bone collapse with subsequent ossification cannot be corrected manually.

Radiography

Early radiographic evaluation of foals with ALDs is important, particularly when incomplete ossification is present. Dorsopalmar views of the carpus and fetlock using 7- × 17-inch film cassettes and a lateromedial view of the tarsus are recommended. Determining the exact site of deviation is described and illustrated in *Large Animal Internal Medicine,* third edition.

Treatment

Once an ALD is recognized, the mare and foal should be confined to a stall until clinical and radiographic examinations are completed. Treatment depends on the site and severity of the deviation and the age of the foal.

Mild deviation

If the deviation is 10 degrees or less and radiographs reveal normal ossification, stall confinement with periods of controlled exercise is recommended. Hoof trimming may also be considered (see main text).

Moderate to severe congenital deformities

In foals with congenital ALDs of more than 10 degrees that are accompanied by incomplete ossification or that fail to improve with 3 to 5 days of controlled exercise, the limb should be externally supported with polyvinyl chloride tube casts, rigid splints, or more sophisticated orthotic devices (see main text).

Severe or unresponsive acquired deformities

Acquired ALDs of the carpus or tarsus and those not responding to restricted exercise within 4 to 6 weeks are candidates for surgery (periosteal stripping, transphyseal bridging). Surgery for correction of ALDs involving the carpus or tarsus generally is best performed before the foal is 3 months old. ALDs of the fetlock should be treated surgically before 6 weeks of age.

SPIDER LAMB SYNDROME *(Text pp. 1094-1096)*

Spider lamb syndrome (ovine hereditary chondrodysplasia) has been reported in Suffolk and Hampshire sheep; it apparently is an autosomal-recessive trait. Affected lambs have multiple appendicular and axial deformities, including kyphosis, scoliosis, concavity of the sternum, lateroventral deviation of the maxilla, and ALDs. Radiographic changes are diagnostic, although serial radiographs may be necessary. The most consistent radiographic lesion (multiple islands of ossification) is found in the olecranon.

SEPTIC ARTHRITIS *(Text pp. 1096-1099)*

Septic (infectious) arthritis is an inflammatory joint disease caused by bacterial, fungal, or viral infection. One or more joints may be involved.

Causes

In septicemic foals the most common isolates are *Actinobacillus equuli, Streptococcus* spp., *Salmonella* spp., *Escherichia coli,* and other enterobacteria. In older horses, septic arthritis is often iatrogenic (e.g., intraarticular injections); staphylococci are the most common isolates. Multiple organisms may be isolated in septic arthritis related to traumatic wounds, often including enterobacteria and anaerobes. In cattle, *Actinomyces pyogenes* is the most common pathogen.

Infectious polyarthritis

Several pathogens can cause polyarthritis in ruminants. *Chlamydia psittaci* polyarthritis occurs both endemically and epidemically in sheep, goats, and calves. *Erysipelothrix rhusiopathiae* commonly causes polyarthritis in lambs 1 to 5 weeks after processing (e.g., tail docking, castration). *Actinobacillus seminis* causes septic polyarthritis in sheep 4 to 8 months old. *Mycoplasma mycoides* subsp. *mycoides* causes polyarthritis in kids (see p. 1100).

Clinical Signs

An important localizing sign is lameness, which progresses to non-weight bearing. Other localizing signs include heat, pain, swelling, and synovial effusion. Fever is not a consistent finding unless polyarthritis is present. Patients with polyarthritis are stiff and lame and often have marked weight loss. Keratoconjunctivitis may also be found in animals with chlamydial polyarthritis.

Diagnosis

In addition to clinical findings, a complete blood count (CBC) may reveal leukocytosis and elevated fibrinogen. Radiography can be useful, although no lesions may be evident for the first 2 to 3 weeks.

Synovial fluid analysis

Samples of joint fluid should be obtained for aerobic and anaerobic culture and for Gram stain. Special culture techniques are needed if *Chlamydia* or *Mycoplasma* spp. infection is suspected. When culture is negative and no bacteria are seen on cytologic examination, supportive findings include synovial fluid nucleated cell count greater than 10,000 cells/μl (more than 80% of which are neutrophils) and a total protein of more than 40 g/L. Normal and abnormal synovial fluid characteristics are summarized in Table 36-1 in *Large Animal Internal Medicine,* third edition.

Treatment

Successful treatment depends on an accurate clinical and microbiologic diagnosis. Effective treatment in horses with septic arthritis must neutralize lysosomal enzymes, drain the joint of purulent exudate, and eliminate fibrin clots. Methods of joint drainage include needle aspiration, through-and-through lavage, distention irrigation, and arthrotomy/arthroscopy with or without synovectomy (see main text). Other supportive treatments include immobilization of the affected limb, analgesics, and intraarticular injection of sodium hyaluronate.

Antimicrobial therapy

Depending on culture and susceptibility results, the following drugs may be effective when used systemically: penicillin G, β-lactamase-resistant penicillins, cephalosporins, ticarcillin, ticarcillin-clavulanic acid, erythromycin, and aminoglycosides. A combination of amikacin and a cephalosporin is recommended for empiric therapy in horses. A 4- to 6-week course of antibiotics is advisable to reduce the risk of recurrence.

Infectious polyarthritis. Chlamydial polyarthritis must be vigorously treated with tetracycline (20 mg/kg of long-acting tetracycline IM or subcutaneously [SC] every 48 hours for three treatments), tylosin (label dose), or erythromycin (label dose). *E. rhusiopathiae* is sensitive to most antibiotics; penicillin is commonly used.

M. MYCOIDES POLYARTHRITIS IN GOATS *(Text pp. 1099-1100)*

M. mycoides subsp. *mycoides* causes a variety of clinical syndromes in goats. In most outbreaks the predominant abnormalities are polyarthritis and pneumonia in kids and mastitis in does. *Mycoplasma* pneumonia in kids is discussed in Chapter 29.

Clinical Signs

Affected kids have multiple warm, swollen joints; fever (can be high); pneumonia; conjunctivitis; and weight loss. Many kids are unable to rise or are very reluctant to move. The febrile phase lasts 1 to 3 days, after which polyarthritic kids are bright, alert, and appetent. Failure to respond to antibiotic therapy or rapid relapse after treatment is common. Morbidity is high, but the mortality rate varies from 15% to more than 90%.

Diagnosis

Most affected kids have a neutrophilic, monocytic leukocytosis (more than 13,000 white blood cells [WBCs]/mm^3) with elevated plasma fibrinogen (greater than 400 mg/dl). Peracutely affected kids have a CBC typical of toxic shock (neutropenia with a degenerative left shift). The joint fluid is increased in volume and contains large fibrin clots with increased numbers of neutrophils and lymphocytes. The organism can usually be cultured on *Mycoplasma* medium from the joint fluid.

Treatment

There is no effective treatment. Antibiotics may effect complete remission, but relapse can be expected. Prevention and control are discussed in *Large Animal Internal Medicine,* third edition.

CAPRINE ARTHRITIS ENCEPHALITIS *(Text pp. 1100-1102)*

Caprine arthritis-encephalitis (CAE) virus infection causes two major forms of disease: leukoencephalomyelitis in kids 2 to 6 months of age (see Chapter 33) and polysynovitis-arthritis in goats 6 months of age or older.

Clinical Signs

The onset of joint disease is insidious, with brief inflammatory episodes and apparent remission. The carpal joints are most commonly involved, followed by the stifle, hock, hip, and atlantooccipital joints. Over time, chronic joint enlargement is evident and is accompanied by weight loss. The affected joints are painful and show a decreased range of motion. Severely affected animals may remain recumbent or walk on their knees, resulting in soft tissue ankylosis of the carpus. Most infected does also have some mammary gland involvement ("hard udder").

Diagnosis

The joint fluid in affected joints may be normal but is usually increased in volume, is brown to red, and has a decreased protein and increased cell count (1000 to 20,000 cells/mm^3 with 90% mononuclear cells, mostly lymphocytes). Animals with positive serologic examination (agar gel immunodiffusion) are infected with the virus. Infection is lifelong, and virus is shed by these individuals regardless of clinical appearance. There is no treatment. Control is discussed in *Large Animal Internal Medicine,* third edition.

OSTEOARTHRITIS *(Text pp. 1102-1104)*

Osteoarthritis encompasses a large group of joint disorders characterized by progressive, permanent deterioration of the articular cartilage. Cartilage damage (ranging from splitting and fragmentation to complete erosion and loss of articular cartilage) is often accompanied by subchondral bone sclerosis, periarticular new bone formation, and synovial inflammation. Factors involved are discussed in *Large Animal Internal Medicine,* third edition.

Clinical Signs

In horses, often the first sign noticed by the owner/caretaker is lameness or stiffness. Affected horses initially may warm out of the lameness or temporarily improve with rest. Flexion and extension of the joint often exacerbate the lameness or elicit a pain response. Other common findings include decreased range of joint motion, palpable osteophytes or enthesiophytes (with chronic bone spavin and ringbone), and subtle gait abnormalities (shortened stride, limb abduction, toe dragging). However, osteoarthritis may be present in the absence of clinical signs. In contrast, food animals typically present in the advanced stages of osteoarthritis.

Diagnosis

Nerve blocks and intraarticular anesthesia can be useful for localizing the lameness. Synovial fluid analysis typically shows only minimal and nonspecific changes. Radiographic changes typical of advanced osteoarthritis include marginal osteophyte proliferation, enthesiophytes, narrowing or obliteration of the joint space, and subchondral bone sclerosis (and occasionally lysis). Scintigraphy is valuable in early cases when radiographic findings are unremarkable.

Treatment

Rest is the simplest recommendation, but it is often the most difficult to enforce. Other treatments for soft tissue changes include physical therapy and controlled exercise, systemic NSAIDs, joint lavage, and topical antiinflammatory products. The most popular intraarticular (IA) or systemic therapies include intraarticular corticosteroids, intraarticular or intramuscular polysulfated glycosaminoglycans, intraarticular or intravenous sodium hyaluronate, and oral methylsulfonylmethane or glycosaminoglycan (see main text).

SPRAINS, SUBLUXATIONS, AND LUXATIONS
(Text pp. 1104-1105)

Sprains are periarticular injuries caused by overstretching or tearing of a ligament. Clinical signs include localized pain, heat, swelling, and altered gait. Ligament rupture may result in non-weight-bearing lameness, edema, bruising or hematoma, joint crepitus, and joint instability (subluxation or luxation). Chronic sprains have minimal inflammatory signs but are characterized by joint capsule thickening and joint instability.

Diagnosis

Palpation may elicit a pain response and signs of joint instability. Although regional anesthesia can help localize a sprain, patients should be moved cautiously to avoid exacerbating the injury. Ultrasonography and magnetic resonance imaging are useful for assessing ligament damage. Radiography aids in the diagnosis of avulsion fractures and subluxation or luxation.

Treatment

For sprains, treatment involves antiinflammatory therapy, confinement, and support or immobilization of the injured joint (bandage, splint, cast), depending on the severity of the injury. Surgical stabilization may be required for severe injuries. The duration of treatment and confinement also depend on the severity of the injury. Return to regular activity should be gradual. Arthrodesis may allow early return to weight bearing and maintenance of most function in low-motion joints (e.g., pastern).

Luxation

Luxations require immediate reduction, either manually (under anesthesia) or surgically. Support of the joint and stall rest are indicated after reduction. Arthrodesis may be necessary to stabilize a joint with severe ligament damage.

ARTHROGRYPOSIS *(Text pp. 1106-1107)*

Arthrogryposis is one of the most common congenital diseases in calves; foals, kids, and lambs are less commonly affected. Possible causes are categorized as infectious (e.g., Akabane, bluetongue, border disease, and Cache Valley viruses), genetic (breeds include Charolais cattle, Norwegian Fjord horses, and Merino and inbred sheep flocks), and toxic (e.g., Sudan grass in horses, lupine alkaloids in cattle and sheep).

Clinical Signs

Arthrogryposis causes varying degrees of rigid and irreducible flexural deformity of both carpi and forelimb fetlock joints and, less often, hyperextension of the tarsus and flexural deformity of the hind fetlocks. Other anatomic and neurologic defects, including hydranencephaly, scoliosis, and cleft palate, are often found.

Treatment

Passive stretching and flexing of the affected limbs and forced extension using bandages and splints or casts may be beneficial in mildly affected animals. Surgical techniques have been described (see main text).

OSTEOMYELITIS *(Text 1107-1110)*

Osteomyelitis is an infectious inflammatory disease of bone and its marrow cavity. It may be acute or chronic and involve the epiphyseal, metaphyseal, or diaphyseal regions of a bone.

Causal Organisms

Most cases of osteomyelitis in large animals are bacterial in origin. The most common aerobic isolates in horses are enterobacteria, streptococci, and staphylococci. *A. pyogenes* is the most common isolate in adult ruminants. Neonates are particularly susceptible to infection by *E. coli* and *Salmonella* spp. Most cases of osteomyelitis include a mixture of anaerobes or a combination of aerobes and anaerobes; *Bacteroides* spp. is the predominant anaerobe.

Clinical Findings

Acute infection

Animals with acute osteomyelitis usually exhibit localized inflammation and soft tissue swelling, may resent palpation of the affected area, and often have an obvious lameness. Fever, anorexia, and depression may be observed. Acute osteomyelitis is rare in adults and usually is associated with direct bacterial inoculation during trauma or open reduction of a fracture.

Neonates. Acute osteomyelitis is seen most often in neonates and is usually secondary, so signs related to the primary focus of infection (e.g., respiratory or gastrointestinal tract, umbilical remnant) may be present. Osteomyelitis in young animals is also commonly associated with septic arthritis (see p. 315).

Chronic infection

In adults, infection is usually localized and the result of direct trauma to the bone. Common clinical signs include firm swelling of the affected area, reluctance to bear weight on the limb, mild to moderate lameness, and the presence of a draining fistulous tract. Drainage may be constant or intermittent and is usually purulent. Fever and depression are usually not observed.

Diagnosis

Diagnosis is based on history, physical examination, and radiographic findings (see main text). Definitive diagnosis is made by culture of deep needle aspirates, sequestra, or necrotic tissue removed during surgical debridement. Culture of draining tracts is not recommended because tract organisms are not usually the pathogens responsible for the bone infection. Synovial fluid cytologic examination and culture and blood culture are also advisable in neonates. Culture for both aerobic and anaerobic bacterial pathogens is indicated in every case of osteomyelitis.

Clinical pathology

The WBC count is usually elevated in animals with acute osteomyelitis, and a degenerative left shift is often present. Initial leukopenia may be observed in neonates. The leukogram tends to return to normal with chronicity. Plasma fibrinogen may be elevated in acute infections.

Treatment

Treatment consists of broad-spectrum systemic antimicrobial therapy and surgical management. Selected early cases may respond to aggressive antimicrobial therapy alone, but once infection is established in the bone, it is difficult to resolve without surgical intervention. Duration of antibiotic therapy depends on the clinical response; 4 to 6 weeks of therapy is usually needed for chronic osteomyelitis.

Regional antibiotic therapy

Localized antibiotic therapy is a useful adjunct to systemic treatment. Methods include regional perfusion, local implantation of antibiotic-impregnated polymethylmethacrylate beads, and autogenous cancellous bone grafts (see main text).

NAVICULAR SYNDROME *(Text pp. 1110-1114)*

Navicular syndrome is a clinical diagnosis based on history, physical findings, and diagnostic regional anesthesia and imaging. Disorders encompassed by navicular syndrome include distal interphalangeal joint synovitis, deep digital flexor tendinitis, desmitis of the collateral or distal impar sesamoidean ligaments, navicular bursitis, and degenerative changes of the navicular bone.

Diagnosis

The most common sign is chronic forelimb lameness of insidious onset that in the early stages improves with exercise. As the condition progresses, lameness is exacerbated by exercise and improves with rest. The condition is generally bilateral, with most cases being asymmetric. The lameness usually can be accentuated by working the horse on a hard surface or on a circle. Over time the affected foot may become narrowed and more upright (contracted).

Manipulations

Application of hoof testers over the center of the frog often produces a pain response. Flexion of the distal limb may exacerbate lameness but is not specific. Elevation of the toe with a wedge-shaped block while holding the other limb off the ground may also accentuate the lameness.

Regional anesthesia

Regional anesthesia is useful for localizing the pain. Blocking the medial and lateral palmar digital nerves typically produces at least 80% improvement, with frequent enhancement of lameness in the contralateral limb, but complete resolution of the lameness usually does not occur. A logical approach is to perform the following blocks, in sequence: (1) palmar digital nerves, (2) distal interphalangeal joint, and (3) navicular bursa (if necessary).

Radiography

Radiography is important in confirming the diagnosis. A minimum of three projections are taken: lateromedial, dorsoproximal-palmarodistal oblique, and palmaroproximal-palmarodistal oblique (flexor, skyline, or caudal tangential) views. Radiographic features of diagnostic relevance are described and illustrated in *Large Animal Internal Medicine,* third edition. Nuclear scintigraphy is useful when radiographic findings do not support the clinical findings.

Treatment

Treatment is directed toward slowing further degeneration and providing pain relief. Initial management should begin with correcting any foot abnormalities, rest, and administration of NSAIDs for 7 to 14 days. Other therapies to consider if signs return with exercise include corrective shoeing, NSAIDs, corticosteroids, polysulfated glycosaminoglycans, isoxsuprine, and pentoxifylline (see main text). Surgery (navicular suspensory desmotomy or palmar digital neurectomy) can be considered with chronicity, marked radiographic changes, or lack of response to medical therapy.

SPONDYLITIS *(Text pp. 1114-1115)*

Spondylitis (vertebral osteomyelitis) is an infectious or inflammatory degenerative disease of one or more adjoining vertebrae. Discospondylitis is concurrent infection of the vertebral body and adjacent intervertebral disc. These are rare but life-threatening conditions. Vertebral osteomyelitis occurs most often in foals and calves; discospondylitis is more prevalent in the cervical or upper thoracic region of adult horses.

Clinical Signs and Diagnosis

An early sign of spondylitis is localized spinal pain, but diagnosis is usually not made until signs of meningitis or spinal cord compression occur (see Chapter 33). Diagnosis is confirmed by radiography, scintigraphy, computed tomography, or ultrasonography. Cytologic examination and culture of fine needle aspirate, blood, or feces are important for selecting appropriate antimicrobial therapy.

Treatment

Successful treatment depends on early diagnosis and appropriate antimicrobial therapy. Surgical curettage with lavage and drainage is recommended if possible. Long-term antibiotic therapy (2 to 6 months) is usually required to eliminate the infection; however, relapse is common.

SPONDYLOSIS *(Text pp. 1115-1116)*

Spondylosis is a degenerative disease of the intervertebral joints. It is most common in adult horses and Holstein bulls. Signs of pain or stiffness are usually elicited on palpation of the paraspinal tissues and spinous processes of the involved region. Neurologic signs may result from nerve root or spinal cord compression (see Chapter 33).

Diagnosis and Treatment

Enthesiophytes on the lumbar vertebral bodies may be palpated rectally and noted on radiography or scintigraphy. Systemic antiinflammatory medication (e.g., NSAIDs, corticosteroids, DMSO), ice packs, and confinement are recommended until the inflammation subsides or until ankylosis forms a stable, nonpainful joint.

LAMINITIS (FOUNDER) *(Text pp. 1116-1124)*

Laminitis is a disease that causes inflammation and degeneration of the dermal and epidermal laminae in the hoof wall of horses and ruminants.

Causes

Overconsumption of grain or other high-carbohydrate feeds (including lush grass) is the most common cause in horses. Other possible causes include digestive disturbances and other disorders that cause endotoxemia, administration of high levels of corticosteroids, severe unilateral lameness with excessive weight bearing in the supporting limb, and black walnut toxicity. In cattle, laminitis is most often seen after calving in fat heifers that have been fed excess concentrates and kept on concrete surfaces.

Clinical Findings

Acute laminitis

The signs of acute laminitis are lameness, depression, anorexia, and reluctance to move. Initially, affected animals often paddle or shift their weight from one foot to the other. Increased pulse strength can be palpated in the digital arteries. Hoof tester examination reveals sensitivity over the sole at the toe, and tapping on the dorsal hoof wall may elicit pain.

The forefeet are usually affected more often and more severely in horses. Horses with laminitis commonly stand with the hindlimbs drawn under the body and the forelimbs forward. In ruminants the hindlimbs are most commonly involved, and affected animals characteristically become recumbent.

Severe cases. When laminar degeneration circumferentially involves the foot, a depression can be palpated along the coronary band, indicating that the distal phalanx has shifted distally with respect to the hoof wall (i.e., severe rotation or sinking of the distal phalanx). In such cases the sole becomes flat or bulges between the toe and apex of the frog. Pulse and respiratory rates are usually increased; other clinical signs reflect the underlying disease process.

Chronic laminitis

Chronic laminitis causes lameness and abnormal foot conformation. The sole is flat or dropped, the white line is widened, and the hoof wall shows signs of uneven growth (e.g., irregular horizontal rings, more closely spaced at the toe). In ruminants the sole softens and assumes a light yellow discoloration. Hemorrhages can often be found in the abaxial white line region, and fissures parallel to the coronary band may be seen in the hoof wall.

Diagnosis

Radiographic examination of the affected digits should be performed in horses. Initial examination should include lateromedial and 65-degree dorsoproximal-palmarodistal projections. Lateromedial views are periodically repeated to check for disease progression. Radiographic signs of laminitis include ventral displacement of the extensor process with respect to the proximal hoof wall, increased distance between the dorsal cortex of the distal phalanx and the surface of the hoof wall, and ventral rotation of the tip of the distal phalanx.

Treatment

Acute laminitis should be considered an emergency. General principles of therapy are aimed at the following:

- Eliminating the cause–3 to 4 L of mineral oil via nasogastric tube for grain overload; removal of retained placenta; hyperimmune serum for endotoxemia
- Promoting digital circulation with acetylpromazine (0.02 to 0.04 mg/kg IM four times daily)
  - Heparin (40 to 100 U/kg SC two or three times daily) may be helpful before lameness develops.
- Reducing tension on the laminae–frog support, sole casts, bedding on sand, raising the heels, trimming the toe (see main text)
- Minimizing digital inflammation and pain
  - In horses, phenylbutazone is given once at up to 8.8 mg/kg intravenously [IV], then 4.4 mg/kg orally [PO] twice daily for several days; the dose is then tapered to 2.2 mg/kg PO twice daily.
  - Flunixin meglumine (1.1 mg/kg IV once per day) may be given concurrently for the first 3 to 4 days.
  - DMSO (0.2 to 1 g/kg IV, diluted to less than 20% solution) may also be given for 2 to 3 days.
  - Aspirin (10 mg/kg PO once per day) is sometimes used for its antiplatelet activities.

Determining the prognosis in horses is outlined in *Large Animal Internal Medicine,* third edition.

FLUOROSIS *(Text pp. 1124-1125)*

Chronic fluoride toxicosis, or fluorosis, occurs with ingestion of excessive fluoride. Cattle are susceptible to dental fluorosis between about 6 months and 3 years of age; the incisors are chalky and mottled. With osteofluorosis the first palpable lesions occur on the medial surface of the proximal metatarsal bones. Later, lesions can be palpated on the mandible, metacarpal bones, and ribs. The bony lesions eventually cause intermittent lameness and stiffness.

Diagnosis

Fluorosis may be suspected from the history, clinical signs, and radiographic findings, which include bone thickening with a roughened, irregular periosteal surface. Urine and bone fluoride concentrations can be useful (see main text). Dietary fluoride analysis is also helpful.

Treatment

There is no specific treatment. Animals removed from the offending diet or water may lose 50% of the fluoride from bone within 2 to 5 years; however, severe dental damage is irreversible.

HYPERTROPHIC OSTEOPATHY *(Text pp. 1125-1126)*

Hypertrophic osteopathy (HO; hypertrophic pulmonary osteopathy, Marie's disease) refers to the formation of irregular subperiosteal new bone on the distal diaphyses of the long bones (especially the metacarpal and metatarsal bones) or on the axial skeleton or facial bones. These changes are most often associated with intrathoracic disease.

Clinical Signs and Diagnosis

Initially the distal limbs are swollen and warm. There may be decreased range of motion and pain on manipulation of the affected joints, with a stiff gait and reluctance to move. If there is an associated pulmonary lesion, respiratory signs may also be present. Radiography reveals generalized soft tissue swelling and periostitis. Thorough evaluation for the presence of a primary pulmonary or intraabdominal lesion is warranted.

Treatment

There is no specific treatment. When HO is recognized early and the underlying primary disease process is treated appropriately, the periosteal reactions disappear.

FESCUE FOOT *(Text pp. 1126-1127)*

Fescue foot affects cattle grazing pastures that contain tall fescue infected with the endophytic fungus *Acremonium coenophialum*. It is characterized by lameness, particularly of the rear limbs, progressing to dry gangrene of the feet and lower legs. The condition usually occurs in the winter. Morbidity generally is low, although up to 30% of the herd may be affected.

Clinical Signs

Signs usually begin with hindlimb lameness. The feet and pasterns become cold and the coronary bands reddened and swollen. As the condition progresses, a sharp line of demarcation develops at the pastern or fetlock, distal to which the skin becomes dry and gangrenous and eventually sloughs. The tips of the ears and tail may also necrose. Affected animals eventually are unable to stand.

Treatment

Affected animals should be removed from the pasture as soon as possible. Antibiotic treatment is valuable in early cases; recovery can occur in 2 weeks. Once the extremities have necrosed, treatment is unsuccessful and euthanasia is recommended.

INTERDIGITAL NECROBACILLOSIS (FOOT ROT) IN CATTLE *(Text pp. 1127-1128)*

Interdigital necrobacillosis, or foot rot, is an infectious disease of cattle characterized by inflammation of the subcutaneous tissues in the interdigital space. It is caused by infection with *Fusobacterium necrophorum* and *Bacteroides melaninogenicus,* acting synergistically, after maceration and trauma to the foot.

Clinical Signs

There is usually a sudden onset of lameness in one or more limbs (most often the hindlimbs). The interdigital space is swollen and painful, and the toes may be spread apart. The coronet and heel bulbs become swollen, and the swelling may extend to the pastern and fetlock. The interdigital space is often necrotic and fissured, with a characteristic foul odor but little pus. In severe cases, fever, inappetence, reduced milk yield, and weight loss occur.

Complications and sequelae. Complications such as septic arthritis, tenosynovitis, or other deep infections of the foot may occur in severe cases. Interdigital hyperplasia and distortion of the horn are possible chronic sequelae.

Treatment

Systemic antimicrobials and local treatment of the interdigital area usually result in rapid healing (2 to 4 days). Suitable antimicrobials include sulfonamides (130 mg/kg IV), oxytetracycline (10 mg/kg IV), and procaine penicillin (20,000 to 40,000 IU/kg IM or SC twice daily). One treatment is often sufficient. Local wound cleaning, curettage of the necrotic tissue, and application of antiseptics or antimicrobials improve the rate of healing. Other methods of management and control are discussed in *Large Animal Internal Medicine,* third edition.

CONTAGIOUS FOOT ROT IN SHEEP *(Text pp. 1129-1130)*

Contagious foot rot in sheep is caused by *Bacteroides nodosus.* The disease occurs in all age groups and causes lameness in one or more feet. Initially, the interdigital skin becomes reddened and swollen. Slight undermining of the sole develops at the heels and progresses to involve the sole and wall. Infected feet have a characteristic foul odor. Some sheep spontaneously rid themselves of infection, some are resistant to infection, and others become chronic carriers.

Treatment

Treatment involves foot trimming, foot bathing, segregation, vaccination, and culling of chronically infected sheep. Systemic or topical antibiotics (tetracyclines or penicillin) may aid in treatment of valuable sheep.

SUBSOLAR ABSCESS *(Text pp. 1130-1131)*

Subsolar abscess is one of the most common causes of lameness in horses and cattle. Clinical signs include lameness, heat, and point-pressure pain. The entry site of contamination is not always apparent, even after careful cleaning and trimming of the foot. If signs point to an infection, additional trimming, hot water soaks, or the use of a poultice is necessary.

Treatment

The principal methods of treating infectious processes in the foot are adequate drainage, removal of separated sole or wall, local disinfection, protective covering, and tetanus prophylaxis. If the area of abscess is small, all that may be required is drainage, packing the area with povidone-iodine-soaked gauze for a few days, and applying a protective bandage. Abscesses that are more extensive must be treated more aggressively (see main text).

ASCENDING HOOF WALL INFECTION (GRAVEL) *(Text p. 1131)*

Gravel is ascending infection starting at the white line and breaking out just above the coronary band or bulbs of the heel. Acute lameness and signs of inflammation often precede rupture of the abscess above the coronary band by 1 to 2 days.

Treatment

In some instances the site of infection can be identified at the white line when the foot is trimmed. The abscess is then drained from the bottom of the foot, flushed with disinfectant, and treated like a solar abscess. If an ascending infection is suspected but cannot be identified, the foot should be soaked and a poultice applied for 2 to 4 days until the abscess appears or the inflammation subsides. In chronic cases in which there is large area of separation under the hoof wall, it may be necessary to remove a portion of the wall to provide adequate drainage and to debride the necrotic soft tissue.

OSTEOMYELITIS OF THE DISTAL PHALANX *(Text p. 1131)*

Infection of the distal phalanx may result from extension of any foot infection. The history is usually one of a long-standing foot lameness, possibly accompanied by episodes of drainage or abscesses that tend to recur. Careful and deep trimming of the foot may reveal a draining tract leading to the bone. Good-quality radiographs are important for detecting osteomyelitis and identifying sequestra. Treatment includes surgical drainage and careful curettage of the infected bone. Aftercare is discussed in *Large Animal Internal Medicine,* third edition.

PUNCTURE WOUNDS OF THE FOOT *(Text pp. 1131-1132)*

Puncture wounds of the foot are relatively common and are usually caused by nails. They are treated by pulling the nail and debriding the puncture wound to its full depth, making the hole large enough to maintain drainage during the healing process. If the nail has penetrated to the coffin bone, the bone should be curetted. Aftercare is the same as described for solar abscess.

Deep Puncture Wounds

In horses, nails that enter the frog have a tendency to be directed toward the navicular bursa. Extreme care must be taken to ensure that the puncture wound has been traced to the deepest point of penetration. If the lameness is not significantly improved 48 to 72 hours after drainage of the infected area, additional exploration is needed (see main text).

QUITTOR *(Text p. 1332)*

Quittor is chronic infection of the medial or lateral collateral cartilage of the distal phalanx in horses. Affected horses often present with lameness and a history of chronic or recurrent draining tracts proximal to the coronary band. The treatment of choice is surgical debridement.

FISTULOUS WITHERS *(Text pp. 1132-1133)*

Fistulous withers is an inflammatory condition of the supraspinous bursa in horses. Some cases are caused by infection with *Brucella abortus* or *Actinomyces bovis.* Contamination with environmental pathogens (e.g., *Streptococcus* spp., *E. coli)* is common once the bursa ruptures.

Clinical Signs

Onset may be abrupt or insidious. Initially the most common signs are pain, heat, and swelling overlying the dorsal spinous processes of T2 to T5. Lethargy, fever, and stiffness may also be present. After several days or weeks the bursa ruptures, discharging serous or purulent fluid through a cutaneous fistula. Apparent healing followed by recurrence is common if untreated.

Diagnosis

Percutaneous aspiration and culture of bursal fluid is useful before the bursa ruptures; later, bacterial contaminants may interfere with isolation of the primary organism. In all cases a serum agglutination titer for *Brucella* spp. should be performed (see main text). Radiography of the dorsal processes of the thoracic vertebrae is also recommended.

Treatment

In unfistulated, non-*Brucella* cases, use of appropriate antimicrobial and antiinflammatory agents is recommended. Fistulated bursae may be treated by flushing the open tract with diluted Betadine solution or mild oxidizing agents in conjunction with parenteral antimicrobial treatment. Refractory cases may require surgical excision and drainage. In *Brucella*-confirmed cases a treatment regimen using a killed *Brucella* vaccine is suggested (see main text).

FLEXURAL LIMB DEFORMITIES (CONTRACTED TENDONS) *(Text pp. 1133-1136)*

Flexural limb deformities are common in young horses and calves. The deformity may be congenital or acquired and may affect the carpal, metacarpophalangeal, or distal interphalangeal joints. Carpal and distal limb flexural contractures in neonatal foals may be associated with rupture of the common digital extensor tendon over the carpus.

Congenital Flexural Deformities

Fetlock

Many foals and calves are born with mild tendon contracture, causing fetlock flexion that resolves spontaneously in the first few hours of life. In mild to moderate cases, manual stretching and splinting are often successful (see main text). More severe flexural deformities that can be manually straightened can be cast for 10 to 14 days. Unresponsive cases in foals can be treated with distal check desmotomy and a full-limb cast. A single dose of oxytetracycline (3 g in 250 ml saline IV) has also been used to treat severe flexural deformities in foals.

Carpus

Flexural deformities of the carpus range from very mild (bucked knees) to very severe. If the limb cannot be straightened manually, the deformity probably involves the joint capsule and intercarpal ligaments rather than or in addition to the musculotendinous unit. Radiographic evaluation of the carpus is recommended to determine whether osseous abnormalities are present.

Treatment. Splinting can be helpful in mild cases. Transection of the palmar aspect of the joint capsule is a salvage option in severely affected foals. If rupture of the common digital extensor tendon has occurred, splints or casts should be applied for 10 to 14 days. Casts for carpal contracture should end just proximal to the fetlock to prevent excessive distal limb laxity.

Acquired Flexural Deformities

Distal interphalangeal joint

Acquired deformity of the distal interphalangeal joint occurs in foals and weanling horses and is characterized by flexion of the joint. The primary structure involved is the deep digital flexor (DDF) unit. The heel is elevated, and a boxy ("club") foot develops; if the distal phalanx is pulled palmarly, the hoof develops a dished appearance. Genetic predisposition to rapid growth, faulty nutrition (mineral imbalance or excessive feeding), pain from other skeletal disorders, and lack of exercise have all been implicated.

Treatment. Initial therapy in mild cases should include dietary management (e.g., reducing caloric intake, balancing mineral intake, weaning) and corrective trimming (e.g., lowering the heels and possibly shoeing to elevate the toe). Glue-on shoes or hoof acrylic may be used to extend the toe, causing stretching of the contracted structures. NSAIDs may be helpful if pain is an underlying cause. Repeated assessment should be made. If substantial improvement is not seen in 3 to 4 weeks, surgical intervention (distal check desmotomy) is advised.

Metacarpophalangeal joint

Deformity of the metacarpophalangeal joint occurs in older growing animals (8 to 18 months of age). Most affected horses are on an elevated plane of nutrition and are growing rapidly. In young ruminants it occurs secondary to limb disuse associated with recumbency. The fetlock at first appears upright and then begins to dorsally subluxate. The predominant structure involved is the superficial digital flexor unit; some cases also involve the DDF unit and the suspensory ligament.

Treatment. Mild cases may be treated with corrective shoeing (raising the heel), bandaging or splinting, balancing and reducing the diet, NSAID therapy, and increasing exercise. If there is insufficient improvement in 3 to 4 weeks, surgery (proximal and possibly distal check desmotomy) is indicated. In ruminants it is often necessary to sever the flexor tendons.

TENDINITIS (BOWED TENDON) *(Text pp. 1137-1138)*

The superficial digital flexor (SDF) tendon is the most commonly injured tendon in horses, with the middle metacarpal region of the forelimb the most common site of injury. Tendinitis in the deep digital flexor tendon (uncommon) usually occurs in the pastern region. Extensor tendon injuries are seen most frequently just distal to the carpus or tarsus. In cattle, rupture of the gastrocnemius (Achilles) tendon/muscle is the most common tendon injury.

Clinical Signs

Tendinitis causes lameness either immediately after severe tendon disruption or within 48 hours in less severe cases. In mild to moderate cases the lameness resolves with 3 to 5 days of rest but recurs when the horse is returned to work. Pain, heat, and swelling are present in the affected region of the tendon.

SDF tendinitis at the level of the palmar annular ligament may be complicated by compression of the swollen tendon, which results in a characteristic notching where the ligament is compressing the swollen tendon. Tendinitis occurring within the digital sheath is often accompanied by inflammation and effusion of the sheath and pain on fetlock flexion.

Diagnosis

Careful palpation of the affected tendon often reveals localized pain and swelling, even in the absence of lameness. Because tendinitis often results in subtle clinical signs, any change should be viewed with suspicion. Definitive diagnosis is made using ultrasonography (see main text).

Treatment

Treatment for mild to moderate tendon damage includes NSAID use, local cold application, and stall rest with gradually increasing hand walking. Systemic polysulfated glycosaminoglycan (500 mg administered at 4-day intervals for a total of seven doses) may be of value in treatment of acute tendinitis. For severe cases in which sufficient tendon damage has occurred to permit partial dropping of the fetlock, a support shoe that extends caudally can be helpful (see main text).

Surgical options

Surgical options include decompression of core lesions through stab incisions (tendon splitting; most useful within 21 days of injury), transection of the palmar annular ligament (for distal SDF lesions), and transection of the accessory ligament of the SDF (superior check desmotomy).

Rehabilitation

Stall rest with hand walking should be continued for 60 days. If, at that time, ultrasonographic examination reveals a reduction in tendon size, partial resolution of core lesions, and an improvement in fiber pattern, exercise can be gradually increased. Ultrasonographic examinations at 60-day intervals allows the amount of exercise to be tailored to tendon healing. Pasture turnout is contraindicated until a substantial amount of healing has occurred and tendon strength is judged to be nearly normal.

SUSPENSORY DESMITIS *(Text pp. 1138-1139)*

Desmitis involving the suspensory ligament (SL) is predominantly an injury of athletic horses. The branches are injured more often than the body or origin of the ligament.

Clinical Signs

Mild to moderate suspensory desmitis causes lameness (average grade II/V) that often persists for months if the horse is continued in work or repeatedly returned to work. SL branch lesions cause readily detectable swelling, heat, and pain on palpation. Lesions in the body or origin of the SL are more difficult to diagnose. Deep palpation for 1 to 2 minutes, followed by observation of the horse in motion, is a useful stress test. Severe suspensory desmitis results in extensive swelling in the metacarpal region, grade IV-V/V lameness, and dropping (hyperextension) of the fetlock.

Concurrent lesions

Of horses with suspensory desmitis, 25% also have apical fractures of the proximal sesamoid bones, avulsion fractures at the proximal palmar aspect of the third metacarpal bone (MCIII), or fractures of the distal third of the small metacarpal (splint) bones. Evidence of these abnormalities may be found on careful palpation.

Diagnosis

Infiltration of local anesthetic directly around the suspensory origin or blocking of the ulnar or tibial nerve may be required to localize the lameness to the proximal suspensory region. Ultrasonography is the most useful tool for diagnosing suspensory desmitis; it can also reveal fractures of the sesamoid or splint bones and proximal palmar avulsion fractures of MCIII. These bony lesions can be confirmed radiographically.

Treatment

Therapy should begin with 3 weeks of NSAIDs, cold therapy, and stall rest with hand walking. If an acute (less than 14 days) core lesion is detected ultrasonographically, decompression of the hematoma by percutaneous ligament splitting is indicated. Rehabilitation is tailored to ligament healing, monitored by ultrasound. Surgery is indicated for apical sesamoid fractures and for some splint bone fractures. Proximal palmar avulsion fractures are treated conservatively.

FRACTURES *(Text pp. 1139-1144)*

Fracture should be considered a differential diagnosis for any patient with a non-weight-bearing lameness. Complete displaced fractures in the proximal limb and incomplete fractures may not be immediately obvious, so thorough evaluation is needed. Horses having a history of trauma to a long bone, such as being kicked by another horse, require radiographs of the bone to determine the presence of an incomplete fracture. Undiagnosed incomplete fractures in such cases often become complete displaced fractures if the animal is allowed unrestricted exercise.

Emergency Treatment

Treatment options for particular fracture types in specific locations are discussed in *Large Animal Internal Medicine,* third edition. Following is an outline of emergency management for complete fractures.

Treatment principles

If the fracture and soft tissues are deemed amenable to repair, emergency treatment is important for a successful outcome. Treatment for shock should be instituted if necessary. When open fractures are being dealt with, broad-spectrum antibiotics and analgesics should be given and local debridement of the wound performed if the animal is tractable. Immobilization is essential.

Shoulder region/femur

Fractures of the scapula, humerus, elbow, or femur do not require splinting. If the triceps apparatus is disabled, a splint that supports the carpus in an extended position should be applied.

Radius/tibia

Fractures of the middle or proximal radius or tibia should be stabilized with a Robert-Jones bandage and a lateral splint that extends from the ground to the withers/hip. A caudal splint should also be applied for radial fractures.

Carpal/tarsal region

Fractures between the distal radius and the distal metacarpus are best immobilized with a Robert-Jones bandage and external splints that extend from the elbow to the hoof. Two splints, placed caudal and lateral, provide adequate support. Fractures of the middle or proximal metatarsus should be splinted with lateral and plantar splints over a light Robert-Jones bandage. The splints should reach the level of the calcaneal tuber.

Distal limb

Splinting of the distal metacarpus/metatarsus and phalanges can consist of a light wrap, splint, and cast material. A splint along the dorsal (metacarpus) or plantar (metatarsus) aspect of the limb should align the bones axially, neutralizing the bending forces at the fracture and at the fetlock joint. In young animals a heavy wrap and splint may be applied without cast material.

SPONTANEOUS FRACTURES IN RUMINANTS *(Text pp. 1144-1145)*

Spontaneous fracture of bone is a syndrome that occurs when underlying bone disease weakens bones to the point where otherwise normally applied stresses result in bone failure. Causes in ruminants include (1) tumors affecting individual bones, (2) osteomyelitis, (3) rickets (osteodystrophy) in young ruminants, (4) osteomalacia in adult ruminants, and (5) osteoporosis associated with copper deficiency (see Chapter 30).

BUCKED SHINS AND METACARPAL STRESS FRACTURES IN HORSES *(Text pp. 1145-1148)*

Bucked shins and stress fractures are acute and chronic manifestations of disease of the dorsal cortex of the MCIII in young racehorses.

Bucked Shins

Bucked shins is a painful condition most commonly involving the mid-diaphyseal dorsal cortex of MCIII in horses in their first year of race training.

Clinical and radiographic findings

Bucked shins usually occurs bilaterally. In most horses the first indication is pain on palpation of MCIII, often before lameness or reluctance to perform fast work is reported. Initially the pain is mild and diffuse. With continued training, soft tissue thickening is palpable and diffuse swelling becomes visible on the dorsum of MCIII. Later, discrete, hard swellings can be palpated. Radiographic abnormalities, which often are absent in acute cases, include indistinct periosteal proliferation and subperiosteal demineralization or lucencies.

Treatment

In mildly and moderately affected horses, the pain subsides with 2 to 4 days of rest. Training should be continued, but at a slower pace to promote adaptation of the bone to racing stresses. Severely affected horses, in which the pain persists after 1 week of rest, often require complete rest for a minimum of 3 months.

Stress Fractures

Stress fractures are incomplete fractures located in the mid-diaphyseal dorsal cortex or, less commonly, in the distal diaphyseal dorsal or dorsolateral cortex of MCIII. They are seen most commonly in 3-year-old horses and occur more frequently in the left than the right metacarpus.

Clinical and radiographic findings

Horses with incomplete cortical fractures are more likely than horses with bucked shins to be lame. The lameness, which may be marked after activity, usually subsides within a few days. With chronicity, a discrete, firm swelling is visible and palpable overlying the fracture and focal pain can usually be elicited by digital palpation. Incomplete cortical fractures can often be detected radiographically or scintigraphically.

Treatment

Horses with incomplete cortical fractures must be rested for 3 to 6 months. Some chronic fractures are refractory to rest alone and require interfragmentary drilling (see main text).

37

Diseases of the Eye

Consulting Editor CECIL P. MOORE

Contributors ERIN CHAMPAGNE • DAVID J. MAGGS • R. DAVID WHITLEY
KRISTINA R. VYGANTAS • JOAN DZIEZYC • NICHOLAS J. MILLICHAMP
MARY BELLE GLAZE • ROBERT V. ENGLISH • MARK P. NASISSE
STEVEN M. ROBERTS

OPHTHALMOLOGIC EXAMINATION *(Text pp. 1149-1157)*

Thorough ophthalmologic examination is essential when evaluating a patient with ocular disease. Examination and ancillary diagnostic procedures are described in *Large Animal Internal Medicine,* third edition.

Nerve Blocks

Examination, sample collection, and certain treatments can be facilitated by blocking the auriculopalpebral and supraorbital (frontal) nerves:

- The auriculopalpebral nerve is blocked over the zygomatic arch to paralyze the orbicularis oculi muscle and allow eyelid manipulation.
- The supraorbital (frontal) nerve is blocked at its exit from the supraorbital process to anesthetize the upper eyelid.
  - A 25-gauge needle is inserted into the supraorbital foramen and 5 ml of lidocaine is injected alongside the nerve.

SIGNS OF OCULAR DISEASE *(Text pp. 1157-1159)*

The five major signs of ocular disease are (1) ocular or periocular asymmetry, (2) ocular color change, (3) ocular discharge, (4) ocular pain, and (5) visual deficits or blindness.

Ocular or Periocular Asymmetry

Asymmetry results from the presence of an ocular surface mass or unilateral changes in anatomy of the orbit, orbital contents, globe, eyelids, or pupils. Specific abnormalities include the following:

- Ocular or periocular mass–squamous cell carcinoma, sarcoid (horses), other neoplasms, parasitic or foreign body granuloma
- Exophthalmos–space-occupying orbital lesion
- Enophthalmos–globe retraction from ocular pain or loss of retrobulbar tissue
- Phthisis bulbi (shrinking of the globe)–chronic uveitis
- Megaloglobus/buphthalmos (stretching of the globe)–glaucoma
- Eyelid abnormalities–entropion, ectropion, blepharitis, conjunctivitis, facial nerve paralysis
- Third eyelid protrusion–retraction of the globe from ocular pain, third eyelid mass, orbital disease, neurologic disorders (e.g., Horner's syndrome, tetanus)
- Congenital abnormalities–congenital strabismus in Jersey, Shorthorn, and Holstein cattle; microphthalmia in cattle and horses

- Anisocoria (pupil asymmetry)–Horner's syndrome, unilateral intraocular disease (e.g., uveitis, glaucoma, retinal lesions), diseases involving the optic nerve or brainstem, and certain drugs (e.g., atropine)

Ocular Color Change

Change in color of the ocular or periocular tissues or the presence of opacities in the cornea, aqueous humor, lens, or vitreous are important features of ocular disease. Color changes must be differentiated from normal congenital differences in ocular pigmentation. Examples of abnormal coloration include the following:

- Hyperemia of conjunctival (surface) or episcleral (deep) blood vessels associated with ocular inflammation–causes are listed in the following section; see Red eyes
- Hemorrhage secondary to trauma or coagulopathies
- Pallor of the conjunctiva–indicates severe anemia
- Yellowing of the sclera and sometimes the iris–indicates icterus

Red eyes

Causes of ocular inflammation include the following:

- Noninfectious conjunctivitis/keratitis–entropion, foreign body, chemical irritation
- Infectious conjunctivitis/keratitis–most likely organisms vary with the animal species
    - *Moraxella,* bovine herpesvirus (infectious bovine rhinotracheitis [IBR]), and bovine viral diarrhea (BVD) virus in cattle
    - *Mycoplasma, Branhamella, Chlamydia* (sheep), and IBR (goats) in small ruminants
    - *Pseudomonas, Streptococcus,* and coliforms in horses
- Uveitis–septicemia, trauma, *Mycoplasma* infection (goats), malignant catarrhal fever (cattle), equine recurrent uveitis (ERU; horses)
- Glaucoma–trauma, *Moraxella* infection, ERU

Hyperemic ocular masses include granulation tissue, healing corneal ulcer, ocular squamous cell carcinoma, and hemangiosarcoma.

Opacity

Causes of ocular opacity vary with the structure involved:

- Cornea–pigmentation (melanosis) secondary to chronic exposure; grayish scars from previous ulcerative keratitis; neovascularization secondary to chronic inflammation; bluish discoloration of corneal edema (keratitis, trauma, ulceration, uveitis, glaucoma)
    - Specific causes of keratitis, uveitis, and glaucoma are listed under Red Eyes.
- Anterior chamber–trauma, uveitis, glaucoma, anterior lens luxation, *Mycoplasma* infection (goats), septicemia, ERU
- Lens–trauma, congenital cataracts, uveitis
- Vitreous–trauma, uveitis, congenital vascular remnants (cattle), ERU, posterior lens luxation, retinal detachment

Ocular Discharge

Ocular discharges are characterized as serous (watery), mucoid (catarrhal), mucopurulent, or hemorrhagic. The type of discharge often indicates the cause:

- Watery (serous)–painful eye, nasolacrimal system blockage or atresia
    - Painful causes include entropion, ectopic or misdirected cilia, foreign body, uveitis, trauma, chemical irritation, and conjunctivitis/keratitis.
- Thick (mucoid or mucopurulent)–foreign body, surface tumors, infectious keratoconjunctivitis, chronic inflammation or blockage of the nasolacrimal duct, secondary bacterial infection, inadequate secretion of tears (keratoconjunctivitis sicca)
- Hemorrhagic–trauma, foreign body, ulcerative conjunctivitis, tumor

Ocular Pain

Blepharospasm, epiphora, photophobia, and periocular hyperesthesia are signs of ocular pain. Specific causes include the following:

- Blunt or penetrating trauma
- Corneal ulceration (often secondary to ocular trauma)
- Uveitis–infectious keratoconjunctivitis, ERU
- Corneal irritation–entropion, trichiasis, distichia, ectopic cilia, foreign material, exposure keratitis

Visual Deficits or Blindness

A functional approach to blindness involves anatomically classifying the cause as follows:

- Obstruction of the ocular media–corneal opacity (see p. 332), hyphema, hypopyon, vitreal exudation or hemorrhage
- Retinopathy–retinal dysplasia, detachment, or degeneration; retinitis/chorioretinitis; microphthalmia; phthisis bulbi; glaucoma
- Central nervous system lesion–optic nerve hypoplasia, optic neuritis, meningitis/encephalitis, trauma, neoplasia, vitamin A deficiency

Assessment of pupillary light reflexes (PLR) assists with localization of the lesion. Animals with lesions involving the retina, optic nerves, optic chiasm, or optic tracts generally do not have a PLR. Patients with more central lesions are likely to exhibit normal PLRs.

OCULAR TRAUMA *(Text pp. 1159-1164)*

Trauma to the Orbit

Orbital injuries in domestic animals frequently include fractures of the orbital rim and zygomatic arch and damage to the supraorbital process of the frontal bone. Fractures of the orbit may be identified by palpation and radiography.

Orbital fractures

Treatment involves antiinflammatory therapy (e.g., ice packs, nonsteroidal antiinflammatory drugs [NSAIDs]) and, if sinus involvement is suspected, systemic antibiotics. If the bone fragments are only minimally displaced, surgical intervention may not be required. If eyelid movement is impaired but the globe is only minimally exposed, a sterile ophthalmic lubricant may be used three or four times daily. In more severe cases, a third eyelid flap or temporary tarsorrhaphy may be required.

Orbital cellulitis or retrobulbar abscess

Orbital cellulitis and exophthalmos may result from traumatic puncture wounds of the eyelids and conjunctiva. Onset of swelling may be sudden; pyrexia, inappetence, and leukocytosis may also be present. Therapy should consist of systemic and topical antibiotics and ophthalmic lubricants to protect the exposed cornea and conjunctiva. The wound or abscess should be debrided or drained to facilitate healing.

Traumatic proptosis

Traumatic proptosis has a guarded to poor prognosis for return of vision. If the globe is ruptured or the extraocular muscles avulsed, the eye should be enucleated. If the extent of the damage cannot be evaluated initially, the globe should be repositioned, a temporary tarsorrhaphy performed, and the globe reevaluated after 7 to 10 days of therapy (topical broad-spectrum antibiotics and atropine).

Trauma to the Eyelids and Conjunctiva

Blepharoedema (simple swelling) usually resolves without therapy, as does chemosis and conjunctival hemorrhage. Recovery may be hastened by use of ice packs and systemic NSAIDs or corticosteroids. If chemosis is severe enough to cause exposure and drying of tissues, topical sterile ophthalmic lubricants or antibiotic ointments are indicated. NOTE: Careful ocular examination should be part of the evaluation of animals with eyelid trauma.

Lacerations

Eyelid lacerations should be promptly repaired to avoid lid distortion with scarring. It is essential to preserve the eyelid margin, so eyelid lacerations should be repaired with minimal debridement; lacerated or displaced tissue should not be excised. In cases of avulsion of part or all of the eyelid, blepharoplastic procedures may be performed to restore functional eyelid margin. Conjunctival lacerations rarely require closure unless they are extensive.

Postoperative care. Tetanus prophylaxis, standard wound hygiene, application of fly repellent and topical ophthalmic antibiotics, and prevention of self-trauma are important. In contaminated wounds, systemic antibiotic therapy is indicated for 5 to 7 days.

Trauma to the Third Eyelid

Lacerations involving the third eyelid should be repaired whenever possible. The margin should be realigned as precisely as possible and the lacerated conjunctiva repaired with absorbable suture material. Topical ophthalmic antibiotics should be used three times a day for 7 to 10 days.

Trauma to the Cornea

Blunt trauma

Blunt trauma to the globe can result in corneal edema (focal, linear, or diffuse). Signs of traumatic uveitis may accompany such an injury. Therapy includes topical application of a hypertonic saline solution or ointment two to four times a day.

Corneal foreign bodies

Most corneal foreign bodies are easily removed with a moistened cotton-tipped applicator or ophthalmic forceps. Sedation, nerve blocks, and topical anesthesia facilitate removal. Samples for culture and sensitivity tests and cytologic examination should be collected and the cornea stained with fluorescein before therapy is initiated. Therapy should include a topical ophthalmic antibiotic (e.g., gentamicin three or four times daily) and atropine (twice daily or as needed).

Corneal lacerations

Nonperforating corneal lacerations are frequently treated as corneal ulcers (see following discussion). Perforating corneal lacerations are repaired surgically. Preoperative preparation includes tetanus prophylaxis (horses and goats), systemic antibiotics, and sample collection for culture and sensitivity. Enucleation should be considered with severe corneoscleral lacerations.

Corneal Ulceration

Treatment of corneal ulceration should be guided by the results of ophthalmic examination, cytologic examination, culture and sensitivity testing of corneal samples, and fluorescein staining. (NOTE: Cultures must be obtained before application of topical anesthetics.)

Medical therapy

Treatment involves removal of the cause (if still present), topical antimicrobials, topical atropine, and, in horses, systemic NSAIDs. Initially, the ulcer may be cleaned with povidone-iodine solution, diluted 50:50 with sterile saline, or collyrium. Subpalpebral lavage systems greatly facilitate delivery of topical medication to the equine eye (see main text).

Antimicrobials. The initial choice of antibiotic should be based on cytologic results. Oxytetracycline combined with polymyxin B may be comparable in efficacy to gentamicin and superior to chloramphenicol. If fungal hyphae are found, therapy with a topical antifungal agent (natamycin, miconazole, itraconazole, ketoconazole) should be instituted immediately.

Surgical therapy

Surgery should be considered in cases of deep corneal ulceration and exposure of Descemet's membrane. Options include conjunctival pedicle flap, keratoplasty, and tarsorrhaphy. Ophthalmic tissue adhesives and soft contact lenses are nonsurgical options for deep corneal ulcers.

Trauma to the Uveal Tract

Signs of inflammation of the iris and ciliary body include ocular pain, miosis, aqueous flare, corneal edema, fibrin in the anterior chamber, hyphema, hypopyon, low intraocular pressure, and synechia formation.

Treatment

Therapy includes the following:

- Topical atropine
- Topical corticosteroids (1% prednisolone acetate or 0.1% dexamethasone) or prostaglandin inhibitors (e.g., 0.03% flurbiprofen [Ocufen])
  - Subconjunctival injection of corticosteroids may also be beneficial.
  - Topical and subconjunctival corticosteroids should be avoided if corneal ulceration or abrasion is present.
- Systemic antiinflammatory medication (NSAIDs or corticosteroids) as needed
- Topical and systemic antibiotic therapy if a penetrating wound is suspected

Hyphema

Stall rest, topical 1% atropine, topical corticosteroids, and systemic antiinflammatory therapy should be instituted. If a penetrating wound is suspected, topical and systemic antibiotic therapy should be included, along with periodic fluorescein staining. Lavage of the anterior chamber with urokinase may be beneficial in horses with total hyphema of more than 24 hours' duration. Diluted tissue plasminogen activator may be injected to dissolve fibrin in the anterior chamber.

Trauma to the Lens

Trauma to the eye may damage the lens and cause lens opacity (cataract), rupture of the lens capsule, or subluxation or luxation. Cataracts may occur acutely or develop weeks after injury. If the remainder of the eye is normal, surgical removal of the lens may improve vision. A luxated lens should be removed if it causes obstructive glaucoma or chronic corneal edema or if it becomes cataractous and reduces vision.

Rupture of the lens capsule

Release of lens proteins after capsule rupture can induce severe granulomatous uveitis. In such cases the eye should be vigorously treated with topical atropine and topical and systemic antiinflammatory drugs. If the globe has been penetrated, topical and systemic antibiotics are indicated. Lens removal is often required.

Trauma Involving the Vitreous

Trauma to the eye may result in hemorrhage into the vitreous or release of inflammatory products that cause vitreal degeneration. Antiinflammatory therapy generally is adequate. Vitrectomy may be beneficial in the management of severe vitreal hemorrhage.

Endophthalmitis

If infectious endophthalmitis is suspected, diagnostic paracentesis of the vitreous or anterior chamber should be performed to obtain samples for cytologic examination and culture and sensitivity. After the samples are obtained, but before removing the needle, gentamicin (400 μg) or cefazolin (2.2 mg) may be injected into the vitreous. Further therapy should be based on culture and sensitivity results and cytologic findings.

Trauma to the Retina

Retinal tears, hemorrhage, edema, and detachment may be caused by trauma. Retinal hemorrhage and edema may respond to systemic and topical corticosteroids.

Trauma to the Optic Nerve

Optic nerve trauma may occur when a horse rears up and strikes its poll. Early examination may reveal only a dilated pupil that may be partially responsive or completely unresponsive to light. Later changes may include optic nerve atrophy and peripapillary retinal pigment changes. Systemic antiinflammatory drugs may be of benefit, but severe damage is often irreversible.

Chemical Injury

Treatment for chemical injury should include lavage with copious amounts of sterile saline. No attempt to neutralize the substance should be made. Subsequent treatment includes topical antimicrobials, atropine, and acetylcysteine (hourly at first) and systemic antiinflammatory drugs. Soft contact lenses can be used to protect the corneal stroma in cases with extensive corneal ulceration.

Thermal Injury

Minor burns to the eyelids should be managed by keeping the injured area moist with antibiotic dressings and protecting the cornea if eyelid dysfunction is present. Injury to the conjunctiva or cornea should be treated with topical antibiotics and systemic antiinflammatory drugs. Full-thickness eyelid burns may require immediate grafting to protect the cornea and minimize scarring. Third eyelid or conjunctival flaps may be required to protect the cornea until eyelid function returns.

INFECTIOUS OCULAR DISEASES IN RUMINANTS
(Text pp. 1164-1173)

Mycoplasmal Keratoconjunctivitis in Goats and Sheep

Several *Mycoplasma* species can cause isolated cases or outbreaks of keratoconjunctivitis in small ruminants. Evidence of other organ involvement may also be seen, such as mastitis and polyarthritis with *Mycoplasma mycoides* subsp. *mycoides* infection in goats and respiratory signs with *Mycoplasma conjunctivae* infection in sheep and goats.

Clinical signs and diagnosis

Ocular signs include lacrimation, conjunctival hyperemia, and occasionally follicular conjunctivitis. Keratitis with neovascularization, and occasionally anterior uveitis, is seen later. Signs are usually unilateral but can be bilateral. *Mycoplasma* spp. can be cultured from conjunctival swabs. Conjunctival scrapings taken early in the disease contain many neutrophils; later, lymphocytes predominate. The organisms are occasionally seen in epithelial cells.

Treatment

Mycoplasmal keratoconjunctivitis is usually transient, with spontaneous recovery occurring in 10 days; some animals have recurring episodes for several weeks. Animals may be treated with topical oxytetracycline or long-acting systemic oxytetracycline.

Chlamydial Keratoconjunctivitis in Sheep

Chlamydia psittaci can cause outbreaks of keratoconjunctivitis in sheep. Early clinical signs include epiphora, chemosis, and conjunctival hyperemia, usually involving both eyes. Later conjunctival follicle formation becomes prominent. Corneal neovascularization may be seen subsequently. In some flocks, outbreaks of polyarthritis also occur; most lambs that develop chlamydial polyarthritis also develop conjunctivitis.

Diagnosis

Early in the disease, conjunctival smears show numerous neutrophils and some lymphocytes; later there are more neutrophils and fewer mononuclear cells. Cytoplasmic chlamydial inclusions are seen in up to 30% of cases. *Chlamydia* spp. can be cultured from conjunctival scrapings and from blood taken from sheep with polyarthritis and conjunctivitis.

Treatment

In uncomplicated cases the disease is self-limiting and eyes return to normal in 2 to 3 weeks. Systemic oxytetracycline and topical tetracycline ophthalmic preparations are effective.

Infectious Bovine Keratoconjunctivitis (Pinkeye)

Infectious bovine keratoconjunctivitis (IBK) is a contagious ocular disease of cattle. It is caused by the gram-negative coccobacillus *Moraxella bovis.*

Clinical signs

The earliest signs are excessive lacrimation, blepharospasm, and photophobia. Conjunctival injection and chemosis quickly develop, followed by keratitis. Initially, an area of corneal opacity and superficial ulceration is seen. The ulcer becomes wider and deeper over the next few days, and signs of anterior uveitis may develop. The ocular discharge becomes mucopurulent.

Clinical course. Circumlimbal corneal vascularization begins to invade the cornea 4 to 7 days after ulceration is first seen. Within 2 to 3 weeks of onset, the cornea is often reepithelialized. After the cornea heals, a faint corneal scar may be detected.

Severe disease. IBK is often severe in younger cattle, with deepening of the corneal ulcer sometimes resulting in corneal perforation. Anterior uveitis with hypopyon is marked.

Diagnosis

Although diagnosis is usually based on clinical signs, affected eyes can be cultured for antibiotic sensitivity testing. *M. bovis* is most readily recovered during the acute stage of the disease.

Treatment

M. bovis is sensitive to a wide range of antibiotics, so most products are effective if administered promptly and frequently. Less labor-intensive options include the following:

- Topical benzathine cloxacillin (375 mg suspended in mineral oil to a final volume of 1 ml) applied twice, 72 hours apart
- Bulbar subconjunctival injection of procaine penicillin G (300,000 U) applied twice, 48 to 72 hours apart
- Long-acting oxytetracycline (20 mg/kg intramuscularly [IM] every 48 hours) until clinical improvement is seen
- Long-acting oxytetracycline (20 mg/kg IM) once, followed by feeding of alfalfa pellets containing oxytetracycline (see main text)
- Florfenicol (40 mg/kg subcutaneously or IM once or followed in 2 days by 20 mg/kg IM)

Secondary uveitis can be treated with 1% atropine applied topically with the antibiotic. Corticosteroids should not be used during the acute ulcerative phase and are of doubtful value in the healing stages. Prevention and control are discussed in *Large Animal Internal Medicine,* third edition.

Infectious Bovine Rhinotracheitis Conjunctivitis

Conjunctivitis is the most common ocular manifestation of IBR. It may occur as an isolated clinical entity or with involvement of other body systems (e.g., respiratory tract).

Clinical signs

The conjunctivitis is frequently bilateral, but it can be unilateral. Excessive lacrimation, initially serous and later mucopurulent, is usually seen without blepharospasm. Chemosis may become severe. The conjunctivae are injected, and petechial hemorrhages may be seen.

Clinical course. Multiple small, white plaques may develop on the conjunctival surfaces 1 to 2 weeks after onset and may later coalesce. During recovery, diphtheritic membranes develop on the conjunctival surfaces secondary to conjunctival necrosis. Perilimbal edema, opacity, and vascularization occur in severe cases; iridocyclitis (miosis) may also occur in severe cases.

Diagnosis

Corneal changes with IBR are differentiated from those of IBK by their peripheral rather than central distribution and the lack of corneal ulceration. The virus can be recovered from infected eyes during the first 7 to 9 days of disease. Serologic examination may be helpful if blood samples can be collected during the acute and convalescent stages. Polymerase chain reaction is also being used.

Treatment

Recovery from conjunctivitis occurs spontaneously within 10 to 20 days. Palliative treatment may be indicated in some cases.

Malignant Catarrhal Fever Keratoconjunctivitis

Ocular involvement is seen in the acute "head and eye" form of malignant catarrhal fever (MCF), the most common presentation of the disease (see Chapter 30). Ocular signs include photophobia, excessive lacrimation, episcleral injection and scleritis, severe conjunctivitis, perilimbal keratitis (corneal edema and vascularization), and anterior uveitis.

Diagnosis and treatment

The absence of central corneal ulceration distinguishes this disease from IBK, and the severity of the ocular lesions is greater than would be expected with IBR. No specific diagnostic tests or treatments are available for MCF. Prognosis for recovery is poor.

Ocular Manifestations of Neonatal Septicemia

Ocular signs of neonatal septicemia include miosis, aqueous flare with fibrin deposition, hypopyon or hyphema, and, in severe cases, panophthalmitis. Bacteria involved include *Escherichia coli, Streptococcus* spp., *Pasteurella* spp., *Salmonella* spp., *Rhodococcus equi, Corynebacterium pyogenes,* and *Klebsiella* spp. Therapy should include systemic antibiotics (based, when possible, on sensitivity testing) and treatment for uveitis.

Miscellaneous Infectious Causes

Other infectious causes of ocular disease in ruminants include *Branhamella (Neisseria) ovis* keratoconjunctivitis (sheep and goats), scrapie-associated retinopathy (sheep and goats), bluetongue-induced retinal dysplasia (sheep) or conjunctivitis (cattle), *Listeria monocytogenes* keratoconjunctivitis (sheep and cattle), IBR keratoconjunctivitis (goats), *Colesiota (Rickettsia)* spp. keratoconjunctivitis (sheep), mycoplasmal conjunctivitis (cattle), *Haemophilus somnus* conjunctivitis and retinitis (cattle), and BVD-induced ocular disease (congenital retinal dysplasia, cataracts, microphthalmia, optic neuritis, and leukocoria). These conditions are briefly discussed in *Large Animal Internal Medicine,* third edition.

INFECTIOUS OCULAR DISEASES IN HORSES
(Text pp. 1173-1179)

Bacterial Keratitis

Bacterial keratitis occurs when a corneal ulcer becomes infected with opportunistic bacteria. The most devastating clinical manifestations are associated with *Pseudomonas* spp. and *Streptococcus* spp. Other isolates include streptococci, staphylococci, *E. coli, Acinetobacter* spp., and *Clostridium* spp.

Clinical signs

Corneal ulcers cause blepharospasm, lacrimation, and photophobia. The conjunctiva is hyperemic, and the ulcerated cornea stains with fluorescein. Signs indicative of infection include a deep ulcer (a crater in the corneal stroma), white or yellowish corneal opacity, and rapid progression ("melting" ulcer). What begins as a small ulcer may progress to corneal perforation within 24 to 48 hours. (Fungal keratitis can have a similar appearance, but most cases of bacterial keratitis present more acutely and have a much more rapid course.)

Stromal abscess. Bacterial keratitis can also present as a stromal abscess, in which cellular infiltrate is seen in the corneal stroma. The overlying damaged epithelium has healed and no longer stains with fluorescein.

Diagnosis

Diagnosis can be made from gram-stained corneal scrapings, which usually show many bacteria (some intracellular) and many neutrophils (some degenerate). NOTE: In any eye in which bacterial infection is suspected, the ulcer should be swabbed for bacterial culture and sensitivity (before topical anesthetic is applied) and the margin scraped for Gram stain and cytologic examination (after application of topical anesthetic).

Treatment

The therapeutic goals are as follows:

- Eliminate the bacteria with appropriate antibiotics (see following discussion).
  - Subpalpebral lavage systems are the best means of delivering the drug (see main text).
- Treat the concurrent uveitis–administer topical atropine (every 1 to 2 hours initially) or topical or systemic NSAIDs.
  - Monitor bowel motility when using atropine frequently.
  - Corticosteroids may compromise healing and predispose to corneal rupture.

Gram-negative infection. Appropriate drugs include gentamicin, tobramycin, amikacin or ticarcillin, and fluoroquinolones (e.g., ciprofloxacin, ofloxacin). Fortified gentamicin solution (add 30 mg gentamicin sulfate to a 5-ml bottle of gentamicin ophthalmic solution) may also be used. The antibiotic should be instilled every 1 to 2 hours.

Gram-positive infection. If gram-positive organisms are seen on the corneal scraping, ticarcillin, cefazolin, penicillin, or ampicillin can be used.

Reevaluation. If the ulcer continues to worsen, antibiotics should be changed on the basis of initial sensitivity results. The cornea should also be recultured because organisms can become resistant to the first antibiotic used.

Surgery. Surgical options include conjunctival pedicle flap, corneoconjunctival transposition, corneal graft (after lamellar keratectomy), and penetrating keratoplasty using donor cornea. Third eyelid flaps should not be used for rapidly progressing or deep ulcers. Keratectomy with a conjunctival flap or penetrating keratoplasty can be used to treat stromal abscesses.

Fungal Keratitis

Fungal keratitis occurs when an ulcerated cornea becomes infected with a mycotic organism. The most common genera isolated are *Aspergillus* and *Fusarium* spp. Horses seem to be uniquely susceptible to fungal keratitis, and even with intensive therapy the prognosis is guarded to poor.

Clinical signs

A common presentation is a corneal ulcer that fails to heal or worsens despite antibiotic or antiinflammatory therapy. The eye is painful and the conjunctiva is hyperemic. Corneal edema and cellular infiltrates (which can be very dense) surround the ulcer. Corneal neovascularization is usually seen. The secondary uveitis can be very severe. Fluorescein stains the ulcerated cornea. In some cases the epithelium heals over the fungal infection, forming a stromal abscess.

Mild form. Fungal keratitis can also present as a chronic, mild corneal disease. Small multifocal, superficial opacities can be seen. Sometimes there are small focal areas of fluorescein uptake; sometimes there is no uptake of stain. Ocular pain typically is mild, with some lacrimation. There is usually neither corneal neovascularization nor uveitis.

Diagnosis

A diagnosis of superficial fungal keratitis is made when fungal hyphae or yeasts are seen on cytologic examination of corneal scrapings. A diagnosis of deep fungal keratitis may be made only with corneal biopsy. Fungal hyphae have a predisposition for Descemet's membrane, which makes preenucleation diagnosis difficult.

Treatment

Treatment includes the use of antifungal agents, such as natamycin (topical), fluconazole (topical, subconjunctival, intravitreal, or systemic), or itraconazole/ DMSO (topical), and standard therapy for uveitis (see p. 335). Therapy usually must be continued for several weeks. Subpalpebral lavage systems are probably the best means of delivering the drug (see main text). Surgery may be indicated for deep fungal keratitis (see main text).

Miscellaneous Infectious Causes

Other infectious causes of ocular disease in horses include leptospirosis (a possible cause of ERU; see following discussion), equine adenovirus, salmonellosis, *Moraxella* spp., equine viral arteritis, *R. equi,* borreliosis, cryptococcosis, equine herpesvirus types 1 and 2, strangles *(Streptococcus equi),* brucellosis, and *Mycobacterium avium.* These conditions are briefly discussed in *Large Animal Internal Medicine,* third edition.

IMMUNE-MEDIATED OCULAR DISEASES *(Text pp. 1182-1188)*

Allergic Blepharoconjunctivitis

Animals with allergic conjunctivitis have acute swelling of the eyelids and conjunctiva, accompanied by serous ocular discharge, mild conjunctival hyperemia, and pruritus. If the stimulus persists, multiple subconjunctival lymphocytic aggregates (tiny, semitransparent follicles) appear within the conjunctival sac.

Diagnosis and treatment

Diagnosis is often presumptive; conjunctival cytologic examination may reveal eosinophils. Ocular signs subside with removal of the offending allergen, but this is often impractical. Individual animals may be treated with a topical ophthalmic corticosteroid preparation. Oral or parenteral flunixin meglumine (1 mg/kg) may be of benefit in horses.

Eosinophilic Keratoconjunctivitis

Eosinophilic keratoconjunctivitis is an uncommon disorder characterized clinically by corneal ulceration and plaque formation in one or both eyes. The cause is unknown.

Clinical signs

Nonspecific signs include blepharospasm, ocular discharge, and conjunctival hyperemia. Perilimbal corneal ulcers appear as raised, white corneal plaques (adherent caseous exudate), often accompanied by corneal edema and superficial vascularization.

Diagnosis

Definitive diagnosis is based on clinical signs and cytologic findings. Eosinophils and neutrophils predominate in corneal scrapings. Light microscopic evaluation of corneal tissue reveals coalescing foci of degenerated collagen fibers in the corneal plaques.

Treatment

Treatment consists of topical 0.05% dexamethasone and antibacterial ointments every 6 hours until clinical signs resolve. Lesions remodel with minimal corneal scarring, but healing may take several weeks. Use of ophthalmic NSAID preparations may increase the severity of clinical signs in horses. Excision of the corneal plaques by superficial keratectomy appears to enhance healing.

Equine Recurrent Uveitis

Equine recurrent uveitis (periodic ophthalmia, moon blindness) refers to a specific clinical pattern of intraocular inflammation in which recurring episodes of acute uveitis are separated by periods of clinical quiescence. Anterior uveitis predominates in the early stages; repeated episodes damage other structures, including the cornea, lens, vitreous, retina, and optic nerve.

Causes

The disorder is undoubtedly immune mediated. Two pathogens frequently incriminated are *Leptospira interrogans* serovar *pomona* and *Onchocerca cervicalis.* Over time the immune response may encompass endogenous ocular self-antigens.

Signs of acute ERU

Acute episodes of ERU are painful, causing blepharospasm and excessive tearing. Affected eyes appear red and cloudy; dilation of subconjunctival vessels near the limbus ("ciliary flush") intensifies the hyperemia. Generalized corneal edema gives the eye a blue-white appearance. The cornea may also exhibit peripheral circumferential vascularization, cellular precipitates on its inner surface, and linear stromal opacities.

Other ocular abnormalities include aqueous opacity (flare, hypopyon, or hyphema), iridocyclitis (dull, edematous iris), myosis (with or without posterior synechiae), decreased intraocular pressure, and retinal changes indicative of chorio-retinitis (see main text).

Signs of chronic ERU

Intraocular damage increases as inflammation recurs. Chronic recurrent uveitis is characterized by widespread posterior synechiae, iris depigmentation/hyperpigmentation, iris atrophy, lens changes (ranging from pigment flecks to dense cataracts), and retinal degeneration. Permanent hypotony is followed by shrinkage of the globe (phthisis bulbi). Conversely, chronic uveitis may result in glaucoma.

Diagnosis

Diagnosis is based on a history of chronic, recurrent ocular disease and the presence of characteristic ocular lesions. Serologic testing for *Leptospira, Brucella,* and *Toxoplasma* spp. may be useful, but negative titers do not exclude a diagnosis of ERU. A positive leptospiral titer at dilutions of 1:400 or more are of clinical importance. A higher titer in the aqueous than in the serum further supports a leptospiral cause for the uveitis. *Onchocerca* microfilariae may be identified in conjunctival biopsies.

Treatment

For acute uveitis, reduction of ocular inflammation using antiinflammatory agents and mydriatics is the primary objective. Following is a recommended treatment strategy for active uveitis:

- Initially rule out corneal ulceration, begin the following medications, and reevaluate in 24 hours.
  - Administer topical prednisolone acetate every 2 to 4 hours and topical 1% atropine two to four times daily until mydriasis.
  - Also give flunixin meglumine (1 mg/kg intravenously [IV] every 12 hours) or ketoprofen (2.2 mg/kg IV every 12 hours).
- If improved, continue topical treatments every 4 hours and flunixin every 24 hours and reevaluate in 48 to 72 hours.
  - If improved, discontinue flunixin, continue topical prednisolone every 4 to 6 hours, and give topical atropine as needed to maintain mydriasis.
  - Monitor horses for reduced gut motility or colic while on atropine therapy.
  - Consider using topical antibiotic ointments during intensive corticosteroid therapy.
- If not improved after 24 hours, rule out corneal ulcer, continue topical treatments every 2 hours, give methylprednisolone sodium succinate (500-mg intravenous bolus), consider the following medications, and reevaluate in 24 hours.
  - Administer subconjunctival steroids (e.g., Depo-Medrol, 10 to 40 mg), topical NSAIDs, and topical 10% phenylephrine if mydriasis is incomplete.
  - Do not use topical NSAIDs if there is corneal ulceration.
  - If not improved in a further 24 hours, reassess the diagnosis, continue the preceding plan, and consider outside consultation.

In general, therapy should be continued for 2 weeks beyond resolution of clinical signs. No therapy is indicated in painless eyes with lesions of chronic end-stage uveitis. Eyes that remain painful or are unresponsive to therapy are candidates for enucleation or evisceration.

Miscellaneous Conditions

In horses, pemphigus can have ocular manifestations. Bovine-specific ophthalmia causes recurrent uveitis in cattle, similar to ERU in horses. These conditions are briefly discussed in *Large Animal Internal Medicine,* third edition.

OCULAR PARASITES *(Text pp. 1189-1191)*

Ocular Onchocerciasis

In horses, ocular disease caused by *O. cervicalis* is the result of aberrant migration of microfilaria into the palpebral, conjunctival, or corneal tissues. The most common manifestations are conjunctivitis and keratoconjunctivitis (often recurrent) concentrated at the temporal limbus.

Clinical signs

Acutely, there is chemosis and conjunctival hyperemia, accompanied by increased lacrimation and blepharospasm. Small, raised, white nodules in the limbal conjunctiva and punctate, subepithelial corneal opacities are commonly present. Corneal lesions are often wedge shaped (widest at the limbus) and are characterized by neovascularization and cellular stromal infiltrates. Uveitis and chorioretinitis may also occur. With chronicity, patches of depigmentation (vitiligo) occur in the perilimbal bulbar conjunctiva.

Diagnosis

Clinical signs are highly suggestive of *Onchocerca* keratoconjunctivitis, but definitive diagnosis requires corneal or conjunctival biopsy (see main text). The presence of eosinophils in corneal and conjunctival scrapings is suggestive of a parasitic etiology, but microfilaria are rarely found.

Treatment

Microfilaricide therapy has been associated with increased ocular inflammation, so treatment is directed at controlling the inflammatory reaction before eliminating the parasite. Corticosteroids may be given topically, subconjunctivally, or systemically. Systemic administration (e.g., prednisolone at 0.5 to 1 mg/kg orally [PO] once per day for 5 to 7 days initially) is indicated for severe uveitis with concurrent *Onchocerca* dermatitis and before larvicidal therapy (see Chapter 38).

Ocular Habronemiasis

Equine ocular habronemiasis occurs when *Habronema muscae, Habronema microstoma,* or *Draschia megastoma* larvae are deposited on ocular tissues by flies attracted to ocular discharge or periocular wounds. Habronemiasis typically is seasonal, occurring in the warmer months.

Clinical signs

Ocular lesions commonly consist of raised, proliferative, nonhealing wounds at the medial canthus. The lesions are friable and pruritic and bleed easily. Lesions often contain small, yellow, caseated nodules ("sulfur granules"). Fistulous tracts and subdermal nodules may develop below the medial canthus. Corneal neovascularization, edema, and ulceration can occur as a result of altered lid function and contact irritation by the mass.

Diagnosis

Demonstration of the larvae in the granulomatous lesions or fistulous tracts is diagnostic. Biopsy specimens of the affected tissue are directly examined for *Habronema* larvae (see main text) and may also be submitted for histopathologic examination.

Treatment

Ivermectin (0.2 mg/kg PO) is the treatment of choice. Lesions begin to regress in 7 days and are usually healed within 4 to 6 weeks. Topical, intralesional, or systemic corticosteroids may be used to decrease the inflammatory response to the larvae but are often not needed. Debridement of granulomatous areas and drainage of fistulous tracts may speed healing.

Ocular Thelaziasis

Most horses and ruminants with *Thelazia* nematodes in the conjunctival sac are asymptomatic, but chronic conjunctivitis, conjunctival cysts, and superficial keratitis can occur. Dacryocystitis from parasite migration into the nasolacrimal system can also occur, most often in cattle.

Diagnosis and treatment

Direct visualization of adult worms (8 to 18 mm long and milky white with transverse striations) in the conjunctival sac or nasolacrimal flushings is diagnostic. Both ivermectin and doramectin (200 µg/kg) are effective. The parasites may also be manually removed with saline flushes or forceps after administration of topical anesthesia.

Ocular Elaeophoriasis

Elaeophoriasis, or "sore head," is a disease of sheep that is caused by the deer nematode *Elaeophora schneideri.* Adult worms in the common carotid and internal maxillary arteries produce microfilaria that migrate into the capillaries of the face and head, including the eye. The disease is most prevalent in the fall and winter in the western parts of the United States.

Clinical signs

Migration of the microfilaria into ocular capillaries causes local inflammation. The uveal tract is affected most often, but affected sheep may develop chronic keratoconjunctivitis. Funduscopic changes indicative of chorioretinitis and optic neuritis are common.

Diagnosis and treatment

Diagnosis depends on demonstration of the microfilaria in skin or conjunctival biopsy specimens. Drugs used for treatment include piperazine (50 mg/kg PO), diethylcarbamazine (DEC, 100 mg/kg PO), and stibophen (35 ml IV). Symptomatic treatment of keratitis and uveitis is indicated. NOTE: Treatment of heavily parasitized animals may cause death from occlusion of the carotid arteries with adult worms.

Miscellaneous Parasites

Parasitic conditions that can have ocular manifestations include nasal bots (sheep), trypanosomiasis, piroplasmosis, toxoplasmosis, and infestation with *Setaria* spp. and *Dirofilaria immitis.* These conditions are briefly discussed in *Large Animal Internal Medicine,* third edition.

OCULAR NEOPLASIA *(Text pp. 1192-1198)*

Despite the variety of primary and secondary neoplasms affecting the ocular and periocular tissues, most tumors have similar effects on the eye, with tissue distortion and loss of function being the initial concerns. Manifestations and differential diagnoses in particular species are listed in Table 37-3 of *Large Animal Internal Medicine,* third edition.

Ocular Squamous Cell Carcinoma

Ocular squamous cell carcinoma (OSCC) is the most common ocular neoplasm in large animals. In cattle it is commonly called cancer eye. The tumor most often involves the conjunctiva or cornea and is most prevalent in animals with unpigmented periocular tissues. Breeds most commonly affected include Hereford cattle and Belgian, Appaloosa, and paint or pinto horses.

Clinical signs and diagnosis

Premalignant squamous cell carcinomas are small, white, elevated, hyperplastic plaques or papilloma-like structures with verrucous surfaces. Malignant tumors are more irregular, nodular, pink, erosive, and necrotic. The gross appearance usually allows presumptive diagnosis, but cytologic or histologic examination may be necessary to differentiate among benign tumors, carcinoma in situ, and invasive squamous cell carcinomas.

Treatment

Treatment options include radiofrequency hyperthermia, cryonecrosis, intralesional injection of biologic response modifiers (e.g., allogeneic OSCC extract, mycobacterial cell wall fraction, *Propionibacterium acnes*), intralesional chemotherapy with cisplatin (sometimes with initial debulking), radiotherapy, and surgical removal (local excision, enucleation, and exenteration with or without salivary gland and lymph node resection).

Ocular Manifestations of Lymphosarcoma

Lymphosarcoma is the most common cause of orbital neoplasia in cattle; it is reported less often in horses and goats. The most consistent sign is exophthalmos with subsequent exposure keratitis and eventual proptosis; the globe itself usually is not involved. Other physical findings often reflect systemic involvement (see Chapter 35).

Diagnosis and treatment

Definitive diagnosis is made from cytologic samples or biopsy specimens (preferred), either from orbital tissue or involved regional lymph nodes. Chemotherapy with corticosteroids, vincristine, and L-asparaginase may induce remission (see main text). Enucleation is palliative.

Equine Sarcoid

Equine sarcoid is a locally aggressive, nonmalignant, fibroblastic skin tumor. The eyelids are a fairly common site of involvement. Tumors of the eyelids may appear smooth and nodular, crusted and nodular, ulcerated, or pedunculated. Treatment options are discussed in Chapter 38.

38

Diseases of the Skin

Consulting Editor STEPHEN D. WHITE

Contributors ANNE G. EVANS • STEVEN L. BERRY • BRADFORD P. SMITH
ANTHONY A. STANNARDT† • DAVID C. VAN METRE • NATHAN M. SLOVIS
JOHANNA L. WATSON

IMMUNE-MEDIATED SKIN DISORDERS *(Text pp. 1200-1202)*

Pemphigus Foliaceus

Pemphigus foliaceus is an autoimmune disorder that affects the skin. It has been reported in horses and goats; Appaloosas appear to be predisposed.

Clinical signs

Lesions usually are first noted on the head, limbs, and ventrum in horses and on the limbs, perineum, and ventrum in goats. In horses, initial lesions may be associated with ventral and rear limb edema, fever, depression, coronary band erosions, and (rarely) urticaria. The disease progresses over days or weeks to involve the entire body.

The primary lesion is a vesicle that ruptures soon after formation, thus resulting in erosions, epidermal collarettes (rings of exfoliating superficial epidermis), scale, and crust. Lesions may or may not be pruritic or painful.

Diagnosis

Diagnosis usually is based on biopsy specimens of lesions submitted for routine histopathologic examination. Direct immunofluorescence can aid in diagnosis, although in horses the test can be negative despite strong clinical and histologic support for a diagnosis of pemphigus foliaceus.

Treatment

Treatment involves immunosuppressive doses of glucocorticoids with or without chrysotherapy (e.g., aurothioglucose; see text). The following regimen is recommended:

- Give oral prednisone or prednisolone (2 mg/kg/day) until signs of active disease disappear (usually 10 to 14 days).
  - If there is no response in 24 to 48 hours, substitute dexamethasone (0.05 to 0.1 mg/kg twice daily) until remission occurs; alternatively, dexamethasone can be used first.
- Gradually reduce the dosage until the minimum daily dose that keeps the disease in remission is reached; double this dose and administer on alternate mornings.
  - Aim for a maintenance dose of oral prednisolone of 0.5 mg/kg alternate mornings.

Many horses require lifelong therapy.

Bullous Pemphigoid

Bullous pemphigoid is a rare autoimmune, vesiculobullous, and ulcerative disorder that has been reported in horses. It is characterized by painful, ulcerative

†Deceased.

lesions of the skin (face and axillae), mucous membranes, and mucocutaneous junctions. The diagnosis is based on histopathologic and, when available, immunofluorescent findings. Therapy with glucocorticoids is indicated but may be unsuccessful.

HYPERSENSITIVITY DISORDERS *(Text pp. 1202-1206)*

Urticaria

Urticaria is characterized by multiple, transient areas of focal dermal edema (wheals) in the skin or mucous membranes. It is more commonly recognized in horses than in ruminants, with the most common causes in all species being drugs and ingestants (see main text).

Clinical signs and diagnosis

Wheals range from 1 to 10 cm in diameter and tend to involve the neck and craniolateral thorax. The animal may or may not be pruritic. Hair loss is not a feature unless there has been serum leakage onto the skin surface. Individual lesions pit with pressure. Clinical trials can be performed to determine whether insects, feeds, or environmental factors are responsible for the urticarial eruption. Intradermal skin testing may be of value with recurrent urticaria (see main text).

Treatment

Avoiding the allergens is the best therapy. When this is not possible or when the allergens cannot be identified, corticosteroids or antihistamines should be used. Prednisone or prednisolone is the preferred corticosteroid in horses. Antihistamine options include the following:

- Hydroxyzine HCl, 200 to 400 mg two or three times daily
- Doxepin (a tricyclic antidepressant with antihistaminic effects), 300 to 600 mg every 12 hours

Hyposensitization, based on results of intradermal skin testing, is an option with urticaria resulting from inhaled allergens.

Anaphylaxis

Anaphylaxis is an acute, transient, life-threatening alteration in vascular permeability and smooth muscle contraction that rapidly occurs after interaction with a variety of possible stimuli. Anaphylaxis typically involves a number of organ systems, including the respiratory and cardiovascular systems. It may or may not be associated with cutaneous manifestations such as urticaria.

Treatment

Epinephrine is indicated for treatment:

- Life-threatening situations–1:10,000 (0.1 mg/ml) epinephrine slowly intravenously (IV) at 0.01 mg/kg (5 ml for an adult horse or cow)
- Less acute situations or when intravenous injection is impossible–5 to 10 ml of 1:1000 (1 mg/ml) epinephrine intramuscularly (IM) or subcutaneously (SC)

In addition, a corticosteroid such as methylprednisolone sodium succinate (1 to 2 mg/kg IV or IM) or dexamethasone (0.25 to 1 mg/kg IV or IM), an antihistamine such as diphenhydramine (0.25 to 1 mg/kg IV or IM), and intravenous polyionic fluids are indicated.

Milk Allergy

Milk allergy is hypersensitivity to systemically released milk proteins. It is most common in dairy cows (particularly Channel Island breeds) during the drying-off period. The principal cutaneous manifestation is urticaria, which can be localized or generalized. Other signs may include muscle tremors, dyspnea, restlessness, ataxia, dullness, and even maniacal behavior.

Diagnosis and treatment

Diagnosis involves injecting cow's milk or α-casein (diluted 1:1000) intradermally and observing an edematous swelling at the site. The urticaria can be treated with antihistamines.

Erythema Multiforme

Erythema multiforme (EM) is an uncommon condition in horses that is characterized by acute onset of asymptomatic skin lesions that form multiple, raised rings. Hair remains on the lesions unless there is serum exudation. In rare cases, EM presents as a severe ulcerative disease.

Treatment

The most important aspect of treatment is elimination of suspected causes. Drugs are probably the most common identifiable cause, although the majority of cases are idiopathic. Because the lesions are mild and spontaneously resolve in 2 to 3 weeks, overuse of systemic steroids is best avoided.

Vasculitis

Vasculitis is discussed in Chapter 35. Cutaneous vasculitis is characterized by purpura, necrosis, and ulceration, most commonly affecting the head and extremities.

Drug Eruption

Compounds most commonly incriminated in drug eruptions include antibacterial agents (especially penicillin and sulfas), phenothiazine tranquilizers, nonsteroidal antiinflammatory drugs (NSAIDs; especially aspirin and phenylbutazone), local anesthetics, and anticonvulsants. Typically, cutaneous lesions are noted 24 to 48 hours after drug administration and subside within 24 to 48 hours after exposure ceases.

Clinical signs

Urticaria and angioedema (subcutaneous edema), diffuse erythema, papular rashes, intense pruritus that is poorly responsive to corticosteroids, sharply demarcated ulcers (secondary to vasculitis), vesicular and bullous eruptions, and photosensitization should arouse clinical suspicion of a drug eruption.

Treatment

In a suspected case, all medications should be discontinued. If lifesaving medications are being administered, a chemically unrelated compound with similar pharmacologic effects should be substituted. Corticosteroids may provide some relief, but drug eruptions typically are minimally responsive to corticosteroids.

Contact Dermatitis

Irritant contact dermatitis is a cutaneous reaction to an irritating concentration of an offending agent that chemically damages the skin. Allergic contact dermatitis represents a cutaneous reaction in a sensitized animal to a nonirritating concentration of the offending agent.

Clinical signs and diagnosis

Predisposed areas include the muzzle, extremities, and areas contacted by tack. Early lesions, which include erythema, edema, and vesiculation, progress to erosions, ulcerations, crusting, and ultimately lichenification and hyperpigmentation. Provocative exposure is the most useful test. It requires avoiding contact with all suspected agents for 7 to 10 days, then sequential reexposure.

Treatment

Chances of exposure to a known or suspected irritant or allergen should be minimized. Pending spontaneous resolution, the affected regions should be gently washed with water.

BACTERIAL DISEASES *(Text pp. 1207-1210)*

Dermatophilosis (Rain Scald, Lumpy Wool, Strawberry Footrot)

Dermatophilosis is a superficial bacterial dermatitis of horses and ruminants caused by the actinomycete *Dermatophilus congolensis.* It is characterized by exudation and crust formation.

Clinical signs

The characteristic lesions are suppurative crusts that mat the hair or wool. Removal of the crusts reveals a moist, gray-pink surface, with the roots of the hairs protruding through the crust. Affected regions typically are painful but not pruritic. Areas predisposed to maceration and trauma, and thus infection, include the distal limbs, muzzle, and dorsum.

Diagnosis

In the acute stages, stained smears of exudate on the underside of the crusts reveal the characteristic bacteria: gram-positive, branching, filamentous bacteria that form parallel rows of cocci ("railroad tracks"). The diagnosis should not be ruled out without first culturing the crusts.

Treatment

Contributing factors, such as moisture and external parasites, should be corrected and infected animals carefully groomed to remove the crusts. Bathing with a povidone-iodine shampoo or chlorhexidine solution daily for 7 days should be followed by treatment once or twice a week until clinical resolution.

Systemic therapy. Systemic therapy is reserved for severe and generalized cases. Penicillin (22,000 IU/kg IM twice daily for 3 to 5 days) is beneficial. Long-acting oxytetracycline (20 mg/kg IM once) is effective in cattle and sheep.

Folliculitis/Furunculosis

Bacterial folliculitis is inflammation of the hair follicles secondary to bacterial infection. When the inflammatory process ruptures the hair follicle and extends into the surrounding dermis and subcutis, the process is called furunculosis. In addition to *D. congolensis,* causative bacteria include *Staphylococcus* spp., *Corynebacterium pseudotuberculosis, Rhodococcus equi* (horses), *Actinomyces (Corynebacterium) pyogenes* (goats), and *Pseudomonas aeruginosa* (goats).

Clinical signs

Clinical signs in horses are typically first noted in the saddle and harness regions, the neck, or the lumbosacral region. The primary lesion is a follicular papule, although the initial sign may be multiple 2- to 3-mm foci of erect hairs. These areas may spontaneously regress or enlarge, exude serum, and scab. The lesions are painful, and hair loss is common. In goats, lesions commonly begin on the udder and spread to the abdomen, thigh, perineum, and face.

Pastern folliculitis. Pastern folliculitis is a special form of folliculitis/furunculosis that occurs in horses. Lesions are limited to the posterior aspect of the pastern or fetlock of one or more limbs. The initial papular lesions may coalesce, resulting in large areas of ulceration and suppuration if left untreated. *Staphylococcus* spp. or β-hemolytic streptococci are usually cultured.

Diagnosis

Gram-stained smears of pustule contents, bacterial culture and sensitivity tests, and biopsies should be performed.

Treatment

The most important aspect of treatment is to correct any predisposing factors. Mild cases of folliculitis may resolve without treatment. More severe cases require topical therapy with antibacterial solutions containing chlorhexidine or iodophors. Small areas may respond to topical application of silver sulfadiazine cream or mupirocin ointment. In addition to topical treatment, furunculosis requires systemic antibiotic therapy based on sensitivity results.

Equine Staphylococcal Cellulitis

Staphylococcal cellulitis is a specific disease entity caused by *Staphylococcus aureus* in Thoroughbred racehorses. The initial sign is acute swelling and lameness involving one or more limbs. Lesions progress rapidly; the overlying skin becomes devitalized and often sloughs. Accompanying systemic signs include fever and tachycardia.

Diagnosis and treatment

Diagnosis is based on results of bacterial culture and biopsy. Treatment should include broad-spectrum antibiotics (e.g., penicillin and gentamicin, trimethoprim-sulfamethoxazole). NSAIDs, hydrotherapy, and support wraps are also beneficial. The prognosis for complete recovery is guarded.

Papillomatous Digital Dermatitis (Hairy Foot Warts)

Papillomatous digital dermatitis (PDD; digital dermatitis, interdigital papillomatosis, hairy foot warts, heel warts) is a contagious dermatitis of the digital skin in cattle. It is primarily a disease of housed dairy cattle.

Etiology

Current evidence indicates that PDD is multifactorial, involving environmental, microbial, host, and management factors. Numerous obligate anaerobes have been associated with PDD. Spirochetes from the genus *Treponema* have been identified most consistently.

Clinical signs

In most cases, lesions occur on the plantar aspect of a hind foot, immediately proximal to the heel bulbs and adjacent to or extending into the interdigital space. Less common sites are the palmar aspect of a forefoot and the dorsal aspect of any foot. PDD lesions in the interdigital space frequently occur over a preexisting fibroma. A foul odor may or may not be present.

Appearance. Most lesions are 2 to 6 cm in diameter, are circular or oval, and have clearly demarcated, raised borders that are often surrounded by hairs that are 2 to 3 times normal length. The surface may have filiform papillae varying in length from 1 mm to 3 cm. Lesions lacking these papillae may have a granular surface. Washed surfaces generally are very painful and are either red and granular or composites of white-yellow, gray, brown, or black papillary areas interspersed with red granular areas. The lesions bleed easily if traumatized.

Lameness. Swelling of the pastern and fetlock is not present in uncomplicated cases. Lameness is a herd characteristic on dairies with a high prevalence of PPD, but it is an inconsistent finding in individual cattle and is not consistently related to lesion size or maturity. If PDD lesions remain untreated, the claws of feet with plantar/palmar lesions may develop a clubbed appearance because the cow prefers to bear weight on the toes.

Treatment

The most commonly used treatments are topical oxytetracycline and lincomycin (with or without spectinomycin) sprayed on the lesions or applied with a bandage. Topical treatments need to be repeated every 45 to 60 days. Parenteral antibiotics (ceftiofur or procaine penicillin G) may be efficacious but require milk withholding. Footbaths containing 5% formalin, lincomycin, oxytetracycline, copper sulfate, or zinc sulfate effectively control PPD in infected herds (see main text).

Interdigital Dermatitis

Nonpapillomatous interdigital dermatitis is denoted by acute or chronic inflammation of the interdigital skin. Diffuse epidermal erosion in the interdigital cleft may be seen in early cases. More chronic cases show hyperkeratosis and roughening of the interdigital skin. A malodorous, gray, serous exudate may be present, and there is mild sensitivity to pressure. Lameness ranges from absent to moderate in severity. This condition is often accompanied by heel cracks, with potential underrunning of the heel horn. It can be treated topically as described for PPD.

VIRAL DISEASES *(Text pp. 1211-1213)*

Papillomatosis (Warts)

Papillomas, or warts, occur in all livestock species and are caused by species-specific papilloma viruses. The growths, which usually occur in young animals, are pale, firm, protruding masses with a dry, horny surface. They may be single or multiple. In most cases, warts are benign and spontaneously regress after 3 to 12 months. In cattle, warts on the teats, penis, or interdigital skin or in the alimentary tract may produce clinical signs of pain or occlusion.

Treatment

Small warts can be crushed, pinched off, or surgically removed. Cryosurgery can be used on larger warts. When show animals are involved or when animals have multiple large papillomas, tissue can be removed and used to make a crude autogenous vaccine (see main text).

Aural Plaques

Aural plaques are gray-white keratinous crusts on the inner surface of the pinna of the ear in horses. They do not appear to cause discomfort, although they persist indefinitely. The crusts can be dislodged, revealing a pink, nonulcerated base. No effective treatment has been found.

Pseudocowpox

Pseudocowpox is a common parapox virus; its impact is most important in dairy cattle. Cyclic waves of reinfection occur in a herd, where it causes minor teat lesions characterized initially by a small papule and followed by crusting and circular spread of the lesion. Deep ulceration is rare. This virus can cause nodular skin lesions in humans.

Bovine Herpes Mammillitis

Bovine mammillitis is caused by bovine herpesvirus type 2. The disease may be epidemic or endemic. The initial lesion is a swollen, edematous, painful teat. Vesicles may be seen, but most vesicles ulcerate almost immediately. The ulcers take 3 to 10 weeks to heal. The virus may also cause oral lesions, udder lesions, or generalized skin disease.

Treatment

Affected animals should be segregated and milked last. In severe cases, secondary infection may be controlled by topical antibiotic creams or parenteral antibiotics.

MYCOTIC DISEASES *(Text pp. 1213-1215)*

Dermatophytosis

Dermatophytosis is infection of the keratinized tissues of the skin by fungi of the genus *Microsporum* or *Trichophyton.* It is relatively common in horses and cattle and relatively rare in sheep and goats. Young animals are most often affected. Dermatophytosis generally is a self-limiting disease, although infection may persist for up to 4 months.

Clinical signs and diagnosis

A key characteristic is the multifocal nature of the lesions, which are most often located on the head, neck, shoulders, and lateral thorax. The primary lesions are alopecia, scaling, and crusting. Pruritus is mild or absent. In cattle the lesions often have excessive amounts of crusting, giving them a wartlike appearance. Direct microscopic examination of infected hairs is of value, but the most reliable method of diagnosis is fungal culture of broken hairs from the periphery of lesions.

Treatment

Dermatophytosis is a spontaneously regressing disease. Nevertheless, fungistatic/fungicidal products are widely used to decrease the spread of the disease. Treatment options include the following:

- Sponge the horse's tack with 50% captan (2 Tbsp/gallon of water) once or twice per week for 1 month or until 2 weeks after clinical cure.
- Shampoo with miconazole or enilconazole rinse (if available).
- Administer 20% sodium iodide (NaI) IV (250 ml/500-kg horse once or twice at a 7-day interval).
  - NaI is contraindicated in pregnant mares.
- Give griseofulvin (100 mg/kg daily for 7 days).

Topical therapy generally is curative. Vaccination against *Trichophyton equinum* may reduce the incidence of new infections.

Mycetomas and Zygomycosis

Mycetomas and zygomycoses are subcutaneous fungal or actinomycotic infections. Common names include phycomycosis, fungal tumor, swamp cancer, Gulf

Coast fungus, Florida horse leech, and bursattee. They are most common in tropical areas and are caused by a variety of fungal agents or by bacteria of the genera *Actinomyces, Nocardia,* and *Actinobacillus.*

Clinical signs and diagnosis

Lesions are usually localized on the limbs, abdomen, neck, or head (including nasal cavity, lips, and trachea) and are characterized by granulation tissue, necrotic draining tracts, and pruritus. Biopsy material contains diagnostic fungal hyphae. Fungi can also be isolated on Sabouraud's dextrose agar. Mixed infections with cutaneous habronemiasis are common.

Treatment

Surgical debridement in conjunction with intravenous amphotericin B is most effective. Amphotericin B is given at a dosage of 150 mg/day IV in 1 L of 5% dextrose. The dosage is increased by 50 mg every 2 days to a maximum of 400 mg/day. Treatment is continued for up to 30 days. Kidney function must be monitored during therapy. Oral potassium iodide (20 g/day) is also recommended. Topical therapy with either etisazole or amphotericin B in DMSO can also be effective.

Sporotrichosis

Sporotrichum schenckii is a yeastlike fungus that causes sporadic infection (usually chronic) of the skin and lymphatics, most commonly in horses. Hard nodules 1 to 5 cm in diameter form, often in lines along lymphatics; they may ulcerate and discharge a creamy exudate.

Diagnosis and treatment

Diagnosis is by culture and biopsy. Treatment involves NaI (40 mg/kg IV as a 20% solution) for 2 to 5 days, followed by oral iodides (either ethylenediamine dihydroiodide or potassium iodide at 2 mg/kg/day orally [PO]) for up to 60 days.

PARASITIC SKIN DISEASES *(Text pp. 1215-1222)*

Pediculosis (Lice)

Lice are host-specific ectoparasites. The hallmark of infestation is pruritus, and many of the clinical changes (patchy alopecia and crusted ulcerations caused by excoriation) are secondary to self-trauma. The neck and tail typically are affected first, but infestation and symptoms may become generalized. The coat becomes dry and scaly. Heavily infested animals may become anemic.

Treatment

Topical insecticide should be applied to infested animals and all in-contact animals every 2 weeks for two or three treatments. Effective topical treatments include coumaphos, crotoxyphos, malathion, pyrethrins, methoxychlor, and lindane. Fomites should also be treated. Ivermectin (0.2 mg/kg twice, 2 weeks apart) may be effective against sucking lice.

Acariasis (Mite Infestation)

There are several genera of mites that can infest livestock. Most cause variable pruritus with consequent patchy alopecia and crusted ulcerations from self-trauma. Predilection sites vary with the species of mite and the host species. Diagnosis is based on finding mites on microscopic examination of skin scrapings or exudate (see main text).

Trombiculidiasis

Trombiculidiasis is caused by the larval stages of several species of mites commonly called harvest mites or "chiggers." Infestation is most common during the late summer and early fall in pastured animals. Lesions consist of crusted papular eruptions on the face, neck, extremities, or thorax. Pruritus is variable. The disorder is self-limiting.

Psoroptic mange

Psoroptic mange is common in cattle and occasionally reported in goats but has been eradicated from horses and sheep in the United States. Infestation is more prevalent in the cooler months. The hallmark in all species is pruritus. In cattle, crusted papular lesions typically are first apparent on the withers but then become generalized. In goats, lesions usually are restricted to the ears, although they may spread to the neck and body. NOTE: Psoroptic mange is a reportable disease.

Chorioptic mange

Chorioptic mange (foot or leg mange) is common in cattle and sheep, uncommon in goats, and seen with variable frequency in horses. Draft horses may be more susceptible than other horses.

Clinical signs. The primary symptom is extreme pruritus, with secondary lesions resulting from self-trauma. The most common areas involved are the distal rear limbs, perineum, tail, and scrotum in cattle; the lower limbs and scrotum in sheep; the lower limbs, hind quarters, and abdomen in goats; and the lower rear limbs in horses. Infestation can become generalized.

Sarcoptic mange

Sarcoptic mange is an uncommon contagious disease caused by *Sarcoptes scabeii.* It can affect horses and ruminants and is transmissible to humans. The hallmark of infestation is pruritus, often with papular eruptions and lesions secondary to self-trauma. The head (especially the ears) and neck are usually the initial areas of involvement, although lesions generalize.

Diagnosis. The ears should be scraped for mites; however, negative skin scrapings do not rule out the disease. NOTE: Sarcoptic mange is a reportable disease.

Demodectic mange

Demodectic mange is rare in livestock. Affected horses develop alopecia and scaling on the head, neck, and withers; pruritus is variable. Goats and cattle develop nodular lesions on the face, neck, and shoulder; in goats the contents may be white and caseous. Sheep tend to develop periocular nodular lesions. Spontaneous resolution may occur in all species.

Treatment of acariasis

Topical application with one of the following compounds usually is curative: 5% lime sulfur, coumaphos, diazinon, dioxathion, malathion, lindane, and toxaphene. Treatment may need to be repeated, at least twice every 5 to 7 days for psoroptic and chorioptic mange and at 10-day intervals for six treatments for sarcoptic mange. Ivermectin is approved for treatment of sarcoptic mange in cattle at a dose of 0.2 mg/kg SC, repeated in 2 weeks.

Culicoides Hypersensitivity

Culicoides hypersensitivity (Queensland itch, sweet itch) is an intensely pruritic, dorsally distributed, seasonal dermatitis affecting horses. It is caused by hypersensitivity to *Culicoides* gnats (biting midges). The disorder is primarily seen in adult horses during the warmer months.

Clinical signs and diagnosis

Lesions are primarily the result of self-trauma and include alopecia, crusting, and scaling. The forehead, neck, withers, shoulder, rump, and tail are most severely affected. The hypersensitivity tends to worsen in successive years. Chronic excoriation results in marked lichenification and scarring. Diagnosis is based on seasonality, history of exposure, distribution of lesions, and response to therapy.

Treatment

The most important aspect of therapy is reduction of exposure. Stabling in an insect-proof stall during peak gnat feeding hours (primarily at dusk) is advisable. Frequent topical application of insect repellents is necessary. Products that contain pyrethrins with synergists and repellents are of most value and should be applied in the late afternoon.

Corticosteroids. Corticosteroids are needed for control in many cases. Prednisone or prednisolone should initially be administered at a dosage of 1 mg/kg/day until the horse is nonpruritic (usually 7 to 10 days). The dosage is then slowly tapered to the lowest alternate morning dosage that controls the symptoms.

Ventral Dermatitis in Horses

Punctate ulcers with areas of alopecia, leukoderma, crusts, and thickened skin develop on the ventral thorax or abdomen of some horses as a result of fly or gnat bites. Serum or blood exudation from the ulcers is usually present. Pruritus is variable. Treatment consists of diligent application of fly repellents around the lesions and antibiotic-corticosteroid creams on the lesion surface. Severely pruritic animals may require systemic corticosteroids for a few days.

Screwworm Infestation

Screwworm flies cause primary myiasis. In the United States there are now only occasional attacks in areas bordering Mexico. Female flies are attracted to fresh wounds or surgical sites, abraded body orifices, areas soiled by discharges or excretions, and navels of newborns.

Clinical signs

Eggs laid around the wound hatch and the feeding larvae burrow deeply into the flesh, creating a cavernous lesion characterized by liquefaction necrosis, profuse brownish exudate, and an objectionable odor. Infestation often culminates in death as a result of secondary bacterial infection and toxemia.

Treatment

Infested wounds must be thoroughly cleansed, debrided, and covered with dressings containing an antiseptic and a larvicide (e.g., 5% lindane or 3% coumaphos ointment or gel). Treatment is repeated twice a week. Ivermectin (injected SC) can clear wounds of larvae within 3 days and prevent reinfestation for 14 days. NOTE: Screwworm myiasis is a reportable disease in the United States; suspect larvae should be preserved in 70% alcohol for positive identification.

Blow Fly Strike

Blow flies are an important ectoparasite of sheep. Female flies are attracted to decaying animal matter, such as wounds infested by screwworms, infected sores, carcasses, and soiled fleece. The larvae feed on necrotic tissue, but they may invade healthy tissue.

Clinical signs and treatment

The most common site of involvement is the breech. Affected sheep are restless and do not feed; some become systemically ill and die. Fly-blown wool is moist and brown, with an obvious odor. Treatment of individual wounds is as described for screwworms.

Cutaneous Onchocerciasis

Cutaneous onchocerciasis is a common dermatitis in adult horses. It is caused by the microfilaria of *Onchocerca cervicalis.* Many horses are infected without demonstrating clinical disease.

Clinical signs

The dermatitis is nonseasonal and generally nonpruritic. Cutaneous lesions include diffuse or patchy alopecia, erythema, and scaling; focal depigmentation is common. Lesions are most common on the ventral midline, face (forehead, lower eyelid), base of the mane, craniomedial proximal forelimbs, and cranial pectoral region. A bull's eye lesion in the center of the forehead is highly suggestive. The lateral limbus of the eye is another predilection site (see Chapter 37).

Diagnosis

Diagnosis is based on the history, clinical findings, exclusion of differential diagnoses, and response to therapy. Because many normal horses have microfilaria without disease, finding microfilaria in biopsy specimens is not diagnostic.

Treatment

Ivermectin (0.2 mg/kg PO) is the treatment of choice; most lesions improve within 2 to 3 weeks. Minor adverse reactions, including fever and swelling of the periorbital, facial, and ventral midline regions, may occur. Severe reactions may be treated with antiinflammatory medications, but most reactions resolve within 24 to 72 hours even without corticosteroids. There is no effective adulticide, so retreatment is recommended at 4-month intervals.

Stephanofilariasis

Cutaneous stephanofilariasis is a filarial dermatitis of cattle. It is caused by *Stephanofilaria* spp. and is most prevalent in the western and southwestern regions of the United States. Clinical signs include ventral midline dermatitis, initially involving a papular eruption. The lesions, which may be mildly pruritic, progress to nodules, alopecia, and crusted ulcers.

Diagnosis and treatment

Diagnosis is based on the history, clinical signs, and finding the nematodes in biopsy specimens or deep skin scrapings (see main text). Topical trichlorfon (6% to 10% in petroleum jelly) applied daily for 7 days is effective, as is 4% fentrothion applied daily for 30 days.

Hypoderma (Warbles)

Infestation with *Hypoderma* spp. larvae is common in cattle and occasionally seen in horses pastured near cattle. Eggs deposited on the body or legs hatch, and the larvae penetrate the skin and migrate to the esophageal wall *(Hypoderma lineatum)* or spinal canal *(Hypoderma bovis).* After several months, they migrate to the subdermal tissues of the back and form a breathing hole through the skin.

Clinical signs

Third-stage larvae form warbles (cystic lesions) along the back. The lesions range from firm to fluctuant, are raised and painful to the touch, and contain a breathing pore that usually exudes serum. Secondary infection can result in large suppurating abscesses. The number of warbles in an infested animal may range from 1 to 300.

Horses. Most infested horses have only one or two warbles. The lesions are small, nodular swellings, usually with a breathing pore, most often in the region of the withers.

Diagnosis

The season, location of the lesions, and presence of a breathing pore are usually diagnostic. Larvae can be recovered by enlarging the breathing pore with a scalpel and extracting the grub.

Treatment

Manual removal of the grubs is recommended in horses and cattle when small numbers of animals are infested with only a few grubs. Care must be taken to remove the larvae in their entirety, because breaking the larva and rupturing the surrounding cyst can result in a severe systemic reaction.

Insecticides. Systemic insecticides are the only means of eliminating the migrating larvae. Rotenone may be used to kill larvae along the back when manual removal or systemic insecticide treatment is not an option. Effective treatment requires direct contact with the grub. Strategic treatment with systemic insecticides is discussed in *Large Animal Internal Medicine,* third edition.

Sheep Keds

The sheep ked, *Melophagus ovinus,* parasitizes sheep and occasionally goats kept under poor management conditions. Infestation is more common in the winter. Clinical signs include pruritus with subsequent self-trauma, wool stains, and in severely parasitized animals, anemia. Multiple firm nodules (cockles) develop where the keds feed.

Diagnosis and treatment

Diagnosis is based on demonstration of the parasite. All sheep in the flock should be sheared and treated with two topical applications of malathion, diazinon, or coumaphos 2 to 3 weeks apart.

Cutaneous Habronemiasis (Summer Sores)

Cutaneous habronemiasis is a granulomatous dermatitis of horses that results from aberrant intradermal migration of the larvae of the nematodes *Habronema muscae, Habronema microstoma,* and *Draschia megastoma.* It is a seasonal disorder occurring when flies (the vector) are active.

Clinical signs

Cutaneous lesions occur when the larvae are deposited in damaged skin or areas of natural body moisture. The most common sites are leg wounds, the medial canthus of the eye, and the urethral process. Lesions consist of ulcerative, nodular, or tumorous masses with multiple yellow, necrotic foci containing mineralized, dead larvae.

Diagnosis

Diagnosis is based on the history, clinical findings, and biopsy results. NOTE: Any ulcerative lesion may be complicated by secondary habronemiasis, and the primary cause may be overlooked if biopsy specimens contain inadequate tissue.

Treatment

Treatment objectives include the following:

- Reduce the size of the lesions with surgical debridement or cryosurgery.
- Reduce the inflammation associated with the lesions.
  - When multiple lesions are present, give prednisone or prednisolone at 1 mg/kg for 10 to 14 days, then at 0.5 mg/kg for another 10 to 14 days.
  - If there are only one or two lesions, inject triamcinolone intralesionally (5 to 15 mg/lesion, not to exceed a total of 20 mg); repeat every 10 to 14 days as necessary.
  - For lesions involving the conjunctiva, use frequent topical applications of a corticosteroid ophthalmic preparation.
  - Topical DMSO-corticosteroid preparations may be of value in other regions.
- Eliminate the adult parasites from the stomach with ivermectin.
  - All horses on the premises should be treated.
- Prevent recurrence by reducing the fly population.

TUMORS AND CYSTS *(Text pp. 1222-1228)*

Squamous Cell Carcinoma

Squamous cell carcinomas occur in all domestic species. Although their gross appearance may vary, these tumors are usually slightly raised, broad based, and white-to-pink in color, with a cobbled or cauliflower-like surface. They commonly occur on the eye in cattle; on the lips, nose, eyelids, eyes, and ears in horses (and the penis and sheath in aged stallions and geldings); and on the ears in sheep. They commonly accompany cutaneous papillomas of the udder and teats in Saanen does.

Treatment

The treatment of choice is wide surgical excision. Other treatment modalities include cryosurgery, radiofrequency hyperthermia, radiation therapy, topical application of 5-fluorouracil, and intralesional cisplatin.

Equine Sarcoid

Equine sarcoids are locally aggressive, fibroblastic tumors. They are the most common skin tumor in horses and are most often located on the head, legs, and ventral abdomen.

Clinical signs

Clinically sarcoids are classified as follows:

- Occult (flat)
- Verrucous (warty)
  - Usually less than 6 cm in diameter, they may be sessile and plaquelike or pedunculated; when sessile, the skin is usually thickened with a dry, rough surface.
  - There may be partial or total alopecia.
- Fibroblastic (proud flesh)
  - Fibroblastic sarcoids range from small dermal/subcutaneous nodules covered by intact epidermis to large tumors with an ulcerated surface.
- Verrucose-fibroblastic–combination of verrucous and fibroblastic

Verrucous and occult sarcoids can transform to fibroblastic sarcoids and show features of both types during their transition phase.

Diagnosis

Diagnosis is made histologically on excisional biopsy specimens (see main text). Some cases of equine sarcoid are complicated by secondary bacterial infection, fungal infection, or habronemiasis and may be overlooked if biopsy specimens do not contain adequate tissue.

Treatment

Therapy is usually reserved for the more aggressive fibroblastic forms; benign neglect may be preferable for static verrucous lesions. Many forms of therapy have been described for equine sarcoids, yet none has proven uniformly successful. Options include surgical excision, cryotherapy, intralesional bacillus Calmette-Guérin (BCG), radiation therapy, and intralesional chemotherapy (cisplatin in sesame oil). These therapies are discussed in *Large Animal Internal Medicine,* third edition.

Mastocytoma

Cutaneous mastocytoma (mastocytosis, mast cell tumor) occurs uncommonly in horses. Males are affected 5 to 10 times more frequently than are females. The tumor is self-limiting, and metastasis has not been reported. Several clinical forms have been recognized:

- Single cutaneous nodule, 2 to 20 cm in diameter, usually on the head of mature horses
  - The tumor surface may be haired, hairless, or ulcerated.
  - This is the most common form.
- Diffuse swelling of a lower limb, usually below the carpus or hock
  - The swelling typically is firm, and the overlying tissue is normal; radiographs often demonstrate multifocal regions of soft tissue mineralization.
- Disseminated, focal mast cell lesions in the skin, present at or shortly after birth (rare)

Histopathologic examination of biopsy specimens is diagnostic. The finding of large numbers of eosinophils in a mastocytoma may be an indication that the mass is undergoing spontaneous regression.

Treatment

Surgical excision results in a low recurrence rate, even with incomplete excision. Intralesional or sublesional corticosteroids may be used in solitary lesions that are difficult to surgically resect. Radiotherapy may also be of value when surgery is not desirable.

Equine Melanoma

Melanomas occur in all domestic animals but are most significant in horses. They are commonly reported in horses with gray or white coats, especially in the Arabian, Lipizaner, and Percheron breeds. The incidence increases with age.

Clinical signs and diagnosis

Melanomas are firm, dome-shaped, gray or black, epidermal or dermal masses. They are usually multiple. Initially the overlying skin is intact, but ulceration may occur with larger, rapidly growing tumors. The perineal region and the root of the tail are the predilection sites; other frequently affected sites include the head (parotid gland, eyelids), udder, scrotum, prepuce, and limbs. Metastasis is rare. Diagnosis is based on cytologic and histologic evaluation.

Treatment

Treatment is indicated only if the tumors are repeatedly traumatized or cause difficulty with urination or defecation. Options include surgical excision, cryotherapy, immunotherapy with intralesional BCG, and oral cimetidine (2.5 mg/kg PO three times daily for 3 months).

Cutaneous Lymphosarcoma

Cutaneous lymphosarcoma is uncommon in horses and extremely rare in cattle. Lymphosarcoma is discussed in Chapter 35.

Cysts

Epidermal cysts

Epidermal cysts can be found anywhere on the body; may be single or multiple, congenital or acquired; and range in size from 0.2 to 3 cm in diameter. They are covered by intact epithelium. Epidermal cysts are benign lesions, although painful inflammatory responses and ulceration may result if the cyst is ruptured. Definite diagnosis is made by excisional biopsy, which is curative.

Dermoid cysts

Dermoid cysts are clinically similar to epidermal cysts but are much less common. In horses they may be single or multiple and are most often observed along the dorsal midline, between the withers and the croup. Surgical excision is diagnostic and curative.

Dentigerous cysts

Dentigerous cysts are a congenital defect in horses. A unilateral, saclike swelling is seen at the base of the ear and may be firmly attached to the conchal cartilage or temporal bone. These cysts contain embryonic teeth and have a tendency to fistulate. Treatment consists of surgical excision.

Wattle cysts

Wattle cysts are found in goats and usually develop at the base of the wattle. Nubians may be predisposed. The cysts are congenital, but they may not be apparent until several months of age. Surgical excision is diagnostic and curative.

FROSTBITE *(Text p. 1228)*

The areas most commonly affected by cold injury include the ears, tail, teats, scrotum, and distal limbs. Frozen tissue must be handled gently and thawed rapidly in warm water as soon as possible. Analgesics should be administered. Damaged areas are best left exposed during healing. Premature debridement should be avoided because more tissue may be vital than is initially apparent. Supportive care and restraint to prevent self-mutilation are important.

SKIN DISORDERS OF UNKNOWN OR GENETIC ORIGIN *(Text pp. 1228-1231)*

Equine Seborrhea

In horses, seborrhea (abnormal keratinization) usually involves the mane and tail or the dorsal aspect of the rear cannons. There is scaling and crusting, little or no pruritus, and variable alopecia. Frequent use of antiseborrheic shampoos (every 2 to 3 days initially) is recommended.

Nodular Necrobiosis (Equine Collagenolytic Granuloma)

Nodular necrobiosis is a common skin disease in horses. Lesions consist of one or more firm dermal nodules, 0.5 to 5 cm in diameter, on the neck, withers, and back. There is no pruritus or pain, and the overlying skin is normal; large lesions occasionally ulcerate. Therapy consists of surgical removal or sublesional/intralesional corticosteroids (e.g., triamcinolone, 5 mg/nodule, not to exceed 20 mg total). Systemic prednisolone can be used when many nodules are present.

Miscellaneous Conditions

The following disorders of pigmentation are briefly discussed in *Large Animal Internal Medicine,* third edition: albinism, Arabian fading syndrome, vitiligo (acquired loss of skin and hair pigment), reticulated leukotrichia in quarter horses, and hyperesthetic leukotrichia. Rare skin conditions that are also briefly discussed are hyperelastosis cutis, cutaneous amyloidosis, and generalized granulomatous disease in horses.

PHOTOSENSITIZATION *(Text pp. 1231-1232)*

Photosensitization is an increased response to sunlight, caused by the presence of a photodynamic agent in the skin. The most common cause in livestock is liver disease; other causes include certain drugs and plants (see main text). Lesions range from urticaria with erythema and swelling to necrosis; they most commonly occur in hairless and unpigmented areas.

Treatment

Therapy involves preventing exposure to sunlight, applying soothing topical creams, and preventing reexposure to the photodynamic agent. Prednisolone (1.1 mg/kg/day PO for 10 days) or topical corticosteroids may be helpful.

39

Endocrine and Metabolic Diseases

Consulting Editor NOËL O. DYBDAL

Contributors SHERRILL A. FLEMING • NANCY L. HESTERS • ELAINE HUNT
J. TRAVIS BLACKWELDER • JAMES P. REYNOLDS

Part I: Endocrine Disorders

PITUITARY GLAND *(Text pp. 1233-1236)*

Pituitary Pars Intermedia Dysfunction (Equine Cushing's Disease)

Hypertrophy, hyperplasia, adenomatous hyperplasia, and functional adenoma of the pituitary pars intermedia in horses represent a pathologic continuum associated with a clinical syndrome historically characterized by hirsutism, polydipsia, polyuria, and hyperglycemia.

Clinical signs

The average age of affected horses and ponies is 19 years (range is 7 to 40 years). Because of the slow onset of the disease and the complex metabolic aberrations possible, a variety of clinical signs are seen. Hirsutism, with a thick, long, curly coat that is sometimes not shed, is the clinical sign most commonly associated with equine Cushing's disease. Other manifestations include chronic or recurrent acute laminitis, sole abscesses, polyuria and polydipsia (PU/PD), hyperhidrosis, tachypnea, muscle wasting, supraorbital swellings (fat pads), and sinusitis secondary to periodontal disease.

Diagnosis

Affected horses often have a normal complete blood count (CBC) and serum chemistry panel; some are hyperglycemic. Hyperlipemia is present in a small number of cases and is a grave prognostic sign. Resting plasma cortisol is generally in the normal range but can be moderately elevated. Resting plasma thyroxine (T_4) and triiodothyronine (T_3) concentrations are normal. An overnight dexamethasone suppression is an excellent screening test:

- A heparinized blood sample is collected between 4 and 6 PM; dexamethasone (40 μg/kg or 2 mg/100 lb) is then given intramuscularly (IM).
- A second heparinized blood sample is collected at noon the following day.

In normal horses, plasma cortisol 19 hours after dexamethasone administration is 1 μg/dl or less. Other tests for equine Cushing's disease are outlined in *Large Animal Internal Medicine,* third edition.

Treatment

The most important consideration in long-term maintenance is excellent management with regular deworming, nutrition, and hoof care and rapid response to any potential for infection. Euglycemic horses often do well with only careful stable management. Therapeutic intervention should be considered in horses that are moderately to severely hyperglycemic (glucose greater than 275 mg/dl); options include the following:

- Pergolide–0.5 to 2 mg/day (for horses) once daily or divided twice daily
- Cyproheptadine–initial dose of 0.25 mg/kg orally (PO) once daily for 8 weeks; increase to twice daily for 4 to 8 weeks if no improvement is seen

Diabetes Insipidus

Diabetes insipidus results from decreased release of antidiuretic hormone (ADH) from the posterior pituitary gland. The most common cause in horses is posterior pituitary destruction secondary to pars intermedia enlargement; however, idiopathic diabetes insipidus has been reported. The clinical presentation is of PU/PD in an otherwise normal animal. Differentiating diabetes insipidus from psychogenic water drinking is discussed in Chapter 32.

ADRENAL GLANDS *(Text pp. 1236-1238)*

Adrenal Exhaustion

Adrenal exhaustion and turn-out or let-down syndrome are poorly documented syndromes in horses; they are ascribed to adrenal insufficiency. Proposed causes include abrupt cessation of corticosteroid or adrenocorticotropic hormone (ACTH) administration, chronic stress, and adrenal damage from shock.

Diagnosis

Adrenal insufficiency should be considered in horses with depression, anorexia, weight loss, hyponatremia, hypochloremia, hyperkalemia, or hypoglycemia, particularly if any of the following factors are present: (1) recent race training or other intensive training, (2) corticosteroid administration, or (3) recent history of severe illness or dehydration. The diagnosis is made using an ACTH challenge test (see main text). Management of adrenal suppression may be required after long-term corticosteroid administration.

Pheochromocytoma

Functional adrenal medullary tumors in horses cause excessive sweating, PU/PD, apprehension, colic, tachycardia, dilated pupils, hyperglycemia, and hypertension. Measurement of blood and urinary catecholamines aid in diagnosis.

THYROID GLAND *(Text pp. 1238-1239)*

Thyroid disease is rarely documented in horses, except for hypothyroidism in foals. Nonfunctional adenomas are a relatively common finding in aged adults.

Neonatal Hypothyroidism

Hypothyroidism in neonates generally is caused by ingestion of excess iodine (usually as kelp-containing feed supplements) or plant goitrogens by the pregnant dam. A common and pathognomonic clinical sign is thyroid enlargement (goiter) in the neonate. Other signs variably include incoordination, poor sucking and righting reflexes, hypothermia, tendon contracture or rupture, and retarded bone development. Foals may be born with no apparent signs, but skeletal (particularly tarsal) lesions appear after a few weeks.

Diagnosis and treatment

A thyroid-stimulating hormone (TSH) response test (5 IU of TSH intravenously [IV]) in day-old foals should produced a doubling in T_3 within 1 to 3 hours. Thyroid hormone therapy is effective only in patients with low plasma thyroid hormone concentrations. The hormone dose should be based on the secretion rate (see main text for calculation).

Hypothyroidism in Adult Horses

Functional hypothyroidism has not been documented in adult horses. A diagnosis of hypothyroidism is often based on low serum total T_4 and T_3 and clinical response to thyroid hormone supplementation. However, numerous factors affect the concentrations of thyroid hormones, including phenylbutazone administration and food deprivation. Thyroid hormone therapy increases the metabolic rate and general activity level of even euthyroid animals, but it eventually leads to iatrogenic hypothyroidism secondary to negative feedback.

Thyroid Carcinomas

Thyroid carcinoma should be considered with any rapidly enlarging mass in the thyroid region. Biopsy is needed for definitive diagnosis. Complete excision is recommended.

PARATHYROID GLANDS *(Text pp. 1239-1240)*

Parathyroid dysfunction should be considered in any animal exhibiting hypercalcemia or Ca/PO_4 imbalance. Secondary hyperparathyroidism can result from nutritional causes (nutritional secondary hyperparathyroidism) or vitamin D toxicosis (both discussed in the following sections).

PANCREAS *(Text p. 1240)*

Diabetes Mellitus

Primary diabetes mellitus is a disorder involving the pancreatic beta cells. It results in decreased insulin levels and therefore insulin-sensitive hyperglycemia. Primary diabetes mellitus in horses is rare and in all reports has been secondary to chronic pancreatitis. Secondary diabetes mellitus encompasses conditions in which hyperglycemia and glucosuria occur because of resistance to the effects of insulin; plasma insulin levels are normal or elevated. Most cases in horses are associated with equine Cushing's disease (see pp. 1233-1236).

Part II: Metabolic Disorders

KETOSIS IN RUMINANTS (ACETONEMIA) *(Text pp. 1241-1246)*

Ketosis is characterized by abnormally increased concentrations of ketone bodies (acetoacetic acid [AcAc], acetone [Ac], and β-hydroxybutyric acid [BHB]) in the tissues and body fluids. Most clinical cases occur in cows in the first 6 weeks after calving, especially high-producing cows that are overconditioned at calving. The incidence of clinical ketosis increases with parity.

Causes

Primary, spontaneous ketosis results from a negative energy balance during late pregnancy and early lactation. Secondary ketosis may result from any disease process occurring in early lactation that reduces feed intake (e.g., metritis, traumatic reticuloperitonitis, abomasal displacements, parturient paresis, retained placenta). It can also result from ingestion of preformed ketones in the diet (e.g., silage that is high in lactic or butyric acid). Cobalt deficiency has also been implicated.

Clinical signs

Signs of clinical ketosis include a gradual loss of appetite and decreases in milk production and body weight. Physical findings include normal vital signs; firm, dry feces; moderate depression; and sometimes reluctance to move. Rumen motility is decreased if the animal has been anorectic for several days. Pica is occasionally seen. The odor of ketones often can be detected on the breath and in the milk. Transient central nervous system (CNS) signs, such as staggering and blindness, may occur. A thorough physical examination allows differentiation of primary and secondary ketosis.

Diagnosis

Laboratory findings in clinical ketosis typically include blood glucose of 20 to 40 mg/dl, total blood ketones greater than 30 mg/dl, total urine ketones greater than 84 mg/dl, and total milk ketones greater than 10 mg/dl. Cows with subclinical ketosis have no clinical signs of ketosis but have low-normal blood glucose, total blood ketones of 10 to 30 mg/dl, and total milk ketones of approximately 2 mg/dl. Values in animals with secondary ketosis usually fall between the ranges for clinical and subclinical ketosis.

Urine ketones. Commercially available urine dipsticks or tablets used for monitoring diabetic humans detect Ac and AcAc in urine. However, normal lactating cows may test positive for urine ketones, so measuring milk ketones is a more reliable test (see main text).

Other biochemical indices. Onset of ketosis may be associated with elevations of liver enzymes and abnormal liver function tests. However, the degree of liver dysfunction is mild compared with that of cows with fatty liver syndrome (see Chapter 31).

Treatment

Treatment of secondary ketosis requires correction of the primary condition and provision of an adequate diet. Several therapeutic options are available for clinical primary ketosis:

- 50% glucose (dextrose), 100 to 500 ml IV, repeated as necessary to prevent relapse
  - Continuous glucose infusion at 0.5 g/min IV until milk ketones are negative; slow infusion of 20 L of 2.5% glucose with 0.45% saline over 24 hours
  - With both intravenous regimens, monitoring for hypoglycemia is required when therapy is discontinued.
- Oral glucose precursors in the feed or as a drench
  - Propylene glycol drench at 225 g (8 oz) twice daily for 2 days, then 110 g (4 oz) sid for 2 days (NOTE: overuse can have a deleterious effect on rumen flora.)
  - Glycerol at 500 g twice daily for up to 10 days
  - Sodium propionate (125 to 250 g), ammonium lactate (120 g), or sodium lactate (360 g) twice daily
- Glucocorticoids–dexamethasone (0.04 mg/kg once) or betamethasone
  - Overdosing may reduce feed intake and exacerbate fatty liver syndrome if present.
- Chloral hydrate 30 g PO, followed by 7 g bid for several days
  - Sedative effects are helpful in cows with nervous ketosis.

Low dosages of long-acting insulin (e.g., human Ultralente recombinant insulin at 0.25 U/kg subcutaneously [SC] once per day or every 48 hours) may be a useful adjunct to intravenous glucose and glucocorticoid therapy.

Supportive care. Nursing care is important. Supportive therapy may include rumen transfaunations; provision of a variety of palatable feeds; exercise; and dietary supplementation with vitamin B_{12}, cobalt, niacin, and nicotinamide. Monensin may have both therapeutic and prophylactic value, although it is currently not approved for use in lactating cows in the United States. Prevention and control are discussed in *Large Animal Internal Medicine,* third edition.

DISORDERS OF CALCIUM METABOLISM *(Text pp. 1248-1253)*

Bovine Parturient Paresis (Milk Fever, Hypocalcemia)

Parturient paresis is acute or peracute flaccid paralysis and somnolence affecting lactating dairy cows. It usually occurs within 48 to 72 hours of parturition and is seen most often in high-producing cows, particularly those fed a high-calcium diet during the dry period. Most cases occur in cows more than 5 years of age; there is a gradual increase in incidence with parity. Parturient paresis should be considered an emergency, necessitating prompt intravenous therapy with calcium solutions.

Clinical signs

There are three clinical stages of parturient paresis:

- Stage 1–the cow is still able to stand but shows signs of hypersensitivity and excitability.
  - Signs include head bobbing, ear twitching, fine tremors over the flank and

loin, slight ataxia when walking, and restlessness and shuffling of the hind feet while standing.
    - Bellowing and open-mouth breathing with tongue extension may also be noted.
- Stage 2–the cow is unable to stand but is able to maintain sternal recumbency.
    - Signs include depression, anorexia, dry muzzle, and hypothermia with cold extremities; if the ambient temperature is greater than 38° C (100° F), the cow may be hyperthermic.
    - Tachycardia with decreased intensity of heart sounds may be found on auscultation.
    - Gastrointestinal stasis (bloat, absence of feces, loss of anal tone); inability to urinate; retained placenta; and dilated, sluggish, or unresponsive pupils may also be found.
    - The cow lies in sternal recumbency with the head tucked into the flank.
- Stage 3–there is continued loss of consciousness to the point of coma.
    - Such animals have complete muscle flaccidity, are unresponsive to stimuli and unable to maintain sternal recumbency, and suffer from severe bloat.
    - The pulse may be nearly undetectable and the heart rate as high as 120 beats/min.
    - Cows in this stage may not survive more than a few hours.

Diagnosis

Because of the urgency of treating acute hypocalcemia, diagnosis and treatment are usually based on clinical signs. Pretreatment blood samples should be taken so that the diagnosis can be confirmed; cows with a serum calcium level less than 7.5 mg/dl are considered hypocalcemic. When hypoalbuminemia is present, a corrected total calcium may be calculated:

$$\text{Corrected Ca} = \text{Measured Ca (mg/dl)} - \text{Albumin (g/dl)} + 3.5$$

Other serum chemistry findings. Cows with parturient paresis are usually hypophosphatemic (as low as 2.1 mg/dl), hypermagnesemic (2.2 to 2.7 mg/dl), and hyperglycemic (95 to 130 mg/dl). A stress leukogram and moderately elevated creatine phosphokinase (CPK) are common findings.

Treatment

The recommended treatment is intravenous calcium gluconate at a rate of 1 g/45 kg (100 lb) body weight. Usually a single 500-ml bottle containing 8 to 11 g of calcium is adequate; in large, heavily lactating cows a second bottle administered SC may be beneficial. Relapse within 24 to 48 hours occurs in up to 30% of cows and requires additional therapy. Incomplete milking can reduce the incidence of relapse.

Precautions. Calcium-containing solutions should be administered slowly (over 10 to 20 minutes) during continuous cardiac auscultation. If severe arrhythmias or bradycardia develop, administration should be stopped. Once the heartbeat has returned to normal, administration may be resumed at a slower rate. Cardiac arrhythmias may be abolished with intravenous atropine or 10% $MgSO_4$ solution (100 to 400 ml IV).

Mild cases. Oral calcium can be used in mild cases. Calcium propionate in a propylene glycol gel is best. The recommended dosage is 50 g of calcium.

Unresponsive cases. Cows that have not responded within 8 to 12 hours after treatment should be reevaluated, and treatment should be repeated if necessary. Injection with 1-α-hydroxycholecalciferol (1 μg/kg, half IV and half IM) is effective in cows that do not respond to calcium therapy; cows generally recover within 12 hours. Cows that show the expected response to calcium therapy but do not stand should be suspected of having secondary complications, such as musculoskeletal trauma or ischemic muscle necrosis.

Prevention of parturient paresis is discussed in *Large Animal Internal Medicine,* third edition.

Hypocalcemia in Sheep and Goats

Sheep

Ewes are most likely to develop hypocalcemia during the last 4 to 6 weeks of pregnancy. Food deprivation or forced exercise may precipitate hypocalcemia. Flaccid paralysis is the primary sign, but tetany is seen in some cases. Pregnancy toxemia (see Chapter 31) and hypocalcemia can be difficult to differentiate on the basis of clinical signs. Testing for urinary ketones is helpful.

Goats

Hypocalcemia can occur during lactation in high-producing dairy goats. It can also occur during late pregnancy, particularly in does carrying multiple fetuses. Hyperexcitability or mild depression and ataxia are the usual signs observed; unlike dairy cows, untreated does may not become recumbent or progress to coma.

Treatment

Administration of intravenous calcium solutions (1 g/45 kg) results in rapid recovery. The same precautions with intravenous calcium administration as discussed for cattle apply.

Hypocalcemia in Horses

Lactation tetany most often occurs in mares approximately 10 days after foaling or 1 to 2 days after weaning. Animals at greatest risk are those maintained on pasture only or used for hard physical labor (e.g., draft mares). Prolonged transportation can also predispose horses to hypocalcemia (transit tetany). Clinical signs include tetany, profuse sweating, anxiety, tachycardia, arrhythmias, and synchronous diaphragmatic flutter. Prolapse of the nictitating membrane is uncommon. Intravenous calcium, as described for cattle, results in rapid recovery.

Nutritional Secondary Hyperparathyroidism

Nutritional secondary hyperparathyroidism (NSH; big head, bran disease, osteodystrophia fibrosa) is induced by an absolute or relative calcium deficiency caused by an excess of dietary phosphorus. It is most common in horses but is now a rare disease. High-phosphorus diets usually consist of grass hay with large amounts of grain or bran. Horses grazing pastures high in oxalates are also predisposed.

Clinical signs

The early stages are characterized by intermittent shifting lameness and stiff, creaking joints. Spontaneous fractures of the sesamoids and phalanges may also occur. As NSH progresses, affected animals develop thickening of the mandible and the facial bones. Visible facial swelling is bilateral but not always symmetric. The bone enlargement is soft initially and hardens later. Difficulty chewing and breathing and epiphora (from occlusion of the lacrimal ducts) can result.

Diagnosis

Serum calcium and phosphorus are usually maintained within normal limits. The worst aberration that is likely to be seen is low-normal calcium and high-normal phosphorus. Serum alkaline phosphatase may be slightly elevated. The most useful measurement is urinary fractional excretion of PO_4; values greater than 4% suggest excess phosphorous intake.

Treatment

Restoring the dietary Ca/PO_4 ratio to between 1:1 and 2:1 usually resolves the lameness in about 8 weeks. However, facial distortion, once present, is likely to be permanent.

Hypercalcemia

Hypercalcemia is most likely to occur in horses. Causes include renal disease (see Chapter 32), certain neoplasms (gastric squamous cell carcinoma, lymphosarcoma), and excess vitamin D.

Excess vitamin D

Hypervitaminosis D can result from oversupplementation or from ingestion of plants such as *Cestrum diurnum* (wild jasmine) and *Solanum sodomaeum* (in Hawaii). It leads to hypercalcemia and hyperphosphatemia. Affected animals have limb stiffness with painful flexor tendons and suspensory ligaments (soft tissue mineralization). Polydipsia and polyuria with low urine specific gravity may also be found. Removal of the vitamin D source results in recovery in mild cases.

DISORDERS OF PHOSPHORUS METABOLISM
(Text pp. 1254-1256)

Chronic Phosphorus Deficiency/Hypophosphatemia

Most cases of phosphorus deficiency are primary (absolute dietary deficiency). Secondary PO_4 deficiency is mediated by other factors (e.g., diets high in calcium or low in vitamin D). Secondary hypophosphatemia is more likely to occur when the dietary PO_4 level is marginal.

Phosphorus deficiency in natural diets is widespread and is dependent on the PO_4 content of the soil. Young, growing animals and pregnant or lactating females are most severely affected.

Clinical signs

The earliest signs of chronic PO_4 deficiency include decreased feed consumption, weight loss, retarded growth, poor milk production, and reduced fertility. As the deficiency progresses, adult animals develop symptoms of osteomalacia, which include stiffness and shifting lameness, and spontaneous fractures that do not heal. These animals often remain recumbent, although they are alert and continue to eat. Rickets develops in young growing animals (see Chapter 36).

Other problems. Animals deficient in PO_4, as well as in other minerals, commonly develop pica, which may lead to traumatic reticuloperitonitis or botulism (from chewing bones). Acute, severe hypophosphatemia can cause recumbency and muscle weakness in late pregnancy and early lactation. Another disease syndrome associated with PO_4 deficiency in dairy cattle is postparturient hemoglobinuria (PPH; see Chapter 35).

Diagnosis

Depressed serum PO_4 (1.5 to 3.5 mg/dl) is associated with PO_4 deficiency. However, serum PO_4 may be maintained within the normal range for a long period after the onset of PO_4 deficiency, so normal serum PO_4 should not be used to rule out PO_4 deficiency. Serum calcium levels are usually unaffected. In severe cases, serum alkaline phosphatase is elevated. A ratio of ash to organic matter in bone of less than 3:1 is the most accurate means of confirming chronic PO_4 deficiency. Hypophosphatemia (less than 1.5 mg/dl) is a common finding in cows with PPH.

Treatment

Treatment consists of supplementing dietary PO_4. Two commonly used supplements are dicalcium phosphate and defluorinated rock phosphate. Others include bone meal, monosodium or disodium phosphate, ammonium phosphate, and phosphoric acid. The Ca/PO_4 ratio of the diet must be monitored when supplements are used; a ratio of 2:1 is considered optimal.

Acute, severe hypophosphatemia. Feed-grade monosodium phosphate (200 to 300 g) in a warm water drench or by stomach tube provides 50 to 60 g of PO_4. Commercial gel and paste preparations containing monosodium phosphate can be used in place of drenches. Options for intravenous administration of PO_4 are discussed in *Large Animal Internal Medicine,* third edition.

DISORDERS OF MAGNESIUM METABOLISM
(Text pp. 1256-1260)

Hypomagnesemia

Hypomagnesemia is magnesium ion deficiency in the blood and cerebrospinal fluid. It affects only ruminant species and is highly fatal. Lactating beef cows (within 60 days of calving) pastured on cool season grasses or cereal crops are most susceptible. Spring-calving cows are classically affected, but mortalities in the fall and winter are common in the southern United States. Lactating ewes and dairy goats are also susceptible. Hypomagnesemia is usually accompanied by hypocalcemia.

Contributing factors

Clinical signs usually are precipitated by lactation, cold stress, transport, or anorexia. Clinical syndromes can be categorized on the basis of predisposing factors: grass tetany (includes wheat, oat, and barley staggers), transport tetany, winter tetany, and tetany in milk-fed calves housed indoors.

Clinical signs

Lactating cows become anorectic and separate from the herd. They are alert and hyperexcitable, and they may charge. Other early signs include markedly erect ears, ear twitching, hyperesthesia, muscle fasciculations, head and neck tremors, and a high-stepping forelimb gait. Nystagmus, exaggerated chewing, salivation, and a snapping eyelid retraction are seen. Hyperthermia, tachypnea, hyperpnea, and tachycardia with loud heart sounds are also found.

Clinical course. Aberrant behavior with bellowing and frenzied galloping progresses to a staggering, uncoordinated gait and lateral recumbency. Violent episodes of opisthotonos and clonic convulsions can be precipitated by any stimuli, and these alternate with periods of tetanic muscle spasms. Death can occur within 30 to 60 minutes of seizure onset. The animal often is simply found dead.

Mild or chronic hypomagnesemia. Mild or chronic lactation tetany is a vague syndrome that may affect many animals in a group. Serum magnesium levels are often low, although no clinical signs are apparent. Inappetence, unthriftiness, declining milk yields, odd facial expressions, and slight changes in behavior may be noted. This form may suddenly progress to the clinical form. Affected cattle are also predisposed to parturient paresis.

Hypomagnesemia in calves. Whole-milk tetany usually occurs in calves 2 to 4 months of age. Clinical signs are similar to those in adults; in addition, the calf's eyes may bulge or be withdrawn and the third eyelid may prolapse. Diarrhea may exacerbate subclinical hypomagnesemia and complicate the clinical picture.

Diagnosis

Because of the need for rapid therapy, diagnosis is often made on the basis of clinical signs and history. Low serum magnesium levels (less than 1.2 mg/dl) confirm the diagnosis. Urine magnesium levels are also low (less than 2.5 mg/dl). A decrease in urine magnesium precedes declining serum levels, which can be helpful in confirming a subclinical or herd problem.

Fractional excretion. One of the best means of diagnosing ongoing or impending hypomagnesemia is with urine fractional excretion of magnesium. Calculating FE is described in Chapter 22. The average FE of magnesium in nonlactating, nonpregnant dairy cows is 6.5% to 8.3 %. Dramatically lowered values suggest inadequate dietary magnesium.

Other laboratory findings. Hypophosphatemia and hypocalcemia are common; in fact, concurrent hypocalcemia is necessary for the expression of tetanic convulsions associated with clinical hypomagnesemia. Serum potassium, CPK, and aspartate aminotransferase may be elevated in recumbent cows. Urine magnesium levels of less than 1 mg/dl and vitreous humor magnesium levels less than 1.4 mg/dl support a postmortem diagnosis of acute, terminal hypomagnesemic tetany.

Treatment

Slow intravenous administration of a commercial calcium borogluconate solution containing 5% magnesium hypophosphate (to provide 2 to 3 g Mg over 10 minutes) is the treatment of choice. The heart should be monitored carefully during treatment. Solutions containing potassium should be avoided. Other options include subcutaneous injection of $MgSO_4$ (200 to 400 ml of a 25% solution) and administration of a magnesium-rich enema (e.g., 60 g $MgCl_2$ in 250 to 500 ml warm water).

CNS signs. Animals should be left undisturbed after magnesium administration. Chloral hydrate (50 mg/kg IV) may prevent convulsions while equilibration of administered magnesium occurs. Tranquilizers can be given IM, but intravenous administration of these drugs should be avoided. Treatment is often unsuccessful if the cow is already comatose.

Relapse. Relapse is common within 3 to 6 hours of treatment, so animals must be monitored after therapy. Relapse may be prevented by subcutaneous administration of 50% $MgSO_4$ solution (125-150 ml), but this hypertonic solution may result in tissue sloughing. An alternative is oral MgO_2 (60 g/day for 5 to 6 days). Supplementation with legume hay may also prevent relapse.

Calves and sheep. Hypomagnesemic calves respond to intravenous therapy with 125 ml of a 6% magnesium borogluconate preparation. Affected sheep benefit from slow intravenous infusion of 50 to 150 ml of a commercial 5% magnesium preparation that also contains calcium.

Prevention and control are discussed in *Large Animal Internal Medicine,* third edition.

Hypermagnesemia

Hypermagnesemia in ruminants has been associated with severe renal insufficiency and with administration of magnesium-containing rumenatorics or laxatives. Clinical signs of hypermagnesemia in humans include hypotension, areflexia, respiratory paralysis, and cardiac arrest. Intravenous calcium gluconate may reverse the effects of hypermagnesemia, but commercial calcium gluconate products for ruminants all contain magnesium.

BOVINE SOMATOTROPIN *(Text pp. 1261-1264)*

Bovine somatotropin (growth hormone) is available for commercial use in dairy cattle. Somatotropin acts in young cattle to promote growth, but in lactating cows it stimulates milk production. The effects of recombinant bovine somatotropin on metabolism, feed intake, milk production, body condition, and fertility, as well as recommendations for its use, are discussed in *Large Animal Internal Medicine,* third edition.

40

Diseases of Muscle

Consulting Editors STEPHANIE J. VALBERG • DAVID R. HODGSON

Contributors SHARON J. SPIER • GARY P. CARLSON • STEVEN M. PARISH
JOHN MAAS • MICHAEL MURPHY • ANDREW DART

EVALUATON OF THE MUSCULAR SYSTEM *(Text pp. 1266-1269)*

Clinical evaluation of the muscular system begins with a thorough history and physical examination. Serum activities of creatine kinase (CK), aspartate aminotransferase (AST), and isoenzymes of lactate dehydrogenase (LDH) and measurement of plasma/serum myoglobin are useful in determining whether muscle cell damage is a predominant feature of a suspected muscle disease. Urinalysis, renal fractional excretions, exercise testing, electromyography (EMG), and muscle biopsy can be helpful in selected cases. These tests are discussed in Chapter 40 of *Large Animal Internal Medicine,* third edition.

DISORDERS OF MUSCLE TONE *(Text pp. 1270-1276)*

Myotonia

Myotonia congenita is characterized by delayed muscle relaxation after mechanical stimulation or voluntary contraction. Among large animal species, it has been reported in horses and goats.

Clinical findings in horses

Myotonia congenita in horses is usually detected in the first year of life. Affected animals commonly have very well-developed muscles and mild pelvic limb stiffness. Bilateral bulging (dimpling) of the thigh and rump muscles often is obvious. Percussion of affected muscles exacerbates the dimpling; the muscles may remain contracted for a minute or more and relax slowly. In most cases, signs do not progress beyond 6 to 12 months of age.

Severe signs of myotonia that progress to marked muscle atrophy have been reported in Quarter Horse foals. Abnormalities in other organ systems (e.g., ocular, reproductive) may also be found.

Clinical findings in goats

Signs in goats are usually seen by 6 weeks of age and vary from stiffness after rest to marked rigidity after visual, tactile, or auditory stimulation. Affected goats are commonly referred to as "fainting goats." The animal remains clinically affected for life, but signs are not progressive.

Diagnosis

Tentative diagnosis can often be made on the basis of age, clinical signs, and prolonged contractions after muscle stimulation. Definitive diagnosis is based on EMG findings (see text). Muscle biopsy may be helpful.

Treatment and prognosis

There is no specific therapy. Phenytoin may provide some relief. Signs may ameliorate somewhat with age in mildly affected animals. In more severely affected horses the condition may progress to the point where the animal is no longer able to move without great pain and difficulty.

Hyperkalemic Periodic Paralysis

Hyperkalemic periodic paralysis (HYPP) is an autosomal dominant disorder affecting quarter horses (purebred and crossbred), American paint horses, and Appaloosas that are descendants of the Quarter Horse sire Impressive. It is characterized by episodes of muscle fasciculations and weakness. Affected horses seem normal between episodes. Typically, episodes become evident by 2 to 3 years of age, but some affected horses never show clinical signs. Precipitating factors include fasting, transport, stress, dietary changes (especially to high-potassium diets), cold weather, pregnancy, and concurrent disease.

Clinical findings

Episodes typically begin with a brief period of myotonia, which may include prolapse of the third eyelid. Sweating and muscle fasciculations are common. Stimulation and attempts to move may exacerbate the fasciculations; some horses develop severe muscle cramping. Muscular weakness during episodes is characteristic and may progress to swaying, staggering, dog-sitting, or recumbency within a few minutes. The horse remains bright and alert but may seem anxious; heart and respiratory rates may be elevated. Respiratory stridor or distress occurs in some affected horses. Episodes usually last from 15 to 60 minutes.

Diagnosis

Episodic muscle tremors and weakness in a quarter horse that is a descendant of Impressive is strongly suggestive of HYPP. In most cases, serum potassium concentrations are elevated during episodes but return to normal as signs abate. DNA testing using EDTA-preserved whole blood is definitive and the test of choice.

Treatment

In mild cases and early in an episode, signs can often be aborted with light exercise or by feeding grain or corn syrup. Other treatment options include epinephrine (3 ml of 1:1000 solution/500 kg intramuscularly [IM]) and acetazolamide (3 mg/kg orally [PO] two or three times daily).

In severe cases, calcium gluconate (0.2 to 0.4 ml/kg of a 23% solution, diluted in 1 L 5% dextrose) often provides immediate improvement. Dextrose (6 ml/kg of 5% solution intravenously [IV]) alone or combined with sodium bicarbonate (1 to 2 mEq/kg) enhances intracellular movement of potassium. Tracheostomy may be necessary in horses with severe upper airway obstruction.

Control

Control is directed at decreasing dietary potassium and increasing renal potassium loss:

- Avoid high-potassium feeds such as alfalfa and brome hays, canola oil, soybean meal or oil, and molasses.
  - Suitable feedstuffs include timothy or bermuda grass hay, grain, and beet pulp.
  - Complete rations for HYPP horses are commercially available.
- Feed the horse several times per day.
- Exercise the horse regularly or allow frequent access to a large paddock or yard.
- Consider giving either acetazolamide (2 to 4 mg/kg PO two or three times daily) or hydrochlorothiazide (0.5 to 1 mg/kg PO twice daily).

Muscle Cramping and Dietary Electrolytes

Some horses develop muscle stiffness and occasional elevations in serum CK when fed a diet deficient in sodium or potassium. Serum electrolyte values may be normal, although renal fractional excretions may reflect chronic deficiency.

Fractional excretion of electrolytes

Renal fractional excretions (FE) can be calculated after collection of blood and urine and analysis for creatinine, potassium, and chloride concentrations:

$$FE_x\ (\%) = \frac{[S_{Cr} \times U_x]}{[U_{Cr} \times S_x]} \times 100$$

where

U = urine
S = serum
X = measured electrolyte
Cr = creatinine

Normal values for FE of electrolytes depend on the horse's diet. Normal ranges for horses consuming grass, hay, and a sweet feed mix with available salt are as follows:

- FE_{Na}–0.04% to 0.08%
- Fe_K–35% to 80%

Treatment and control

Supplementation of the equine diet with salt is a necessity. Adding 1 to 2 oz of loose salt to the grain is often the best means of supplementing salt in horses. Some horses require more salt to maintain an adequate sodium balance.

Exhaustion in Endurance Horses

Muscle cramping in horses is common during prolonged exercise in hot, humid weather. Affected horses are stiff and have painful cramping in the locomotor muscles. Exhausted horses are also dull, depressed, dehydrated, tachycardic, tachypneic, and hyperthermic. Myoglobinuria generally is not a feature, nor are there marked elevations in serum CK or AST. Common electrolyte abnormalities include hypochloremic metabolic alkalosis, hypokalemia, hypomagnesemia, and hypocalcemia. Synchronous diaphragmatic flutter may therefore be seen.

Treatment and control

In mild cases, signs abate with rest or light exercise. If metabolic derangements are present, treatment for these disorders (e.g., oral or intravenous polyionic fluids) and cooling are indicated. Administration of solutions containing sodium bicarbonate are contraindicated. Addition of 2 oz sodium chloride and 1 oz potassium chloride to the feed each day is recommended for horses with recurrent cramping.

Synchronous Diaphragmatic Flutter

Synchronous diaphragmatic flutter (SDF), or "thumps," usually occurs in horses with derangements in fluid and electrolyte balance. Inciting causes include endurance exercise, hypocalcemia, digestive disturbances, and furosemide therapy.

Clinical and laboratory findings

The classic sign of SDF is twitching in the flank region as the diaphragm contracts synchronously with the heart. Exhausted endurance horses with SDF may also demonstrate dehydration, inappropriate sweating responses, persistent hyperthermia, depression, anorexia, and ileus. The most consistent metabolic derangement is low serum ionized calcium with hypochloremic metabolic alkalosis.

Treatment and control

In most cases, SDF abates when the underlying cause resolves. Most horses rapidly respond to intravenous calcium solutions (see following discussion). Electrolyte supplementation and some dietary manipulations (e.g., reduction in calcium intake a few days before an endurance ride, restriction of alfalfa) may reduce the incidence in endurance horses with recurrent SDF.

Hypocalcemia in Horses

Hypocalcemia (lactation tetany, transport tetany, eclampsia) is relatively rare in horses. Inciting factors include heavy lactation, prolonged transport, hard work, and ingestion of blister beetles (cantharidin toxicosis; see Chapter 30).

Clinical findings

Signs variably include increased muscle tone, stiff and stilted gait, rear limb ataxia, muscle fasciculations (especially temporal, masseter, and triceps), trismus ("lockjaw"), dysphagia, salivation, anxiety, profuse sweating, tachycardia, hyperthermia, arrhythmias, SDF, convulsions, coma, and death. In lactating mares the signs may be progressive over 24 to 48 hours. An important differential diagnosis is tetanus.

Diagnosis

Clinical signs are often highly suggestive of hypocalcemia and are related to the serum calcium concentration:

- More than 8 mg/dl–signs may be limited to increased excitability
- From 5 to 8 mg/dl–tetanic spasms and incoordination
- Less than 5 mg/dl–recumbency and stupor

Treatment and control

Treatment involves intravenous administration of calcium solutions, such as those recommended for treatment of parturient paresis in cattle. Administration at a dose rate of 250 to 500 ml/500 kg, diluted 1:4 with saline or dextrose and given slowly IV, often results in full recovery. Infusion should be stopped temporarily if there is an alteration in heart rate or rhythm during administration. Treatment may be repeated in 15 to 30 minutes if no response is seen after the first infusion. In some cases, complete recovery takes several days. Relapse can occur.

Ear Tick–Associated Muscle Cramping

Infestations of the ear tick *Otobius megnini* can cause intermittent severe muscle cramping involving the pectoral, triceps, abdominal, or semitendinosus/semimembranosus muscles in horses. The cramps last from minutes to a few hours and cause severe pain that often resembles colic. Percussion of the affected muscles results in a myotonic cramp. Serum CK activities are elevated (4000 to 170,000 IU/L). The ticks can be identified in the external ear canal. Local treatment using pyrethrins and piperonyl butoxide results in recovery within 12 to 36 hours.

NONEXERTIONAL RHABDOMYOLYSIS *(Text pp. 1276-1285)*

Rhabdomyolysis unassociated with exertion can be divided into three broad categories:

- Inflammatory myopathies–clostridial myonecrosis, myopathies associated with *Streptococcus equi* infection, virus-associated myopathy, *Sarcocystis* infection
- Nutritional and toxic myopathies–nutritional myodegeneration, toxic myopathies
- Traumatic rhabdomyolysis–compartment (downer, muscle crush) syndrome in cattle, postanesthetic localized myoneuropathy, generalized anesthetic reactions

The specific conditions listed are discussed in the following sections.

Clostridial Myonecrosis

Acute myonecrosis may be caused by various species of clostridial organisms. Synonyms include blackleg, malignant edema, false blackleg, and gas gangrene. Clostridial organisms may enter the body via the gastrointestinal (GI) tract and lodge in the muscle and other tissues in the dormant spore form. When local tissue conditions are suitable, the spores rapidly germinate. Most reports of clostridial myonecrosis in horses show an association with puncture wounds or intramuscular injections.

Clinical findings

Clostridial myonecrosis is highly fatal and rapidly progressive, with development of tremors, ataxia, dyspnea, recumbency, coma, and death within 12 to 24 hours. Many affected animals are found prostrate or dead. Animals that are still alive usually are severely depressed, febrile, tachypneic, anorectic, and lame.

Crepitus may be detectable, indicating subcutaneous gas production. If a wound is present, there may be a malodorous, serosanguineous discharge.

Diagnosis

Hematologic and serum biochemical analyses usually reflect a generalized state of debilitation and toxemia. Elevations in serum CK and AST are typically found but often do not reflect the magnitude of the muscle damage. Diagnosis can be made from direct smears and fluorescent antibody testing of tissue aspirates, as well as by anaerobic bacterial culture.

Treatment and prognosis

Although clostridial myonecrosis is often fatal, aggressive therapy may be successful in individual cases. Successful treatment involves the following:

- Antibiotic therapy–penicillin at 44,000 U/kg IV every 2 to 4 hours until the animal is stable (1 to 5 days)
  - Thereafter, continue treatment every 6 hours or switch to procaine penicillin (15 to 20 mg/kg IM bid) or metronidazole (15 mg/kg PO three or four times daily).
- Aggressive surgical debridement (including fenestration or fasciotomy)
- Supportive care–fluid therapy, analgesics, and possibly corticosteroids (e.g., short-term treatment with dexamethasone, prednisolone, or hydrocortisone)

The prognosis for survival is guarded to poor in all cases. If treatment is attempted, the owner should be made aware that extensive skin sloughing may occur and will complicate recovery. Prevention of clostridial diseases is discussed in *Large Animal Internal Medicine,* third edition.

Myopathies Associated With *S. equi* Infection

Vasculopathy

Some horses exposed to *S. equi* or vaccinated against strangles within the previous 4 weeks develop a severe vasculopathy characterized by infarction of skeletal muscle, skin, GI tract, and lungs. Presenting signs may include colic or severe lameness. Leukocytosis, hyperfibrinogenemia, hypoproteinemia, and extreme elevations in serum CK and AST are present. Treatment with penicillin and dexamethasone (0.12 to 0.2 mg/kg IV), followed by tapering doses of prednisone (1 mg/kg initially), is effective in some cases. Without aggressive corticosteroid therapy, affected horses usually die from intestinal infarction.

Severe rhabdomyolysis

Some Quarter Horses exposed to *S. equi* develop severe rhabdomyolysis characterized by malaise and rapid atrophy of the lumbar and gluteal muscles. There may be no signs of strangles, but mild to moderate elevations in serum CK and AST (1000 to 40,000 IU/L) are seen. Diagnosis is based on a history of exposure to *S. equi,* elevated serum CK, and muscle biopsy. Treatment involves antibiotic therapy and immunosuppressive therapy (e.g., prednisone at 1 mg/kg for 7 to 10 days, then tapered down over 1 month). Some horses require prolonged therapy.

Virus-Associated Myopathy

Necrosis of skeletal or cardiac muscle often occurs in association with some viral diseases, including equine influenza, equine infectious anemia, bovine ephemeral fever, malignant catarrhal fever, bovine virus diarrhea, bluetongue, and foot-and-mouth disease.

Sarcocystosis

Cysts of the sporozoan parasite *Sarcocystis* are commonly seen in histologic sections of heart and in esophageal and skeletal muscle of clinically normal ruminants and horses. However, these agents cause multisystemic dysfunction in heavily infected animals.

Clinical findings

Clinical infection causes fever, anorexia, salivation, weight loss, weakness, muscle fasciculations, severe depression, and sometimes death. Fever is the earliest sign and is biphasic (at 15 to 19 days and at 25 to 42 days postinfection). During the second febrile episode, affected animals commonly develop other clinical problems, the most prominent being anemia. Extravascular hemolysis occurs, and hemorrhage into many tissues is common. Mortality is greatest during this phase of the disease. Surviving animals often continue to be inappetant and have decreased weight gain; muscle atrophy; and hair loss on the neck, rump, and tail.

Diagnosis

Diagnosis of sarcocystosis relies on the history, clinical signs, laboratory evaluations, and muscle biopsy. Laboratory findings during the second febrile phase may include elevations in serum urea nitrogen, bilirubin, sorbitol dehydrogenase, CK, AST, and LDH. If animals survive, these indices usually return to normal in about 2 weeks.

Treatment

Specific treatment is effective only in the early stages. Experimentally, treatment with amprolium or an ionophore antibiotic before the second febrile episode can prevent development of clinical sarcocystosis in cattle.

Nutritional Myodegeneration

Nutritional myodegeneration (NMD; white muscle disease, stiff lamb disease, nutritional muscular dystrophy) is a myodegenerative disease of cardiac and skeletal muscle caused by a dietary deficiency of selenium or vitamin E. Bilaterally symmetrical myodegeneration is a consistent finding and is characterized grossly by pale discoloration and dry appearance of affected muscle, white streaks in muscle bundles, calcification, and intramuscular edema.

Epidemiology

NMD is most common in young, rapidly growing calves, lambs, kids, and foals, particularly those born to dams that consumed selenium-deficient diets during pregnancy. Forages and grains produced in the northeastern and eastern seaboards and northwestern regions of the United States are most likely to be selenium deficient. Other factors influencing the selenium content of feedstuffs are discussed in Chapter 40 of *Large Animal Internal Medicine,* third edition.

Clinical findings

There are two distinct clinical syndromes:

- Cardiac–acute or peracute signs of myocardial decompensation
  - Onset usually is sudden; the animal is found either severely debilitated or dead.
  - Signs include depression, dyspnea, foamy nasal discharge (may be blood tinged), profound weakness, recumbency, and a rapid and often irregular heartbeat.
  - Rectal temperature usually is normal but may be elevated by muscular effort,
  - Death commonly occurs in less than 24 hours despite therapy.
- Skeletal–slower onset of muscle weakness or stiffness
  - Affected animals may be recumbent and unable to stand; those able to stand show muscle weakness, trembling of limb muscles, or stiffness.
  - Limb muscles may appear swollen and may be hard and painful on palpation.
  - If the diaphragm and intercostal muscles are affected, the animal may show respiratory distress and increased abdominal effort when breathing.
  - The muscles of the tongue may be involved, resulting in dysphagia (the predominant manifestation in some cases, especially in foals and lambs).
  - Rectal temperature is normal or moderately elevated.
  - Some animals exhibit apparent abdominal pain with violent thrashing.

Diagnosis

Significantly elevated serum CK, AST, and LDH activities occur during the acute phase of myodegeneration. Other abnormal findings in foals include variable hyperkalemia, hyperphosphatemia, hyponatremia, and hypochloremia. Myoglobinuria is often found in foals and yearling cattle with NMD; it is less common in young calves.

Selenium and vitamin E status. The selenium status of an animal can be determined by laboratory analysis of whole blood or tissue. Whole-blood selenium concentrations greater than 0.07 ppm (μg/g) and red cell glutathione peroxidase concentrations greater than 30 U/mg Hb/min (cattle), greater than 60 U/mg Hb/min (sheep), and greater than 20 U/mg Hb/min (horses) are considered adequate. The critical concentration of vitamin E (α-tocopherol) in plasma is 1.1 to 2 ppm (μg/g) in large animals. Vitamin E in plasma samples deteriorates rapidly, so samples must be put on ice immediately, protected from light, and frozen if analysis is to be delayed.

Treatment and prognosis

In the cardiac form, myocardial damage is often extensive, so treatment is rarely successful. The skeletal form generally is more amenable to treatment, although the prognosis for clinical recovery is guarded. Therapy involves the following:

- Rest
- Injectable selenium at 0.055 to 0.067 mg Se/kg body weight (2.5 to 3 mg/45 kg) IM or subcutaneously (SC)
- Oral vitamin E (even if the injectable selenium product contains vitamin E)
    - For calves, 15 to 60 mg DL-α-tocopheryl acetate/kg dry feed
    - For foals, 600 to 1800 mg DL-α-tocopheryl acetate/day
    - Oral α-tocopherol can also be given at 2.2 to 6.6 IU/kg (1 to 3 IU/lb) body weight
- Supportive care–adequate dietary energy intake, attention to fluid and electrolyte balance, and antibiotics if secondary infections such as pneumonia are a concern

Animals with skeletal NMD often respond favorably to treatment and rest, with improvement evident after a few days. Prevention of NMD is discussed in *Large Animal Internal Medicine,* third edition.

Toxic Causes of Rhabdomyolysis

Ingestion of toxic substances in feed or forage is a common cause of rhabdomyolysis. Common feed toxins include gossypol and ionophores (e.g., monensin, lasalocid, naracin, salinomycin). Two common forage toxins are *Cassia* spp. (e.g., *Cassia obtusifolia* [sicklepod]) and tremetone-containing plants (e.g., *Eupatorium rugosum* [white snakeroot] and *Isocoma wrightii* [rayless goldenrod]). A number of horses have died from rhabdomyolysis while grazing pastures, but a cause for this pasture myopathy has not been identified. Toxicants are discussed in Chapter 50.

Compartment, Downer, or Muscle Crush Syndrome in Cattle

Muscle damage commonly accompanies downer syndrome in large animals (see Chapter 33). Weakness and signs of peroneal or tibial nerve paralysis commonly accompany this type of injury. Mild elevations in serum CK can be expected in recumbent cows, but elevations greater than 5000 U/L usually indicate traumatic muscle damage. Treatment involves correction of the underlying cause of recumbency, nonsteroidal antiinflammatory drugs (NSAIDs), and good nursing care, which may include fluid therapy if renal function is impaired, adequate bedding and footing, and frequent lifting or rolling of the animal.

Postanesthetic Localized Myoneuropathy

Localized myopathy can occur in muscles that are in contact with a hard surface during anesthesia or those in which the arterial supply is compromised through positional occlusion. Commonly affected muscles include the triceps, deltoid, masseter, and hindlimb extensors; if the horse has been in dorsal recumbency, the hindlimb adductor and gluteal muscles are often affected. Injury may also occur to nerves in these areas, resulting in temporary radial or femoral nerve paralysis.

Clinical and laboratory findings

Clinical signs may be apparent on recovery from anesthesia or may be delayed for up to 60 minutes after recovery. Affected muscles are swollen, hot, and painful on deep palpation, and the horse is often reluctant to bear weight on the affected limb. Weakness of affected muscles is common, particularly with peripheral nerve involvement. In some horses the condition limits the animal's ability to stand. Laboratory findings include elevations in serum CK (often tens of thousands of IU/L) and subsequently AST and LDH.

Treatment

Horses with only minor localized signs usually have an uncomplicated recovery with little or no treatment. Supportive care and use of NSAIDs, DMSO, and dantrolene sodium (2 to 4 mg/kg PO) often are sufficient in mild to moderate cases. Treatment of more severe cases is as described below for generalized reactions.

Generalized Anesthetic Reactions

Postanesthetic reactions involving multiple muscle groups can result in anxiety, tachycardia, tachypnea, profuse sweating, and myoglobinuria. Affected horses may be unable to rise and may struggle violently. In some cases a progressive rise in body temperature and muscle contractures develop during anesthesia, and a fulminant metabolic and respiratory acidosis may be noted. These animals can die within a matter of hours.

Treatment

Therapy should include the following:

- Pain relief–detomidine with butorphanol; NSAIDs
- Correction of fluid and electrolyte abnormalities–volume expansion; sodium bicarbonate (1 to 2 mEq/kg slowly IV) if necessary to correct metabolic acidosis
- Prevention of other problems–sedation to limit self-inflicted trauma, dantrolene sodium (2 to 4 mg/kg PO two or three times daily) to limit further muscle damage, diuresis to prevent renal toxicity
- Intensive nursing care–good padding and eye protection, frequent turning of recumbent animals, caloric supplementation

If hyperthermia and contracture develop during anesthesia, discontinue anesthesia and cool the animal with alcohol or cold-water baths. If available, lyophilized dantrolene sodium solution (1 mg/kg) may be given IV.

EXERTIONAL MYOPATHIES IN HORSES *(Text pp. 1285-1290)*

Myopathies associated with exertion can be grouped into two broad categories:

- Local muscle strain–lumbar and gluteal muscles, adductor muscles, semitendinosus/semimembranosus muscles
- Exertional rhabdomyolysis (ER)–sporadic ER, polysaccharide storage myopathy, recurrent ER

The specific conditions listed are discussed in the following sections.

Lumbar, Gluteal, or Adductor Muscle Strain

Strain of the lumbar and gluteal muscles is common in jumpers, dressage, and harness horses. Lameness is often mild, but the horse usually is reluctant to engage its hindquarters. Tearing of the gracilis muscle on the medial thigh causes severe pain. Deep palpation of the affected muscles results in pain and, with lumbar or gluteal muscle strain, dorsiflexion of the spine. Ultrasonography can reveal the extent of fiber disruption with gracilis tears.

Treatment

Treatment of muscle strain consists of rest and NSAID therapy. Hand walking once the initial stiffness has dissipated may be beneficial. Massage and heat therapy may aid the healing process. Exercise should be resumed gradually and preceded by an appropriate warm-up period.

Semitendinosus/Semimembranosus Muscle Strain

The semitendinosus/semimembranosus muscles are most often damaged in horses that perform abrupt turns and sliding stops (e.g., working Quarter Horses). Damage may also occur in horses caught in a rope or fence (and that struggle violently) and as a result of intramuscular injection in this site. Fibrotic myopathy results in chronic cases. A congenital form of fibrotic myopathy has been described. Affected animals are usually less than 12 months of age when characteristic signs are first noticed.

Clinical findings

In acute cases, affected muscles are painful on deep palpation and may appear warm. In chronic cases, hardened areas representing fibrosis and ossification may be felt within the muscle. In these cases the stride has a shortened anterior phase and a characteristic hoof-slapping gait that is most apparent at the walk. Pain is not a feature of chronic fibrotic myopathy, and manipulative tests have little, if any, effect on the degree of dysfunction.

Diagnosis and treatment

The diagnosis can be confirmed by ultrasonography, thermography, or scintigraphy. Several surgical procedures for correction of fibrotic myopathy have been described. They involve either excision or transection of the fibrotic muscle or tenotomy of the tibial insertion of the semimembranosus tendon.

Exertional Rhabdomyolysis: General Discussion

ER is probably the most common muscle disorder in horses. It is a complex syndrome with many possible causes, depending on whether the episodes are sporadic or chronic/recurrent. Current research suggests that horses with repeated episodes are susceptible to ER because of an inherent disorder of muscle function. Two heritable causes of chronic ER have recently been identified: polysaccharide storage myopathy and recurrent ER.

Clinical findings

Horses experiencing ER develop a stiff, stilted gait with excessive sweating and tachypnea during or after exercise. Most commonly, signs are seen after only 15 to 30 minutes of light exercise. After exercise the horse may stretch out as if to urinate, become reluctant to move, and, in severe cases, show signs of colic or become recumbent. Firm, painful muscles may be palpated over the back and hindlimb muscles. Attempts to move more severely affected animals may result in extreme pain, obvious anxiety, and possible exacerbation of the condition. Myoglobinuria is common in more severely affected horses.

Sporadic Exertional Rhabdomyolysis

Causes of sporadic ER include overexertion (e.g., excessive exercise relative to training status, endurance exercise), dietary imbalances (e.g., excess soluble carbohydrates, inadequate sodium or potassium, high-calcium/low-phosphorus diet, inadequate vitamin E/selenium), viral respiratory infections (e.g., equine herpesvirus type 1, influenza), and hormonal influences (e.g., estrus in fillies and mares).

Diagnosis

Most cases can be diagnosed on the basis of the history and clinical signs. Elevations in serum CK (often in the tens or hundreds of thousands IU/L), AST, and LDH are common. The degree of elevation reflects the extent of myonecrosis and the time elapsed between rhabdomyolysis and blood collection. Myoglobinuria is found in more severely affected horses.

Treatment

The aims of treatment for severely affected animals include the following:

- Relieve anxiety and muscle pain
  - Acetylpromazine is helpful in relieving anxiety and may increase muscle blood flow, but it is contraindicated in dehydrated horses.
  - Detomidine provides better sedation and analgesia in horses with extreme pain.
  - NSAIDs, DMSO (less than 20% solution IV), and corticosteroids have also been advocated.
- Correct fluid and acid-base deficits with balanced electrolyte solutions (IV and via nasogastric tube)

  - Assessment of packed cell volume, total plasma protein, and serum electrolytes direct fluid therapy.
  - Bicarbonate therapy is inappropriate in endurance horses with ER.
- Prevent renal compromise by inducing diuresis
  - Fluid therapy with Ringer's lactate, saline, or 2.5% dextrose in 0.45% saline should be maintained until the urine is clear.
  - In severely affected animals the blood urea nitrogen and serum creatinine should be monitored.
  - Diuretics are contraindicated in most cases.
- Limit further muscle damage by restricting exercise
  - Rest with hand walking once the initial stiffness has abated is of prime importance.
  - Horses with chronic ER appear to benefit from an early return to regular exercise.
  - Horses with ER as a result of overexertion may benefit from a longer rest period with regular access to a paddock; training should be resumed gradually.

Because the inciting cause is usually temporary, most horses respond to a few weeks of rest, dietary adjustments (see main text), and a gradual increase in training.

Polysaccharide Storage Myopathy

Polysaccharide storage myopathy (PSSM) is a cause of chronic ER that is characterized by the accumulation of glycogen and an abnormal polysaccharide in the muscle. PSSM has been identified in Quarter Horses and related breeds (paints, Appaloosas), draft horses, Warmbloods, and a few Thoroughbreds. The condition appears to be an inherited trait in Quarter Horses.

Clinical findings

Horses with PSSM often have a calm and sedate demeanor. Most have a history of numerous episodes of ER, beginning at the commencement of training. Mildly affected horses may have only one or two episodes per year. Classic signs of mild rhabdomyolysis are seen. Exercise intolerance, muscle atrophy, renal failure, and respiratory distress are less common presenting complaints. PSSM may also cause severe rhabdomyolysis in weanling and yearling Quarter Horses and paints without a history of exertion but often with concurrent pneumonia.

Draft horses with PSSM have either recurrent episodes of ER or weakness and muscle atrophy. Serum CK and AST are often only modestly elevated in weak horses, and difficulty rising is often described. Gait abnormalities, including a "shivers"-like gait and difficulty backing, have been associated with this condition.

Diagnosis

Elevations in serum CK are usually present and may persist for long periods, even with rest. The diagnosis is based on histopathologic examination of muscle biopsy specimens using special stains.

Treatment and prevention

Treatment of horses with acute rhabdomyolysis is as described for sporadic ER. Prevention of further episodes relies on eliminating grain from the diet (and supplementing the diet with fat if necessary) and a gradual training program that includes daily exercise and ample turnout. Details are given in Chapter 40 of *Large Animal Internal Medicine,* third edition.

Recurrent Exertional Rhabdomyolysis

Recurrent exertional rhabdomyolysis (RER) refers to a specific subset of Thoroughbred and probably Standardbred and Arabian horses that have intermittent episodes of ER. These horses likely have an inherited defect in the regulation of muscle contraction. Pedigree analysis in Thoroughbreds suggests that RER is an autosomal dominant trait. Factors that can trigger ER in susceptible horses include gender (more common in fillies), temperament (more common in nervous horses), excitement, lameness, high-grain diet, and exercise duration or intensity.

Clinical findings and diagnosis

Episodes often occur in horses once they become fit and are often associated with excitement at the time of exercise. A history of poor performance and elevated serum CK and AST may be the only presenting complaints. Characteristic findings on histopathologic examination of muscle biopsy specimens support the diagnosis.

Prevention

Prevention of further episodes of RER in susceptible horses includes implementing a standardized daily routine, providing an environment that minimizes stress, daily exercise (turnout, longeing, or riding), and dietary modifications to limit soluble carbohydrate intake (see text). Small doses of acetylpromazine (2 to 5 mg) 30 minutes before exercise can be helpful in excitable horses. Other drugs that may help limit repeated episodes include dantrolene (2 to 4 mg/kg PO, given 1 hour before exercise) and phenytoin (6 to 8 mg/kg PO for 3 to 5 days, increased in 1-mg/kg increments every 3 days until ER is prevented or the horse appears drowsy).

HEREDITARY/CONGENITAL MYOPATHIES *(Text pp. 1290-1291)*

Glycogen Branching Enzyme Deficiency

Glycogen branching enzyme deficiency (GBED) is a newly recognized disorder that causes muscle weakness in quarter horse foals and related breeds. Most foals diagnosed with GBED have presented with weakness and flexor contracture of all limbs at birth. Persistent leukopenia; recurrent hypoglycemia; and high serum CK, AST, and GGT activities are found in affected foals. All foals have died (apparently from cardiac arrhythmia) or were euthanized.

Other Conditions

The following conditions are briefly discussed in *Large Animal Internal Medicine,* third edition: exercise intolerance associated with a mitochondrial myopathy in an Arabian filly, phosphorylase deficiency in Charolais cattle, and myofiber hyperplasia (double muscling) in cattle.

41

Diseases of the Reproductive System

Consulting Editors BRAD SEGUIN • MATS H.T. TROEDSSON

Contributors MAARTEN DROST • PHILIP G.A. THOMAS • R. NEIL HOOPER
TERRY L. BLANCHARD • DICKSON D. VARNER

Part I: Female Reproductive Disorders

ESTROUS CYCLE ABNORMALITIES *(Text pp. 1292-1295)*

This section examines conditions that affect normal cyclicity of ovarian function or normal manifestations of estrous behavior. Anestrus is discussed separately in the following section.

Cystic Follicular Degeneration in Cows

Follicular cysts are single, multiple, or multilocular structures on one or both ovaries that arise because of failure of ovulation. Conditions around the time of calving, such as retained placenta, metritis, and hypocalcemia, increase the prevalence of cystic follicular degeneration (CFD).

Clinical findings

Most cows with CFD are anestrous; up to 30% display frequent or intense estrus (nymphomania). Rectal examination of the ovaries reveals large (often greater than 50 mm diameter), fluid-filled structures raised above the surface of the ovary. The uterus typically is flaccid. In neglected cases, mucometra may develop and must be differentiated from pregnancy.

Diagnosis

Diagnosis is based on the history and clinical findings. Sequential examinations may be necessary to differentiate between ovarian cysts and corpora lutea (CLs). Ultrasonography is useful; unlike most CLs, follicular cysts are thin-walled structures. The progesterone concentrations in milk and plasma are low in cows with CFD.

Treatment

Spontaneous recovery occurs in up to 60% of cows that develop CFD before the first ovulation after calving but in only about 20% that develop CFD after this time. The goal in treating CFD is to induce luteinization. Two hormonal methods are described:

- Human chorionic gonadotropin (hCG)–dosages range from 5000 IU (intravenously [IV] or intramuscularly [IM]) to 10,000 IU (IM)
  - Most cows establish a normal estrous cycle within 3 to 4 weeks of treatment.
- Gonadotropin-releasing hormone (GnRH)–100 µg IM, followed in 10 to 14 days by a luteolytic dose of prostaglandin
  - With this regimen, it is not critical whether the cyst is follicular or luteal, or even whether the structure is a large, smooth corpus luteum (CL) with a fluid-filled cavity.

- An alternative is to just use GnRH and let the cow return to estrus (this takes 18 to 24 days).

Because accurate physical diagnosis can be a problem, measurement of milk or plasma progesterone allows the selection of hCG or GnRH for treatment of follicular cysts and prostaglandin for treatment of partially luteinized cysts. Thin-walled follicular cysts may be manually ruptured, either inadvertently or intentionally.

Ovarian Cysts in Ewes and Does

In ewes and does, shortened interestrous intervals and nymphomania during the breeding season have been attributed to ovarian cysts. Treatment with hCG or GnRH has been suggested.

Behavioral Nymphomania in Mares

Abnormal estrous behavior and aggression may be demonstrated by otherwise normal mares at any stage of the estrous cycle, but initially during estrus. Exogenous progestins have been used to limited effect. Short-term dexamethasone treatment (5 to 10 mg) may alleviate signs for 3 to 4 days. Bilateral ovariectomy is necessary in some mares.

ANESTRUS *(Text pp. 1295-1299)*

Common causes of anestrus include the following:

- Any species–pregnancy, unobserved estrus, pyometra, undernutrition, granulosa-theca cell tumor
- Mares–seasonal anestrus, prolonged diestrus, gonadal dysgenesis
- Cows–cystic follicular degeneration, mummified fetus, ovarian hypoplasia, freemartinism

Specific conditions are discussed in the following sections.

Lack of Behavioral Estrus

Absence of behavioral estrus is most often the result of inadequate estrus detection methods. Management recommendations for improving estrus detection in mares, cows, ewes, and does are discussed in *Large Animal Internal Medicine,* third edition.

Seasonal Anestrus in Mares

Seasonal anestrus occurs in most mares in late fall and winter. As day length increases in early spring, mares demonstrate estrous behavior of varying levels for 1 month or more. Transrectal palpation and ultrasonography reveal multiple ovarian follicles up to 30 mm in diameter. The uterus usually is flaccid.

Advancing the onset of regular cyclicity

Most mares ovulate and begin regular cyclicity without treatment as day length increases. Methods to advance the onset of regular ovulation in nonpregnant mares include the following:

- Artificial lighting–16 hours of light and 8 hours of dark each 24-hour period (see main text)
- GnRH
  - Administering twice-daily injections of GnRH induces ovulation in most mares in 2 to 3 weeks.
- Dopamine antagonists–domperidone, sulpiride (see main text)
- Exogenous progestins–progesterone in oil (150 to 300 mg IM) or altrenogest (0.044 mg/kg orally [PO]) daily for 10 to 14 days
  - Ovulation occurs within 10 days of cessation.
  - To be effective, mares must be in mid- to late transition and have at least a 25-mm follicle.
- hCG
  - This may reduce the time to first ovulation in transitional mares, particularly when used with lights or progestin therapy.

Prolonged Luteal Phase in Mares

The CL continues to function in the following situations: (1) pregnancy, (2) embryonic loss between day 14 and 30, (3) endometrial infection and inflammation, (4) late diestrous ovulation, and (5) nonsteroidal antiinflammatory drug (NSAID) therapy. Spontaneous persistence has also been proposed. Examination reveals that the tubular tract has tone and the cervix is closed. Ultrasonography of the ovaries reveals luteal tissue; plasma progesterone is greater than 1 ng/ml. After pregnancy has been ruled out, luteolysis can be achieved with prostaglandin $F_{2\alpha}$ ($PGF_{2\alpha}$) (e.g., dinoprost tromethamine 10 mg IM).

Pseudopregnancy in Mares

Embryonic loss between days 35 and 150 of gestation induces anestrus in mares. Despite fetal loss, the endometrial cups persist until 100 to 150 days postconception. Cyclic activity is not reestablished until they regress. Daily injections of prostaglandin may cause luteal regression in pseudopregnant mares.

Prolonged Luteal Function in Cows

Several conditions affecting the uterus can result in prolonged luteal function, persistently elevated progesterone levels, and anestrus in cows. Common causes include pregnancy, pyometra, and mummified fetus. These conditions can usually be differentiated by rectal palpation. In all three conditions, plasma progesterone remains higher than 1 ng/ml until spontaneous luteolysis occurs or the condition is treated.

Treatment

Unwanted pregnancy can be terminated with PGF (25 mg dinoprost trimethamine, 500 μg cloprostenol, or 1 mg fenprostalene) between 7 and 150 days of gestation, and after 150 days with a combination of PGF and dexamethasone (20 mg). PGF is also the treatment of choice for pyometra in cows. Mummified fetuses are usually expelled 3 to 5 days after treatment with PGF. Vaginal examination should be performed after treatment and the mummified fetus delivered by gentle traction if necessary.

OTHER OVARIAN ABNORMALITIES IN MARES *(Text pp. 1299-1301)*

Abnormally Small Ovaries

The most common causes of bilaterally small ovaries in mares are (1) severe malnutrition, (2) hypothalamopituitary dysfunction, (3) immaturity, (4) seasonal anestrus, (5) advanced age, (6) use of anabolic steroids, and (7) gonadal dysgenesis (chromosomal abnormalities).

Abnormally Large Ovaries

Granulosa-theca cell tumor

Granulosa-theca cell tumor is the most common ovarian tumor in mares. It is usually benign. Affected mares may show anestrus, constant estrus, irregular estrus, or stallion-like behavior, and are infertile. The affected ovary is large, firm, and often multicystic; the contralateral ovary usually is small and inactive, and the uterus is flaccid. Plasma inhibin and testosterone concentrations are elevated in 90% and 55% of cases, respectively. Plasma testosterone may be 100 to 200 pg/ml in mares with stallion-like behavior. Surgical removal of the affected ovary usually results in return to cyclicity within a year.

Cystadenoma

Cystadenomas are rare, benign, hormonally inactive tumors found at the ovulation fossa. The tumor is unilateral. Its appearance is similar to that of a granulosa-theca cell tumor (multicystic); however, the contralateral ovary is normal. Surgical removal is recommended.

Germ cell tumors

Dysgerminomas and teratomas are rare ovarian tumors of germ cell origin. Both tumors are unilateral and hormonally inactive. The affected ovary is enlarged and multicystic. Teratomas do not cause clinical signs. Dysgerminomas are malignant and often metastasize to the peritoneal and thoracic cavities. Surgical removal is recommended for both tumors. The prognosis is usually good for mares with teratomas but poor for those with dysgerminomas.

Ovarian hematoma

Hemorrhage into the follicular cavity is a normal occurrence at ovulation. Occasionally, the hemorrhage is severe, resulting in the formation of an ovarian hematoma that may be 10 cm or more in diameter. Transrectal palpation and ultrasonography reveal an enlarged ovary that initially is irregularly hypoechoic and then echogenic with organization of the hematoma. The ovulation fossa usually remains distinguishable, and the contralateral ovary remains active. Affected mares continue to cycle normally. Ovarian hematomas spontaneously regress over weeks or months.

Pregnancy

Multiple secondary CLs form in pregnant mares between 40 and 180 days of gestation, resulting in bilaterally enlarged ovaries that may be mistaken for ovarian disease.

Anovulatory hemorrhagic follicles

Hemorrhage into a preovulatory follicle in association with ovulation failure may result in the formation of a hemorrhagic follicle. These follicles are large (up to 6 cm) and on ultrasound contain free-floating echogenic material that swirls during ballottement. Over time the structure takes on a gelatinous consistency. Anovulatory hemorrhagic follicles regress spontaneously and are often undetectable after 1 month.

OTHER OVARIAN ABNORMALITIES IN RUMINANTS *(Text pp. 1301-1302)*

Ovarian Hypoplasia

Ovarian hypoplasia occurs sporadically as an autosomal recessive trait. The condition has incomplete penetrance, so it may be partial or complete and unilateral or bilateral. Individuals affected with complete bilateral ovarian hypoplasia are sterile; those with partial or unilateral hypoplasia may be subfertile. There is no effective treatment.

Freemartinism

A freemartin is a genetic female, born co-twin with a male, that is sterile as a result of arrested development of the reproductive tract. The ovaries are hypoplastic. Abnormalities of the tubular genital organs vary in severity; most freemartins lack a cervix. The condition is more common in cattle than in sheep and goats.

Intersex does

Intersexes are common among Saanen, Toggenburg, and Alpine goats, especially in polled goats. The phenotype of affected animals may approach that of either sex.

Ovarian Enlargement

Although rare, a variety of ovarian neoplasms have been described in ruminants. They include granulosa-theca cell tumors, dysgerminomas, interstitial cell tumors, and teratomas. Other causes of ovarian enlargement include ovarian cysts, ovarian abscesses, and paraovarian cysts.

Granulosa cell tumor in cows

Granulosa-theca cell tumors in cows are characterized by unilateral ovarian enlargement (greater than 10 cm diameter). The surface may be smooth or coarsely lobulated. Function of the contralateral ovary may be suppressed. The behavior of affected cows ranges from anestrus to nymphomania or malelike behavior. Udder development and lactation may occur in affected heifers. Treatment is surgical removal of the affected ovary.

Ovulation tags in cows

Ovulation tags result from follicle rupture and associated blood loss during ovulation. Most ovulation tags resolve spontaneously and have no effect on fertility. Severe ovarian hemorrhage and subsequent adhesions between the ovary and adjacent structures may follow manipulation of the ovaries and can interfere with subsequent ovarian function.

SALPINGITIS *(Text pp. 1302-1303)*

Most cases of salpingitis (inflammation of the oviducts) follow uterine infections. The usual history is one of infertility. Additional history may include uterine infection or traumatic therapy (e.g., uterine irrigation) or administration of exogenous estrogen. Easy identification of the oviduct by transrectal palpation may be indicative of salpingitis. Diagnosis is made by exploratory laparotomy, peritoneoscopy, or necropsy. Embryo recovery is objective evidence that one or both oviducts are patent. Treatment of salpingitis is unlikely to be successful.

RETAINED FETAL MEMBRANES *(Text pp. 1303-1304)*

Fetal membranes are considered retained if they have not been passed by 3 hours after foaling in mares and by 12 hours after delivery of the last fetus in ruminants. Retention of the fetal membranes (RFM) is more common after abortion, dystocia, cesarean section, or fetotomy.

Clinical Findings

Retained fetal membranes are usually visible at the vulva. However, small tags of placental tissue may remain attached without being apparent; in mares this can result in severe metritis, endotoxemia, and laminitis hours or days postpartum. In contrast, most affected cows show no obvious signs other than a transient decrease in appetite and milk production.

Treatment

Mares

Early intervention is essential in mares. Treatment should begin if the membranes are not passed within 3 hours of foaling. Recommendations include the following:

- Oxytocin–IV (5 to 20 IU every 15 to 30 minutes), IM (20 to 40 IU every 30 to 60 minutes), or slow intravenous infusion (30 to 80 IU in 500 ml warm saline, given over 30 to 60 minutes)
  - Overdosage may cause abdominal pain.
- Placental infusion–if chorioallantois is intact, fill cavity with 3 to 4 gallons warm saline or water; hold opening closed until mare exerts abdominal pressure
- Systemic broad-spectrum antibacterials
- NSAIDs (phenylbutazone or flunixin meglumine)
- Tetanus prophylaxis and additional prophylaxis/therapy for laminitis if indicated

Manual removal of the membranes is contraindicated. Some cases of RFM are refractory to treatment, and the membranes may remain firmly attached for several days. Continuation of therapy with oxytocin, antibiotics, and NSAIDs is indicated until the placenta is expelled.

Cows

Specific treatment in cows varies with the clinical presentation:

- Manual removal–indicated only when gentle traction is sufficient to withdraw membranes from genital canal
  - Attempts at manual removal are contraindicated if there are signs of septicemia.
- Intravenous calcium solutions–indicated in cases of RFM secondary to hypocalcemia
- Systemic and intrauterine antibiotics–indicated when cow is febrile, inappetant, or has drop in milk production

◦ Intrauterine tetracycline (e.g., 4 to 6 g/day of oxytetracycline until the placenta is expelled) may reduce the incidence of metritis, but pyometra may develop in treated cows.

Ewes and does

Attempts to manually remove the placenta should be limited to gentle traction on exposed membranes. Treatment with intrauterine and systemic antibiotics, oxytocin (10 to 20 IU twice daily until the placenta is expelled), and NSAIDs is suggested. Tetanus prophylaxis is indicated.

ENDOMETRITIS IN MARES *(Text pp. 1301-1307)*

Persistent endometritis is a major cause of reduced fertility in mares. Based on pathogenesis, persistent endometritis can be divided into four categories:

- Sexually transmitted diseases–notably, contagious equine metritis (CEM; *Taylorella equigenitalis* infection)
- Persistent uterine infection–most common isolates are β-hemolytic streptococci *(Streptococcus zooepidemicus, Streptococcus equisimilus), Escherichia coli, Pseudomonas aeruginosa,* and *Klebsiella pneumoniae*
- Persistent breeding-induced endometritis (sperm-induced inflammation)
- Chronic degenerative endometritis (endometriosis)–common in older, multiparous mares

Diagnostic Approach

History and clinical findings

Infertility following breeding to a fertile stallion is a consistent historical feature. Mares with severe endometritis may have shortened interestrous intervals and vaginal discharge. Other possible findings include defects of the vulva or cervix, cervical discharge, and vaginitis. Accumulation of uterine fluid may be found on transrectal palpation or ultrasonography.

Microbiology

Aerobic culture of the uterine lumen is necessary to identify potential pathogens and determine their antibiotic sensitivity. Samples collected with a guarded swab should be taken during estrus and either plated immediately on solid media or transported to the laboratory in nonnutritive media. NOTE: Culture alone is not diagnostic; results should be interpreted in light of clinical, histologic, and cytologic findings.

Endometrial cytology

Endometritis is rapidly and accurately diagnosed by examination of exfoliated endometrial cells, collected using a guarded swab. Air-dried smears are stained with new methylene blue or modified Wright-Giemsa. More than 1 neutrophil/10 epithelial cells is consistent with a diagnosis of endometritis. Eosinophils may be associated with fungal endometritis or pneumovagina. Urine crystals indicate urovagina.

Endometrial biopsy

Endometrial biopsy is an accurate diagnostic and prognostic tool. It should be performed during the breeding season. Interpretation is discussed in *Large Animal Internal Medicine,* third edition.

Ultrasonography

The presence of free intraluminal fluid before breeding strongly suggests susceptibility to persistent endometritis. If fluid is present 12 hours or more after breeding, the mare should be considered to have persistent mating-induced endometritis. Increased echogenicity indicates the presence of inflammatory cells and debris.

Hysteroscopy

Endoscopic examination of the uterine lumen allows evaluation of the degree of inflammation and identification of other luminal abnormalities (e.g., adhesions, masses, endometrial cysts).

Treatment

Sexually transmitted diseases

Mares with CEM should be treated with intrauterine infusions of antibiotics (based on sensitivity tests), uterine lavage (if inflammatory debris or luminal fluid is present), and daily application of 4% chlorhexidine or nitrofurazone ointment to the vulva and clitoris for 5 days. Control measures are discussed in *Large Animal Internal Medicine,* third edition.

Persistent uterine infection

The first therapeutic concern is to remove any predisposing causes (e.g., perform Caslick's surgery, repair cervical damage or perineal lacerations, correct urovagina). In some mares, spontaneous recovery occurs with sexual rest. Antimicrobials may be administered by either local or systemic routes, basing drug selection on sensitivity results (see following discussion). Uterine lavage (30 to 60 ml total, daily for 4 to 6 days) should be performed before local therapy. Mares should be treated during estrus using strict aseptic techniques. Follow-up cultures are recommended.

Antibacterial drugs used for intrauterine administration in mares with bacterial endometritis include the following:

- Gram-negative spectrum–amikacin* (2 g), ampicillin† (3 g), carbenicillin‡ (2 to 6 g), gentamicin (1 to 3 g)
- *E. coli*–kanamycin (1-3 g), neomycin (3-4 g)
- *S. zooepidemicus*–potassium penicillin G (5 million U), ceftiofur (1 g)
- *Pseudomonas* spp.–potassium penicillin G (1 million U)
- Broad-spectrum–polymyxin B (6 g), ticarcillin (6 g), ticarcillin/clavulanic acid (6 g/200 mg), ceftiofur (1 g)

Antimycotic drugs used for intrauterine administration in mares with fungal endometritis include the following:

- Nystatin–500,000 U (dissolve in 30 ml 0.9% saline) daily for 1 week
- Clotrimazole–500 mg (suspension or cream) daily for 1 week
- Miconazole–500 mg; effective against yeast
- Amphotericin B–200 to 250 mg daily for 1 week
- Vinegar–2% solution (20 ml vinegar in 1 L 0.9% saline)

Persistent breeding-induced endometritis

Treatment is aimed at assisting the uterus to clear contaminants and inflammatory products using one of the following procedures:

- Uterine lavage–1 to 2 L sterile normal saline 6 to 24 hours after each breeding/insemination
  - Therapy should begin no sooner than 4 hours after breeding and should not continue beyond 4 days after ovulation.
- Uterotonic drugs–oxytocin (10 to 20 U IV) or $PGF_{2\alpha}$ (5 to 10 mg IM) given 6 to 12 hours after breeding.
  - Oxytocin may also be given after uterine lavage.

Chronic degenerative endometritis

Consistent results have not been reported for any treatment. Intrauterine infusion of DMSO improves the biopsy score in some mares.

METRITIS AND PYOMETRA IN MARES *(Text pp. 1307-1308)*

Metritis

Metritis (inflammation of all layers of the uterine wall) most often occurs in the first 2 weeks after foaling and commonly follows abortion, dystocia, and RFM. Endotoxemia and laminitis are common sequelae. Discharge from the cervix

---

*Buffer with equal volume of 7.5% bicarbonate.
†May irritate the endometrium.
‡Spermicidal.

(and in some cases the vulva) is usually fluid and red-brown; it may be fetid. Endotoxemia causes depression and leukopenia (neutropenia).

Treatment and prognosis

Treatment includes broad-spectrum systemic antibiotics, antiinflammatory drugs, gentle uterine lavage, and fluid therapy. Vigorous lavage should be avoided. The prognosis is guarded once endotoxemia and laminitis develop.

Pyometra

Pyometra (accumulation of purulent exudate in the uterine lumen) may be caused by a variety of bacteria, including *E. coli, Pseudomonas* spp., and *Streptococcus* spp. However, cultures may be negative. The interestrous interval may be shortened, prolonged, or normal. A purulent vaginal or cervical discharge is sometimes apparent. Transrectal palpation and ultrasonography reveal a fluid-filled uterus. The uterine wall may be thin and flaccid or thickened.

Treatment and prognosis

Treatment involves correction of any predisposing causes, fluid evacuation, and local antibiotic therapy. Prognosis for return to normal fertility is guarded to poor, so endometrial biopsy should precede vigorous treatment. Hysterectomy is an option if treatment is unsuccessful and the discharge is unacceptable or adhesions impair athletic ability.

UTERINE INFECTION IN RUMINANTS *(Text pp. 1308-1309)*

A variety of microorganisms contaminate the bovine uterus peripartum. Most are transient, being eliminated during involution in normal cows. *Actinomyces pyogenes* can persist and act with *Fusobacterium necrophorum* and *Bacteroides* spp. to cause uterine infections. Coliforms, *P. aeruginosa,* hemolytic streptococci, and various anaerobes also are frequently isolated from cases of postpartum uterine disease. Uterine infections may follow dystocia and RFM in ewes and does, but they usually do not cause infertility. In ewes, RFM and metritis follow abortions caused by *Listeria monocytogenes, Campylobacter fetus* subsp. *fetus,* and *Chlamydia psittaci.*

Postpartum Metritis in Cows

In cows with postpartum metritis, variable amounts of lochia are felt in the uterus during rectal palpation. Vaginal discharge is usually present, but it may become obvious only during palpation. Septic metritis is characterized by signs of toxemia that may include fever, depression, inappetence or anorexia, and laminitis. Milk yield is depressed, and the cow may be unwilling or unable to rise. Tenesmus is seen in some cases. Discharges associated with septic metritis vary from scant white mucus to copious amounts of red-black, watery, malodorous fluid. Perimetritis and peritonitis complicate some cases of septic metritis (see following discussion).

Endometritis in Cows

Endometritis is usually observed 2 to 8 weeks after calving. Discharge ranges from white pus to estrual mucus. The history may indicate that the cow has failed to conceive after several services but is otherwise healthy. Uterine culture usually is not performed on individual cases, but it may be indicated when the incidence of postpartum metritis/endometritis suddenly rises on a farm.

Pyometra in Cows

Pyometra is most likely to develop in cows that ovulate before invading microorganisms are cleared from the postpartum uterus. It rarely endangers the life or general health of the cow. Pyometra that develops after breeding may be caused by *Tritrichomonas foetus.*

Treatment of Uterine Infections

Treatment may include the following:

- Intrauterine antibiotics–penicillin (1 million IU) or oxytetracycline (4 to 6 g)

  - Penicillin is unlikely to be effective during the first month after calving (see main text).
  - Adequate withdrawal times must be observed when using intrauterine antibiotic therapy because milk residues can result.
- Intrauterine antiseptics–diluted povidone-iodine solution (1 part povidone-iodine stock solution and 10 to 20 parts saline)
  - This solution is bactericidal and fungicidal.
- Uterine lavage–saline infused in 0.5- to 1-L increments and allowed to reflux through catheter; lavage is repeated until returning fluid is no longer turbid
- Prostaglandin therapy–may be sufficient in mild cases of endometritis or in combination with intrauterine or systemic therapy
  - Prostaglandin therapy is the treatment of choice for pyometra in cows; treatment may be repeated in 6 to 12 hours.

Septic metritis

Large doses of broad-spectrum systemic antibiotics are indicated, along with fluids and other supportive therapy. Attempts to remove RFMs or irrigate the uterus are contraindicated during the acute phase.

PERIMETRITIS *(Text pp. 1309-1310)*

Perimetritis (inflammation of the peritoneal surface of the uterus) may occur as a sequela to severe uterine infections, uterine rupture, vaginal perforation during mating, traumatic insemination or obstetric procedures, or cesarean section. Perimetritis may be accompanied by localized or diffuse peritonitis and results in adhesions between the uterus and other organs.

Clinical and Laboratory Findings

Associated peritonitis may cause fever, depression, inappetence or anorexia, gut stasis, and signs of abdominal pain (colic in mares, teeth grinding in cows). Laboratory findings include leukopenia (neutropenia with a degenerative left shift) and peritoneal fluid abnormalities (cytologic and bacteriologic).

Treatment and Prognosis

The cause should be treated if possible (e.g., suture uterine tears, treat septic metritis as described earlier). Broad-spectrum systemic antibiotics should be administered; intravenous fluids and antiinflammatory drugs may also be indicated. The prognosis depends on the severity of the lesions. Fatalities can occur despite prompt treatment. In general, the prognosis for fertility in surviving animals is fair at best.

UTERINE PROLAPSE *(Text pp. 1310-1311)*

Uterine prolapse occurs when the previously gravid uterine horn becomes invaginated after delivery of the fetus and protrudes from the vulva. It is an uncommon sequel to normal foaling, dystocia, or RFM in mares. In ruminants, predisposing factors include dystocia, hypocalcemia, and, in does (and probably in ewes), lack of exercise.

Mares

Eversion of the previously gravid uterine horn is accompanied by pain and abdominal straining. Systemic signs rapidly develop if eversion progresses to complete uterine prolapse.

Treatment and prognosis

The prolapsed uterus should be cleaned with saline and replaced as rapidly as possible. Sedation and epidural anesthesia aid replacement of the uterus. Correct positioning of the uterus is important to prevent recurrence. Broad-spectrum antibiotics, antiinflammatory drugs, and intravenous fluids should be administered. After replacement, treatment with oxytocin (10 to 20 U IM) facilitates uterine involution. The prognosis depends on the development of sequelae (e.g., uterine tears, metritis, endometrial damage).

Ruminants

Signs that may accompany uterine prolapse include straining, abdominal pain, restlessness, anorexia, tachycardia, and tachypnea. Parturient paresis is common in affected dairy cows. In most patients these signs are transitory, but shock develops in some cases.

Treatment

Replacement of the prolapsed uterus is performed as follows:

1. Treat the hypocalcemia if the cow is recumbent and semicomatose (otherwise wait until after the uterus is replaced).
2. Remove the fetal membranes if they can be easily separated from the endometrium (otherwise leave them attached).
3. Clean the prolapsed tissue with a mild presurgical scrub.
4. If the prolapsed tissue is highly edematous, lubricate the tissue with an emollient ointment and vigorously but carefully massage the tissue from the ovarian pole toward the cervical pole.
5. Replace the uterus, beginning at the cervical pole; ensure that the uterine horns are fully inverted and in a normal position. (NOTE: Replacement is facilitated by epidural anesthesia or administration of clenbuterol.)
6. Begin broad-spectrum antibiotic therapy.

Oxytocin is often administered after the uterus has been replaced. Temporary closure of the vulva with heavy sutures is commonly performed but may not be necessary. If replacement of the uterus is impossible or if the tissue is severely traumatized, amputation may be necessary.

Prognosis

The prognosis for survival is favorable. However, the calving interval is prolonged and the incidence of infertility is higher than in cows that calve without this complication. Barring hypocalcemia, the risk of uterine prolapse at subsequent calvings is not increased.

OTHER UTERINE ABNORMALITIES *(Text pp. 1310-1312)*

Endometrial Cysts in Mares

Endometrial cysts and lymphatic lacunae are common degenerative changes of the endometrium in older mares (more than 11 years). The cysts may mimic pregnancy during transrectal palpation or ultrasonography; however, sequential examination reveals that the cysts remain static in size. Cysts may also be identified by hysteroscopy. Lymphatic lacunae cause enlargement of the uterus and thickening of the wall.

Treatment

No treatment is required unless the cysts are suspected of interfering with pregnancy. Treatment options include endoscopy-guided laser ablation, needle aspiration, mechanical rupture, uterine curettage, and intrauterine infusion of hypertonic saline. However, the cysts often recur.

Uterine Tumors

Uterine tumors in livestock are uncommon. They include leiomyomas, lymphosarcomas (multicentric form in cows), and various carcinomas and sarcomas. Small tumors may escape detection; larger ones may be examined by rectal palpation in mares and cows. Solitary leiomyomas thought to interfere with fertility may be removed. Other forms of uterine neoplasia are usually not treated, and the prognosis generally is poor.

Segmental Defects (White Heifer Disease)

Segmental aplasia occurs sporadically in all cattle breeds. Defects range from nearly complete absence of tubular genital organs to an imperforate hymen that blocks drainage of secretions from a normal genital tract. In most cases the cranial parts of the genital tract (ovaries, uterine tubes, and cranial part of the uterine horns) are normal. The only form of segmental aplasia amenable to treatment is that in which an imperforate hymen occludes an otherwise normal tract.

Hydrometra (Pseudopregnancy in Goats)

Hydrometra is characterized by accumulation of several liters of clear fluid in the uterus, abdominal distention, and anestrus. It occurs sporadically in goats, and when it develops after mating, does are often assumed to be pregnant. The condition can be differentiated from pregnancy by the inability to detect a fetus with ballottement or ultrasonography in late pregnancy. Accumulated fluid is expelled 150 days after the infertile mating. If treatment is desired, PGF (2 to 3 mg dinoprost or 100 to 150 μg cloprostenol) can be used.

Paramesonephric Duct Abnormalities

Aplasia of one paramesonephric duct leads to development of only one uterine horn (uterus unicornis). Subfertility results from prolonged periods of anestrus as a result of a persistent CL on the ovary ipsilateral to the missing uterine horn. Prostaglandin therapy or unilateral ovariectomy may improve fertility. Incomplete fusion of the paramesonephric ducts may result in duplication of various parts of the caudal tubular tract (cervix and vagina).

CERVICAL ABNORMALITIES *(Text p. 1312)*

Cervicitis

Inflammation of the cervix usually results from trauma associated with dystocia and obstetric procedures. Hyperemia and edema may be apparent on speculum examination in acute cases. In more chronic cases, digital examination may reveal luminal adhesions or anatomic defects.

Treatment and prognosis

Most cases resolve spontaneously when coexisting endometritis and vaginitis improve. Exudate can be flushed from the cervical canal with warm saline lavages and a nonirritating antibiotic ointment applied to the affected tissue. Treatment with systemic antibiotics is indicated in cases complicated by anaerobic infection. The prognosis in cases of simple cervicitis is fair to good. However, cervical damage is a serious threat to reproductive performance in mares.

Cervical Lacerations in Mares

Cervical lacerations are most often seen after dystocia. They may result in adhesions and a nonpatent cervix or in failure to seal the uterus during diestrus or pregnancy. Cervical lacerations are diagnosed by vaginoscopy and digital examination of the cervix. Adequacy of cervical closure is best evaluated during diestrus.

Treatment and prognosis

If cervical lacerations are diagnosed shortly after parturition, antimicrobial ointment should be applied frequently. Early adhesions should be broken down as often as necessary until the cervix has healed. Surgical correction is indicated when the laceration results in an incompetent cervix. However, the condition is likely to recur at the next parturition.

VAGINAL AND VULVAR ABNORMALITIES *(Text pp. 1312-1315)*

Pneumovagina in Mares

Pneumovagina is characterized by aspiration of air and feces into the vagina secondary to changes in perineal conformation. Vaginitis, cervicitis, and endometritis often result. Pneumovagina is corrected by surgical closure of the dorsal vulva (Caslick's surgery). Secondary problems (e.g., endometritis) should be treated as described in the relevant sections.

Urovagina in Mares

Urovagina is characterized by pooling of urine in the cranial vagina. Urine is spermicidal and may cause cervicitis and endometritis. In mild cases a history of infertility may be the only indication of urovagina. In more severe cases, urine dribbles from the vulva at rest or during exercise. In some mares, urovagina occurs intermittently or only during estrus. Speculum examination reveals variable vaginitis and cervicitis and a pool of urine in the ventral vaginal fornix. Surgical correction (urethral extension, vaginoplasty) is indicated.

Vaginitis

Vaginitis may occur as a result of ascending infection or exposure to irritants, or it can be secondary to pneumovagina, urovagina, perineal laceration, rectovaginal fistula, breeding, endometritis, abortion, parturition, or dystocia. Signs vary from hyperemia on speculum examination to mucopurulent vulvar discharge. Severe trauma and infection may be followed by necrotic vaginitis with tenesmus, fetid discharge, elevated tail, swollen vulva, and systemic signs.

Treatment and prognosis

The inciting cause should be treated. Mild cases recover spontaneously, whereas moderate cases require lavage with diluted antiseptic or antibiotic solutions. In mares, Caslick's surgery may be necessary to prevent aspiration of air. Severe, necrotic vaginitis is treated with systemic antibiotics and antiinflammatory agents. Vaginal adhesions and stenosis may follow vaginitis. Local application of antibiotic and steroid-impregnated ointments may help prevent adhesions.

Infectious Pustular Vulvovaginitis in Cows

Infectious pustular vulvovaginitis (IPV) is caused by bovine herpesvirus type 1. The incubation period is short (1 to 3 days), and infection spreads rapidly through a herd. Initially, IPV causes a mucopurulent vaginal discharge and inflammation of the vaginal and vulvar mucosae. Pustules develop and progress from small ulcers to painful coalescing erosions. Signs subside in 10 to 30 days. Treatment is usually not required, although lavage with diluted antiseptic and application of emollients have been recommended. Mating should be suspended until the disease subsides.

Vaginal Varicose Veins in Mares

Vaginal varicose veins are common in older mares. Affected mares may exhibit vaginal hemorrhage, although clinical signs are absent in most cases. Vaginoscopy reveals varicose veins in the vagina or the vestibulovaginal transverse fold. Treatment is not required in most cases. Ligation of the veins may be necessary in cases with severe bleeding.

Equine Coital Exanthema

Coital exanthema is a recurrent dermatitis of the genital region of horses caused by equine herpesvirus type 3 (EHV-3). The disease affects the vulva and perineum of mares and the penis and prepuce of stallions and usually is mild and transient. Lesions are initially small papules that rapidly progress to pustules and then ulcers. The ulcers usually heal within 14 days, leaving depigmented spots. Treatment is unnecessary unless secondary bacterial infection occurs. The disease does not affect fertility, but genital contact should be prevented until lesions have healed.

Granular Vulvitis

Granular vulvitis may occur in females of all livestock species but is of most significance in cattle. It is characterized by raised granules or papules in the vulvar mucosa, accompanied by mucopurulent discharge that subsides after 3 to 10 days. The chronic form, in which lesions are mild and there is little or no discharge, may persist for several months; thus the disease becomes endemic in some herds. Infertility can be a feature of this syndrome.

Diagnosis

Samples for culture should be obtained from the vulva, cervicovaginal mucus, and uterus. *Haemophilus somnus, Mycoplasma bovigenitalium,* and *Ureaplasma diversum* have been implicated in cattle. Use of transport medium for shipping of samples is mandatory.

Treatment

Most cases of nonspecific vulvitis resolve spontaneously. Natural breeding should be suspended. Intrauterine infusion of tetracycline or spectinomycin 24 hours after breeding is recommended in cows. Treatment of vulvar lesions with tetracycline or spectinomycin has also been suggested.

Ulcerative Dermatosis in Sheep

Ulcerative dermatosis is a venereal disease of sheep caused by a parapox virus. It is characterized by ulceration of the skin and mucous membranes of the vulva in ewes and the penis and prepuce in rams. Lesions also occur on the lips, nares, feet, and legs. The lesions are painful, and affected animals avoid coitus. The disease subsides in 7 to 10 days. No specific treatment is available. Symptomatic treatment with local astringent and antiseptic ointments has been suggested.

Miscellaneous Conditions

Other conditions of the tubular genital organs briefly discussed in *Large Animal Internal Medicine,* third edition, include abnormal labial approximation, persistent hymen, clitoral hypertrophy, vulvar neoplasia, and ectopic mammary tissue.

INFECTIOUS CAUSES OF INFERTILITY AND ABORTION *(Text pp. 1315-1328)*

There are many infectious causes of abortion in livestock. Following are the major causes in each species, with expected gross fetal and placental findings and recommended diagnostic tests. Affected females should be separated from pregnant animals and all fetal and placental tissues removed from the environs. Several of the infectious agents have zoonotic potential, so care should be taken when handling these animals and materials. Other control measures are discussed in *Large Animal Internal Medicine,* third edition.

Abortion in Cows

Major causes of abortion/infertility in cows include the following (in alphabetical order):

- *Aspergillus* spp. and other fungi–abortion typically occurs in late pregnancy, often near term
  - Placentitis with necrosis and leathery thickening of the fetal membranes is characteristic.
  - With aspergillosis, fetal autolysis is minimal; the fetus may be emaciated, dehydrated, and have dry, scaly skin lesions.
  - Diagnosis is based on histopathologic examination and fungal culture (fetus or placenta).
- Bluetongue–abortion can occur at any stage
  - Diagnosis is based on pathologic findings (anomalies of the skeletal and nervous systems), virus isolation, and fetal serologic examination (see Chapters 30 and 33).
- Bovine herpesvirus type 1 (IBR)–abortion usually occurs between 5 and 9 months
  - Autolysis usually obscures any gross lesions in the fetus; the placenta is grossly normal.
  - Diagnosis is based on histopathologic examination, virus isolation (placenta or fetal lung), and fluorescent antibody tests of fetal kidney.
  - The disease may be controlled by vaccination.

- Bovine virus diarrhea virus–abortion can occur at any stage of pregnancy
    - The aborted fetus may be mummified, autolyzed, or fresh and may have a variety of dysplastic lesions (especially skeletal and central nervous system [CNS]).
    - Diagnosis is based on pathologic findings, fluorescent antibody tests on fetal tissues (kidney, lung, lymph node), fetal serologic examination, and serologic survey of the herd.
    - The disease may be controlled by vaccination.
- *Brucella abortus* (brucellosis)–abortions typically occur in third trimester
    - Autolysis often obscures gross fetal lesions (fibrinous serositis, flocculent abomasal contents, bronchopneumonia).
    - Placentitis is a consistent finding; the cotyledons are necrotic and the intercotyledonary placenta is thickened and opaque, with accumulation of odorless, flocculent, yellow-brown exudate.
    - Diagnosis is based on culture (fetal lung or abomasum, placenta, milk, or uterine secretions) and maternal serologic examination (positive card test or titer of 1:100 or more on plate or tube agglutination).
    - Lameness, mastitis, or orchitis may be present in infected herds.
    - In the United States, regulations require quarantine and elimination of all reactors from a herd with a diagnosed case of brucellosis (see main text).
- *Campylobacter fetus* subsp. *venerealis* (vibriosis)–usually causes early embryonic death
    - Autolysis of abortuses usually is minimal; fetal dehydration and fibrinous serositis and necrotizing placentitis may be apparent grossly.
    - Diagnosis is based on pathologic findings, demonstration of the organism (curved rod with darting, corkscrew motility) on dark-field microscopy, or culture.
    - The vaginal mucus agglutination test is used to survey herds for infection.
    - Heifers should be vaccinated with a killed bacterin before breeding (see main text).
- Epizootic bovine (foothill) abortion–abortion usually occurs in third trimester in first-calf heifers and newly introduced cows in the foothills of the Central Valley in California
    - Diagnosis is based on fetal pathologic findings (lymphadenopathy, splenomegaly, hepatopathy).
    - Chlortetracycline (2 to 5 g/day in feed) reduces the rate of abortion.
- *H. somnus*–abortion with necrotizing placentitis can occur at any stage
    - Diagnosis is based on histopathologic examination, culture, and serologic testing (fourfold or greater change in titer).
- *Leptospira interrogans* (leptospirosis)–abortion usually occurs between 5 and 9 months
    - The aborted fetus is usually autolyzed, icteric, and edematous.
    - Diagnosis is based on fetal and maternal serologic examination.
    - Leptospires may be isolated or demonstrated by dark-field microscopy, fluorescent antibody staining, or histologic examination of fetal or placental tissues or the dam's urine.
    - Single titers of 1:800 or more in unvaccinated animals, seroconversion, or fourfold changes in titers in paired sera indicate leptospirosis in the herd.
    - In abortion outbreaks, pregnant cows can be vaccinated with killed bacterin and treated with oxytetracycline.
- *L. monocytogenes* (listeriosis)–abortion usually occurs in eighth or ninth month
    - Placentitis may be evident (small, gray-white foci in cotyledons, exudation between cotyledons); most abortuses have similar foci in their livers.
    - Diagnosis is based on histopathologic examination and culture.
    - Tetracycline may be used in remaining pregnant animals in the herd.
- *Neospora caninum* (neosporosis)–abortion typically occurs midgestation
    - There are no consistent gross fetal lesions.

  - Diagnosis is based on histopathologic evaluation and serologic survey of the herd.
- Salmonellosis–abortion with placentitis and fetal autolysis typically occurs in third trimester
  - Diagnosis is based on culture or fluorescent antibody tests of impression smears from sections of placental or fetal tissue.
- *Sarcocystis cruzi*–abortion usually occurs in third trimester
  - Diagnosis is based on histopathologic examination or fluorescent antibody testing of placental caruncles.
- *T. foetus* (trichomoniasis)–abortions occur in first half of pregnancy
  - There are no specific gross lesions in the aborted fetus or placenta; placentitis is a consistent microscopic lesion.
  - Diagnosis is made by identifying or culturing trichomonads from cervico-vaginal mucus, uterine exudate, placental fluids, or fetal abomasal contents (see main text).

Abortion in Ewes and Does

Major causes of abortion in ewes and does include the following (in alphabetical order):

- Bluetongue–as described for cattle
- Border disease–abortion can occur at any stage
  - Diagnosis is based on pathologic findings (skeletal and CNS dysplasia, abnormal fleece), virus isolation, and serologic examination.
- *C. fetus* subsp. *fetus* (vibriosis)–abortion usually occurs in last 6 weeks
  - Gross lesions include placentitis (cotyledonary necrosis and intercotyledonary edema) and fetal edema, fibrinous polyserositis, and foci of hepatic necrosis.
  - Diagnosis is based on pathologic findings, culture, and microscopic demonstration of the organism.
  - Infected ewes may have fever, diarrhea, depression, and vaginal discharge several days before parturition/abortion.
  - Outbreaks can be controlled with procaine penicillin G (22,000 IU/kg) plus dihydrostreptomycin (11 to 22 mg/kg) IM once per day or with in-feed oxytetracycline (75 mg/head/day).
  - The disease can be controlled by vaccination (see main text).
- *Chlamydia psittaci* (enzootic abortion of ewes)–abortion usually occurs in fourth or fifth month
  - Placentitis is the most consistent finding; the cotyledons are necrotic and the intercotyledonary placenta is thickened, with accumulation of red exudate.
  - Diagnosis is based on histopathologic examination, demonstration of the organisms in placental impression smears, fluorescent antibody tests on placenta or fetal tissues, culture, and serologic findings (acute and convalescent titers; maternal titers greater than 1:32 indicate recent infection).
  - The dam may have a serosanguineous vaginal discharge for several days before and after parturition; other animals in the flock may be affected by arthritis or pneumonia.
  - Oxytetracycline (80 to 450 mg/head/day in feed or water or long-acting oxytetracycline at 20 mg/kg subcutaneously [SC] twice a week until the fifth month) reduces the number of abortions.
- *Coxiella burnetii* (Q fever)–abortions usually occur near term
  - There are no specific gross fetal lesions, but the placenta is thickened with white, chalky plaques and red-brown exudate, especially in intercotyledonary areas.
  - Diagnosis is based on characteristic placental lesions, with large numbers of rickettsia on placental impression smears, and a rising maternal titer.
  - Pregnant animals can be treated with tetracycline to reduce the chances of abortion.

- *Toxoplasma gondii* (toxoplasmosis)–abortion can occur at any stage of pregnancy
  - The most characteristic gross lesion is small, white, chalky foci of necrosis and calcification in the placental cotyledons; the intercotyledonary areas are grossly normal.
  - Diagnosis is based on demonstration of the organism or antigen (fetal heart, lung, brain, spinal cord, skeletal muscle, or placenta) and on fetal serologic examination (fetal serum, pleural, or amniotic fluid).

Abortion in Mares

Major causes of abortion/infertility in mares include the following (in alphabetical order):

- *Aspergillus* spp. and other fungi (as described for cows)
- Equine herpesvirus type 1–abortion typically occurs between 7 months and term
  - The aborted fetus is fresh; findings often include fluid accumulations in body cavities, pulmonary congestion and edema, hepatomegaly with 1-mm white lesions, subcutaneous edema, and icterus.
  - The placenta may be normal or edematous.
  - Diagnosis is based on histopathologic examination (fetal lung, liver, adrenal cortex, and lymphoid tissues), virus isolation (fetal tissues, maternal blood), fluorescent antibody tests (fetal tissues), and fetal serologic findings.
  - The disease can be controlled by vaccination (see main text).
- Equine viral arteritis–abortion usually occurs between 5 and 10 months
  - There are no characteristic lesions in the aborted fetus or placenta.
  - Diagnosis is based on histopathologic examination, virus isolation, polymerase chain reaction, and serologic findings.
  - Control using vaccination is discussed in the text.
- Leptospirosis–abortion usually occurs between seventh month and term
  - Gross fetal lesions include icterus and autolysis.
  - Diagnosis is based on culture, immunofluorescence, and serologic findings.
- Nocardioform *actinomycete*–abortion usually occurs in mid- to late gestation
  - Characteristic placental lesions are located ventrally in the uterine body and at the base of the horns; diagnosis is based on culture.
- *S. zooepidemicus*–abortion can occur at any stage of pregnancy
  - Ascending placentitis is concentrated around the cervical star; the fetus is autolyzed.
  - Diagnosis is based on histopathologic examination and culture (abortus or uterine discharge).

Abortion caused by endotoxemia

Gram-negative septicemia and endotoxemia can cause luteolysis and abortion during the first 2 months of gestation, when pregnancy is still dependent on the CL. Experimentally, altrenogest (0.44 mg/kg PO once per day) prevents endotoxin-induced abortion. In early pregnancy (before day 80), measuring serum progesterone is useful in determining whether progestagen therapy is indicated. If serum progesterone is less than 1 ng/ml, progestagen therapy should continue until day 100.

Placentitis in Mares

Bacterial and fungal abortions in mares are primarily caused by ascending infections that enter through the cervix and cause placentitis and subsequent fetal infection. Bacteria most commonly cultured include *Streptococcus* spp., *E. coli*, *Pseudomonas* spp., *Klebsiella* spp., and *Staphylococcus* spp. Nocardioform *actinomycete* is an important cause of placentitis in mares in central Kentucky.

Clinical findings

Mares that abort from placentitis often show signs of impending abortion, including premature udder development and vaginal discharge. Transrectal ultrasonography of the placenta in the area near the cervix may show thickening of the uterus and placenta, placental edema, and separation of the placenta from the endometrium. With nocardioform placentitis, placental lesions are located ventrally in the uterine body and at the base of the horns. Transabdominal ultrasonography may be needed to identify this condition before abortion.

Diagnosis

Placental lesions tend to be most severe between the "cervical star" and base of the horns. Affected areas are edematous, thickened, and discolored, with a mucoid or fibronecrotic exudate. In cases of mycotic placentitis, the placenta is characteristically thickened and leathery, with well-demarcated lesions. Microorganisms can be isolated from the placenta and various fetal organs, most consistently the stomach.

Treatment

Pregnant mares showing signs of placentitis should be treated with broad-spectrum antimicrobials and antiinflammatory drugs. Drugs that cause uterine quiescence (e.g., altrenogest 0.44 mg/kg PO once per day or clenbuterol 0.5 mg/kg IM or IV) should be considered. However, the disease process often is too advanced for treatment to be effective once clinical signs are observed. Treatments for endometritis (see pp. 1306-1307) should be instituted after abortion that results from placentitis.

Other Causes of Abortion

The following infectious causes of abortion are also discussed in *Large Animal Internal Medicine,* third edition: *Brucella melitensis* (mostly goats and sheep), *Brucella ovis* (sheep), *Campylobacter jejuni* (sheep), *Mycoplasma* and *Ureaplasma* spp. (ruminants), *Sarcocystis* spp. (ruminants), equine infectious anemia (horses), *Ehrlichia risticii* (horses), trypanosomiasis (dourine; horses), and various bacterial infections (all species).

Part II: Male Reproductive Disorders

PENILE INJURY *(Text pp. 1332-1333)*

Stallions

Penile injuries include cutaneous abrasions, lacerations, and hematomas. Paraphimosis occurs when swelling is sufficient to prevent retraction of the penis through the prepucial ring. Immediate treatment is directed toward reducing inflammation and edema and controlling infection (see Paraphimosis). Sexual rest is indicated until the lesions have healed.

Bulls

Penile injury during mating can result in hematoma formation, which restricts full retraction of the penis and results in prolapse of the prepuce. Possible sequelae include abscess, restriction of penile extension or full erection, and deviation of the penis. Surgical intervention may be required to optimize the chances of full recovery (see main text). Regardless of whether surgical or conservative management is selected, the bull should be treated with systemic antibiotics (e.g., penicillin) and given sexual rest for at least 2 months.

PREPUCIAL INJURY AND PHIMOSIS *(Text pp. 1333-1334)*

Phimosis refers to stenosis of the prepucial orifice that prevents extension of the penis. It is usually a sequel to prepucial injury that results in cicatrix formation.

Stallions

Acute posthitis (inflammation of the prepuce) often accompanies prepucial injury or infections such as equine coital exanthema. Edema may be severe enough to cause temporary phimosis and prolapse of the external prepuce. Stricture formation may permanently narrow the prepucial orifice. Options for reducing prepucial edema include cold therapy (ice pack, cold hosing), massage using emollient antibiotic preparations, administration of diuretics, and exercise. Systemic antibiotics and NSAIDs are indicated, as is sexual rest.

Bulls

Breeds with pendulous sheaths are more prone to prepucial injury. The polled gene is linked to weak or failed development of the prepucial muscles and habitual prepucial eversion. Common prepucial injuries are contusions, abrasions, lacerations, and frostbite. Minor injuries may resolve spontaneously, but more extensive injuries may progress to abscess and stricture.

Treatment

Initial treatment should include systemic antibiotics, hydrotherapy, massage with emollient creams, and attempts to return the prepuce to the prepucial cavity. If the prolapsed prepuce can be replaced, a retention technique (e.g., purse-string suture) should be used to prevent reprolapse, being careful not to restrict urination. If the prolapsed prepuce cannot be returned to the sheath, it should be coated in emollient ointment and a protective dressing and gently supported against the abdominal wall. The dressing should be changed daily. Once sufficient healing has occurred, the necessity for surgery is determined by extending the penis.

PARAPHIMOSIS *(Text pp. 1334-1335)*

Stallions

Paraphimosis refers to the inability to retract the penis into the preputial cavity. Causes include severe injury to the penis or prepuce, debility, exhaustion, and penile paralysis or priapism (e.g., caused by spinal cord disease or injury, use of phenothiazine tranquilizers). Prolonged penile prolapse or priapism usually results in extensive penile trauma.

Treatment

Principles of treatment are similar to those described for prepucial injuries. To maintain the penis within the prepuce, a temporary purse-string suture can be placed near the prepucial orifice. If the penis cannot be returned to the prepuce, external support should be applied. Chronic, refractory penile prolapse results in severe balanoposthitis that may require circumcision or penile amputation.

In cases of drug-induced priapism seen within 4 hours of occurrence, benzotropine mesylate (8 mg slowly IV) may cause detumescence, allowing penile retraction. Flushing the corpus cavernosum penis with heparinized Ringer's solution through a 12-gauge needle has been recommended for horses with priapism of 12 to 24 hours' duration that has not responded to other treatment.

Bulls

Paraphimosis is less common than phimosis in bulls. Causes include penile tumors, parasitic invasion, spinal cord disease or injury, and penile or prepucial injury. Exposed portions of the penis should be cleansed and protected by a bandage soaked in an oily antibiotic preparation. The penis should be returned to the sheath as soon as possible and mechanically restrained if necessary. Otherwise, the prolapsed penis should be supported close to the abdomen. If the ability to retract the penis does not return in a few days, the prognosis for recovery is poor.

URETHRAL INJURY AND URETHRITIS *(Text pp. 1335-1336)*

Stallions

Causes of urethral injury or inflammation include trauma, calculi, parasitic invasion (e.g., *Habronema* spp.), and bacterial infection (e.g., *Pseudomonas* spp.). Urethral inflammation may result in fibrous strictures. The following diagnostic procedures may be helpful: culture of the urethra, urine, and semen; urinalysis; transrectal palpation of the bladder; endoscopy; biopsy of lesions; ultrasonography; and contrast radiography (to identify strictures in the distal urethra).

Treatment

Any inciting factors (e.g., tight stallion ring) must be corrected and ability to void urine established. Systemic antibiotics are indicated, particularly in cases complicated by secondary bacterial infection. Severe urethritis may be treated by infusion of oily antibiotic preparations through a sterile urethral catheter (see main text). Inflammation of the urethral process may respond to topical antibiotic salves. Parasitic granulomas that do not respond to ivermectin may require surgical removal. Treatment of proximally located urethral lesions are discussed in the text. Sexual rest is indicated in all cases of urethritis.

Bulls

Urolithiasis is the primary problem affecting the urethra in bulls. It is discussed in Chapter 32.

BALANOPOSTHITIS *(Text pp. 1336-1337)*

Stallions

Inflammation of the penis (balanitis) and prepuce (posthitis) often occur together. The lesion may be caused by trauma, equine herpesvirus type 3 (equine coital exanthema), bacteria, or parasites.

Equine coital exanthema

EHV-3 infection is characterized by vesicles up to 1.5 cm in diameter that develop first on the penis and then on the prepuce. The vesicles progress to circumscribed pustules that slough and ulcerate. Some affected stallions refuse to breed mares. Systemic signs, such as dullness, anorexia, and fever, may also be seen. Healing occurs in a few weeks, often leaving depigmented spots. Local treatment with antibiotic ointments may minimize secondary bacterial infection and discomfort.

Bacterial balanoposthitis

Documentation of bacterial balanoposthitis requires isolation of a pathogen, preferably in large numbers and in relatively pure culture. Samples for culture should be retrieved from the fossa glandis, penile body, and folds of the external prepuce before the penis is cleaned. Colonization with *Pseudomonas* or *Klebsiella* spp. can be treated as follows:

- Thoroughly wash the penis and prepuce daily with an iodine-based surgical scrub.
- Rinse with copious quantities of water containing dilute disinfectant.
  - 10 ml concentrated HCl per gallon of water for *Pseudomonas;* 40 ml 5.25% Na-hypochlorite bleach per gallon of water for *Klebsiella*
- Dry the penis and apply a generous amount of 1% silver sulfadiazine cream.

The procedure is repeated daily for 1 to 2 weeks and followed by serial cultures. Breeding management using antibiotic-containing semen extender is discussed in *Large Animal Internal Medicine,* third edition.

Bulls

Most cases of balanoposthitis in bulls are caused by trauma. Injuries to the penis or prepuce predispose to infection, particularly when deeper tissues are exposed. Pain and prepucial discharge may be evident. Because many potentially pathogenic organisms inhabit the prepuce, culture is likely to be unhelpful or misleading. Treatment is as described for prepucial injuries.

Infectious balanoposthitis

Balanoposthitis may also be caused by bovine herpesvirus type 1 (infectious bovine rhinotracheitis-infectious pustular vulvovaginitis, or IBR-IPV), tuberculosis (rare), or screwworm infestation. With IBR-IPV, sexual rest for 6 to 8 weeks is recommended. Control measures are discussed in *Large Animal Internal Medicine,* third edition.

Rams and Bucks

Balanoposthitis (pizzle rot, sheath rot, ulcerative posthitis) commonly affects the penis and prepuce of male small ruminants. It is discussed in Chapter 32.

OTHER CONDITIONS INVOLVING THE PENIS AND PREPUCE *(Text pp. 1337-1338)*

Persistent Frenulum and Penile Deviations in Bulls

Phallocamposis (deviation of the erect penis) is relatively common in bulls. The most common cause is persistent penile frenulum (a band between the prepuce and the tip of the penis). Less commonly, penile deviation is the result of prepucial or penile injury. Diagnosis is based on physical examination of the extended penis, preferably by observation during natural mating. Persistent penile frenulum is easily corrected by severing the band. Other deviations require surgical correction.

Tumors

Squamous cell carcinoma

The most common genital neoplasm in horses is squamous cell carcinoma. The tumor usually involves the glans penis but may also involve the shaft of the penis and the prepuce. It often causes ulcerative lesions that have a fetid discharge. Most do not metastasize, but the tumor can spread to the inguinal lymph nodes or to the abdominal or thoracic organs. Treatment with cryosurgery or hyperthermia is usually recommended.

Fibropapilloma

Fibropapilloma is the only tumor that frequently invades the bovine penis. The tumor usually affects young bulls and may be single or multiple. Many of these tumors spontaneously regress within a few months. Surgical removal may be indicated, but fibropapillomas can recur.

Habronemiasis in Stallions

Habronema larvae commonly invade the urethral process, glans penis, and preputial ring of stallions. Diagnosis and treatment of habronemiasis is discussed in Chapter 38.

SEMINAL ABNORMALITIES *(Text pp. 1338-1339)*

Hemospermia

Hemospermia is contamination of the ejaculate with blood. Specific causes include penile lacerations, cutaneous habronemiasis, urethritis, urethral lacerations, and infection or inflammation of the accessory genital glands. Stallions with overt hemospermia are subfertile. Treatment depends on the underlying cause.

Urospermia in Stallions

Urospermia is an uncommon and perplexing disorder of breeding stallions. Affected stallions generally exhibit normal libido and mating ability, but the semen becomes contaminated with urine during ejaculation. The problem may be incessant or intermittent. Gross contamination of the ejaculate with urine is easily detected by its color and odor. Elevated concentrations of urea nitrogen or creatinine document the presence of urine in the ejaculate.

Treatment

Treatment is often unrewarding. Management strategies for limiting the incidence and impact of urospermia are discussed in *Large Animal Internal Medicine,* third edition. Imipramine (100 to 500 mg PO twice daily) has been useful for controlling urospermia in some stallions.

SCROTUM AND TESTES *(Text pp. 1339-1342)*

Scrotal Injury, Hydrocele, and Hematocele

Scrotal edema usually results from scrotal injury. Possible causes of hydrocele (accumulation of serous fluid in the vaginal tunic) include ascites, peritonitis, and local lymphedema. Hematocele (accumulation of blood in the testicular tunics) usually results from scrotal trauma. In any case, accumulation of fluid (whether edema, peritoneal fluid, or blood) in the scrotum can result in thermal testicular degeneration and infertility. Diagnosis is made by physical examination and ultrasonography. Sterile tap is useful in determining the character of the fluid.

Treatment

Acute scrotal injury is treated with cold therapy. Lacerations and abrasions should be treated with topical antibiotic ointments. Systemic antibiotics and antiinflammatory drugs may also be indicated. Hydrocele is managed by correcting the underlying cause. Exercise may aid in control of fluid accumulation in stallions. Hematocele carries a poor prognosis for return of testicular function, so surgical removal of the clot and the affected testis may be indicated to minimize damage and speed recovery of the remaining testis.

Scrotal Dermatitis or Abscess

The scrotal skin is vulnerable to dermatitis. Causes include environmental contaminants, bacteria, fungi, parasites, and frostbite. Thermal degeneration of the testes may result and may be temporary or permanent. Semen quality should be periodically evaluated after skin lesions have resolved. Scrotal abscesses are common in small ruminants and are most often caused by shearing injuries or penetrating wounds. Treatment involves removal of the affected testis.

Testicular Hypoplasia

Testicular hypoplasia may be unilateral or bilateral. Dimensions vary with species and age:

- Scrotal width in stallions should be more than 8 cm by 3 years of age.
- Scrotal circumference in beef bulls should be 32 cm or more by 12 months of age.
- Scrotal circumference in rams should be more than 30 cm by 12 months and more than 32 cm at maturity.

Ejaculate from animals with testicular hypoplasia may be azoospermic or contain low numbers of spermatozoa with numerous morphologic defects. There is no effective treatment.

Cryptorchidism

Most cases of cryptorchidism (incomplete testicular descent) are unilateral. When deep palpation of the superficial inguinal rings does not reveal the testis in the canal, rectal palpation can be performed in stallions and bulls in an attempt to locate the testis.

Hormone assays

Equine cryptorchids have high basal concentrations of testosterone (usually greater than 100 pg/ml) and respond to hCG (10,000 to 12,000 U IV) with a significant elevation in testosterone within 60 minutes if testicular tissue is present. Geldings and "false rigs" (geldings with malelike behavior) have low basal concentrations of testosterone (less than 40 pg/ml) and do not respond to hCG stimulation. Finding high plasma conjugated estrogens (greater than 400 ng/ml) in a single sample is almost as reliable in diagnosing cryptorchidism in horses as is hCG stimulation.

Treatment

Stimulation of testicular descent with repeated injections of GnRH, sometimes combined with hCG, has been attempted. Surgical removal of both testes is usually recommended.

Testicular Degeneration

Testicular degeneration has several possible causes, including infection, trauma, testicular hyperthermia, and spermatic cord torsion. Diagnosis is based on physical examination and semen evaluation; plasma hormone concentrations may also be helpful (see main text). Differentiation from testicular hypoplasia can be difficult without a complete history. In some cases, degeneration is temporary (once the cause has been corrected) and semen quality improves after 2 to 5 months. However, once testicular degeneration has occurred, treatment is usually of no benefit.

Orchitis

Orchitis (inflammation of the testis) is most often caused by infection or trauma. Orchitic testes are hot, swollen, and painful. Abscesses sometimes develop, occasionally culminating in purulent liquefaction of the parenchyma. Periorchitis may occur simultaneously. Testicular atrophy and fibrosis follow as the condition becomes chronic. Acutely affected animals may refuse to mate, and ejaculates contain numerous white blood cells. Decreased sperm motility and increased morphologic abnormalities are evident.

Treatment

Treatment consists of cold therapy and systemic antiinflammatory drugs. Bacterial orchitis is treated with antibiotics selected by in vitro sensitivity and continued for 1 to 2 weeks beyond resolution of testicular swelling and pain.

Testicular Neoplasia

Primary testicular tumors are uncommon in large animals. Seminomas are the most common testicular tumor in stallions. Interstitial (Leydig) cell tumors have been reported in stallions and bulls. Teratomas are sometimes found in cryptorchid testes. Testicular tumors should be surgically removed.

SPERMATIC CORD *(Text pp. 1342-1343)*

Torsion of the Spermatic Cord

Torsion of the spermatic cord occurs more commonly in stallions than in other large animals. If rotation is less than 180 degrees, torsion is often transient and does not interfere with testicular function or cause pain. Torsion of sufficient degree to result in vascular compromise causes pain, tachycardia, unilateral scrotal swelling, and increased testicular temperature. Affected testes are painful and quickly become soft and friable.

Diagnosis

Diagnosis is made by finding a displaced epididymal tail and scrotal ligament on palpation of the scrotum. In torsions that result in vascular compromise, the condition must be differentiated from a strangulated scrotal hernia by rectal palpation of the inguinal rings.

Treatment

Manual correction can be attempted, although it is not always possible and recurrence is likely. Surgical correction is indicated if manual correction is unsuccessful. NSAIDs and analgesics may be administered to control pain. If hemorrhage or necrosis of the testis is evident, removal is indicated to prevent permanent damage to the contralateral testis.

Varicocele

Varicoceles are abnormally distended and tortuous veins of the pampiniform plexus. They can result in infertility by disturbing local thermoregulation. Diagnosis is made by palpating the dilated, tortuous veins ("bag of worms") within the spermatic cord. Confirmation can be made using ultrasonography (see main text). Thrombosis of a varicocele necessitates unilateral castration.

EPIDIDYMIS AND ACCESSORY SEX GLANDS *(Text pp. 1343-1344)*

Epididymitis

Epididymitis is caused by infection or trauma. It commonly occurs secondary to orchitis or infection of the accessory sex glands. Clinical findings include changes in shape and texture (e.g., enlarged epididymal tail) and painful swellings of the epididymis and adhesions between the epididymis and scrotal tunic. The clinical course varies from acute swelling and edema to chronic abscesses, periorchitis, and fibrosis. Abnormal sperm morphology (especially detached heads) and leukocytes in the ejaculate may be seen before lesions are palpable.

Treatment

Infectious causes are treated with systemic antibiotics selected by in vitro sensitivity and continued for 1 to 2 weeks after inflammatory cells disappear from the semen. In unilateral cases, removal of the testis, epididymis, and spermatic cord on the affected side may salvage some valuable animals for breeding. Testicular atrophy is a common sequel to epididymitis.

Efferent Duct Blockage (Sperm Stasis)

Blockage of the efferent ducts sometimes occurs in stallions. Azoospermia results if the condition is bilateral. On palpation the ampullae are tense. Rectal massage of the ampullae followed by sexual stimulation and semen collection may be effective. Regular semen collection helps prevent recurrence. Sperm granulomas resulting from accumulation of spermatozoa in blind efferent ducts are a common cause of infertility in bucks.

Seminal Vesiculitis

Inflammation of the vesicular glands is relatively common in bulls, especially young bulls fed high-energy rations and housed together. Seminal vesiculitis is uncommon in stallions.

Clinical findings

Most affected bulls exhibit few signs other than deterioration of semen quality (poor sperm motility, increased morphologic defects, elevated pH). In severe cases, pelvic inflammation and peritonitis result in reluctance to move, stiff gait, tense abdomen, and refusal to mate. During the acute phase the vesicular glands may not be significantly enlarged, but if inflammation becomes chronic, the glands become enlarged (losing their lobularity) and fibrotic. In stallions with seminal vesiculitis, the glands may be of normal size or enlarged and painful when rectally palpated. The stallion may refuse to cover or may be unable to ejaculate.

Diagnosis

The semen may contain numerous neutrophils and blood. Bacterial pathogens are readily recovered from the semen, but special collection techniques are necessary to pinpoint the seminal vesicles as the site of infection (see main text).

Treatment

Infections are treated with antibiotics selected by culture and in vitro sensitivity and administered for 2 to 4 weeks. Mild cases may recover spontaneously in 2 to 3 months. A technique used with some success in stallions involves repeated irrigation of the seminal vesicles through a catheter guided into the vesicles by endoscopy (see main text).

PART VI

Preventive and Therapeutic Strategies

42

Principles of Antimicrobial Therapy

Consulting Editors GORDON W. BRUMBAUGH • VERNON C. LANGSTON

Contributor DWIGHT C. HIRSH

PRINCIPLES OF THERAPY *(Text pp. 1349-1359)*

The principles of antimicrobial therapy can be summarized as follows:

1. Consider the patient.
2. Document the infection.
3. Determine in vitro microbial susceptibility.
4. Use an appropriate dosage regimen.
5. Monitor results of treatment.
6. Investigate causes of therapeutic failure.
7. Restrict concomitant use of antimicrobial drugs.
8. Attend adverse reactions to drugs.

These points are discussed in detail in *Large Animal Internal Medicine,* third edition. Items 2, 5, 6, and 7 are briefly discussed in the following sections.

Document the Infection

Without evidence of involvement of a susceptible etiologic agent, use of an antimicrobial drug is irrational and exposes the patient to unnecessary risks. Steps necessary to document an infection include the following:

- Develop a reasonable suspicion of infection based on clinical signs and knowledge of the disease process.
- Carefully collect and submit a representative sample of material from the lesion.
  - Microscopically examine a stained smear for organisms (see following discussion).
  - Demonstrate and identify the infectious agent in vitro or find serologic evidence of antibodies produced against the agent.
- Interpret the results of all diagnostic procedures.
  - It is important to decide if the isolated organisms could be responsible for the patient's condition; if they are commensal, resident flora; or if they are merely contaminants.

Examining smears

The following methods are useful for identifying infectious organisms or inflammatory cells:

- Gram stain–bacteria
- Wright stain (Diff-Quik)–cytologic examination
- Acid-fast stain–mycobacteria
- Methylene blue and potassium hydroxide preparations–fungi
- India ink preparations–cryptococci
- Dark-field microscopic examination–spirochetes
- Fresh wet mounts–motile organisms (trichomonads)

Gram or Wright stain will demonstrate the presence of most microorganisms. Newer techniques of DNA typing, or polymerase chain reaction, are available for identifying some organisms.

Prior antimicrobial therapy

If the patient has received antimicrobial drugs, sample collection should be delayed until the drugs are eliminated from the animal's body. A fairly reliable rule of thumb is to wait 18 to 36 hours after the last dose of a drug (longer for repository formulations). If the patient's condition does not permit a delay, the probability of isolating organisms from body fluids can be increased by passing the sample through an antibiotic removal device.

Monitor Results of Therapy

Clinical signs, hematologic changes, radiologic findings, results of microbiologic tests, and monitored concentrations of drugs are useful in assessing the response to therapy. Therapeutic drug monitoring is most applicable in patients (1) receiving aminoglycosides, (2) with impaired function of organs involved in drug elimination or biotransformation, or (3) receiving more than one drug.

Treatment Failure

When response to treatment is not as expected, the cause should be sought and the problem corrected. Possible causes include the following:

- Incorrect diagnosis
- Inappropriate drug or dosage regimen, inadequate compliance to the drug regimen
- Interaction between drugs, drug toxicity, inactive drug
- Impaired host defense mechanisms
- Development of drug resistance
- Superinfection
- Irreversible condition of the patient

Concommitant Use of Antimicrobial Drugs

Fixed-drug combinations or concomitant use of two or more antimicrobial drugs is occasionally appropriate. Examples include penicillin or a cephalosporin with an aminoglycoside, erythromycin with rifampin, and trimethoprim with a sulfonamide. However, in most instances, one drug with a specific antimicrobial spectrum provides adequate therapy and reduces the potential for adverse effects or selection of resistant organisms.

Indications

Concomitant use of antimicrobial drugs should be limited to the following situations:

- To provide synergy against infecting organisms (e.g., trimethoprim-sulfonamide)
- To prevent bacterial resistance to antimicrobial drugs (e.g., rifampin-erythromycin)
- To extend the antimicrobial spectrum as initial therapy for life-threatening conditions (e.g., penicillin-aminoglycoside)
- To treat documented mixed bacterial infections

Extralabel Drug Use

Veterinarians often encounter infectious conditions for which the drug of choice is not approved by the U.S. Food and Drug Administration's Center for Veterinary Medicine (FDA-CVM). In these situations, treatment must be based on experience, established practices, and scientifically substantiated facts. Guidelines include the following:

- A valid licensed veterinarian-client-patient relationship
- A medical diagnosis
- A situation in which approved use of a drug has proven ineffective in animals being treated or for which no available drug is specifically labeled

- Acceptable labeling of the prescribed drug
- Proper identification of treated animals and observation of extended withdrawal times

PROPHYLACTIC USE OF ANTIMICROBIAL DRUGS
(Text pp. 1360-1363)

Although indiscriminate use of antimicrobial drugs to prevent disease is unjustifiable, prophylactic use is appropriate in certain circumstances. When antimicrobial drugs are used prophylactically, there are several principles that should be followed:

1. The risk of infection must be sufficient to warrant prophylactic antimicrobial use. Risk of infection is related to virulence of the organism, amount of exposure (size of inoculum and duration), and the host's defense status.
2. Therapy should be directed at a specific pathogen, rather than at all possible organisms. Organisms that are likely to cause infection and their antimicrobial susceptibility should be known or accurately predicted.
3. The drug must reach the site of potential infection and reach inhibitory concentrations before the onset of infection.
4. As much as possible, drugs used prophylactically should not be those that would be used therapeutically if an infection develops.
5. The duration of antimicrobial prophylaxis should be as brief as possible (e.g., 3 to 6 hours postoperatively). If host defenses are temporarily deficient or if exposure is prolonged, administration may need to be extended.
6. Antimicrobial drugs chosen for prophylaxis should present minimal risk of adverse effects.
7. In theory the selected dosage regimen should achieve bactericidal rather than bacteriostatic concentrations at the site of infection.

HOSPITAL-ACQUIRED (NOSOCOMIAL) INFECTIONS
(Text pp. 1363-1369)

All animals are at risk of acquiring an infectious disease after entering the hospital environment. An animal with a communicable infectious disease should be kept completely isolated from other animals in the hospital. Diseases for which isolation in a separate barn is indicated include salmonellosis, anthrax, and leptospirosis (all species); tuberculosis (ruminants); brucellosis (cattle, goats); scabies (cattle); and strangles (horses).

Prevention and Control of Nosocomial Disease

The contaminated environment should be thoroughly cleaned and disinfected (see Chapter 43). The area should then be sampled and cultured. More specific recommendations are given in *Large Animal Internal Medicine,* third edition.

Rational Use of Antimicrobics in a Hospital Setting

Rational use of antimicrobics in this setting involves the following:

- Determining that an infectious process is present, threatens the well-being of the patient, and will not resolve without intervention
- Choosing an antimicrobial that is effective against the microorganisms most likely to be isolated from the site involved
  - Nosocomial agents, especially enterobacteria, are likely to be quite resistant to antimicrobic drugs.

Prophylactic use in this setting should follow the aforementioned guidelines.

43

Disinfectants and Control of Environmental Contamination

Consulting Editor SUSAN L. EWART

Contributor ROBERT L. JONES

Controlling the spread of infection involves a combination of judicious segregation of animals and the use of chemicals that kill microorganisms or their spores in the environment. No single agent or procedure is adequate for all purposes. Factors to consider in the selection of disinfectants include the type of pathogen to be targeted, the extent of microbial killing required, the nature of the item to be treated, and the cost and ease of using the available agents.

CONTROLLING CONTAMINATION AND PREPARING FOR DISINFECTION *(Text pp. 1372-1374)*

Cleaning of contaminated items and proper disposal of contaminated material are essential prerequisites to disinfection because organic matter considerably reduces the efficacy of most disinfectants. Preparation involves the following:

- Control of animal movement (e.g., segregation or depopulation)
- Carcass disposal by rendering, burial, or incineration
- Pest control
- Proper handling of manure and other organic materials (e.g., feed, bedding, soil)
- Surface preparation and cleaning

Cleaning can be accomplished by using water, pressure (e.g., a high-pressure washer at 90 to 120 psi), heat (hot water or steam), and detergents. Any porous materials (e.g., wood, straw, feed) that cannot be thoroughly cleaned should be removed and buried, burned, or fumigated with formaldehyde vapor (see main text). Contaminated dirt cannot be treated effectively except by burning or deep burial. All cleaning equipment must also be cleaned and disinfected.

DISINFECTION *(Text pp. 1374-1379)*

Disinfectants are biocides that are applied directly to inanimate objects. Disinfectants usually destroy most harmful microorganisms but ordinarily do not kill bacterial spores.

Selecting a Disinfectant

There is no single multipurpose disinfectant available for all applications. The interplay of physical conditions (e.g., heat, sunlight, desiccation), mechanical cleaning, time, and composition of surfaces to be disinfected must be considered when selecting a disinfectant. Knowledge of the microorganisms that are causing a risk of disease also influences the choice of disinfectant. The properties of the various disinfectants are discussed in *Large Animal Internal Medicine,* third edition.

Microbial Susceptibility

In general, the following groups of microorganisms are susceptible to the listed disinfectants:

- Most viruses–alcohols, aldehydes, chlorhexidine (not adenoviruses or rotaviruses), chlorine, iodophors, substituted phenolics, and quaternary ammonium compounds (QACs)
  - Parvoviruses are susceptible to aldehydes, chlorine, and QACs.
- Most bacteria–same as for most viruses
  - Chlorhexidine is ineffective against *Staphylococcus* spp. and *Pseudomonas aeruginosa.*
- Bacterial endospores (*Clostridium* and *Bacillus* spp.)–aldehydes and chlorine
- *Mycoplasma* spp. and some filamentous fungi–same as for most viruses
- *Mycobacterium* spp., yeasts, algae, some dimorphic and filamentous fungi–same as for most viruses, with the exception of chlorhexidine

44

Use of Biologics in the Prevention of Infectious Diseases

Consulting Editors W. DAVID WILSON • NANCY E. EAST
JOAN DEAN ROWE • VICTOR S. CORTESE

Contributors ROBERT W. FULTON • JOHN A. ELLIS • ANTHONY W. CONFER
GERALD E. DUHAMEL • CHARLES A. HJERPE • J. GLENN SONGER
DEREK MOSIER

EQUINE VACCINATION AND INFECTIOUS DISEASE CONTROL *(Text pp. 1381-1397)*

Recommended vaccination schedules for horses are shown in Table 44-1 of *Large Animal Internal Medicine,* third edition. Guidelines for use of the most commonly indicated equine vaccines are provided in Table 44-2 of the text.

Tetanus

All horses should be actively immunized against tetanus using tetanus toxoid. Following are the current recommendations:

- Primary immunization–two doses of toxoid (intramuscularly [IM]) should be given 3 to 6 weeks apart, followed by annual booster.
- Pregnant mares–the annual booster should be given 4 to 6 weeks before foaling.
- Foals–the primary series should consist of 3 doses of toxoid given at 4- to 6-week intervals beginning at 6 months of age.
    - Begin the series at 3 to 4 months of age in foals born to nonvaccinated mares.

Vaccinated horses that sustain a wound or have surgery more than 6 months after their previous tetanus booster should be revaccinated with tetanus toxoid.

Tetanus antitoxin

Administration of tetanus antitoxin to unvaccinated horses induces immediate passive protection that lasts up to 3 weeks. A small but significant number of horses experience serum sickness and fatal hepatic failure (serum hepatitis) several weeks after receiving tetanus antitoxin. Indications for administration of tetanus antitoxin include the following:

- Nonvaccinated horse that sustains an injury
- Foal born to a nonvaccinated mare

In these instances, tetanus antitoxin and tetanus toxoid should be given concurrently in separate syringes at different sites. Second and third doses of toxoid should be administered at 4- to 6-week intervals to complete the primary series.

Encephalomyelitis

All horses in North America should be immunized against eastern (EEE) and western (WEE) equine encephalitis. Horses residing in or traveling to areas where there is a risk of exposure to Venezuelan (VEE) equine encephalitis should also be immunized against VEE. Vaccination with one of several available inactivated bivalent (EEE and WEE) or trivalent (EEE, WEE, and VEE) vaccines provides effective control. Recommendations are as follows:

- Primary immunization–administer three doses (IM) 4 to 6 weeks apart, followed by annual booster.
  - Revaccination is best performed in the spring, before the peak insect vector season.
  - Vaccination every 6 months is practiced by many veterinarians in southern states in which mosquitoes are active year round.
- Pregnant mares–give the booster 4 to 6 weeks before foaling.
- Foals–begin primary immunization at 6 months of age; give a booster at 12 months of age, then annual or semiannual boosters thereafter.
  - In foals born late in the breeding season, primary vaccination can be delayed until the following spring in climates where mosquitoes die off in the winter.
  - In areas where there is a high risk of exposure to EEE, the initial series should begin at 3 to 4 months of age.

Influenza

All horses should be vaccinated against equine influenza unless the facility is totally closed. Recommended vaccination protocols depend on the product: modified live virus (MLV) or inactivated virus vaccines.

MLV intranasal vaccine

The MLV intranasal vaccine is currently licensed for use in nonpregnant animals more than 11 months of age. Recommendations are as followed:

- Primary immunization–give a single dose intranasally (IN), followed by boosters every 6 months.
  - There may be an advantage to giving two initial doses at an interval of 3 months.
- Foals–give the first dose at 11 months of age.
  - If the first dose is given before 11 months of age, give a second dose at 11 months.

Until more safety data are available, it is recommended that inactivated influenza vaccines be used for prefoaling boosters in pregnant mares.

Inactivated vaccines

Recommendations for use of inactivated influenza vaccines, which are given by intramuscular injection, are as follows:

- Primary immunization–give three doses (IM) 3 to 6 weeks apart, followed by boosters every 3 to 12 months, depending on the risk.
  - Revaccination every 3 to 4 months is recommended for young horses in competition.
  - Mature performance, show, or pleasure horses constantly at risk of exposure should be revaccinated every 3 to 6 months.
- Pregnant mares–give a booster using a killed virus vaccine 4 to 6 weeks before foaling.
  - All mature horses on the breeding farm should be regularly revaccinated at an interval appropriate for their risk of exposure.
- Foals–timing of the primary vaccination series (three doses 4-6 weeks apart) depends on the mare's vaccination status.
  - In foals born to vaccinated mares and not exposed to horses from other premises, primary vaccination can be delayed until the foal is 9 months of age.
  - In foals born to nonvaccinated mares, primary vaccination should begin at 6 months.

Influenza outbreaks

Definitive diagnosis of equine influenza should be pursued during outbreaks of suspected viral respiratory disease. Same-day diagnosis can be accomplished using enzyme-linked immunosorbent assay test kits marketed for human use (see main text). Vaccination of healthy horses in the face of an outbreak is often a useful supplement to isolating infected and in-contact horses. The intranasal vaccine is likely to induce more rapid and complete protection than that induced by inactivated vaccines.

Equine Herpesvirus (Rhinopneumonitis)

The principal indication for use of equine herpesvirus (EHV) vaccines is prevention of EHV-1-induced abortion in pregnant mares. Bivalent inactivated EHV-1/EHV-4 vaccines and modified live EHV-1 vaccines are often used as an aid to prevention of respiratory tract disease (rhinopneumonitis) in foals, weanlings, yearlings, and young performance and show horses.

Breeding stock

Of the vaccines currently licensed for use in pregnant mares in the United States, only inactivated monovalent EHV-1 vaccines (Pneumabort-K + 1b and Prodigy) containing abortogenic strains of EHV-1 carry a label claim for preventing abortion. Recommendations are as follows:

- Pregnant mares–vaccinate during the fifth, seventh, and ninth months of gestation.
  - Many veterinarians also recommend a dose during the third month of gestation.
- Barren mares and stallions–vaccinate before the start of the breeding season and thereafter at intervals of 6 months.

Young horses

The role of EHV-1 and EHV-4 in causing clinically important respiratory disease is uncertain, and there is a lack of published data regarding the efficacy of available vaccines in preventing infection and establishment of latency. Thus there appears to be little rationale to support the common practice of frequent revaccination of young horses against EHV-1 and EHV-4. Frequent vaccination of nonpregnant mature horses (except those on breeding farms) with EHV vaccines generally is not indicated.

Streptococcus equi Infection (Strangles)

Vaccination against *Streptococcus equi* is not routinely recommended except on premises where strangles is a persistent problem or for horses that are expected to be at high risk of exposure. Recommendations depend on the product.

Inactivated vaccines

Recommendations for use of inactivated strangles vaccines, which are given IM, are as follows:

- Primary immunization–give two or three doses 2 to 4 weeks apart, followed by annual revaccination
  - Efficacy may be improved by using a primary series of three doses with boosters at 6-month intervals.
- Pregnant mares–give an M-protein vaccine 4 to 6 weeks before foaling.
- Foals–begin initial series (three doses 3 to 6 weeks apart) at 4 to 6 months of age, followed by semiannual or annual boosters.

MLV intranasal vaccine

The modified live intranasal strangles vaccine generally is preferred for primary vaccination of foals and weanlings and for routine use in older horses at high risk for infection. The recommended protocol is as follows:

- Primary immunization–two doses (IN) 2 to 3 weeks apart, with annual or semiannual boosters thereafter, depending on the risk of infection.
- Foals–begin primary series at 4 to 6 months of age; give a third dose 3 months later.

- ◦ Can be given to foals as young as 5 to 6 weeks of age during outbreaks; a third dose should be given 2 to 4 weeks before the foal is weaned.

The intranasal vaccine is preferred over inactivated vaccines for use in an outbreak. It is safe for use in mares at all stages of pregnancy; however, an inactivated M-protein vaccine should be used for prefoaling boosters to maximize passive transfer of specific immunoglobulins to the foal.

Adverse effects

The following adverse effects have been reported with the inactivated strangles vaccines:

- Injection site reactions–swelling and muscle pain (which may manifest as lameness)
    - Most common adverse effect and most likely with the whole-cell bacterin
- Systemic signs–uncommon; include fever, depression, and inappetence
- Sterile or infected abscesses at the injection site
- Purpura hemorrhagica–manifested as edema with or without petechial hemorrhages on mucosal surfaces in the weeks after vaccination

The following adverse effects have been reported with the MLV intranasal strangles vaccine:

- Injection site abscesses–if the intranasal product is inadvertently injected IM, or if other vaccines are administered IM immediately after intranasal administration of the MLV vaccine
- Nasal discharge, submandibular or retropharyngeal lymphadenopathy with or without abscesses
- Limb edema
- Internal abscesses (bastard strangles)
- Purpura hemorrhagica

Most adverse events have occurred on farms with endemic or epidemic strangles.

Rabies

All horses kept in areas where rabies is endemic in the wildlife population are at risk and should be vaccinated against rabies. Recommendations are as follows:

- Primary immunization–one dose (IM), followed by annual boosters
- Brood mares–vaccinate before breeding
- Foals–timing depends on vaccination status of mare
    - In foals born to nonvaccinated mares, begin vaccination at 3 months of age; give a booster at 12 months of age and annual boosters thereafter.
    - In foals born to vaccinated mares, give the first dose no earlier than 6 months of age; give a second dose 1 month later, a third dose at 12 months of age, then annual boosters.

Equine Monocytic Ehrlichiosis (Potomac Horse Fever)

Currently available Potomac horse fever vaccines are limited in their ability to provide protection against field infection. Nevertheless, the severity of the disease may be attenuated and mortality may be reduced in vaccinated horses. If vaccination is elected, recommendations are as follows:

- Primary immunization–give two doses 3 to 4 weeks apart, then boosters every 6 to 12 months.
    - Revaccination in late spring, about 1 month before the first cases are expected, followed by a second dose 4 months later, is a reasonable strategy.
    - Revaccination can be administered at 4-month intervals in endemic areas with high risk of exposure.
- Pregnant mares–a booster can be given 4 to 6 weeks before foaling.
- Foals–primary immunization (using a series of three doses) can begin after 5 months of age.

Botulism

A toxoid directed against *Clostridium botulinum* type B is licensed for use in horses in the United States. Its main indication is for prevention of shaker foal syndrome, a significant problem in foals between 2 weeks and 8 months of age in Kentucky and the mid-Atlantic states. Vaccination protocols are as follows:

- Pregnant mares–give the initial series of three doses 4 weeks apart, timed so that the last dose is given 4 to 6 weeks before foaling.
  - In subsequent years, give a booster annually 4 to 6 weeks before foaling.
- Foals–begin the primary series at 2 to 3 months of age.

Treatment of botulism using botulinum antitoxin is discussed in Chapter 33.

Equine Viral Arteritis

Vaccination of stallions, nonpregnant mares, and prepubertal colts is a safe and effective means of controlling equine viral arteritis (EVA). A modified live vaccine is licensed for commercial use, with the primary indications being (1) to prevent infection and establishment of the carrier state in previously unexposed stallions and (2) to protect nonpregnant mares being bred to carrier stallions. Primary immunization involves administration of a single dose of vaccine, with annual boosters thereafter.

Specific recommendations

Specific recommendations are as follows:

- Breeding stallions–give annual revaccination 28 days before the start of breeding season.
- Mares being bred to carrier stallions–revaccinate annually at least 21 days before breeding.
  - Isolate mares for 21 days after breeding.
- Pregnant mares–MLV vaccine is not recommended for use in pregnant mares, especially during the last 2 months of gestation.
  - Foaling mares should be vaccinated after foaling, before being rebred.
- Young intact males–vaccination between 8 and 12 months of age is strongly encouraged in breeds or in areas in which equine arteritis virus is prevalent.
  - Routine vaccination of Standardbred colts is a logical approach to reducing the number of stallions that later become chronic carriers.
  - MLV vaccine is not recommended for use in foals less than 6 weeks of age.

NOTE: Vaccination against EVA may complicate testing of horses for export (see main text).

Rotaviral Diarrhea

An inactivated rotavirus A vaccine is conditionally licensed in the United States for administration to pregnant mares as an aid to prevention of rotaviral diarrhea in their foals. The recommendation is for three doses to be given at 8, 9, and 10 months of gestation during each pregnancy.

Anthrax

A live spore vaccine has been used to vaccinate horses against anthrax. A primary series of two doses (subcutaneously) 2 to 3 weeks apart is followed by annual revaccination. Adverse systemic or local effects occasionally occur. Vaccination of pregnant mares is not recommended.

VACCINATION PROGRAMS FOR SHEEP AND GOATS *(Text pp. 1399-1403)*

Several vaccines are labeled for sheep or goats, and some cattle vaccines are used off-label in these species. Available vaccines for use in sheep and goats are listed in Table 44-3 of *Large Animal Internal Medicine,* third edition. The subcutaneous route of administration is preferred for all listed products. The preferred site is the neck or behind the elbow.

Universal Recommendations

All sheep and goats should be vaccinated against *Clostridium perfringens* types C and D and tetanus. It is recommended that pregnant ewes and does be revaccinated annually, about 4 weeks before parturition, with a combined *C. perfringens* types C and D and tetanus toxoid.

Sheep

Other recommended vaccines in sheep include those immunizing against footrot, *Chlamydia psittaci* (enzootic abortion of ewes), *Campylobacter* spp. (vibriosis), bluetongue virus, and other clostridial agents as needed. Vaccination schedules and flock management calendars for ewes and lambs (Table 44-4) and rams (Table 44-5) in North America are given in *Large Animal Internal Medicine,* third edition.

Dairy Goats

Other recommended vaccines in goats include those immunizing against contagious ecthyma virus (if premises are infected), *C. psittaci,* and other clostridial agents as needed. Vaccination schedules and flock management calendars for does and bucks (Table 44-6) and kids (Table 44-7) are given in *Large Animal Internal Medicine,* third edition.

BOVINE VACCINES AND HERD VACCINATION PROGRAMS *(Text pp. 1403-1435)*

A list of currently available vaccines approved for use in cattle is given in Table 44-8 of *Large Animal Internal Medicine,* third edition. Considerations for designing a herd vaccination program are discussed in the text.

General Recommendations

Beef cattle

The following vaccines are highly recommended for the particular types of beef cattle listed:

- Adult cattle–infectious bovine rhinotracheitis (IBR), bovine viral diarrhea (BVD), *Leptospira pomona* (cows only), and *Campylobacter* spp.
  - *Campylobacter* bacterin is recommended except in closed herds in which the disease can be reliably excluded by isolation from other potentially infected herds.
- Calves (less than 12 months of age)–IBR, BVD, bovine respiratory syncytial virus (BRSV), parainfluenza type 3 (PI-3), *L. pomona,* and brucellosis (replacement heifers only)
- Replacement heifers–IBR, BVD, *L. pomona,* and *Campylobacter* spp. (with the aforementioned exceptions)
- Stocker cattle–IBR, BVD, BRSV, PI-3, *Pasteurella haemolytica,* and *L. pomona*
- Cattle entering a feedlot–modified live IBR (essential) and BVD (recommended), *P. haemolytica* ("One-Shot," Pfizer), and *L. pomona*

Dairy cattle

The following vaccines are highly recommended for the particular types of dairy cattle listed:

- Adult cows–IBR, BVD, and *L. pomona*
  - *Leptospira hardjo* bacterin is highly recommended in infected herds.
  - *Clostridium haemolyticum* and *Clostridium novyi* bacterins and anthrax vaccines are highly recommended for dairy cows grazing in endemic areas.
- Adult bulls–IBR, BVD, and *Campylobacter* spp.
  - Inactivated anaplasmosis vaccine, *C. haemolyticum* and *C. novyi* bacterins, and anthrax vaccines are highly recommended for bulls grazing in endemic areas.
- Calves (less than 12 months of age)–IBR, BVD, BRSV, PI-3, *L. pomona,* and brucellosis
  - Blackleg, *C. haemolyticum,* and *C. novyi* bacterins, and anthrax vaccines are highly recommended for calves grazing in endemic areas.
  - A modified live anaplasmosis vaccine is highly recommended for calves in herds in which adult cows are grazing in endemic areas.

- Yearling replacement heifers–IBR, BVD, and *L. pomona*
  - *Campylobacter* bacterin is highly recommended for heifers to be bred by natural service.
  - *L. hardjo* bacterin is highly recommended for heifers in infected herds.
  - Blackleg, *C. haemolyticum,* and *C. novyi* bacterins and anaplasmosis and anthrax vaccines are highly recommended for heifers grazing in endemic areas.

Infectious Bovine Rhinotracheitis

Five types of IBR vaccine are available: (1) MLV, administered IM; (2) MLV, administered IN; (3) chemically altered virus for parenteral use; (4) inactivated virus; and (5) combination parenteral MLV and inactivated virus. General guidelines for use are discussed in *Large Animal Internal Medicine,* third edition.

Calves

Calves may be vaccinated at or 30 days before weaning. If vaccinated earlier than 6 months of age, calves should be revaccinated. MLV vaccines (whether parenteral or intranasal) require only one dose, whereas the chemically altered live virus and inactivated vaccines require two doses.

Breeding cows and heifers

Yearling heifers should be vaccinated at least 1 month before breeding. Any of the vaccine types may be used; however, if two doses are required, the second dose should be given at least 1 month before breeding. Pregnant cows may be vaccinated with a product labeled for such use (MLV intranasal, chemically altered live virus, or inactivated virus vaccines).

Stocker/feeder cattle

Cattle to be shipped to pasture after weaning or to feedyards should be vaccinated 2 to 3 weeks before shipment. Any of the types of IBRV vaccine may be used; however, those requiring only one dose may be best. Cattle entering the feedyard usually receive the MLV parenteral or intranasal vaccine because of its rapid onset of immunity.

Bovine Virus Diarrhea Virus

Three kinds of BVDV vaccines are currently available: (1) MLV, (2) temperature-sensitive virus (available in Europe only), and (3) inactivated virus. The MLV vaccines have demonstrated advantages over the newer inactivated BVDV vaccines (see main text). However, the MLV vaccines cause mild immunosuppression for a short time after administration, they have been associated with postvaccinal mucosal disease, and they are not recommended for use in pregnant cattle.

Vaccination programs

All herds should be vaccinated against BVDV. Following are some general considerations for devising a BVDV vaccination program:

1. Use vaccines with proven protection against both types 1 and 2 BVDV.
2. Institute a virus isolation and cull program along with a vaccination program that includes administration of at least one MLV vaccine to all replacement animals.
3. Either increase the frequency of vaccination with killed vaccine to two or three times a year or give a MLV vaccine to open cows 3 weeks before breeding.
4. If an early BVDV problem does not exist, waiting to administer the first BVDV vaccine until 5 to 6 months of age increases the number of animals responding to vaccination.

These and other recommendations are discussed in *Large Animal Internal Medicine,* third edition.

Bovine Respiratory Syncytial Virus

Administration of BRSV vaccines to cows in late gestation is a rational strategy for dealing with BRSV-induced respiratory disease in young (1- to 3-month-old) calves in problem herds. Several parenteral MLV and inactivated BRSV vaccines are commercially available; most are formulated in combination with other viral respiratory pathogens.

Parainfluenza Type 3 Virus

Currently, there are five types of commercially available PI-3 virus vaccines: (1) MLV for intramuscular injection, (2) MLV temperature-sensitive for intramuscular injection, (3) MLV for intranasal administration, (4) MLV temperature-sensitive for intranasal administration, and (5) inactivated virus. All PI-3 vaccines available in North America are combined (at a minimum) with a BHV-1 vaccine. Calves vaccinated parenterally before 8 months of age should be revaccinated after reaching 8 or 9 months of age.

Pasteurella haemolytica

P. haemolytica vaccines are often combined with viral vaccines, *Haemophilus somnus* or *Pasteurella multocida* bacterins, and occasionally *Clostridium* spp. biologics. Use of these products in herd vaccination programs are discussed in *Large Animal Internal Medicine,* third edition.

Other Respiratory Vaccines

Indications and recommendations for use of *P. multocida* and *H. somnus* vaccines are discussed in *Large Animal Internal Medicine,* third edition.

Brucella abortus

The legal use of *Brucella abortus* vaccines is limited to heifer calves between 4 and 12 months of age. Because the strain 19 vaccine may cause clinical illness, septicemia, and occasional deaths, vaccination of sick, unhealthy, or stressed cattle should be avoided. The control program should include testing and culling of all positive animals.

Leptospira interrogans

Leptospira spp. vaccinations (initial and booster) help prepare the heifer for entry into the breeding herd. Current bacterins contain either *L. pomona* antigen only or a combination of *Leptospira* antigens. Other important serovars are *L. hardjo, L. grippotyphosa, L. canicola,* and *L. icterohaemorrhagiae.* Although many *Leptospira* bacterins are labeled for a single initial dose, a booster dose approximately 1 month later is recommended. Most manufacturers specify annual revaccination, but more frequent revaccination is often needed to control leptospiral abortions.

Bovine Genital Campylobacteriosis

Use of *Campylobacter (Vibrio) fetus* bacterins is recommended in all breeding herds that use bulls. In heifer herds using virgin bulls, or 100% artificial insemination bred herds, vaccination against *Vibrio* is not necessary. Specific recommendations vary with the product:

- Oil-adjuvant bacterin–administer no earlier than 4 months before the breeding season.
- $Al(OH)_3$-adsorbed bacterin–give a priming dose at least 6 weeks before the immunizing (booster) dose, which should be given 10 days before the start of the breeding season.

Campylobacteriosis is most effectively controlled when all breeding-age animals, including bulls (see main text), are included in the vaccination program.

Bovine Trichomoniasis

The efficacy of *Tritrichomas* vaccines is questionable, but they appear to decrease reproductive losses. Heifers, cows, and breeding bulls should be vaccinated twice at 2- to 4-week intervals, the second dose given 4 weeks before the start of the breeding season. In subsequent years a single booster vaccination should be given 4 weeks before the start of the breeding season. Vaccination must be coupled with other control measures, such as culturing, culling, and treatment.

Neonatal Enteric Disease Vaccines

Following is a brief discussion of vaccines directed against neonatal enteric diseases. However, it is worth noting that vaccination programs for neonatal enteric disease are rarely successful in the absence of good sanitation and management practices.

Rotavirus and coronavirus vaccines

Two approaches are widely used in an attempt to protect calves against rotavirus and coronavirus infection and diarrhea:

- Parenteral vaccination of pregnant cows
- Oral vaccination of neonatal calves (ideally before they receive colostrum)

Protocols for specific products are given in *Large Animal Internal Medicine,* third edition.

Enterotoxigenic *Escherichia coli*

Control of *Escherichia coli* infection in neonatal calves is aimed at controlling calf exposure to the pathogen and vaccinating the cow in late gestation to increase the colostral antibody levels against this pathogen. The protocol depends on the product:

- Oil-adjuvant bacterin–single intramuscular dose 2 weeks to 6 months before calving; repeated annually
- Non-oil-adjuvant bacterins–two intramuscular or subcutaneous doses 2 to 4 weeks apart, the second dose given 2 to 3 weeks before calving; in subsequent years, a single booster 2 to 3 weeks before calving

Salmonella vaccines

Vaccination of cattle 3 months of age or older with two doses of killed *Salmonella* bacterin can be useful for preventing salmonellosis. Vaccination of adult cows is often used in dairies for control of calfhood salmonellosis (see main text).

Clostridial Vaccines

The following clostridial vaccines are briefly discussed in *Large Animal Internal Medicine,* third edition: *Clostridium chauvoei* (blackleg) bacterins, *Clostridium septicum* (malignant edema) bacterins, *C. novyi* types A and B (bighead and infectious necrotic hepatitis) bacterins, *C. haemolyticum* (*C. novyi* type D; bacillary hemoglobinuria) bacterins, *C. botulinum* (botulism) toxoids, *Clostridium tetani* (tetanus) toxoids, *C. perfringens* toxoids, and *Clostridium sordelli* bacterins. General recommendations for use are summarized in Table 44-12 of *Large Animal Internal Medicine,* third edition.

Miscellaneous Bovine Vaccines

Vaccines against the following agents or diseases may be indicated in certain herds or areas: gram-negative core antigen (for prevention of coliform mastitis and calf scours), anaplasmosis, infectious bovine keratoconjunctivitis, staphylococcal mastitis, anthrax, interdigital necrobacillosis, papillomatous digital dermatitis (foot warts), rabies, and fibropapillomas (warts). Use of these vaccines is discussed in *Large Animal Internal Medicine,* third edition.

45

Parasite Control Programs

Consulting Editor CHRISTINE A. UHLINGER

Contributors CRAIG R. REINEMEYER • JOSEPH DiPIETRO

Design of parasite control programs, anthelmintic drugs, and the life cycles of each of the parasites discussed in the following sections are covered in *Large Animal Internal Medicine,* third edition.

EQUINE STRONGYLE DISEASE *(Text pp. 1438-1443)*

Horses of all ages are susceptible to strongylosis, but young and parasite-naive animals are most susceptible. Strongylosis in horses causes a wide spectrum of effects, from inapparent infection to sudden death. Although *Strongylus vulgaris* is considered the most pathogenic of the strongyle species, small strongyle disease (cyathostomiasis) is emerging as an important clinical syndrome. In most adult horses, cyathostomes account for 85% to 100% of the animal's total gastrointestinal (GI) nematode burden.

Clinical Manifestations

Large strongyles

Access to large numbers of infective larvae can cause an acute syndrome of fever, inappetence, diarrhea, lethargy, dehydration, weight loss, and colic. Recurrent episodes of mild to moderate colic or diarrhea (acute or chronic) may be seen throughout the migration phase of large strongyle infection. Less severely affected horses may exhibit dullness, progressive weight loss, and loss of bloom (or intermittent colic); mild anemia may also be found.

Atypical manifestations. Other reported findings include sudden death from coronary arterial thrombosis or renal infarction; hindlimb lameness from aortoiliac thrombosis; and neurologic dysfunction from aberrant migration of larvae through the central nervous system.

Small strongyles (cyathostomes)

Cyathostomiasis causes a variety of clinical syndromes. The most consistent finding is weight loss. Diarrhea is a common feature, although it is not always present. Clinical presentations include the following:

- Sudden onset of diarrhea (which can become chronic) and marked weight loss; colic, subcutaneous edema, and pyrexia may also be seen.
  - Some severely affected horses are unresponsive to therapy and die within 2 to 3 weeks.
- Seasonal diarrhea in young horses (seen in late winter/spring in temperate climates)
- Rapid weight loss, severe peripheral edema, and pyrexia without diarrhea in young horses
- Loss of vigor, depressed growth, intermittent soft feces, and inappetence in foals
- Recurrent diarrhea in aged horses or ponies

- Weight loss of several months' duration before the onset of diarrhea
- Vague malaise with decreased appetite, lethargy, and reduced performance
- Various forms of colic (ranging from mild medical colic to severe colic caused by cecocecal intussusception, nonstrangulating infarction, or cecal tympany)

A feature in many cases is a history of regular anthelmintic treatment.

Prevention and Control

Pasture hygiene and management are important in the control of equine strongylosis. Twice-weekly removal of manure from paddocks and pastures is critical in intensive management systems. Other strategies for minimizing reinfestation during grazing are discussed in the text.

Anthelmintic drugs

The following anthelmintics are effective against equine strongyles:

- Luminal stages–ivermectin (0.2 mg/kg), moxidectin (0.4 mg/kg), benzimidazoles* (5 to 10 mg/kg, depending on the product), febantel* (5 to 6 mg/kg), pyrantel pamoate (6.6 mg/kg), dichlorvos (30 to 35 mg/kg)
  - Piperazine (110 to 200 mg/kg) may be effective against cyathostomes.
  - Pyrantel tartrate (2.65 mg/kg daily) prevents infection by newly acquired infective larvae.
- Migrating large strongyle larvae–ivermectin (0.2 mg/kg), moxidectin (0.4 mg/kg), fenbendazole (7.5 to 10 mg/kg daily for 5 days), oxibendazole (20 mg/kg daily for 5 days)
- Mucosal cyathostome larvae–moxidectin, fenbendazole, or oxibendazole at the dosages specified for migrating large strongyle larvae

Products should be selected that are effective against small strongyles. No single schedule controls parasites on all farms; the program must be tailored to the management unit. Evaluation of strongyle control programs is discussed in *Large Animal Internal Medicine,* third edition.

Clinical Management

Diagnosis

Definitive antemortem diagnosis of strongylosis can be difficult. In many cases, diagnosis is based on clinical presentation and response to therapy. Fecal egg counts more than 1000 eggs per gram (EPG) are indicative of parasitism, but many animals show signs of disease in the prepatent phase of infection. When present, hypoalbuminemia, eosinophilia, anemia, and hyperglobulinemia (particularly β-globulins or IgG[T]) are supportive of the diagnosis.

Treatment

For many animals, appropriate anthelmintic treatment is sufficient to resolve the clinical signs associated with strongyle infection. However, unless the animal's grazing environment is properly managed, the problem may recur. All animals sharing the pasture must be treated unless pyrantel tartrate is administered daily used.

Larvicidal therapy. Animals heavily infected with strongyles or those with chronic colic or nonresponsive diarrhea may require larvicidal treatment with one of the following regimens:

- Fenbendazole–7.5 to 10 mg/kg daily for 5 days or 50 mg/kg daily for 3 days
- Moxidectin–0.4 mg/kg once
- Ivermectin–0.2 mg/kg once (ineffective against encysted cyathostomes)

Occasionally, the larvicidal regimen is given in combination with antiinflammatory agents (e.g., dexamethasone for larval cyathostomosis). After treatment the animal must be returned to noncontaminated pasture.

---

*Note: many of the small strongyles are now resistant to benzimidazoles and febantel.

EQUINE ASCARID INFECTION *(Text pp. 1443-1445)*

Infection with *Parascaris equorum* is common in foals. Ascarid infection should be included in the list of differential diagnoses for foals exhibiting ill thrift, coughing, pneumonia, and colic. Ascarids can be difficult to eradicate from premises and may cause disease in each foal crop.

Clinical Manifestations

Coughing and mucopurulent nasal discharge occur during larval migration through the lung. Respiratory signs may be very mild or may be associated with depression and anorexia. Fever is often absent unless secondary bacterial pneumonia develops. Other manifestations of roundworm infection include ill thrift, rough hair coat, hypoproteinemia, poor weight gain, and debility. Adult worms in the gut may cause ileus or impaction that may lead to intestinal rupture.

Prevention and Control

Management practices that enhance parasite control in young horses include good sanitation in foaling facilities, frequent removal of manure from stalls and paddocks, use of feeders and waterers that minimize the potential for fecal contamination, and avoidance of overgrazing and mixing of foals with yearlings.

Anthelmintics

Piperazine, benzimidazoles, pyrantel, organophosphates, ivermectin, and moxidectin all have some efficacy against ascarids. However, few of these drugs are highly effective against migratory stages at normal doses. Ivermectin is highly effective against larval stages, but its efficacy is short lived. Reinfection can occur as early as 2 weeks after treatment if the foal remains in a contaminated environment. Daily pyrantel tartrate therapy is prophylactic and can be used as soon as foals reliably consume grain.

Clinical Management

Diagnosis

McMaster's fecal analysis may reveal the presence of the thick-walled ascarid eggs; counts greater than 100 EPG indicate that treatment is warranted. In the absence of a positive fecal examination, diagnosis is often made on the basis of clinical signs and farm history. Parasitized animals may exhibit eosinophilia in a blood sample or in tracheal wash cytologic examination.

Treatment

Heavily parasitized foals present a therapeutic challenge. Too sudden or rapid a kill may result in fatal bowel obstruction with dead worms or a toxic response to large numbers of disintegrating worms. It may be prudent to pretreat such foals with a benzimidazole chosen for its relatively low efficacy (e.g., fenbendazole at 5 mg/kg) and follow up with ivermectin. Some veterinarians administer mineral oil after anthelmintic administration to ease the passage of adult worms. Organophosphates and piperazine are contraindicated in heavily infected foals.

Verminous pneumonia. Foals suspected of verminous pneumonia should be treated with a larvicidal regimen of fenbendazole (see p. 1444). Antibiotic coverage is generally recommended.

EQUINE TAPEWORM INFECTION *(Text pp. 1445-1446)*

Most horses tolerate a low level of tapeworm infection without exhibiting clinical signs. However, tapeworm infection can alter bowel motility, increasing the risk for spasmodic colic; ileal impaction; and intussusceptions involving the ileum, cecum, and cecocolic junction. Heavy infections may also be associated with nonspecific GI disturbances and ill thrift. Heavy infections appear to be more common in young horses.

Management

Diagnosis

The presence of the distinctive angulated eggs during microscopic fecal examination constitutes a definitive diagnosis of infection. However, discharge of proglottids is sporadic, so the absence of eggs does not rule out infection. An enzyme-linked immunosorbent assay (ELISA) has been developed for diagnosis of tapeworm infection.

Treatment

Pyrantel pamoate at 13.2 mg/kg or 19.8 mg/kg orally (PO) (i.e., two to three times the standard dose) is effective against *Anoplocephala perfoliata* but not against *Anoplocephala mamillana.* Daily feeding of pyrantel tartrate at 2.65 mg/kg/day is highly effective at suppressing fecal egg output. Praziquantel at 0.75 to 1.0 mg/kg PO is highly effective against both *A. perfoliata* and *A. mamillana.* NOTE: Praziquantel is not approved for use in horses in most countries.

GASTROINTESTINAL NEMATODE INFECTIONS IN SHEEP AND GOATS *(Text pp. 1447-1449)*

GI nematode infections in sheep and goats are responsible for severe clinical syndromes and profound production losses. Young animals, parturient ewes and does, and animals on substandard planes of nutrition are most susceptible. Goats are more susceptible to GI nematodes than are sheep.

Parasites

The parasites of primary importance in sheep and goats are *Haemonchus contortus, Ostertagia* (or *Teladorsagia*) spp., and *Trichostrongylus* spp. *H. contortus* usually is the most significant pathogen in wet, temperate climates. *Ostertagia circumcincta* may predominate in northern or arid climates.

Clinical Manifestations

Most GI nematode infections in small ruminants are associated with altered gut function, anorexia, ill thrift, weight loss, and hypoproteinemia. Diarrhea is a variable sign. Animals may die suddenly without overt clinical signs or may exhibit chronic wasting. Most animals acquire mixed infections of nematodes. Clinical signs may therefore reflect the effects of more than one species of parasite.

Haemonchus

Clinical signs of infection with *Haemonchus* spp. are caused by blood loss and abomasitis. Severely affected animals become hypoproteinemic and exhibit edematous swellings under the jaw and ventrum. Blood loss may be severe enough to cause sudden collapse and death. In these cases the animal may die before the infection is patent. Diarrhea is an inconsistent finding.

Chronic parasitism. In chronic cases the animals become anorectic, anemic, and debilitated; the wool becomes brittle and may fall out in patches. In addition, parasitized animals are more susceptible to diseases from other agents; pneumonia is common in debilitated animals.

Ostertagia

Clinical disease associated with this parasite appears to be less common in small ruminants than in cattle (see p. 1447). Infection may cause two separate syndromes:

- Type I infections–heavy burdens of L_3 larvae acquired in the fall or early spring cause diarrhea, anorexia, and weight loss, most often in young animals.
- Type II infections–emergence of arrested larvae in the spring or early fall causes anorexia, hypoproteinemia, and submandibular edema.

Prevention and Control

Anthelmintic resistance among GI nematodes is now widespread in sheep and goats. Sustainable control requires an integrated management system that incorporates strategic anthelmintic use, selective breeding, and nutritional and environmental management (see main text).

Anthelmintics

The most widely used anthelmintics in small ruminants are the benzimidazoles, levamisole, and avermectins. Drugs and dosages are listed in Table 45-1.

Maximizing anthelmintic efficacy

The following strategies are recommended for maximizing efficacy and limiting anthelmintic resistance in sheep and goats:

- Use the full therapeutic dose on all members of the group.
- Rotate anthelmintic classes annually.
- Limit dosing frequency by using strategic treatments in an integrated pasture management system (e.g., "dose and move"; time treatment for seasonal peaks in larval numbers).
- Avoid introducing resistant nematodes with newly acquired animals.

TABLE 45-1

Efficacy of Various Anthelmintics Against Gastrointestinal Nematodes in Ruminants

	Dosage (mg/kg)*			
Drug	Sheep†	Cattle	Adults	Hypobiotic larvae
BENZIMIDAZOLES				
Albendazole	5-7.5	7.5 to 10	+	+
Febantel	5	7.5 to 10	+	+/–
Fenbendazole	5	7.5 to 10	+	+/–
Mebendazole	15-20		+	+/–
Netobimin	7.5	7.5	+	+
Oxfendazole	5	7.5	+	+
Oxibendazole	15	15	+	+/–
Ricobendazole	5		+	–
LEVAMISOLE/MORANTEL				
Levamisole	5-7.55	5 to 7.5‡	+	+/–
Morantel	5-12.5	10	+	–
Pyrantel	25	12.5	+	–
AVERMECTINS/MILBEMYCINS				
Ivermectin	0.2	0.2§	+	+
Doramectin	0.2	0.2§	+	+
Eprinomectin		0.5‖	+	+
Moxidectin	0.2	0.2§	+	+
OTHER DRUGS				
Closantel	5-10		+¶	–
Nitroxynil	10		+¶	–

+, Highly effective; +/–, moderately effective or effective according to some authors; –, ineffective.

*All dosages are for oral administration unless otherwise indicated.

†Goats must be given higher dosages for equal efficacy.

‡10 mg/kg for topical administration.

§0.2 mg/kg for PO, SC, or IM administration; 0.5 mg/kg topically ("pouron").

‖Available only for topical administration at 0.5 mg/kg; not recommended for sheep.

¶Effective against *H. contortus* only

Note: administration of some of these products may constitute extralabel use in sheep and goats; follow manufacturers' guidelines for meat and milk withdrawal in cattle.

- Do not graze sheep and goats on the same farm.
- Periodically check anthelmintic efficacy with fecal egg counts.

Clinical Management

Diagnosis

Internal parasites should be suspected in cases of diarrhea, poor condition, anemia, or acute collapse in small ruminants. Necropsy and histologic section are the most reliable methods of diagnosis. It is unwise to base a diagnosis solely on the results of fecal examination.

Treatment

Most animals respond to appropriate anthelmintic treatment. In severely affected animals, any additional therapy is supportive and symptomatic (e.g., fluids for animals with diarrhea). Transfusions have been attempted in anemic animals. However, the stress of treatment may kill severely parasitized animals.

GASTROINTESTINAL NEMATODE INFECTIONS IN CATTLE *(Text pp. 1450-1452)*

Cattle are susceptible to infection with a variety of nematode parasites, including *Ostertagia, Haemonchus, Cooperia, Trichostrongylus,* and *Nematodirus* spp. Mixed infections are common. *Ostertagia ostertagi* is the target of most parasite control programs for cattle. In general, anthelmintic programs designed to minimize *Ostertagia* infections also successfully control other GI nematode parasites.

Clinical Manifestations

Clinical manifestations of infection with *Ostertagia* and other nematode parasites in young cattle range from poor growth and ill thrift to serious clinical illness and even death. A feature of *Ostertagia* infection is inappetence, which results in decreased growth and weight gain and delayed onset of puberty. Clinical ostertagiasis is classified as types I and II.

Type I ostertagiasis

Type I ostertagiasis is associated with ingestion of large numbers of infective larvae while on pasture. It manifests as diarrhea, anorexia, and severe production losses in calves during their first grazing season.

Type II ostertagiasis

Type II ostertagiasis is caused by the emergence of previously hypobiotic larvae. It is usually seen in cattle 1 to 2 years of age. Although it is most common in pastured animals, type II disease can also be seen in feedlot and housed animals that have previously grazed infected pasture. Anorexia, ill thrift, and hypoproteinemia are consistent signs. Fever, diarrhea, anemia, and submandibular edema may also be seen. The prognosis for recovery is guarded because of the widespread destruction of abomasal glands.

Control of GI Nematodes

Anthelmintics

Adult *Ostertagia* and other GI nematodes are susceptible to most of the commonly used anthelmintics. Drugs and dosages are listed in Table 45-1. The newer avermectins and moxidectin are particularly effective against both adult and larval stages of the various GI nematodes, including inhibited L_4 larvae.

Treatment intervals

Options for preventing clinical disease and maximizing gains in first-season grazing calves using strategic anthelmintic treatments include the following:

- Two treatments with an avermectin or moxidectin early in the grazing season
- "Dose and move" just before the anticipated peak in pasture infectivity (e.g., early to mid-summer in temperate climates)
- Use of an intraruminal sustained-release device at turnout or weaning
- Treatment during peak pasture infectivity (e.g., summer and early autumn in temperate climates)

Type II ostertagiasis

Hypobiotic larvae can be difficult to eliminate. The avermectins/moxidectin and albendazole are effective against arrested larvae and are useful in the treatment and prevention of type II ostertagiasis (see main text).

Clinical Management

Diagnosis

Antemortem, the history and clinical signs are most useful in suggesting a diagnosis of ostertagiasis. Fecal egg counts can be misleading because they are neither specific nor sensitive for the disease. Serum pepsinogen levels and specific ELISAs for *Ostertagia* spp. can be helpful if available.

Postmortem diagnosis. The most reliable method of diagnosis is necropsy. The abomasal mucosa looks like Moroccan leather (pathognomonic for *Ostertagia* infection). Histologic section and abomasal wall digestion techniques can be used to confirm the presence of larvae.

Treatment

Animals should be treated with an avermectin or moxidectin and moved to a less contaminated environment at the first indication of clinical signs. All animals in the group should be treated. Severely affected animals may need treatment with fluids, plasma transfusions, and supportive therapy to survive. Recovered animals often fail to thrive.

LUNGWORM INFECTION IN LARGE ANIMALS
(Text pp. 1452-1455)

Lungworms, in particular *Dictyocaulus* spp., are nematode parasites that reside in the lung as adults. Clinical disease occurs most frequently in pastured calves, lambs, and kids in the first year of life. The disease is also reported in housed cattle, related either to heavily contaminated bedding or to synchronous maturation of large numbers of hypobiotic larvae. Outbreaks of acute lungworm disease occasionally are seen in adult cattle on pasture. Horses appear to be susceptible to *Dictyocaulus arnfieldi* infection at any age.

Clinical Manifestations

Clinical signs of lungworm infection ("husk") can occur within a week or two of susceptible animals being introduced to contaminated pasture. However, clinical disease is most often seen 2 to 4 months into the grazing season. Affected animals develop either an acute or subacute form of the disease, depending on the number of larvae ingested and the animal's level of immunity.

Acute disease

In calves, acute verminous pneumonia causes dyspnea, cough, and high fever. The animal may expectorate froth. Mortality rates are high, and animals may die before a patent infection has been established. (Note the similarity between this presentation and that of bacterial pneumonia or shipping fever.)

Subacute or chronic disease

The subacute or chronic manifestation of disease is more common. In all species the primary signs are coughing, dyspnea, and loss of condition. The animals show elevated respiratory rates but initially are afebrile; however, affected animals are susceptible to bacterial pneumonia. Signs of reinfection syndrome in adult cattle include cough, tachypnea, and a sudden drop in milk production about 2 weeks after exposure to heavily contaminated pastures.

Lungworm infection in horses

In horses, lungworm infection typically causes a syndrome similar to chronic obstructive pulmonary disease. Donkeys, the source of infection in most cases, remain asymptomatic. Horse and pony foals also may not exhibit overt signs of lungworm infection.

Control

Management strategies designed to decrease exposure to infective larvae are most effective in preventing lungworm disease (see main text). Strategic anthelmintic use, such as treatment at turnout and again 8 weeks later, can substantially reduce pasture infectivity with lungworm larvae.

Anthelmintics

A number of anthelmintics are effective against lungworm. The avermectins/milbemycins are particularly effective against both adult and larval stages and have prolonged residual activity. Anthelmintic options include the following:

- Avermectins/milbemycins–ivermectin, abamectin, doramectin, eprinomectin, moxidectin
  - 0.2 mg/kg PO, subcutaneously (SC), intramuscularly (route depends on product and species); 0.5 mg/kg topically ("pour-on"); intraruminal sustained-release device (ivermectin)
- Albendazole–5 mg/kg PO (sheep, goats); 7.5 to 10 mg/kg PO (cattle)
- Fenbendazole–5 mg/kg PO (sheep, goats); 5 to 10 mg/kg PO (cattle); 30 mg/kg PO (horses); intraruminal sustained-release device (cattle)
- Levamisole–7.5 to 10 mg/kg PO, SC (ruminants); 10 mg/kg topically ("pour-on")

Other anthelmintics (mebendazole, netobimin, oxfendazole, diethylcarbamazine) are listed in Table 45-4 of *Large Animal Internal Medicine,* third edition.

Clinical Management

Diagnosis

Lungworm infestation is often diagnosed on the basis of farm history, seasonal prevalence, and clinical presentation. In ruminants the presence of larvae in fresh feces using the Baermann technique is suggestive of lungworm infection. However, in acute outbreaks, animals may succumb before infections are patent, and an allergic form of the disease may persist even after the worms have been killed or expelled.

Transtracheal wash. Finding a large number of eosinophils on transtracheal wash is supportive of verminous pneumonia; eggs or larvae are occasionally seen with patent infections. This procedure can also help rule out bacterial pneumonia. Because lungworm infections generally do not become patent in horses, transtracheal wash or bronchoalveolar lavage is important in establishing a diagnosis of lungworm disease in this species.

Serology. An ELISA and an indirect hemagglutination assay (IHA) have been developed for detection of *Dictyocaulus viviparus* infection in cattle. The specificity of both assays reportedly is greater than 99%, but the sensitivity of the ELISA is much higher than that of the IHA.

Treatment

Removal of the adult parasites with anthelmintics may result in recovery. However, if the infection is heavy and lung damage is severe, anthelmintic treatment is unlikely to result in complete recovery. In some cases, anthelmintic treatment worsens the signs, and some heavily infected animals die. In severely affected individuals, antihistamines and antibiotics should be included in the therapeutic regimen.

COCCIDIOSIS IN FOOD ANIMALS *(Text pp. 1455-1457)*

Coccidiosis is caused by intracellular parasites, including members of the genera *Isospora* and *Eimeria.* Coccidiosis causes serious economic losses in food animals.

Populations at Risk

Most animals infected with coccidia do not exhibit signs of illness, and after an initial period of infection the host is essentially immune to coccidiosis. Consequently, coccidiosis is primarily a disease of young, nonimmune animals crowded together in unsanitary housing or lots. Outbreaks are often associated with the stress of shipping, weaning, and dietary changes. Corticosteroid treatment, concurrent illness, and severe cold can also precipitate an acute form of coccidiosis. Kids are especially susceptible to coccidiosis.

Clinical Manifestations

Clinical coccidiosis typically is manifested by profuse diarrhea containing mucus and blood. Dehydration may occur, but most animals continue to drink and meet their fluid requirements. The animals typically strain to defecate, which may result in rectal prolapse. Affected animals are often anorectic. In dairy calves the classical signs of dysentery and tenesmus are uncommon. Rather, the predominant signs are loose manure, poor condition, poor growth, and poor hair coat.

Severe cases

Sudden death may occur in kids and lambs, although in most outbreaks the case fatality rate is low. Animals that develop "nervous" coccidiosis may exhibit muscle tremors, hyperesthesia, convulsions, nystagmus, and blindness. The mortality rate is high.

Recovery

Gut function does not return to normal for several weeks, and appetite may be suppressed concurrently. Thus coccidiosis is associated with weakness, ill thrift, and poor weight gain. Diarrhea in kids can become chronic (often without blood) and results in stunting and wasting.

Control

The most important preventive strategies are directed at decreasing exposure to oocysts. This is usually accomplished by standard management techniques: decreasing stocking rates, minimizing stress, and providing clean housing and feed. Exposure to sunlight and low humidity and treatment with formaldehyde, ammonia, or methyl bromide kills the oocysts.

Drug therapy

A variety of drugs have been used to prevent or treat coccidiosis. Treatment options (in mg/kg body weight PO) include the following:

- Amprolium–10 mg/kg for 5 days (calves); 25 to 40 mg/kg for 5 days (lambs, kids); or 65 mg/kg once
- Monensin–2 mg/kg for 20 days (lambs)
- Nitrofurazone–10 to 15 mg/kg for 5 to 7 days
  - Can also be delivered in feed at 0.04% or in water at 0.0133% for 7 days
- Sulfamethazine–110 mg/kg for 5 days; 140 mg/kg for 3 days; or 140 mg/kg once, then 70 mg/kg for 5 to 7 days
- Sulfaquinoxaline–10 to 20 mg/kg for 5 to 7 days
- Toltrazuril–20 mg/kg once

Drug regimens for prevention are given in Table 45-5 of *Large Animal Internal Medicine,* third edition.

Clinical Management

Diagnosis

Young, diarrheic animals passing large numbers of oocysts are not difficult to diagnose. However, making a diagnosis on the basis of oocyst counts alone can be misleading (see main text). Definitive diagnosis may be made at necropsy.

Treatment

Drugs used for treatment are listed in Table 45-5 on p. 1457. Supportive therapy, when indicated, is primarily directed at replacing fluid losses and supporting the animal until the gut epithelium regenerates.

46

Nutrition of the Sick Animal

Consulting Editors RAYMOND W. SWEENEY • PAMELA A. WILKINS

Although it is generally accepted that sick animals have increased nutritional requirements, these requirements have not been quantitated for specific conditions. Therefore the clinician should ensure that nutritional intake is at least 100% of maintenance requirements. Supplementation may be necessary if weight loss ensues.

ORAL SUPPLEMENTATION *(Text p. 1458)*

If the appetite is poor, the patient should be offered a variety of highly palatable feeds. Fresh silage and dried brewer's grain often appeal to hypophagic cattle, and many sick horses and ruminants benefit from grazing if grass is available.

LIQUID DIETS FOR HORSES *(Text p. 1459)*

If the aforementioned measures fail, force-feeding of a liquid diet by intragastric administration should be considered. Dysphagic animals require a liquid diet as the sole source of nutrition.

Adult Horses

Liquid diets for adult horses may be divided into three categories:

- Blender diets–finely ground whole food suspended in water
  - For example, grind one third of the daily ration in a blender (with water) or soak pellets in water to create a slurry; feed three times daily to horses that require complete feeding and one or two times daily if only partial supplementation is needed.
- Composition diets–a mix of highly digestible whole protein, fats, and carbohydrates
  - Commercial liquid diets (e.g., Osmolite HN) are available.
  - A homemade diet consisting of dehydrated cottage cheese, dextrose, and alfalfa meal in water is described in the text.
  - Composition diets may cause mild, self-limiting diarrhea, so they should be gradually introduced over 4 to 7 days.
- Elemental diets–contain hydrolyzed protein and free amino acids
  - These diets are expensive and rarely indicated.

Young Foals

Orphan or critically ill foals may be fed mare's milk (200 ml/kg divided into 6 to 10 feedings). If mare's milk is unavailable, goat's milk or a commercially available milk replacer (e.g., Mare's Match, Udder Delight) may be substituted. Indigestion (mild colic, gastric distention, flatulence) may be observed when the foal is on a diet other than mare's milk. If indigestion occurs, both the frequency and volume of feeding should be decreased until the indigestion resolves.

LIQUID DIETS FOR RUMINANTS *(Text pp. 1459-1460)*

Hypophagic adult cattle may be force-fed a suspension of alfalfa meal and dried brewer's grain (3 to 5 kg each in 20 L water) two or three times a day, either orally or intraruminally. Cattle with omasal transport failure require intraabomasal feedings of a liquid diet via stomach tube placed into the abomasum through a rumenotomy incision or temporary rumenostomy. Liquid composition diets as described for horses are preferred but should be introduced gradually.

INTRAVENOUS FEEDING *(Text p. 1460)*

Intravenous feeding–partial or total parenteral nutrition–is a means of providing nutritional support that does not require the patient to have a functional digestive tract. It should be reserved for cases in which bowel rest is necessary. Parenteral nutrition solutions provide an energy source (usually glucose and lipids) and protein hydrolysates or free amino acids. Formulas for parenteral nutrition solutions in foals, calves, and adult horses are given in *Large Animal Internal Medicine,* third edition. Practical considerations and precautions are also discussed in the text.

PART VII

Congenital, Hereditary, Immunologic, and Toxic Disorders

47

Congenital Defects and Hereditary Disorders in Ruminants

Consulting Editor GEORGE SAPERSTEIN

Contributor EUGENE C. WHITE

Congenital defects and inherited disorders are abnormalities of structure, formation, or function that are present at birth. Most are first diagnosed in newborn animals, but some, although present at birth, are not detected until later in life.

CAUSES OF CONGENITAL DEFECTS AND DISORDERS *(Text pp. 1466-1467)*

Many congenital defects and disorders have no clearly established cause. Others are caused by environmental and/or genetic factors. Teratogens include toxic plants, infectious agents, drugs, trace elements, deficiencies, and physical agents such as (e.g., irradiation, hyperthermia, and embryo manipulation). Teratogenicity often follows seasonal patterns or known stressful conditions, may be linked to maternal disease, and does not follow a familial pattern.

Toxic Plants

The following congenital defects in ruminants have been associated with certain toxic plants:

- Arthrogryposis in calves–*Lupinus* spp., when ingested by pregnant cows between days 40 and 100 of gestation; Sudan grass; and poison hemlock *(Conium maculatum),* when ingested between days 50 and 70 of gestation
  - Joint contracture may be accompanied by spinal deviations (torticollis, scoliosis, kyphosis) and/or cleft palate.
- Congenital limb defects in calves and lambs–locoweed (*Oxytropis* and *Astragalus* spp.)
  - *Trachymene* spp. may cause bent legs in lambs.
- Cyclops–*Veratrum californicum* when grazed in early pregnancy by ewes or does
  - This plant can also cause malformations of the skull or brain, and hypoplasia of the metacarpal and metatarsal bones in kids.

Other plants suspected of causing congenital defects include *Senecio, Indigofera, Spicata, Cycadales, Blighia, Papaveraceae, Colchicum,* and *Vinca,* spp. and tobacco and related plants.

Viral Infections

The following viruses can cause multiple congenital defects:

- Akabane virus–causes arthrogryposis and hydranencephaly

- Bovine virus diarrhea (BVD) virus–induces a variety of congenital defects, including cerebellar hypoplasia, ocular defects, brachygnathia, alopecia, dysmyelinogenesis, internal hydrocephalus, dysmaturity, and impaired immunologic competence
- Border disease virus–causes hypomyelinogenesis congenita and dysmorphogenesis of the skeleton and skin and/or fleece in lambs ("hairy shaker" lambs)
- Bluetongue virus–experimentally, is thought to causes arthrogryposis, campylognathia (wry jaw), prognathia with doming of the cranium, and hydranencephaly
- Cache Valley virus–causes arthrogryposis and various CNS central nervous system defects (micrencephaly, hydranencephaly, cerebellar hypoplasia, and mycromyelia)

SPECIFIC CONDITIONS *(Text pp. 1469-1553)*

Tables 47-1 to 47-56 in *Large Animal Internal Medicine III,* third edition, list congenital defects and inherited disorders in cattle, sheep, and goats, according to the body part or system primarily affected. A brief description of the condition is followed by notes on its etiology (including breeds affected), frequency, diagnosis, and any associated defects.

IDENTIFYING INHERITED DISORDERS *(Text p. 1467)*

Diagnosis of genetic defects is based on the rule that genetic diseases run in families. Thus, hereditary defects occur in typical intergenerational patterns and intragenerational frequencies. Recognizing these requires enumerating normal and abnormal offspring and identifying their familial relationships. Patterns of inheritance (recessive, dominant, incompletely dominant, "overdominant") are discussed in *Large Animal Internal Medicine III,* third edition.

CONTROL *(Text pp. 1467-1469)*

When a defective animal is submitted, the following information should be obtained:

- History–breed, age of parents, parentage of affected and unaffected herd/flockmates, congenital defects observed previously, and history of any similar congenital defects in neighboring flocks
  - Records should be analyzed for evidence of inbreeding and for characteristic intergenerational transmission patterns and intragenerational frequencies.
- Environmental factors–geographic region, season, type of pasture, soil type, possible exposure to teratogenic plants.
- Management–feeding and management practices, breeding records, maternal medical and vaccination records, disease status of the herd/flock, periods of stress, drugs administered

Serum samples should be submitted to check for BVD virus and other viral antibodies. Samples of brain and other tissues can be submitted for virus isolation and histopathologic examination.

Genetic Testing

Although dominant defects can be eliminated simply by not breeding affected animals, eradicating deleterious recessives requires identification of carriers. There are currently three methods for determination of genotype in common usage:

- Test mating (e.g., sire testing)
- Biochemical testing (primarily used for storage and metabolic disorders)
- DNA-based testing (e.g., polymerase chain reaction)

Recommendations for Breeding Programs

When animals with inherited disorders are identified, the following procedures are recommended: (1) blood typing to verify parentage, especially where artificial insemination (AI) sires are involved; (2) certified statement regarding occurrence of the disorder by veterinarian or third-party witness; (3) extended pedigree chart; (4) laboratory examination by a pathologist, when applicable; (5) decision withheld until all reasonable doubt has been eliminated (for bulls, usually two or more thoroughly documented cases, or sire testing; see main text); and (6) subsequent notification of AI or other concerned organizations (e.g., breed registry) with recommended courses of action, if any.

48

Congenital Defects and Hereditary Diseases in the Horse

Consulting Editor GEORGE SAPERSTEIN

ENVIRONMENTAL FACTORS *(Text p. 1556)*

Very little is known about environmental causes of congenital defects in horses. Although teratogens are difficult to identify, they often follow seasonal patterns or known stressful conditions; they may be linked to maternal disease; and they do not follow a familial pattern as do genetic diseases. The following environmental factors have been incriminated in congenital disorders in horses:

- Hybrid Sudan grass pasture–arthrogryposis
- *Astragalus mollisimus*–congenital limb defects
- Cambendazole–limb deformities and multiple facial and skull defects
- Griseofulvin–microphthalmia, brachygnathia, and palatocheiloschisis when given during the second month of gestation
- Combination of sulfadiazine, pyrimethamine, and folic acid–bone marrow aplasia or hypoplasia, renal nephrosis or hypoplasia, and skin lesions
  - This drug combination is commonly used to treat equine protozoal myeloencephalitis.
- Hypothyroidism–multiple musculoskeletal abnormalities, including forelimb contracture, ruptured common digital extensor tendon, short face, skeletal hypoplasia, and combinations of these defects
- Limited in utero space–could cause various congenital defects of the head, neck, and limbs

No teratogenic viral infections have been described in horses.

GENETIC FACTORS *(Text pp. 1556-1557)*

Genetically induced congenital defects occur in typical intergenerational patterns and intragenerational frequencies. Recognizing these requires enumerating normal and abnormal offspring and identifying their familial relationships. Breeding trials are necessary to confirm inheritance patterns.

Diagnosis and Control

Accurate diagnosis of genetic diseases and defects includes understanding hereditary patterns of disease. DNA-based testing procedures are becoming more important in identifying carriers of defective genes for such diseases as hyperkalemic periodic paralysis and severe combined immunodeficiency. Most breed associations have programs for controlling undesirable traits and genetic defects. Producers need to be provided with genetic disease information and counseling so that they can practice selective breeding to minimize losses from genetic interaction.

SPECIFIC CONDITIONS *(Text pp. 1557-1584)*

Tables 48-1 to 48-15 in *Large Animal Internal Medicine,* third edition, list congenital defects and inherited disorders in horses according to the body part or system primarily affected. A brief description of the condition is followed by notes on its etiology (including breeds affected), frequency, diagnosis, and any associated defects.

49

Immunologic Disorders

Consulting Editors STEVEN M. PARISH • MELISSA T. HINES

Contributors JILL McCLURE BLACKMER • DEBRA C. SELLON
GEORGE M. BARRINGTON • JAMES F. EVERMANN

Part I: Equine Immunodeficiency Diseases

Clinical features generally associated with immunodeficiencies include the following:

- Onset of infection in the first 6 weeks of life
- Repeated infections that respond poorly to standard therapy
- Increased susceptibility to organisms with low pathogenicity
- Infection with organisms rarely observed in immunocompetent individuals
- Systemic illness after administration of attenuated live vaccines
- Failure to respond to vaccination
- Persistent marked abnormalities in leukocyte numbers

Because the clinical signs are nonspecific, laboratory or in vivo testing is necessary to confirm the presence of immunodeficiency and to differentiate the various syndromes (see main text).

FAILURE OF PASSIVE TRANSFER *(Text pp. 1592-1594)*

Failure of passive transfer (FPT) may occur in the following circumstances:

- Ingestion of poor-quality colostrum–low immunoglobulin (Ig) content
  - Lactation before parturition, premature foaling, and a defect in the mare's ability to concentrate Ig in the colostrum can each result in low colostral Ig content.
- Failure to ingest a sufficient quantity of colostrum
  - Foals that are orphaned or rejected at birth, too weak to stand, or unable or lack the desire to nurse are unlikely to ingest sufficient colostrum to prevent FPT.
- Failure to absorb colostral immunoglobulins from the gastrointestinal tract

Clinical Signs

FPT itself produces no clinical signs and cannot be detected by physical examination. However, bacterial infections in the first 2 weeks of life, particularly septicemia, septic arthritis, pneumonia, and enteritis, are strongly suggestive of FPT (see Chapter 19).

Diagnosis

FPT is diagnosed by demonstration of low serum IgG in the foal as early as 6 to 12 hours after birth. Routine measurement of serum IgG in apparently healthy foals is usually recommended at 18 to 24 hours of age. Rapid methods for IgG quantitation include zinc sulfate turbidity, latex agglutination, and enzyme immunoassay (see main text).

Interpretation

Generally accepted interpretation of serum IgG concentration is as follows:

- 400 to 800 mg/dl–adequate passive transfer
  - In relatively clean environments, 400 mg/dl may be adequate for healthy foals, but that amount may be inadequate for foals heavily exposed to pathogens or already showing signs of infection.
- 200 to 400 mg/dl–partial FPT
- Less than 200 mg/dl–complete FPT

Treatment

Treatment of FPT depends on the degree of failure, the foal's environment, age of the foal, and the presence of secondary infection. Treatment goals are as follows:

- Minimize exposure to pathogens
- Supply immunoglobulins using oral colostrum or intravenous plasma
- Manage secondary infections if present

Some foals with partial FPT do well without treatment if exposure to potential pathogens is minimized and they have no preexisting infections. Foals with other risk factors for septicemia, such as prematurity, dysmaturity, or placentitis, should receive intravenous plasma if the serum IgG is less than 800 mg/dl at 18 to 24 hours of age.

Supplemental colostrum

If FPT is anticipated or is diagnosed within a few hours of birth, 2 to 3 L (for a 45-kg foal) of good-quality colostrum should be given (see following discussion) or equine plasma should be administered orally (same volume or greater). Suitable substitutes for equine colostrum include commercial lyophilized equine IgG (50 to 70 g IgG) and, in an emergency, bovine colostrum. Recheck the serum IgG level at 24 hours of age and give intravenous plasma if it remains low.

Intravenous plasma

At least 20 ml/kg of plasma (1 L for a 45-kg foal) must be given intravenously to raise the serum IgG by 200 to 300 mg/dl. Often, two to three times this amount is needed to raise levels to 400 to 800 mg/dl. If the foal is clinically ill, additional plasma is usually required. Serum IgG levels should be rechecked after transfusion and more plasma given if necessary.

Predicting FPT

Evaluation of colostral IgG content is valuable in predicting FPT. The quantity of Ig in colostrum may be estimated by single radial immunodiffusion, refractometry, glutaraldehyde coagulation, or specific gravity (SG; measured with a colostrometer). Colostral IgG levels should be at least 3000 mg/dl, which corresponds to an SG of 1.060 or more; levels of 6000 mg/dl or more are desirable. If colostral SG is less than 1.060, some degree of FPT might be anticipated.

SEVERE COMBINED IMMUNODEFICIENCY *(Text pp. 1585-1596)*

Severe combined immunodeficiency (SCID) is a lethal, inherited condition in which both T- and B-cell function is absent. The condition primarily affects Arabians and part Arabians, in which it is an autosomal recessive trait. Carriers are asymptomatic but can be identified by genetic testing.

Clinical Signs

Homozygous foals generally appear normal at birth, but they typically develop infectious diseases between birth and 2 months of age and invariably die before 5 months of age. A variety of bacterial, viral, parasitic, and fungal agents may be involved, some of which rarely cause disease in immunocompetent animals (e.g., *Pneumocystis carinii* and adenovirus). Many body systems may be involved, but pneumonia is particularly common.

Diagnosis

Definitive diagnosis is made by demonstrating that the foal is homozygous for the defective SCID gene. Blood or cheek swabs may be submitted for DNA testing to determine whether a horse is clear, heterozygous, or homozygous for the gene defect.

Other diagnostic criteria

In the absence of genetic testing, the criteria required to confirm a diagnosis of SCID include the following: (1) persistent lymphopenia (less than 1000/μl), (2) absence of serum IgM in presuckle samples or samples collected after 3 weeks of age, and (3) thymic hypoplasia and characteristic histopathologic changes in lymphoid tissue. The total white blood cell count may be low, normal, or elevated, depending on the neutrophil response.

Treatment and Control

There is no treatment at this time. Affected foals invariably die despite intensive therapy (e.g., antimicrobials, plasma, isolation). Control through identification of carrier animals and selective breeding is discussed in *Large Animal Internal Medicine,* third edition.

SELECTIVE IgM DEFICIENCY *(Text pp. 1596-1597)*

Selective IgM deficiency is characterized by undetectable or decreased serum IgM levels with normal or elevated levels of other immunoglobulin classes. It is most often reported in Arabians and quarter horses. Three presentations have been described:

- Foals with severe infectious pneumonia (often caused by *Klebsiella* spp.), arthritis, or enteritis resulting in death before 10 months of age
  - This is the most common presentation.
- Foals with a history of infections that respond to antimicrobial therapy but recur when treatment is stopped
  - These foals do poorly and are stunted, although they may survive for 1 to 2 years.
- Older horses (usually 2 to 5 years of age at initial diagnosis) that do not necessarily have problems with recurrent infections but may ultimately develop lymphosarcoma

The only significant immunologic abnormality is low or undetectable serum IgM (see main text). This condition has an unfavorable prognosis, and most cases eventually succumb to infection despite appropriate antimicrobial therapy.

OTHER IMMUNOLOGIC DISORDERS IN HORSES *(Text pp. 1597-1600)*

The following uncommon or rare immunodeficiency disorders are briefly discussed in *Large Animal Internal Medicine,* third edition:

- Transient hypogammaglobulinemia–characterized by delayed onset of immunoglobulin synthesis by the neonate, resulting in recurrent bacterial and viral infections
  - The cardinal feature is low immunoglobulin levels, particularly IgG and IgG(T), at 2 to 4 months of age.
- Agammaglobulinemia–involves persistently decreased production of all classes of immunoglobulins
  - Blood lymphocyte counts are within normal range.
- Anemia, immunodeficiency, and peripheral ganglionopathy in Fell pony foals (see main text)
- Unclassified immunodeficiencies–diverse group of conditions with little in common except propensity for patients to develop infections; in foals, perinatal infection with equine herpesvirus type 1 and oral candidiasis and

septicemia; in adults, acquired immunodeficiency syndrome, plasma cell myeloma, and nonspecific immune suppression

Part II: Ruminant Immunodeficiency Diseases

FAILURE OF PASSIVE TRANSFER *(Text pp. 1600-1602)*

Failure of newborn ruminants to obtain and absorb colostral immunoglobulins is often associated with increased morbidity and mortality from bacteremia and common neonatal diseases. Septic arthritis, meningitis, and panophthalmitis commonly develop in neonates with FPT that survive the initial challenge of bacteremia.

Diagnosis

The following methods are available for evaluating passive transfer of immunoglobulins:

- Single radial immunodiffusion (SRID)–serum concentrations for IgG, IgM, and IgA of less than 1000 mg/dl, 80 mg/dl, and 22 mg/dl, respectively, at 48 hours are consistent with FPT
- Zinc sulfate turbidity (see main text)
- Sodium sulfite precipitation (Bova-S; see main text)
- Glutaraldehyde coagulation test (see main text)
- Refractometer (total serum solids)–in the absence of dehydration, serum total protein greater than 5 g/dl is indicative of successful passive transfer; values less than 4.5 g/dl are consistent with FPT
- γ-Glutamyltransferase–serum levels less than 300 U/L within 48 hours after birth are consistent with FPT

Treatment

When FPT is diagnosed, serum or plasma should be given at a rate of 20 to 40 ml/kg intravenously (or intraperitoneally if intravenous administration is not possible). Although absorption has ceased, continued feeding of colostrum may provide some local immune protection in the gut. Prevention of FPT is discussed in *Large Animal Internal Medicine,* third edition.

MISCELLANEOUS IMMUNODEFICIENCY CONDITIONS *(Text pp. 1602-1604)*

The following conditions are briefly discussed in the text:

- Lethal trait A46–reported in black pied Danish cattle of Friesian descent
  - Causes skin disease and increased susceptibility to infection.
- Selective IgG_2 deficiency–reported in red Danish cattle
  - Animals are susceptible to gangrenous mastitis and other pyogenic infections.
- Chédiak-Higashi syndrome–reported in Hereford cattle
  - Causes partial albinism, coagulation defects, and increased susceptibility to infection.
- Bovine leukocyte adhesion deficiency (BLAD)–reported in Holstein calves
  - Causes chronic bacterial infections, persistent mature neutrophilia (greater than 40,000/μl), and premature death.
- Viral- and bacterial-induced immunodeficiency–implicated pathogens include bovine viral diarrhea virus (chronic bovine virus diarrhea syndrome) and *Mycobacterium johnei* (Johne's disease).
- Combined immunodeficiency–reported in an Angus calf
- Pregnancy-associated immunodeficiency–increased susceptibility to infection or recrudescence of infection during late pregnancy and early lactation

Part III: Allogenic Incompatibilities

BLOOD TYPING *(Text pp. 1604-1608)*

Blood typing is useful for animal identification, pedigree analysis, prediction of potential for neonatal isoerythrolysis, and crossmatching for blood transfusion. The principles are discussed in *Large Animal Internal Medicine,* third edition. Samples required include serum and whole blood that is preserved in acid-citrate-dextrose anticoagulant. Addresses of laboratories that provide large animal blood typing services are listed in the text.

NEONATAL ISOERYTHROLYSIS IN HORSES *(Text pp. 1608-1611)*

Neonatal isoerythrolysis (NI) is characterized by the destruction of red blood cells (RBCs) in the circulation of a foal by alloantibodies of maternal origin absorbed from colostrum. Mares that are negative for the blood group factors Aa and Qa, and all mule pregnancies, are considered at risk. The prevalence of NI in Thoroughbreds is about 1% and in standardbreds about 2%. Although NI is more common in multiparous mares, it can occur with the first pregnancy.

Clinical Signs

Affected foals are born healthy and usually begin to show signs of NI at 24 to 36 hours of age. Progressive lethargy and weakness are early signs. The mucous membranes initially are pale but may then become icteric; in peracute cases, death may precede the development of icterus. Breathing becomes rapid and shallow, and the foal may yawn repeatedly. The heart rate is elevated. Seizurelike activity may occur as the anemia becomes more severe.

Diagnosis

Affected foals are anemic; packed cell volume (PCV) values often decline into the teens. Hemoglobinemia and hemoglobinuria may be present. Bilirubin (mainly unconjugated) is increased; total bilirubin levels may approach 20 mg/dl in severe cases. Affected foals, especially mule foals, may also be thrombocytopenic. Definitive diagnosis requires demonstration of significant amounts of antibody in the colostrum (or mare's serum) directed against the foal's RBCs (see main text).

Treatment

Treatment consists of supportive care:

- Minimize stress and restrict exercise.
- Give intravenous fluids to induce diuresis.
- Give a blood transfusion if the anemia becomes severe (PCV less than 15%).

Transfusion with 1 to 4 L washed RBCs or whole blood is usually adequate; repeated transfusion may be required if the anemia continues to worsen.

Washed RBCs

Washed RBCs from the dam are preferred for transfusion. In the absence of a large-volume centrifuge, the procedure involves the following steps:

- Collect 3 to 4 L (up to 8 L) of blood from the mare into acid-citrate-dextrose or sodium citrate.
- Allow the blood to settle for 1 to 2 hours, then aseptically draw off the plasma and add a similar or greater volume of sterile isotonic saline.
- Mix, then allow the blood to settle again.
- Draw off the saline, resuspend the RBCs in an equal volume of isotonic saline, and either administer the blood to the foal or wash the RBCs again before administration.

Whole blood transfusion

An alternative to washed RBCs is whole blood from a donor horse that is unlikely to have the RBC antigen to which the alloantibodies in the colostrum (and now the foal's plasma) are directed. Crossmatching is important (see main text). In the case of mule foals, blood from any horse not previously sensitized by pregnancy to a donkey usually is safe.

Withholding milk

By the time the problem is recognized (usually when the foal is at least 24 hours of age), the bulk of colostral antibody has been depleted from the mare's milk and the absorptive ability of the foal's gut is diminished. Thus withholding milk at this point is of questionable benefit.

Prevention

With an unknown or incompatible mating, serum from at-risk mares should be screened for anti-RBC antibodies within 30 days before foaling:

- Serum and anticoagulated blood samples are submitted to a screening laboratory (see main text).
- If anti-RBC antibody is detected, the colostrum should be checked for reactivity against the foal's RBCs before allowing the foal to ingest colostrum.
    - Alternatively, another source of colostrum should be provided to the foal.

A field method of screening colostrum is described in the text.

NEONATAL ISOERYTHROLYSIS IN RUMINANTS
(Text pp. 1611-1612)

NI does not occur naturally in cattle, sheep, or goats. Its occurrence in cattle has been associated with administration of vaccines derived from blood (e.g., anaplasmosis and babesiosis vaccines).

50

Disorders Caused by Toxicants

Consulting Editor FRANCIS D. GALEY

Contributor KONNIE H. PLUMLEE

DIAGNOSING TOXICOSIS *(Text pp. 1614-1615)*

When one is faced with a disorder possibly caused by a toxicant, samples of blood, serum, urine, body fluids, and ingesta should be obtained for clinical pathologic and toxicologic analyses. Complete necropsies should be performed on dead animals and appropriate tissues fixed for histologic examination. Separate fresh tissue samples should be frozen for toxicologic analyses. Environmental samples should also be collected for testing (see main text).

TOXIC PLANTS *(Text pp. 1616-1627)*

Locoweed

Genera: *Astragalus* (locoweeds); *Oxytropis* (crazyweed)
Distribution: from the Rocky Mountains and Texas to California
Conditions conducive to toxicity: locoweed is unpalatable and is ingested when other feed is lacking (although animals can acquire a taste for the plant); remains toxic when dried
Livestock affected: all species
Clinical findings:

- Ingestion causes gradual onset of signs related to production/metabolism and the central nervous, reproductive, and cardiovascular systems.
- Affected animals become emaciated, lethargic, dull, and ataxic, with an impaired sense of direction; despite being depressed, they are nervous and may react violently to stimulation.
  - Horses do not recover from the tendency to react uncharacteristically to stimuli.
- Reproductive consequences include altered breeding behavior (prolonged estrus, decreased libido), inhibition of spermatogenesis, abortion, weak and docile newborns, and congenital flexural limb deformities.
- Ingestion predisposes calves to development of right-sided congestive heart failure at high altitudes (high mountain disease).

Diagnosis: history of exposure and clinical signs; possible clinical pathologic evidence of liver damage and mild renal damage
Treatment: no specific treatment; exposure should be prevented and adequate nutrition provided

Pyrrolizidine Alkaloids

Genera: *Senecio* (tansy ragwort and groundsel); *Crotalaria* (rattlebox); *Cynoglossum* (houndstongue); *Amsinckia* (fiddleneck); *Heliotropium* (heliotrope); *Echium* (Patterson's curse, Salvation Jane)

Distribution: *S. jacobea* (tansy ragwort) is found in the northwestern United States; *S. vulgaris* (common groundsel) is found throughout the western United States; *Crotalaria* is present in the Midwest; *Cynoglossum* is primarily found in the Rocky Mountain region; *Amsinckia* is found in California

Conditions conducive to toxicity: these plants are unpalatable, so most poisonings occur when animals are forced to graze the plant or when the plant is masked in hay (e.g., *Senecio* and *Amsinckia*) or grain (e.g., *Crotalaria*); toxicity is retained with drying

Livestock affected: all species; small ruminants are more resistant than cattle and horses

Clinical findings:

- Affected animals usually present with signs and lesions compatible with liver failure; pulmonary disease has also been reported for *Crotalaria* poisoning.
- Signs may be delayed for months after ingestion, appearing after the liver damage has become chronic; emaciation and hepatoencephalopathy are common.
- Ingestion of pyrrolizidine alkaloids enhances the toxicity of copper in sheep (see p. 1617).

Diagnosis: history of exposure, clinical and pathologic evidence of liver failure, and classic histopathologic lesions (see main text)

Treatment: treat for liver failure (see Chapter 31) and prevent further exposure to the plant; prognosis in advanced cases is poor

Larkspur

Genera: *Delphinium* (tall and low larkspurs); *Aconitum* (monkshood)

Distribution: losses in cattle are important in the western United States, especially in mountain ranges

Conditions conducive to toxicity: larkspurs are palatable and appear in early spring; although dried plants may be toxic, toxins are highest in early spring leaf growth; calves are often affected when they graze with nurse cows on edges of meadows

Livestock affected: all species are susceptible, but cattle are most sensitive

Clinical findings:

- Stiffness and weakness, abdominal pain, collapse, and death (may be sudden) from aspiration of regurgitation or respiratory paralysis appear within 3 to 8 hours after exposure.
- Recovery may occur in sublethal cases within 1 to 2 days.

Diagnosis: history of sudden death with rapid bloating on rangeland in early spring, evidence of plant consumption, and lack of other findings

Treatment: no specific treatment

Nicotinic-Acting Alkaloids

Genera: *Nicotiana* (tobacco, tree tobacco); *Lupinus* (lupines); *Cytisus scoparus* (Scottish broom); *Laburnum anagyroides* (golden chain); *Thermopsis montana* (mountain thermopsis); *Lobelia* (Indian tobaccos); *Conium maculatum* (poison hemlock)

Distribution: lupines and thermopsis are found in climax/grassy habitats; poison hemlock and tree tobacco are found in disturbed soils

Conditions conducive to toxicity: plants are bitter and ingested only when animals are forced to do so, or when they are hidden in hay or forage; plants are toxic when dry (except for poison hemlock)

Livestock affected: all species; acute toxicosis is more common in sheep, whereas teratogenesis is more likely in cattle; cattle are more sensitive to acute effects of poison hemlock than horses or sheep

Clinical findings:

- Acute toxicosis is characterized by ataxia, weakness, tremors, and initial central nervous system (CNS) stimulation followed by lethargy, increased salivation, respiratory distress, bloating, and death from respiratory paralysis.

- Teratogenic signs vary with the period of exposure, but include cleft palate and arthrogryposis.

Diagnosis:
- Diagnosis of acute toxicosis depends on identification of the plant and appropriate signs.
- Thermopsis may cause elevations in creatine kinase (CK) and aspartate aminotransferase (AST).
- Alkaloids in urine and serum may be detected by chemical assay for poison hemlock, tree tobacco, and some lupines.

Treatment: symptomatic; exposure to plants should be eliminated

Steroidal Alkaloids

Genera: *Zigadenus* (deathcamas); *Veratrum* (false hellabore, skunk cabbage); *Solanum* (nightshades); *Lycopersicon* (tomatoes)

Distribution: deathcamas and *Veratrum* spp. are found in moist meadows at upper elevations; *Solanum* spp. are found throughout the United States

Conditions conducive to toxicity: deathcamas is most hazardous in early spring because it is among the first plants present; alkaloids resist drying

Livestock affected: all species; sheep are most commonly poisoned by *Veratrum* spp. and deathcamas

Clinical findings:
- Deathcamas and false hellabore–cause hypotension; ingestion of as little as 0.6% of body weight can cause ataxia, stiffness, tremors, increased salivation, vomiting, and prostration
  - Death may occur within 1.5 to 8 hours of exposure.
- Veratrum–teratogenic when grazed by ewes around day 14 (cyclopia, microphthalmia, cleft palate, and other craniofacial deformities) and day 30 (limb defects) of gestation
- Solanaceous plants (nightshades, tomatoes, potatoes)–vary in toxicity and effect
  - Signs include gastrointestinal (GI) irritation, ileus (in horses), diarrhea or constipation, lethargy, increased salivation, dyspnea, tremors, paralysis, and death.
  - Some *Solanum* spp. accumulate nitrate or have other toxic factors such as vitamin D.

Diagnosis: clinical findings and evidence of plant consumption

Treatment: no specific treatment

Tropane Alkaloids

Genera: *Datura* (jimsonweed); *Atropa belladonna* (belladonna)

Conditions conducive to toxicity: jimsonweed prefers disturbed soils such as barnyards; although *Datura* is bitter and unpalatable, herbicide application or overgrazing may encourage consumption; grain contaminated with *Datura* seeds is toxic

Clinical findings: GI atony, anorexia, tachycardia, tachypnea, mydriasis, thirst, diarrhea, excess urination, disturbed vision, and delirium; death is uncommon

Diagnosis: tropane alkaloids can be identified in urine, ingesta, and plant material

Treatment: no specific treatment

Yew

Genera: *Taxus cuspidata* (Japanese yew); *T. baccata* (English yew)

Distribution: found throughout the United States in hedges and yards

Conditions conducive to toxicity: yew poisoning often results from accidental ingestion of hedge clippings; toxicity is retained in dry plants

Livestock affected: all species; yew is extremely toxic (greater than 0.1% body weight can kill a horse)

Clinical findings: collapse and sudden death, occasionally preceded by tremors and weakness

Diagnosis: history of exposure to yew clippings and sudden death; finding leaf parts (flattened needles) in ingesta
Treatment: no specific treatment

Phalaris (Canary Grass)

Genus: *Phalaris* (canary grass)
Livestock affected: cattle and sheep (more likely to be affected)
Clinical findings:

- Cardiac failure and sudden death
  - Chronic, low-level exposure in sheep may cause ataxia (grass staggers), hopping gait, tremors, excitability, head nodding, convulsions, and eventually paddling and death.
  - Onset of signs may be delayed up to 40 days after exposure has ended.

Diagnosis: sudden death or staggers in sheep that have previously grazed canary grass pasture; characteristic bluish-gray discoloration of brainstem (see main text)
Treatment: no specific treatment; supplementation with cobalt may help prevent toxicosis

Cardiac Glycosides

Genera: *Nerium oleander* (oleander); *Thevetia peruviana* (yellow oleander); *Digitalis purpurea* (foxglove); *Rhododendron* (azaleas); *Kalmia* (laurels); *Convallaria* (lily-of-the-valley); *Pieris japonica* (Japanese pieris); *Asclepias* (milkweeds); *Apocynum* (dogbanes)
Conditions conducive to toxicity: although plants are bitter, dried leaves and flowers are readily ingested; discarded lawn clippings that contain oleander leaves are a common source of livestock poisoning
Livestock affected: all species
Clinical findings:

- Signs include abdominal pain, nausea, weakness, anorexia, rumen atony, increased salivation, bradycardia (or tachycardia later in the syndrome), heart block, and ventricular arrhythmias.
- Onset of signs may be delayed by several hours after ingestion; death (which may be sudden) usually occurs within 36 hours after ingestion but may take up to 14 days.

Diagnosis:

- Toxicosis may cause hypertension, hypoxemia, acidemia, hemoconcentration, hyperkalemia, hyperchloremia, and elevations of serum creatinine and glucose.
- Diagnosis depends on identification of the plant and evidence of its consumption.
- Laboratory assays are available for detection of exposure to oleander and *Digitalis.*

Treatment:

- Eliminate exposure to the plant and administer cholestyramine resins or activated charcoal (repeated administration suggested).
- Avoid fluids containing calcium and potassium.
- Atropine may be useful if bradycardia or heart block is present (use with care in horses).
  - β-Adrenergic blocking agents and antiarrhythmic drugs can be used for cardiac arrhythmias, but otherwise β-blockers should be avoided.
- Avoid stress.

Photosensitizing Saponins

Genera: *Tribulus terrestris* (puncture vine); *Panicum coloratum* (kleingrass); *Brachiaria decumbens* (signalgrass); *Nolina texana* (sachuista); *Agave; Narthecium ossifragum*
Conditions conducive to toxicity: most hazardous when grazed during stages of early, rapid growth; mature plants are often grazed without incident

Livestock affected: all species
Clinical findings:
- Anorexia, weight loss, icterus, hepatoencephalopathy, and secondary photosensitization (evidence of liver damage)
  - *N. ossifragum*, like other lilies, may cause chronic renal failure in ruminants.

Diagnosis: serum chemistry alterations reflect liver damage
Treatment: remove animals from offending pastures, at least until grass matures

Cyanogenic Glycosides

Genera: *Linum* (flax); *Prunus* (cherries, apricots, peaches); *Sorghum* (sorghum/Sudan grass); *Triglochin* (arrow grass); *Trifolium repens* (white clover); *Zea maize* (corn)
Conditions conducive to toxicity: many listed plants may be grazed safely; however, cyanide is released when plants are damaged by maceration, drought, frost, wilting, and stunting; toxicity wanes with drying
Livestock affected: all species
Clinical findings:
- Cyanide toxicosis is very rapid in onset, often resulting in sudden death.
- Clinical signs, when observed, include dyspnea, excitement, tremors, salivation, gasping, and clonic convulsions.
- Animals grazing *Sorghum* spp. may develop ataxia, urinary incontinence, and cystitis.

Diagnosis:
- Blood from animals with cyanide toxicosis is cherry red.
- Diagnosis is supported by evidence of cyanide in forage and samples from affected animals.
  - Samples for cyanide analysis should be frozen immediately and kept frozen until analyzed.

Treatment: judicious use of sodium nitrite (16 mg/kg intravenously [IV], to form a small amount of methemoglobin) and sodium thiosulfate (30 to 40 mg/kg IV)

Nitrotoxins

Genera: *Astragalus* (milk vetches); *Coronilia varia* (crown vetch); *Indigofera spicata* (indigo)
Livestock affected: all species; cattle and sheep are most at risk
Clinical findings:
- Acute toxicosis–rapid onset of ataxia, distress, dyspnea, cyanosis, weakness, collapse, and death within 4 to 12 hours
  - Sudden death can occur in sheep.
- Chronic toxicosis–respiratory distress, weakness (especially pelvic limbs), fetlock knuckling, goose stepping, and knocking together of hind feet when walking ("cracker heels")
  - Salivation, constipation, and diarrhea have also been reported.

Diagnosis: nitro-compound toxicity is distinct from nitrite poisoning; usually, less than 33% methemoglobin is formed after exposure to nitro compounds
Treatment: no specific treatment; affected animals may linger for months, but severely affected individuals seldom recover

Bracken Fern

Genera: *Pteridium aquilinum* (bracken fern); *Chelianthes humilis* (rock fern); *Equisetum arvense* (horsetail)
Conditions conducive to toxicity:
- Grazing of fresh, young fronds when other forage is not yet available is hazardous for cattle and horses; plowed-up rhizomes and hay containing bracken can also be toxic.
- Signs suddenly appear after animals have grazed approximately their body weight in plant material over several months.

Livestock affected: all species

Clinical findings:
- Cattle–widespread hemorrhages and hematuria caused by severe bone marrow depression and tumors in the bladder and other organs (hematopoietic and digestive system)
  - Reduced fertility may occur in chronic cases.
- Horses–toxicosis results in thiamine deficiency, manifested as weight loss, ataxia, lethargy, a braced stance with an arched back, tremors, and recumbency
  - Death may occur within days or weeks after onset of signs.

Diagnosis:
- Cattle with bracken toxicosis have a normocytic, normochromic anemia; neutropenia; and lymphocytosis; severe thrombocytopenia and hemorrhage occur with bone marrow failure.
  - Urine from affected animals is hemorrhagic, with high levels of calcium and protein.
- Horses with bracken toxicosis have low serum levels of thiamine.

Treatment: no specific treatment for ruminants with bracken poisoning; horses not in terminal state may respond well to large doses of parenteral thiamine

Phytoestrogens

Genera: *Medicago sativa* (alfalfa); *Trifolium subterraneum* (subterranean clover); *Trifolium pratense* (red clover)
Livestock affected: ruminants
Clinical findings:
- Infertility and hyperestrogenism or antiestrogenism
  - Signs of hyperestrogenism include nymphomania, cystic ovaries, swollen genitalia, and in males, development of female characteristics.
  - Antiestrogenic signs include gonadal hypoplasia and anestrus.

Diagnosis: demonstration of estrogens in forages and in plasma or urine
Treatment: removal from offending forages

Other Toxic Glycosides

The following plants contain various other toxic glycosides:
- *Melilotus alba and Melilotus offinalis*–white and yellow sweet clovers (contain dicumarol)
  - Toxicosis leads to widespread, vitamin K-responsive hemorrhage, which is especially hazardous during late-term pregnancy (hemorrhagic abortions).
  - Dicumarol can be assayed in feed and animal samples.
- *Xanthium* spp.–cocklebur and spiny clotburs
  - Sprouts, burrs, or mature plant in hay can cause massive liver necrosis in cattle.
  - Signs include depression, dyspnea, weakness, convulsions with opisthotonus, and death; severe hypoglycemia may be found.
- *Ammi majus* (Bishop's weed); *Cymopterus watsonii* (spring parsley); *Thamnosa* spp. (Dutchman's breeches); *Cooperia pedunculata*–primary photosensitizing agents
- *Cestrum diurnum, Solanum malacoxylon, Trisetum flavescens*–calcinogenic glycosides
  - Ingestion causes weight loss, lameness, stiffness, abnormal posturing, and increases in serum calcium and phosphate in cattle and horses.
  - Lesions involve widespread calcification of tissues, including the cardiovascular system, tendons, lungs, and kidney.
- *Medicago* spp. (alfalfa); *Saponaria* spp.; *Gutierrezia sarothrae* (broom snakeweed); *Sesbania vesicaria* (bladderpod)–contain plant saponins
  - Signs in cattle include gastroenteritis with diarrhea, poor weight gains, and ill thrift.
  - Midsummer alfalfa cuttings tend to have the highest saponin levels.
  - Broom snakeweed also has an abortifacient factor.

- *Aesculus* spp. (buckeye or horse chestnut)–young growth and seeds contain toxic levels of the glycoside aesculin
  - Ingestion causes ataxia, twitching, and excitability or sluggishness in livestock.
- *Ranunculus* spp. (buttercups); *Ceratocephalus testiculatus* (bur buttercup)–contain a potent GI irritant that becomes nontoxic when plant is crushed or dried
  - Ingestion of this bitter plant by cattle and sheep results in watery diarrhea, weakness, and dyspnea; death may occur in severe cases.
- *Brassica* (turnips, mustards, cabbages)–toxins cause GI irritation; some also have goitrogenic effects in both adults and neonates
- *Cycas* and *Macrozamia* spp.–cycads have a variety of glycosides, including a hepatogastrointestinal toxin and carcinogen
  - Toxicity causes depression, anorexia, and weight loss in ruminants.
  - Zamia staggers is characterized by weight loss, swaying, weakness, and rear limb ataxia.
  - Cycad toxins may also harm pancreatic beta cells, potentially leading to diabetes mellitus.

Gossypol (Cottonseed)

Source: gossypol is a yellow pigment found in the glands of cottonseed *(Gossypium)*

Conditions conducive to toxicity: both whole cottonseed and cottonseed meal can be toxic; solvent extraction of cottonseed may leave high levels of free (toxic) pigment

Livestock affected: all species; ruminants are more resistant than horses

Clinical findings:

- Acute toxicosis results in severe dyspnea, weakness, and death (can be sudden).
  - Signs may appear suddenly after stress, making toxicosis resemble acute shipping fever.
- Adult ruminants may have decreased milk production, anorexia, dyspnea, weakness, gastroenteritis, and reproductive failure (lack of spermatogenesis in bulls).
- Low levels of gossypol in a ration limited in iron or protein may cause ill thrift and poor weight gains in cattle less than 1 year old.

Diagnosis:

- Analysis of feed for free and bound gossypol levels
  - High-pressure liquid chromatography (HPLC) can detect gossypol in some animal-related samples.
- Postmortem findings (see main text)

Treatment: no specific treatment; feeding vitamin E may help control some gossypol effects in young animals

Oak

Genus: *Quercus* (oak)

Conditions conducive to toxicity: toxicity is more likely in spring (during budding stage) and in fall (acorns)

Livestock affected: all species

Clinical findings: signs generally appear after 3 days of ingestion; losses result from gastroenteritis, renal failure, liver damage, death, and fetal deformities (cattle) Oak toxicosis is discussed further in Chapter 30.

Soluble Oxalates

Genera: *Halogeton glomeratus* (halogeton or barilla); *Sarcobatus vermiculatus* (greasewood); *Rumex crispus* (curly dock); *Setaria; Rheum* (rhubarb); *Oxalis* (sorrel or soursob); *Kochia scoparia* (fireweed, summer cypress)

Distribution: the plants grow in disturbed or arid soils

Conditions conducive to toxicity: rumen flora adapt to oxalate in forage if animals are gradually acclimated over at least 4 days, so poisoning occurs when hungry

animals that are unaccustomed to oxalates ingest these bitter plants in large quantities
Livestock affected: all species; sheep are most often affected
Clinical findings:
- Signs include dyspnea, ataxia, rumen stasis and bloat, depression, weakness, coma, and death.
- Horses chronically grazing setaria develop bighead from a low calcium/phosphorus ratio.

Diagnosis: evidence of hypocalcemia or uremia; analytic tests are available for oxalate in plant and animal samples
Treatment: symptomatic therapy for gastroenteritis, shock, and renal failure

White Snakeroot

Genera: *Eupatorium rugosum* (white snakeroot); *Haplopappus* spp.
Distribution: white snakeroot is a perennial that grows in shady, wooded areas in the Midwest
Conditions conducive to toxicity: hazard to grazing animals is highest when other forages have dried during winter or conditions force overgrazing; toxic fresh or dried
Livestock affected: all species, although lactating animals are resistant
Clinical findings:
- Toxicosis causes cardiac and skeletal muscle damage and ketosis.
- Clinical signs include weight loss, tremors and stiffness, ataxia, depression, cardiac arrhythmias, recumbency, and death; sudden death is possible.

Diagnosis: ketosis, increased serum CK, lactate dehydrogenase (LDH), alkaline phosphatase (AP), and AST; differential diagnoses include selenium deficiency and ionophore toxicosis
Treatment: supportive

Other Toxic Alcohols/Acids

The following plants contain other toxic alcohols or acids:
- *Agropyron desertorum* (crested wheatgrass)
  - Lush, early growth of many forages, including crested wheatgrass, can contain acidic compounds that sequester magnesium.
  - Ingestion during this lush stage can lead to hypomagnesemia in cattle (see Chapter 39).
- *Pinus ponderosa* (Ponderosa pine); *Pinus radiata* (Monterey pine); *Juniperus communis* (juniper)–ingestion by cows during late pregnancy causes abortion or birth of weak calves
  - Other signs include lethargy and digestive upsets.
  - Abortions are characterized by retained placentas and metritis (can be fatal).
- *Cicuta* (water hemlock); *Asclepias* (narrow-leafed milkweeds)–contain convulsant resins
  - Ingestion of less than 0.5% of body weight may be lethal.
  - Signs in all species may appear within 15 minutes of ingestion and include nervousness, salivation, weakness, tremors, violent convulsions, and death.
  - Administration of sodium pentobarbital at the onset of signs can result in recovery
- *Hypericum perforatum* (St. John's wort); *Fagopyrum esculentum* (buckwheat)–primary photosensitizing toxins (see Chapter 38).
- *Tetradymia* (horsebrush) with *Artemisia* (black or big sage)
  - Ingestion of horsebrush plus black sage can cause hepatogenous photosensitization in sheep.

Nitrates

Genera: *Sorghum* (sorghum/Sudan grass); *Avena* (oat); *Amaranthus* (pigweed); *Beta* (beets); *Solanum* (nightshades); *Zea maize* (corn)

Conditions conducive to toxicity: drought, plant stress, rapid growth spurts, some herbicides, low light, and fertilization can lead to nitrate accumulation
Livestock affected: ruminants are ten times more sensitive to nitrates than are horses
Clinical findings:
- Signs appear within 4 hours of exposure and include polypnea, dyspnea, weakness, tremors, exercise intolerance, terminal convulsions, and death (often within hours).
- Mildly affected cattle may recover spontaneously; abortion may occur in mild or subclinical cases within 5 days of exposure.

Diagnosis:
- Chocolate-brown blood; more than 45 ppm of nitrate in ocular fluid or serum
- Identification of a toxic level of nitrate in forage or water
  - Forages with 1% or more (dry weight) nitrate may be lethal in cattle not acclimated to nitrate.
  - Acute toxicosis can result from nitrate in water at levels greater than 0.12%.

Treatment: methylene blue (5 to 15 ml of 1% solution IV)

Selenium Indicators

The plants listed here are called *selenium indicators* because of their requirement for high selenium levels in soil. Although the plants are not palatable because of a garlicky odor, they indicate the presence of selenium. In arid, alkaline soil, selenium may also be accumulated in toxic levels in a variety of common forage plants and consumable weeds (e.g., alfalfa, *Asteraceae, Castilleja, Atriplex*).
Genera: *Stanleya pinnata* (prince's plume); *Astragalus bisulcatus* (two-grooved milk vetch); *Xylorrhiza* (woody asters)
Livestock affected: all species
Clinical findings:
- Signs of acute selenium toxicosis include weakness, dyspnea, bloating, abdominal pain with diarrhea, paresis, shock, and death from respiratory failure.
  - Acute selenosis occurs with ingestion of indicator plants containing 10,000 ppm or more of selenium.
- Horses with chronic alkali disease (5 to 50 ppm of selenium in forage) develop ill thrift, anemia, stiffness, lameness, loss of mane and tail, and deformities and sloughing of the hooves.
- Cattle with chronic selenosis may develop hoof lesions or immune incompetence, and if pregnant, they may give birth to nonviable calves.

Diagnosis:
- Selenium in feed more than 2 ppm (dry weight); selenium in whole blood or liver more than 1 ppm
  - After exposure is terminated, tissue levels may fall back to normal well before clinical signs dissipate, leading to a false-negative result.
  - Hair testing may be useful for diagnosis of chronic selenosis.

Treatment: no specific treatment; feeding proteins that are high in sulfur-containing amino acids may be beneficial

Sulfur-Containing Plants

Genera: *Brassica rapus* (turnip); *Kochia scoparia* (fireweed, summer cypress)
Livestock affected: primarily ruminants
Clinical findings:
- Ruminal or intestinal microbes may produce excess sulfide, rapid absorption of which can cause polioencephalomalacia (characteristic CNS disease with blindness; see Chapter 33).
- High levels of sulfur may also contribute to copper deficiency in ruminants.

Diagnosis: testing of all potential sources of sulfur, including feed, pasture, and water
Treatment: no specific treatment

Pneumotoxic Plants

Genera: *Perilla frutescens* (perilla mint); rapidly growing forages; moldy sweet potato; moldy green beans

Conditions conducive to toxicity: lush forage, seed and flowering stage of perilla mint (even when dried), and moldy sweet potatoes and green beans

Livestock affected: ruminants, especially cattle moved from dry feed to lush pasture

Clinical findings:

- Signs include sudden onset of polypnea, severe dyspnea with an expiratory grunt, frothing at the mouth, and open mouth breathing; affected animals may be found dead (see Chapter 29).
- Affected cattle have wet, heavy lungs with variable amounts of emphysema.

Treatment: no specific treatment

Hemolytic Toxins

Genera: *Allium* (onions, garlic, chives); *Brassica* (kale, beets, rape, cabbage, turnips); *Acer rubrum* (red maple)

Livestock affected: all species (*Allium* and *Brassica);* horses (red maple)

Clinical findings: lethargy, anorexia, dyspnea, coffee-colored urine, icterus, hypoxic abortion, and shock; death results from respiratory failure secondary to anemia

Diagnosis: hemolytic anemia with hemoglobinuria and Heinz bodies; increased AST, sorbitol dehydrogenase, plasma protein, and bilirubin

Treatment: see Chapter 35 (Heinz Body Hemolytic Anemia)

Pigweed

Amaranthus retroflexus (pigweed) contains a renal toxin, in addition to potentially high levels of nitrate. Cattle may develop signs of renal failure, including weakness, tremors, ataxia, recumbency, and death, after grazing the plant for 5 to 10 days. Serum potassium, blood urea nitrogen (BUN), and creatinine concentrations are increased.

Senna

Cassia spp. (senna) are annual shrubs found in the southeastern United States that contain an unknown myotoxin. Signs of toxicosis can occur in all livestock species and include anorexia, ataxia, weakness, weight loss, and recumbency. Abnormalities may include increases in CK and AST, and myoglobinuria.

Yellow Star Thistle

Centaurea solstialis (yellow star thistle) and *Centaurea repens* (Russian knapweed) contain potent neurotoxins. Prolonged ingestion of large amounts of these plants by horses may result in neurotoxicity (see Chapter 33). The principal sign is dysphagia characterized by dystonia of the lips and tongue. Lethargy and aimless walking are also reported.

Sneezeweed

Genera: *Helenium* spp. (sneezeweed) and *Hymenoxys richardsoni* (bitter rubberweed)

Distribution: Rocky Mountains and southwestern United States

Conditions conducive to toxicity: the plants are unpalatable but may be ingested by sheep or goats in winter when other forage is limited

Clinical findings: the toxins are extremely irritating to the nose, eyes, and GI tract; severe gastroenteritis with vomiting often results in aspiration pneumonia

Diagnosis: increases in serum γ-glutamyl transferase (GGT), AST, creatinine, and BUN

Treatment: administration of thiol-containing substances (e.g., cysteine, protein, methionine) and antioxidants is protective

Black Walnut

Horses exposed to fresh black walnut *(Juglans nigra)* experience transient leukopenia, limb edema, and severe laminitis. As little as 5% in shavings used as bedding is toxic. Treatment involves removal of the shavings and traditional therapy for acute laminitis. *Berteroa incana* (hoary alyssum), a potential contaminant of alfalfa hay, can also cause fever, limb edema, and laminitis in horses.

Coyotillo

Genera: *Karwinskia humboldtiana* (coyotillo); *Rhamnus* sp. (buckthorn)
Distribution: woody shrubs found in southwestern United States
Conditions conducive to toxicity: toxicosis can occur when other forages are scarce
Livestock affected: ruminants
Clinical findings:

- Ingestion of small amounts of the fruit and seeds leads to weakness, incoordination, and eventually paralysis; onset of signs is delayed for days or weeks after exposure.
- Ingestion of the green parts of the plant may lead to wasting, weakness, and death.

Plants Causing Stringhalt

Hypochoeris (flatweed or smooth catsear) and *Lathyrus* (pea) contain neurotoxins. In horses, toxicosis may cause outbreaks of Australian stringhalt, a distal axonopathy characterized by an unusual gait in which the hock is hyperflexed during movement.

Avocado

Genus: *Persea americana* (avocado)
Conditions conducive to toxicity: primarily the Guatemalan varieties of avocado
Livestock affected: all species
Clinical findings:

- Plant matter from avocado trees causes aseptic mastitis, myocardial necrosis (with widespread edema), and skeletal muscle lesions with edema.
- Signs in horses include edema of the lips, tongue, mouth, and neck; lethargy; and colic.
- Increases in serum CK, AST, and LDH may be found.

Castor Bean and Black Locust

Genera: *Ricinus communis* (castor bean); *Robinia pseudoacacia* (black locust); *Abrus precatorius* (rosary pea)
Conditions conducive to toxicity: seeds, cakes, and foliage are toxic
Livestock affected: all species
Clinical findings: violent gastroenteritis, weakness, and death

Hairy Vetch

Genus: *Vicia villosa* (hairy vetch)
Conditions conducive to toxicity: systemic granulomatous disease may develop in cattle and horses grazing hairy vetch when it is green (prior sensitization may be required); dried seeds may cause convulsions in cattle
Livestock affected: primarily cattle and horses
Clinical findings:

- Initially, affected animals are presented for listlessness and welts on the skin, with alopecia and peeling around the nares; horses may have lymphadenopathy and dependent edema.
- Affected animals may develop wasting, diarrhea, lymphocytosis, and hyperproteinemia; the mortality rate may be high.

Blue-Green Algae

Conditions conducive to toxicity: potentially toxic blue-green algae (cyanobacteria) may form on stagnant bodies of water under conditions of heat, eutrophication (high nitrogen and nutrients), low flow rates, and concentrating wind

Livestock affected: all species

Clinical findings:

- Hepatotoxic algae can cause death within 1 hour of exposure, from hypovolemia and shock secondary to blood loss into the disintegrated liver and embolism of hepatocytes in the lung.
  - Lower dosages lead to characteristic signs of liver failure.
- A toxic dose of anatoxin-a causes tremors, collapse, dyspnea, convulsions, and death within minutes; respiratory paralysis is persistent and unresponsive to assisted ventilation.
- Anatoxin-a(s) causes cholinesterase inhibition, manifested as diarrhea, tremors, hypersalivation, dyspnea, paresis, opisthotonos, cyanosis, convulsions, and death.

Diagnosis:

- Hepatotoxic blue-green algae cause elevations in serum AST, GGT, AP, LDH, bilirubin, creatinine, and BUN.
- Animals with anatoxin-a(s) toxicosis have a decrease in peripheral cholinesterase.
- If blue-green algae toxicosis is suspected, samples of ingesta and bloom can be mixed with 10% neutral-buffered formalin for visual identification.
  - Samples should be accompanied by at least 20 L refrigerated fresh bloom material.

Treatment: supportive; exposed animals might benefit from oral adsorbents such as activated charcoal

MYCOTOXINS *(Text pp. 1627-1630)*

Mycotoxins may be found in cereal grains, other crop feeds such as beans, and forages. Ingestion of mycotoxins can cause acute and chronic poisoning, immunosuppression, loss of production, carcinogenicity, and teratogenicity. A given fungus may not always be toxic (many are ubiquitous); diagnosis requires identification of the toxins. Samples of feed for mycotoxin assays should be representative of the lot and frozen for storage.

Aflatoxins

Genera: many, including *Aspergillus, Penicillium, Rhizopus, Mucor,* and *Streptomyces*

Conditions conducive to toxicity:

- Colonization and toxin production can occur in grains, cottonseed, and peanuts in all phases from growth through harvest.
- Aflatoxins are produced in soybeans and small grains mainly during storage.
- Aflatoxin production is encouraged when warm, moist conditions are combined with crop damage (e.g., drought, storm).

Livestock affected: all species

Clinical findings:

- Signs of peracute toxicosis include hemorrhage, bloody diarrhea, and sudden death.
- Subacute toxicosis may lead to hepatic failure with icterus, anorexia, ataxia, reproductive failure (e.g., abortion), weakness and tremors, slowed rumen motility, coma, and death.
  - Impairment of immune function may also occur with moderate levels of aflatoxin.
- Chronic toxicity is associated with decreased growth rates, decreased feed efficiency, rough hair coat, ill thrift, increased incidence of disease, and liver damage.
  - Carcinogenesis may occur at low levels.

Diagnosis:
- Lesions of acute toxicosis include hemorrhages and prolonged prothrombin times.
- Testing of feed and liver for aflatoxins supports the diagnosis (see main text for values).

Treatment: supportive

Trichothecenes

The trichothecene mycotoxins of major agricultural concern include deoxynivalenol (DON or vomitoxin), T-2 toxin, stachybotryotoxin, and diacetoxyscirpenol (DAS).

Genera: *Fusarium, Myrothecium, Stachybotrys atra, Trichothecium roseum,* and others

Conditions conducive to toxicity: trichothecenes are produced in grains and some forages; fungal growth and toxin production is favored by undulating cool temperatures

Livestock affected: all species; ruminants are much less sensitive than horses

Clinical findings: dose-dependent signs include feed refusal, reduced weight gain, severe gastroenteritis with vomiting and diarrhea, coagulopathy and shock, skin necrosis (from direct contact), decreased reproductive performance, and immunosuppression

Diagnosis:
- Clinical pathologic changes in severe cases reflect shock or hemorrhagic gastroenteritis (decreases in packed cell volume; white blood cell count; and serum glucose, calcium, and phosphate).
    - Bilirubin may be increased (anorexia); AST and LDH may be transiently increased.
- Diagnosis is aided by finding the toxin in feed.

Treatment: oral adsorbents such as activated charcoal; therapy for the shock; broad-spectrum antibiotics to minimize complications of skin lesions and gastroenteritis

Fumonisin

Genus: *Fusarium moniliforme*

Conditions conducive to toxicity: fumonisins are mainly produced on corn, especially screenings

Livestock affected: horses

Clinical findings:
- Clinical signs appear suddenly after 7 to 90 days of ingesting toxic corn/screenings.
- Signs may include depression, confusion, ataxia, sweating, apparent blindness, head pressing, recumbency, convulsions, and death within 5 days of onset.
    - This condition is known as *moldy corn poisoning* or *equine leukoencephalomalacia.*
- Morbidity generally is low, but mortality rates are high.

Diagnosis:
- Transient increases in serum liver enzymes
- Pathognomonic CNS lesion, characterized by liquefactive necrosis of white matter of the brain, leaving fluid-filled cavities
- Levels of fumonisin B_1 10 ppm or more in corn-based concentrates or screenings
    - *F. moniliforme* is ubiquitous in the environment, so its presence in feed is not diagnostic.
    - Elevation of the sphinganine/sphingosine ratio in the urine is a very sensitive indicator of exposure to fumonisins.

Treatment: supportive

Grassland Staggers

Staggers in livestock is often caused by ingestion of forages that contain tremorogenic mycotoxins.

Genera:

- Perennial ryegrass *(Lolium perenne)* infested with *Neotyphodium* (formerly *Acremonium*) *lolia* in leaf sheaths
- Dallisgrass *(Paspalum dilatatum)* infested with the seed fungus *Claviceps paspali*
- Bermuda grass *(Cynodon dactylon;* mold unknown)
- *Phalaris* spp. (discussed earlier)
- Annual grasses (e.g., annual ryegrass, blowgrass [*Agrostis*], *Polypogon*) infested with a nematode that is subsequently infected by the bacterium *Clavibacter toxicus*

Conditions conducive to toxicity:

- Perennial ryegrass is most hazardous late in the grazing season, when grass is grazed low to the ground (more of a hazard for sheep); dried grass and seeds may retain toxicity.
- Dallisgrass is hazardous when ergotized seed heads are grazed (more of a hazard for cattle).
- Annual ryegrass toxicosis is most likely when grazing moist stubble and floodplains ("floodplain staggers").

Livestock affected: all species

Clinical findings:

- Signs appear within 7 days of initial grazing.
- Affected animals appear normal at rest or may have a fine head tremor; when stimulated, they have a characteristic stiff, spastic gait, followed by spasms and tetanic seizures.
- Recovery may occur within 2 weeks following removal from the offending forage.
- Annual ryegrass toxicity causes ataxia, convulsions, and other signs consistent with grassland staggers; death often occurs within 24 hours.

Diagnosis: rule out other tremorogenic syndromes; for perennial ryegrass, identification of the fungus or toxin in the plant

Treatment: alternate forage should be provided until new pasture growth is available

Fescue Toxicosis

Genera:

- Tall fescue grass *(Festuca arundinacea)* infested by *Neotyphodium coenophialum*
- Strains of perennial ryegrass *(Lolium perenne)* infested by *N. lolia*

Conditions conducive to toxicity: toxicity of tall fescue depends on the ambient weather and reproductive stage of exposed animals (see following discussion)

Livestock affected: all species

Clinical findings:

- During warm conditions, cattle, sheep, and horses suffer from summer syndrome, characterized by hyperthermia, lethargy, ill thrift, and heat intolerance.
- During cool conditions, cattle may develop ergot-type lesions of dry gangrene in the distal extremities ("fescue foot").
- Tall fescue toxicosis also causes reproductive failure, characterized by agalactia, prolonged gestation, weak births or stillbirths, and thickened placentas in horses and cattle.

Diagnosis: aided by demonstration of the endophyte or toxins in grass

Treatment: supportive; pregnant animals should be removed from tall fescue pastures 30 to 60 days before parturition; treatment with dopamine antagonists such as domperidone is being investigated

Other Mycotoxins

The following mycotoxins can also cause disease in large animal species:

- Ergot–parasitism of developing grass/grain flowers by *Claviceps purpurea,* resulting in production of various ergot alkaloids
  - Several grasses and grains (rye, triticale, wheat, oat, sorghum, barley) may be affected; the fungus causes formation of dark sclerotia on the seed heads.
  - Signs variably include ataxia, convulsions, lameness, dyspnea, diarrhea, dry gangrene of the extremities, abortion, neonatal mortality, reduced lactation, poor weight gains, and lowered feed intake.
- Zearalenone–an estrogenic mycotoxin produced in corn and other grains by various *Fusarium* spp.
  - Causes chronic hyperestrogenism with vulvar swelling, rectal prolapse, mammary enlargement, reduced fertility, and feminization in cattle.
  - Dairy cows are most sensitive.
- Slaframine–a mycotoxin produced by black batch mold contamination of red clover
  - Slaframine causes salivation, diarrhea, and bloat in cattle and horses.
- Ochratoxin–a nephrotoxin; horses are more sensitive than ruminants
  - Liver damage, enteritis, reduced growth rates, and abortion have also been reported.

ZOOTOXINS *(Text pp. 1630-1631)*

Venomous Snakes

Pit vipers (rattlesnakes, copperheads, cottonmouths) are the snakes most often involved in livestock envenomation. Their toxins include proteolytic enzymes, coagulation/hemorrhagic toxins, myotoxins, and in the Mojave rattlesnake, a potent paralytic neurotoxin.

Clinical findings

The effects of pit viper envenomation include extensive local edema and necrosis around the bite and, in systemically affected animals, anaphylactoid reactions with hemolysis and shock. Systemic effects vary somewhat with the crotalid species: hemolysis with eastern diamondback rattlesnakes, cardiovascular shock with western diamondbacks, and neurotoxicity (respiratory distress and other signs of neurologic paralysis) with Mojave rattlesnakes.

Clinical pathology

Common abnormalities include hemolysis, hypofibrinogenemia, thrombocytopenia, prolonged clotting times, and elevated CK. The urine may contain protein, glucose, and blood.

Treatment

Initial treatment in animals bitten near the nose involves maintenance of airway patency. Other treatments include broad-spectrum antibiotics, tetanus prophylaxis, nonsteroidal antiinflammatory drugs (NSAIDs), and local wound care and debridement. Corticosteroids and fluid therapy are rarely indicated.

Blister Beetles

Alfalfa and other blooming hays may attract blister beetles, which contain cantharidin, a potent vesicant toxin that causes necrosis of all mucous membranes to which it comes into contact.

Conditions conducive to toxicity: hays grown in the midwestern states; beetles retain toxicity in dried hay

Livestock affected: horses and ruminants; most cases have been reported in horses

Clinical findings: colic, gastroenteritis, nonspecific neurologic signs, polyuria, cystitis, shock, and death

Diagnosis:
- Laboratory evidence of dehydration, shock, and renal damage; decreased serum levels of protein, calcium, and magnesium
- Identification of beetles in hay or ingesta and chemical analysis for cantharidin in beetles, ingesta, blood, and urine

Treatment: aggressive symptomatic therapy for shock and renal failure

METALS AND OTHER INORGANIC COMPOUNDS *(Text pp. 1637-1640)*

Arsenic

Arsenic-containing compounds are used as rodenticides, insecticides, and herbicides, as well as medications (e.g., tonics, feed additives). The inorganic and the aliphatic organic arsenic compounds irritate the GI tract, resulting in necrotic lesions. Arsenic also acts directly on capillaries, potentially resulting in shock and sudden death.

Clinical findings

Clinical signs and lesions are similar for all arsenic compounds, except for the phenylarsonic compounds used as feed additives, which cause peripheral nerve degeneration in monogastric animals. All the other arsenic compounds can cause peracute, acute, or subacute conditions:
- Peracutely ill animals die from cardiovascular collapse and usually present as sudden deaths.
- Acute toxicosis is seen 3 to 12 hours after ingestion; the most prominent sign in acute or subacute cases is diarrhea (often hemorrhagic).
  - Other clinical signs include anorexia, dehydration, weakness, colic, and agalactia.

Diagnosis

Diagnosis of acute arsenic toxicosis generally is made by finding elevated levels of arsenic in the liver, kidney, and GI contents. Urine and whole blood are the best samples to collect from live animals. In cases of chronic toxicosis, arsenic levels in hair can be used as a retrospective diagnostic tool; deposition in hair is evident 2 weeks after exposure.

Treatment

Treatment is dictated by the type and severity of clinical signs. If toxicosis is caused by a trivalent inorganic or an aliphatic organic arsenic, British anti-lewisite (BAL) can be used as a specific antidote. A loading dose of 4 to 5 mg/kg is given intramuscularly (IM), followed by 2 to 3 mg/kg every 4 hours for 24 hours, then 1 mg/kg every 4 hours for the next 48 hours. Adverse effects include hypertension, tremors, convulsions, and coma.

Other chelators. Sodium thiosulfate (30 to 40 mg/kg IV or 60 to 80 mg/kg orally [PO] two or three times daily for 3-4 days) is a safe chelator in large animals. D-Penicillamine is an effective arsenic chelator in humans. Dimercapto succinic acid (DMSA) is a newer chelator used in human and small animal medicine.

Copper

Tolerance for copper varies widely among livestock species. Sheep are more susceptible to copper toxicity than are cattle; horses are least susceptible. Copper toxicity can be acute or chronic.

Acute copper toxicity

Acute toxicosis results from administration of soluble copper salts (e.g., injection of copper disodium edetate as treatment for copper deficiency). Signs include dyspnea, head pressing, ataxia, and circling.

Mechanisms of chronic copper toxicity

Chronic toxicosis can be categorized as simple, hepatogenous, or phytogenous:
- Simple toxicosis is caused by ingestion of excessive copper in relation to the levels of dietary molybdenum or sulfate.

  - Sheep are often poisoned when fed rations intended for cattle or horses; llamas have developed copper toxicosis when fed cattle feed.
- Hepatogenous toxicosis occurs when plant toxins damage the hepatic parenchyma, causing the liver to have an increased avidity for copper.
  - The plants most often incriminated are those containing pyrrolizidine alkaloids, such as *Senecio* spp. (tansy ragwort, groundsels) and *Heliotropium europaeum* (heliotrope).
- Phytogenous toxicosis occurs when animals graze plants with elevated copper/molybdenum ratios for prolonged periods, such as subterranean clover.

In any case, copper accumulates in hepatic lysosomes over several weeks or months. This phase is followed by a sudden release of copper from the liver into the bloodstream, either spontaneously or after some type of stress to the animal. Acute intravascular hemolysis ensues and leads to anemia and hemoglobinuric nephrosis.

Clinical signs of chronic copper toxicity

The first signs of chronic copper toxicosis are depression, anorexia, and weakness, which often have a sudden onset. The feces may be watery, dark, or blood tinged, especially in cattle. Evidence of a hemolytic crisis is apparent. Affected animals have anemia, methemoglobinemia, and hemoglobinuria, and the mucous membranes are icteric or muddy brown.

Diagnosis of chronic copper toxicity

Animals with toxic levels of copper in their livers can have normal or even low levels of copper in their serum, so serum copper is an unreliable method of monitoring for chronic copper toxicity. If an animal is suspected to have died from chronic copper toxicosis, copper levels should be measured in fresh liver and kidney and samples of each organ submitted in formalin for histopathologic examination.

Treatment of copper toxicity

Treatment options include the following:

- Ammonium molybdate (50 to 500 mg) and Na-thiosulfate (300 to 1000 mg) PO once per day for 3 weeks
- Ammonium tetrathiomolybdate (1.7 mg/kg IV or 3.4 mg/kg subcutaneously [SC]) on alternate days for three treatments
- D-Penicillamine (26 mg/kg PO once per day) for 6 days

Treatment is often unsuccessful once an animal has an acute hemolytic crisis.

Fluoride

Most cases of fluorosis are caused by exposure to industrial emissions; fluorosis has also occurred after volcanic eruptions. Horses and sheep tolerate higher levels of fluoride than cattle.

Clinical findings

Fluorosis primarily affects developing bones and teeth:

- The main clinical signs are weight loss and lameness (especially of the forelimbs); palpation of the long bones results in intense pain.
  - Radiographs reveal sclerosis, porosis, periosteal and endosteal hyperostosis, and osteophytosis.
- Characteristic dental lesions include hypoplasia, dysplasia, and yellow-brown discoloration of the enamel, which may be eroded or pitted and have a chalky appearance.
  - The molars may become so abraded and painful that animals have trouble with mastication and drinking cold water.

Diagnosis and treatment

Osteofluorosis is associated with increased serum alkaline phosphatase activity; urine, serum, and bone have elevated levels of fluoride. These findings, in conjunction with clinical and radiographic findings, are used to make a diagnosis. There is no specific treatment, and affected animals do not recover completely.

Iodine

Oversupplementation of iodine can result in toxicosis. Clinical signs include a nonproductive cough, lacrimation, serous nasal discharge, scaly hair coat, and hyperthermia. Other signs include decreased milk production and decreased rate of gain. Young animals seem to be more susceptible. Excess supplementation in mares has been associated with goiter in foals.

Diagnosis and treatment

Serum biochemical changes are inconclusive; the diagnosis can be confirmed only with serum or milk analysis. Treatment is restricted to removal of the iodine source. Respiratory signs disappear 1 to 4 weeks after the iodine source is removed.

Iron

Most cases of iron overload have occurred in neonatal foals given oral ferrous fumarate before 3 days of age. Clinical signs in neonatal foals include depression, icterus, head pressing, and disorientation. Adult horses develop anorexia, icterus, and sometimes petechial hemorrhages. Signs of iron toxicosis in calves include trembling, vocalizing, bruxism, colic, and convulsions.

Diagnosis

Diagnosis usually is based on clinical signs and a history of recent iron supplementation. Serum levels of free (unbound) iron may be elevated. Clinical pathologic findings, if abnormal, relate to cholestatic liver failure (elevated levels of GGT, AP, bile acids, and unconjugated bilirubin). Coagulopathies are demonstrated by abnormal coagulation profiles, thrombocytopenia, and elevated fibrinogen and fructose diphosphate. Liver iron concentrations range from normal to several thousand parts per million.

Treatment

Treatment is limited to supportive care. Repeated phlebotomy or chelation therapy with deferoxamine is used to treat iron overload in humans and small animals.

Mercury

Sources of mercury toxicosis include ingestion of seed treated with organic mercurial fungicides and topical application or ingestion of inorganic mercurials used as counterirritants (especially if used concurrently with DMSO).

Clinical findings

Ulceration of the mouth, esophagus, and the rest of the GI tract may be accompanied by diarrhea and anorexia. If the animal survives, toxic nephrosis occurs. Anorexia, gastroenteritis, weight loss, nephritis, and alopecia have been reported in animals chronically exposed to small doses of mercury.

Diagnosis

Diagnosis is based on the history; clinical presentation; and mercury levels in liver, kidney, brain, whole blood, or urine. Clinical pathologic examination may reveal elevated serum creatinine and BUN, as well as proteinuria, glucosuria, and isosthenuria, depending on the stage of the disease.

Treatment

Chelation therapy can be done using BAL or sodium thiosulfate, as described for arsenic toxicosis. Remaining topical mercurials should be washed off the skin. Supportive care is necessary for gastroenteritis and kidney failure.

Other Toxic Metals

Lead toxicosis is discussed in Chapter 33. Excess dietary molybdenum (copper deficiency) is discussed in Chapter 30. Sodium (salt) toxicosis is discussed in Chapter 33. Excess dietary sulfate is discussed with copper deficiency in Chapter 30 and with polioencephalomalacia in Chapter 33. Excess dietary zinc is discussed with osteochondrosis in Chapter 36.

INSECTICIDES *(Text pp. 1640-1642)*

Anticholinesterases

Anticholinesterase insecticides include organophosphates and carbamates. Their mechanism of action is to bind with and inhibit acetylcholinesterase. Carbamates bind the enzyme reversibly, so their inhibition of acetylcholinesterase is temporary. Organophosphates bind irreversibly, so their duration of action is longer than for carbamates.

Clinical findings

Clinical signs of toxicosis are described by the acronym SLUD: salivation, lacrimation, urination, and defecation. In addition, miosis, diarrhea, muscle tremors, seizures, dyspnea, or bloating may be seen. Death can occur within minutes, depending on the toxicity of the compound and the amount ingested.

Diagnosis

Measuring the cholinesterase activity in blood/serum, retina, or brain tissue can be used to make a presumptive diagnosis. The blood sample should be refrigerated after collection. An insecticide screen can be performed on GI contents or liver. These samples should be stored in glass or metal (e.g., foil) and frozen as soon as possible after collection.

Treatment

Treatment for anticholinesterase toxicosis includes the following:

- Supportive care
- Activated charcoal–1 to 2 lb (0.5 to 1 kg) PO for 500-kg animal
  - This should be given even if the route of exposure was not oral.
- Atropine–0.25 to 0.50 mg/kg; one fourth of the initial dose IV and the rest SC or IM
  - Repeat if clinical signs recur; monitor GI motility in horses.
- 2-Pyridine aldoxime methiodide (2-PAM)–20 mg/kg IV or 10 to 15 mg/kg SC twice daily
  - This is indicated only for organophosphate toxicosis; it is not necessary for carbamate toxicosis.

If the route of exposure was dermal, the animal should be washed with soap and water.

Chlorpyrifos

Chlorpyrifos is a chlorinated organophosphate used topically for lice and fly control in cattle. It causes delayed toxicosis in bulls and some exotic breeds of cattle. The manufacturer recommends not treating bulls more than 8 months old. Clinical signs, which do not appear until 2 to 7 days after exposure, include depression, weakness, muscle fasciculations, anorexia, rumen stasis, and rumen distention. Treatment includes the following:

- Wash the animal with detergent and water immediately.
- Give activated charcoal PO.
- Treat rumen stasis as indicated (often requires removal of rumen contents by a large-bore stomach tube or rumenotomy).
  - Atropine may be contraindicated in animals with rumen stasis.
- Give 2-PAM (can be effective if given within 4 days of insecticide exposure).

Haloxon

Haloxon reportedly causes toxicity in sheep that have a familial absence of a plasma A-esterase. Clinical signs occur 5 to 90 days after exposure; the predominant signs are hindlimb ataxia or paresis. Haloxon has also been associated with bilateral laryngeal paralysis in Arabian and part Arabian foals.

Organochlorine Insecticides

Chlorinated hydrocarbons are used to control insects and other pests. Examples include DDT, aldrin, heptachlor, and lindane. Organochlorines persist in fat and are excreted in milk.

Clinical findings

Initial clinical signs may include apprehension, hypersensitivity, and a belligerent attitude. Intermittent convulsions are the major manifestation in most cases.

Fasciculations of the face and cervical muscles are followed by spasms of the eyelids, forequarters, and finally hindquarters. Ataxia, hypersalivation, and diarrhea have been reported.

Diagnosis

Fatty samples such as brain, fat, milk, and liver should be submitted for analysis. The compounds may also be found in whole blood and GI contents. Samples should be put in glass or metal containers and frozen (with the exception of blood, which should be refrigerated).

Treatment

Treatment is symptomatic. The animal should be washed with water and detergent if the exposure was dermal. Activated charcoal is beneficial if given immediately after oral exposure. Convulsing animals require treatment with sedatives and muscle relaxants.

HERBICIDES *(Text pp. 1642-1643)*

Paraquat

Paraquat is a concern only when the animal ingests a concentrated form of the herbicide or grazes a field that is still wet from paraquat application. Acute signs generally occur 1 to 3 days after ingestion and involve anorexia, depression, and diarrhea. Several days later the animal develops respiratory distress, dyspnea, and pneumomediastinum. Death may be delayed until several weeks after ingestion.

Treatment

Fuller's earth or bentonite should be given PO as soon as possible after exposure (certainly within 24 hours of ingestion). Oxygen therapy reportedly worsens the lung damage. Regardless of therapy, the prognosis is poor.

Chlorophenoxy Acids

Chlorophenoxy acids include the compounds 2,4-D; 2,4,5-T; and silvex. They are relatively nontoxic unless ingested in a concentrated form. However, indirect toxicosis may occur because of altered metabolism of the sprayed plants; toxic plants that are normally untouched by grazing animals may become more palatable, and altered plant metabolism may cause some plants to accumulate higher levels of nitrate or cyanide or increase the level of their inherent toxins.

Clinical findings and treatment

Clinical signs of chlorophenoxy acid toxicosis include depression, anorexia, abdominal pain, diarrhea, and weakness (especially in the hindlimbs). Treatment consists of activated charcoal and supportive care. Animals should be removed from treated pastures for at least 7 days after application to reduce the occurrence of plant toxicosis.

Triazines

Products in this group of herbicides include atrazine, simazine, and propazine. Affected sheep exhibit generalized muscle tremors, which progress to mild tetany and hindlimb collapse or a short, prancing gait. Cattle develop diarrhea, followed by salivation, ataxia, and stiffness. Treatment with activated charcoal once a day for 4 days after exposure has reportedly decreased death losses. Livestock should be held off pastures treated with simazine for 30 days.

RODENTICIDES AND OTHER PESTICIDES *(Text pp. 1643-1644)*

Anticoagulant Rodenticides

Anticoagulant rodenticides include warfarin and the second-generation compounds brodifacoum and bromadiolone. The latter compounds tend to be more toxic and have longer half-lives.

Clinical findings

Clinical signs may not be noticed until 3 to 5 days after ingestion. Affected animals may present with melena, epistaxis, hematuria, or excessive bleeding from a wound or injection site. Often, hemorrhaging occurs in body cavities, and the animal may present with nondescript signs such as depression, weakness, pallor, colic, dyspnea, or fever. Sudden death is also a possibility.

Diagnosis

Diagnosis is based on history, clinical signs, clinical pathologic findings, and response to treatment. The degree of anemia varies with the severity of the hemorrhage. A coagulation panel reveals prolongation of prothrombin time (PT), partial thromboplastin time, and activated coagulation time. Fibrinogen, fibrinogen degradation products, and platelet count are not directly affected. Liver, GI contents, and unclotted blood can be tested for anticoagulant rodenticides.

Treatment

Treatment involves the following:

- Administer vitamin K_1, 300 to 500 mg (for an adult horse) SC every 4 to 6 hours
  - PT should return to normal within 24 hours.
  - Warfarin toxicosis may have to be treated for only a few days, whereas toxicosis from other compounds may have to be treated for several weeks.
  - To monitor duration of treatment after the animal has stabilized, discontinue vitamin K therapy for 48 hours and retest PT.
- Activated charcoal can be given PO to decrease further absorption of rodenticides.
- Whole blood or plasma transfusion may be needed initially in severe cases.

Note: Vitamin K_3 should not be used (see pp. 1645-1646).

Strychnine

Clinical signs of strychnine ingestion include sweating, incoordination, recumbency, and tonic-clonic seizures that are induced by loud noises, touch, or bright light. Signs appear within 10 minutes to 2 hours after ingestion. Diagnosis is based on clinical signs and detection of strychnine in urine or serum. Stomach contents, liver, kidney, and urine should be collected postmortem and analyzed for strychnine.

Treatment

Treatment includes oral administration of activated charcoal, and control of seizures with anticonvulsants and rigidity with muscle relaxants. The animal should be protected from excessive light and noise.

Zinc Phosphide

Clinical signs of zinc phosphide ingestion are similar to those caused by strychnine or the anticholinesterase insecticides. Diagnosis is based on detecting phosphine gas in the stomach contents. Because the gas rapidly dissipates in air, the collected stomach contents should be placed in an airtight container and immediately frozen.

Treatment

Treatment is supportive after activated charcoal therapy. It may be helpful to add an antacid to the activated charcoal to reduce the amount of phosphine gas that is produced.

Metaldehyde

Clinical signs of metaldehyde ingestion can occur immediately or be delayed for up to 3 hours after ingestion. Affected animals have convulsions (continuous or intermittent). Between convulsions the animal may have muscle tremors and anxiety and may be hyperesthetic. Hyperthermia is common. Other findings include tachycardia, defective vision, hyperpnea, hypersalivation, ataxia, cyanosis, acidosis, diarrhea, and dehydration. Death usually results from respiratory failure and occurs 4 to 24 hours after ingestion.

Diagnosis and treatment

Diagnosis is based on testing of the GI contents or serum for metaldehyde. No antidote is available. Activated charcoal should be given to prevent further absorption from the GI tract. Tranquilizers should be used to control seizures.

INDUSTRIAL TOXICANTS *(Text pp. 1644-1645)*

Petroleum

Most cases of petroleum toxicosis occur when the animal's water supply is contaminated. Clinical signs vary but usually include anorexia, depression, GI stasis, bloat, and either diarrhea or constipation. Oil may be seen in the feces within days after ingestion. The most common cause of death is aspiration pneumonia after regurgitation of the hydrocarbons. Some petroleum products contain heavy metals, such as lead, so concurrent toxicosis can occur.

Diagnosis

Diagnosis is based on the history, clinical findings, and detection of hydrocarbons in tissues. The product may be visible on the animal, as well as in the GI contents and lungs. Collecting suspect source material is important because these toxicoses may become legal cases.

Treatment

The primary aim of treatment is to prevent aspiration pneumonia, which is best achieved by performing a rumenotomy and removing the contaminated ingesta. If surgery is not feasible, activated charcoal should be administered, followed by a cathartic. Supportive care is needed for GI stasis and diarrhea or constipation. Giving vegetable oil (500 to 1000 ml PO) may increase the viscosity of the ingested petroleum within the rumen and reduce the occurrence of aspiration pneumonia. The prognosis generally is good unless the animal aspirates or severely bloats.

Ethylene Glycol

The most common cause of ethylene glycol toxicosis is ingestion of antifreeze. Ruminants may be more resistant than horses. Toxicosis results in initial inebriation, followed by metabolic acidosis and renal damage.

Clinical findings

Clinical signs in ruminants include ataxia, depression, hypersalivation, and absence of a menace response. Signs may progress to recumbency and clonic-tonic seizures in pygmy goats.

Diagnosis

Clinical pathologic changes include azotemia, metabolic acidosis, and hyperosmolality. Rumen or stomach contents can be analyzed for ethylene glycol. It is absorbed within 48 hours after ingestion in horses but may be detected in the rumen contents for up to 4 days after the onset of clinical signs. Urine, serum, and ocular fluid can also be analyzed for glycolic acid.

Treatment

The classic treatment is 20% ethanol, 5 ml/kg at 4- to 8-hour intervals. However, it is effective only if initiated within a few hours of ingestion. Treatment with activated charcoal may be beneficial in ruminants, even after the appearance of clinical signs.

Chlorinated Naphthalene

Chlorinated naphthalene is used in wood preservatives, asphalt roofing, insulating waxes, sealing compounds, and condensers. Initial signs of toxicosis include weight loss, anorexia, depression, and excessive salivation (papular stomatitis) and lacrimation. Several weeks later, nonpruritic thickening and fissuring of the skin occurs involving the withers, neck, head, trunk, and medial thighs. Diarrhea may occur late in the disease.

Diagnosis and treatment

Diagnosis is based on clinical signs and low serum vitamin A. Suspected source material can be analyzed for chlorinated naphthalene. Treatment with vitamin A may minimize some clinical signs, but it is usually unsuccessful, especially after the appearance of skin lesions.

Pentachlorophenol

Pentachlorophenol (PCP) is primarily used as a wood preservative. Horses have developed toxicosis when bedded on wood shavings that contain PCP.

Clinical findings

Signs vary with the stage of disease and with the species:

- Acute signs in cattle include weight loss, depression, anorexia, intense thirst, and decreased milk production.
- Chronic signs in cattle include dyspnea, hyperkeratosis, liver damage, and abortion.
- Horses develop anorexia, dependent edema, weight loss, and alopecia, and the skin has cracks and fissures that exude serum; horses may also develop colic or recurrent hoof problems.

Diagnosis and treatment

In horses, clinical pathologic findings reveal hepatic changes, anemia, and thrombocytopenia. Liver, kidney, and serum can be analyzed for PCP. Because of the rapid rate of excretion, serum PCP concentrations may be useful only during acute toxicosis. No antidote exists, and treatment usually is unsuccessful.

Phosphatic Fertilizers

Toxicosis with "superphosphate" fertilizers usually occurs after a short pasture has been top-dressed. Sheep may develop ataxia, bruxism, depression, and diarrhea.

Diagnosis and treatment

Diagnosis is based on history, clinical signs, and postmortem lesions (see main text). Affected animals are hypocalcemic, probably because of renal failure; however, hyperphosphatemia does not occur until oliguria develops and the animal is near death. Treatment is limited to supportive care, which generally is successful if the disease is diagnosed early.

Boron Fertilizer

Sodium borate is only mildly toxic; toxicosis usually occurs only if animals eat concentrated fertilizer. Clinical signs in cattle include weakness, depression, muscle fasciculations, seizures, and a spastic gait. Most animals develop diarrhea and become dehydrated. In goats given a sublethal dose, seizurelike activity mostly consisted of ear flicking and chomping motions; tremors, star-gazing, head jerking, and extensor rigidity were also noted.

Diagnosis and treatment

Liver, kidney, and rumen contents can be analyzed for boron content. Treatment is limited to supportive care.

THERAPEUTIC AGENTS *(Text pp. 1645-1646)*

Vitamin K_3

Vitamin K_3 is toxic to horses. Within 4 to 48 hours of administration, the horse becomes depressed, anorectic, and weak and may develop muscle stiffness, laminitis, or colic. Renal failure results, with some patients becoming hypercalcemic. Treatment should include diuresis and maintenance of serum electrolyte concentrations.

Propylene Glycol

Propylene glycol is used as a vehicle for drugs with poor water solubility, for treatment of bovine ketosis, and in some new antifreeze products. Toxicosis has been reported when cows are overdosed or when horses are accidentally dosed with propylene glycol.

Clinical findings

In cattle, ataxia develops in 2 to 4 hours and resolves by 24 hours after dosing. The cattle also become depressed and temporarily recumbent. Serum and cerebrospinal fluid osmolality increase. A horse mistakenly given propylene glycol developed ataxia and depression in 10 to 15 minutes. Pain and excessive sweating and salivation occurred but disappeared within 5 minutes. The animal developed rapid, shallow breathing and cyanosis and died of respiratory distress the next day.

Diagnosis and treatment

Serum and urine can be analyzed for the presence of propylene glycol. If acidosis occurs, sodium bicarbonate may be useful if given early in the disease.

Phenothiazine Toxicosis in Ruminants

Phenothiazine causes primary photosensitization in ruminants. Most cases occur in young or debilitated animals. Clinical signs begin with erythema and edema of unpigmented areas, combined with varying amounts of pruritus, photophobia, and pain. Vesicles and bullae form and progress to oozing, necrosis, and ulceration of the skin. Black cattle usually do not slough their skin but can develop epiphora, corneal edema, and blindness.

Diagnosis and treatment

Diagnosis is based on a history of phenothiazine consumption and on clinical signs. Treatment is limited to supportive care (antibiotics, antiinflammatory drugs, protection from direct sunlight).

Phenothiazine Toxicosis in Horses

In horses, phenothiazine acts as an oxidant and causes Heinz body hemolytic anemia. Clinical signs include anorexia, depression, weakness, icterus, anemia, and hemoglobinuria. Colic, diarrhea, fever, and dependent edema are less frequently reported. Treatment is supportive. Blood transfusion may be necessary if the anemia reaches a critical level.

FEED ADDITIVES *(Text pp. 1646-1647)*

Urea/Nonprotein Nitrogen

Clinical signs of urea or nonprotein nitrogen (NPN) toxicity in ruminants include weakness, dyspnea, salivation, bruxism, bloat, and convulsions. Because death can occur in a few hours, some animals may simply be found dead.

Diagnosis

The rumen pH is greater than 8.0, but rumen pH can decrease with time after death. Feed material and rumen contents can be analyzed for urea. However, a diagnosis should not be based solely on the urea level in the rumen; ammonia levels in the rumen contents, blood, or eye should also be used. Because ammonia is volatile, the samples should be frozen immediately after collection.

Treatment

Treatment is aimed at decreasing the absorption of ammonia from the rumen. In adult cattle, 20 to 30 L cold water with 2 to 6 L 5% acetic acid (vinegar) should be given PO and rumenotomy considered to remove the remaining NPN source.

Ammoniated Feed

Molasses, hay, and silage may be treated with aqueous or anhydrous ammonia to increase the dietary quality for ruminants. However, under certain conditions these ammoniated feeds can cause "bovine bonkers," a disease characterized by hyperexcitability. Conditions that predispose to toxicosis are ammoniating feedstuffs with more than 20% moisture, treating feedstuffs that contain ample soluble sugars (e.g., good-quality hay), overapplying the ammonia, or treating the forage during high ambient temperatures.

Clinical findings

The most striking clinical sign is hyperexcitability. Affected animals suddenly stampede and collide with other animals or with buildings and fences. Other signs include ear twitching, mydriasis, trembling, salivation, increased urination and defecation, and bellowing.

Diagnosis and treatment

Diagnosis is based on clinical signs and a history of consumption of ammoniated feed. Treatment is limited to sedation. Thiamine has been used with variable results. Most animals spontaneously recover once the ammoniated feed source is removed.

Ionophores

Ionophore antibiotics (e.g., monensin, salinomycin, narasin, lasalocid) are used as coccidiostats and feed additives for poultry and cattle. Toxicosis can result from calculation or mixing errors or from use in inappropriate species (e.g., in cattle and sheep fed treated poultry litter and horses fed cattle rations containing ionophores). Horses are most sensitive to ionophores.

Clinical findings and diagnosis

Clinical findings vary with the species and stage of disease:

- Acute signs in horses include colic, anorexia, weakness, and ataxia.
  - Serum CK significantly increases within 24 hours; AST and AP increase to a lesser degree, and unconjugated serum bilirubin may be slightly increased.
- If horses survive the acute episode, they often suffer from delayed toxicosis related to marked cardiac myopathy and fibrosis.
  - The most noticeable sign is exercise intolerance; affected animals may collapse and die during exercise.
- In ruminants, ionophore toxicity affects both the cardiac and skeletal muscles.
  - Signs in feedlot cattle include anorexia, pica, diarrhea, hind limb ataxia, and dyspnea.
  - In dairy calves, signs include weakness, tachypnea, nasal discharge, and reddened nose.
  - Sheep develop depression, anorexia, diarrhea, and stiffness.

Diagnosis is based on clinical signs and postmortem lesions (see main text). The feed source can be analyzed for ionophores; testing of tissue or serum is unreliable.

Treatment

There is no antidote. Mineral oil or activated charcoal may decrease further absorption of the toxicant. Large volumes of intravenous fluids are needed to treat dehydration and shock. Serum electrolyte levels should be monitored frequently and the fluid electrolytes adjusted accordingly.

INDEX

Page numbers followed by t indicate tables.

E

F

Q

R